MEDICINE

An Illustrated History

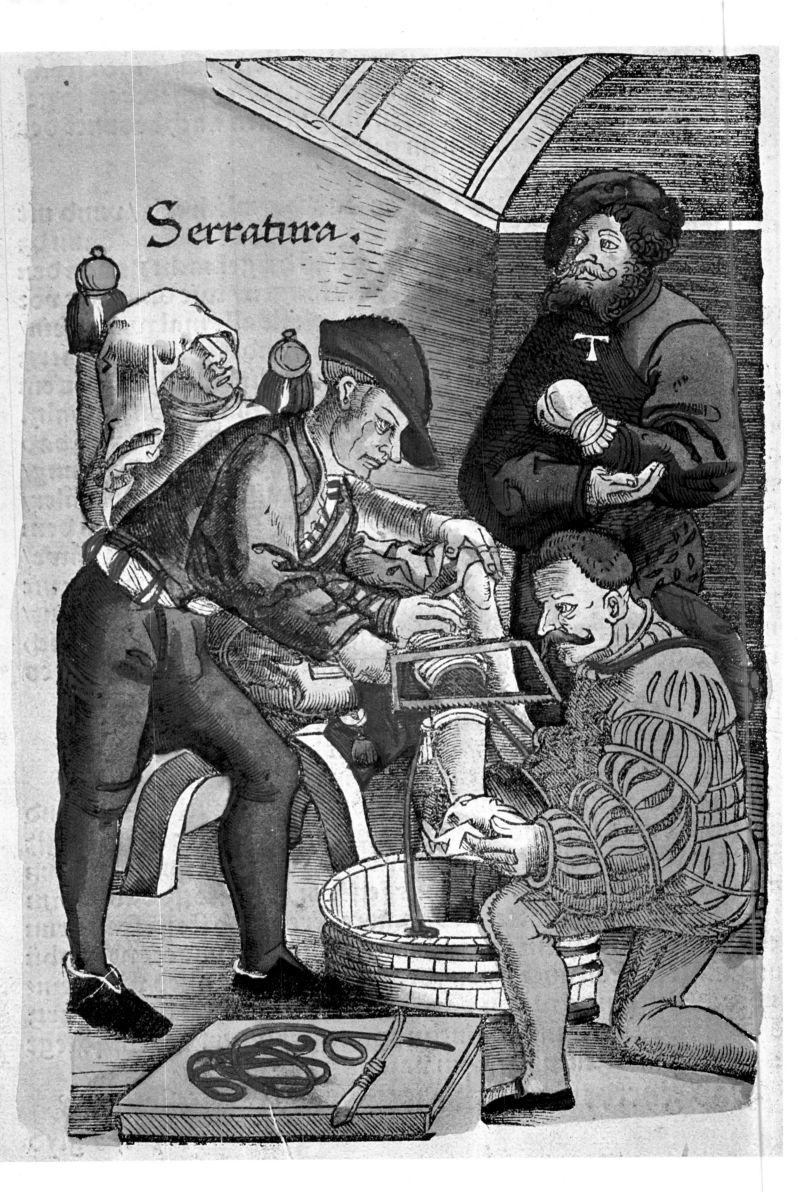

Serratura.

MEDICINE

An Illustrated History

by

ALBERT S. LYONS, M.D., F.A.C.S.

*Clinical Professor of Surgery, Archivist, and
Coordinator of History of Medicine,
Mount Sinai School of Medicine*

and

R. JOSEPH PETRUCELLI, II, M.D.

*Assistant Professor of Physiology and Biophysics,
Lecturer in Medicine,
Mount Sinai School of Medicine*

with special sections by
Juan Bosch, M.D., John Duffy, Ph.D., Melvyn Keiner, M.A. Ed., M.A.,
Morris H. Saffron, M.D., Ph.D.

and contributions by
Alan H. Barnert, M.D., Edgar M. Bick, M.D., Lewis Burrows, M.D.,
Callisto Danese, M.D., J. Lester Gabrilove, M.D.,
Stephen A. Geller, M.D., Kurt Hirschhorn, M.D.,
Horace L. Hodes, M.D., David Kairys, M.D., Arnold M. Katz, M.D.,
J. Michael Kehoe, D.V.M., Ph.D., Jack Klatell, D.D.S.,
David B. Sachar, M.D., Norman Simon, M.D.

HARRY N. ABRAMS, INC., PUBLISHERS, NEW YORK

FOR BARBARA

ACKNOWLEDGMENTS

Hosts of people are owed a large debt of gratitude: John Scarborough for unstinting advice and painstaking review of the chapters on Greece and Rome; David Cowen for detailed modifications and corrections of the items dealing with pharmacy; George and Marion Howe of the Chait Galleries who volunteered much valuable information.

Numerous others who helped generously with materials, background information, and translation include Saul Benison, David Berman, Edward Bottone, Lester Blum, Sylvia Dannett, Kurt Deuschle, David Dreiling, Leslie Falk, Bernard Friedman, Joseph Goldman, Ezra Greenspan, Bruce Hanna, Thomas Haviland, Louise Heinze, Charlotte Isler, Robert Joy, Arieh Kaynan, Fouad Lajam, Julius Leichtling, Robert Litwak, Fazlollah Moqtaderi, Helmuth Nathan, William Ober, Peter Olch, Angelos Papatestas, Demetrius Pertsemlidis, Stuart Quan, Philip and Faith Reichert, Theodore Robinson, Joachim Ronall, Richard Rosenfield, George Schreiber, Mahendra Sheth, Adolfh Singer, Alex Steigman, Gordon Stone, Tibor Szabo, Hans Tauber, Gail Weissman, Carol Ann Wilson, Lawrence Wisham, and Alice Yohalem.

Of course, no one except the authors bears the slightest responsibility for any of the errors, omissions, or statements which appear in the text and picture captions.

Special thanks are due to Professor John Duffy for his ready assent to the fragmentation of his text on American medicine and its dispersal throughout other chapters, at the request of the publisher.

In addition we mention Henry Sigerist, George Rosen, Henry Viets, and George James, all now deceased, whose writings and personalities had educational and inspirational influences on the authors.

Also acknowledged here is the exceptional and cheerful assistance of Alice Weaver, Sali Morgenstern, Elliott Zak, and Marilyn Gardner at the New York Academy of Medicine; of Lucinda Keister at the National Library of Medicine; of Maureen Jones and staff in the Medical Arts Department at the Mount Sinai Medical Center; and especially of Claire Hirschfield in the Mount Sinai Archive. We thank Lita Annenberg Hazen for her generous support of the Archive and the history of medicine program.

Our editor Walton Rawls, a man of knowledge, reliability, perceptiveness, and patience, was a joy to work with. Abundant expressions of gratitude and admiration go to Barbara Lyons, who conscientiously found all the pictures requested or innovatively substituted others when they were not available, and who acted as consultant and sounding board throughout the writing of the book. Finally, the entire personnel at Harry N. Abrams, Inc., in one way or another, warmly supported all our endeavors.

Editor: WALTON RAWLS
Designer: JOHN S. LYNCH
Photo Editor: BARBARA LYONS

Library of Congress Cataloging in Publication Data
Lyons, Albert S
  Medicine: an illustrated history
  Bibliography: p.
  Includes index.
  1. Medicine—History. I. Petrucelli, Joseph, joint
author. II. Title. [DNLM: 1. History of medicine.
WZ40 L992h]
R131.L95   610.9   77-12912
ISBN 0-8109-1054-3

Library of Congress Catalogue Card Number: 77-12912

Published in 1978 by Harry N. Abrams, Incorporated,
New York   All rights reserved. No part of the contents
of this book may be reproduced without the written
permission of the publishers

Printed and bound in Japan

Frontispiece

1 *Colored woodcut showing amputation, from Hans
von Gersdorff*, Feldtbuch der Wundartzney
(1540). *Smith, Kline, and French Collection,
Philadelphia Museum of Art*

Page 10-11

2 *Japanese woodblock print illustrating Chinese tale
of Hua T'o operating on arm of General Kuan
Kung as he ignores pain and concentrates on a
game, eschewing anesthetics available at time.
National Library of Medicine, Bethesda*

Facing page (detail)

847 *Painting (1882) by Robert Hinckley of the
first successful public demonstration of surgical
anesthesia, October 16, 1846, at the Massachusetts
General Hospital. Francis A. Countway Library of
Medicine, Boston Medical Library, Cambridge*

2984

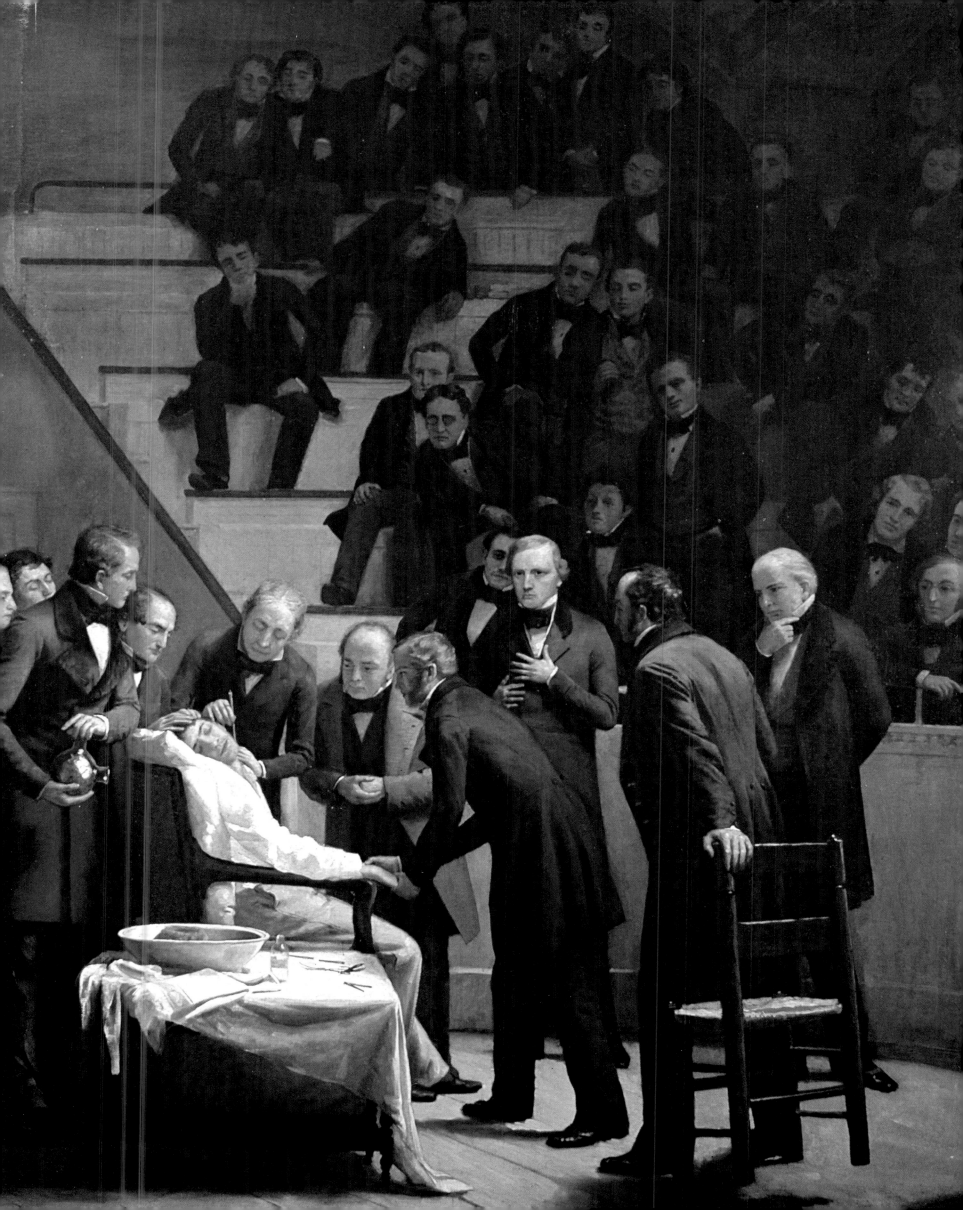

INTRODUCTION

O PPOSING forces are pulling the medical profession in different directions. The
physician is asked to act more responsively to the patient's needs by visiting
his home, giving him more time, maintaining and even raising standards
of practice—in short, to increase his professionalization. At the same time, the
physician is increasingly cast as a tradesman, a "provider" of health care, taxed as a
commercial entrepreneur, put under pressure to shorten his course of study, advertise
the cost of his wares, and submit his performance to auditing by lay examining
groups. Educators, consumers, and legislators urge the physician to broaden his
interests and become holistic in caring for each patient, but simultaneously—notably
in the United States—they threaten him with recertification tests which emphasize his
technical information, not his cultural breadth. Indeed, many of the same medical
institutions which profess an interest in "humanism" offer no courses in history, art,
philosophy, or sociology. Furthermore, medical schools, while asking universities to
send them well-rounded premedical students, actually tend to judge applicants'
suitability on the basis of grades in the sciences, not in the arts.

Political and economic events clearly indicate to the medical student and the
public that society is likely to expect the physician of the future to concern himself
with social justice, the environment, and governmental regulation. Yet, even when an
attempt is made in courses offered in community medicine to deal with these subjects,
they usually focus on the "here and now," not the historical underpinning. Thus,
both the young graduate and the experienced practitioner often find themselves
self-righteously in opposition to what they assume is a brand-new intrusion by outside
forces into their profession; or else they plunge into the "new order," joining hands
with those who condemn the practicing physicians as narrow-minded, ineffectual
mercenaries. They behave as if none of these confrontations had ever happened before.

The student, practitioner, and public marvel at the contemporary medical scene
with its enlarged scientific understanding, remarkable diagnostic tools, effective
therapeutic methods, and broadened attitudes toward the whole patient. Nevertheless,
they are apt to view today's practices either as having always been there or contrarily
as if they were unexpected bright meteors suddenly dropped from a dark sky. Usually,
neither the practitioner nor his patient understands how the doctor came to be
whatever he is; how his methods developed from the past; how his present ethical
principles were reached. Surely it would help to see these developments in historical
context.

Through the many pictures, the captions, and the text, we hope that this book
will introduce the subject and help suggest that medicine is more than just medicines;
that healing and healers comprise more than one discipline. Indeed, we hope it is

apparent that the development of medicine has not been an uninterrupted straight line of progress; that philosophy, history, and medicine have always been interrelated; that society and the profession have exerted mutual influences on each other. Furthermore, one may see that the effectiveness of any one doctor in relation to his patients was—and still is—more a function of his own qualities and abilities than of any philosophy.

George Rosen, the noted medical historian, aptly deplored what he called "iatrohistory"—a summarizing of the story of medicine as if it were merely a series of contributions by physicians. Furthermore, Richard H. Shyrock stated, "Medical history involves social and economic as well as biological content and presents one of the central themes in human experiences." While recognizing that the happenings in society were at least as important to medicine and its practitioners as whatever occurred in the profession itself, one may also perceive that medical ideas, discoveries, and practices had significant impact on society. Where possible, we have tried to give the reader a fair chance to perceive that contrary interpretations of ideas and events exist and that our own views are open to challenge. Nevertheless, we have used reasonable care in assembling information in hopes of presenting an unprejudiced overview of the concepts, healers, methods, and diseases which occupied the minds of people of the past. Our illustrated survey is therefore more an introduction than a study. We have frequently consulted primary works, either in the original or translation, but most of our sources have been secondary—the writings of others. Although we have aimed at avoiding conclusions based on scanty evidences, we have surely sometimes subscribed to one series of opinions over another without having ourselves engaged in the investigation upon which the opinions were based.

We have also tried to present past doctrines on their own terms, using current knowledge only as a means of understanding or guessing at how the past methods functioned. We acknowledge probable failures here, but mostly, we believe, because of technique not intentions. All of us in any century are just as encased in the beliefs and practices of our times as were our progenitors in theirs. The tradition-shattering anatomist Andreas Vesalius still subscribed to the ancient doctrine of the four humors; Ambroise Paré while pioneering in the management of wounds also believed in witches; the revolutionary experimentalist William Harvey proved the circulation of the blood, yet accepted "vital spirits" as a contribution to the heart.

To which erroneous doctrines do we in the twentieth century still cling? If we knew with certainty that they were wrong, we would discard them. Instead we search and wait and hope.

Albert S. Lyons

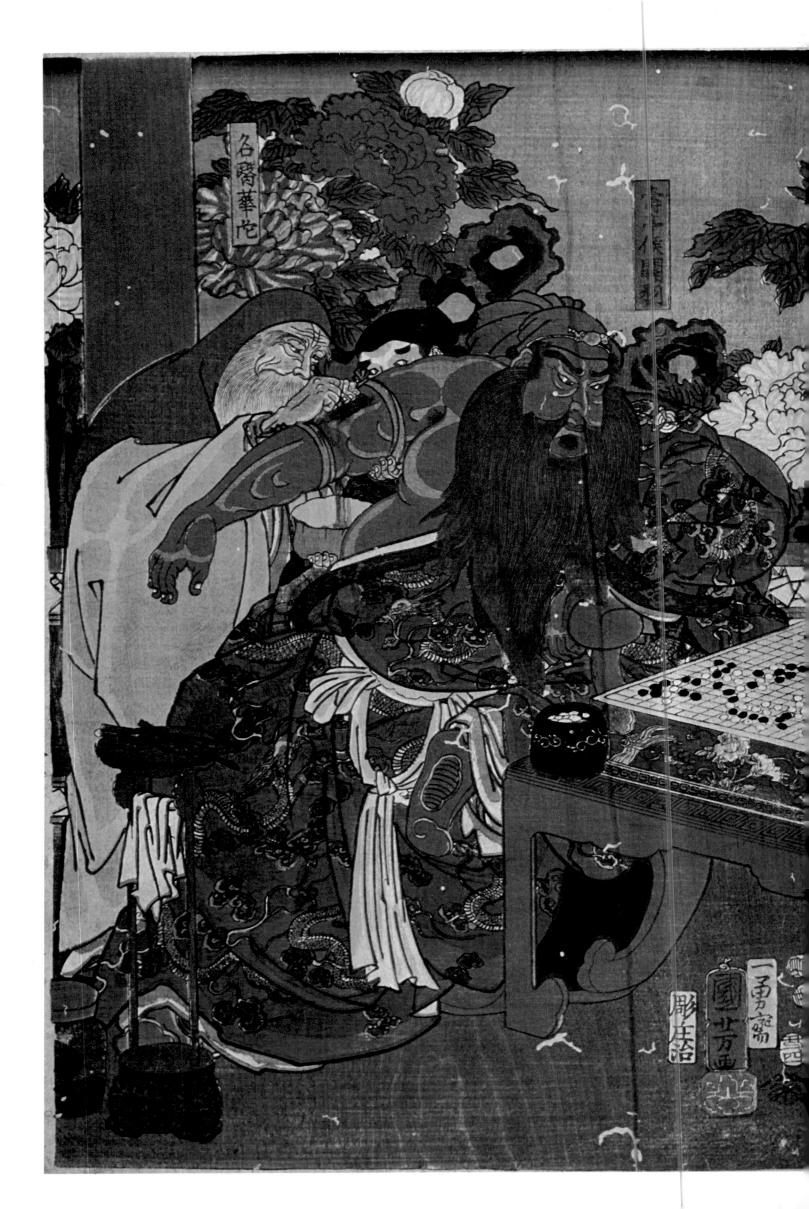

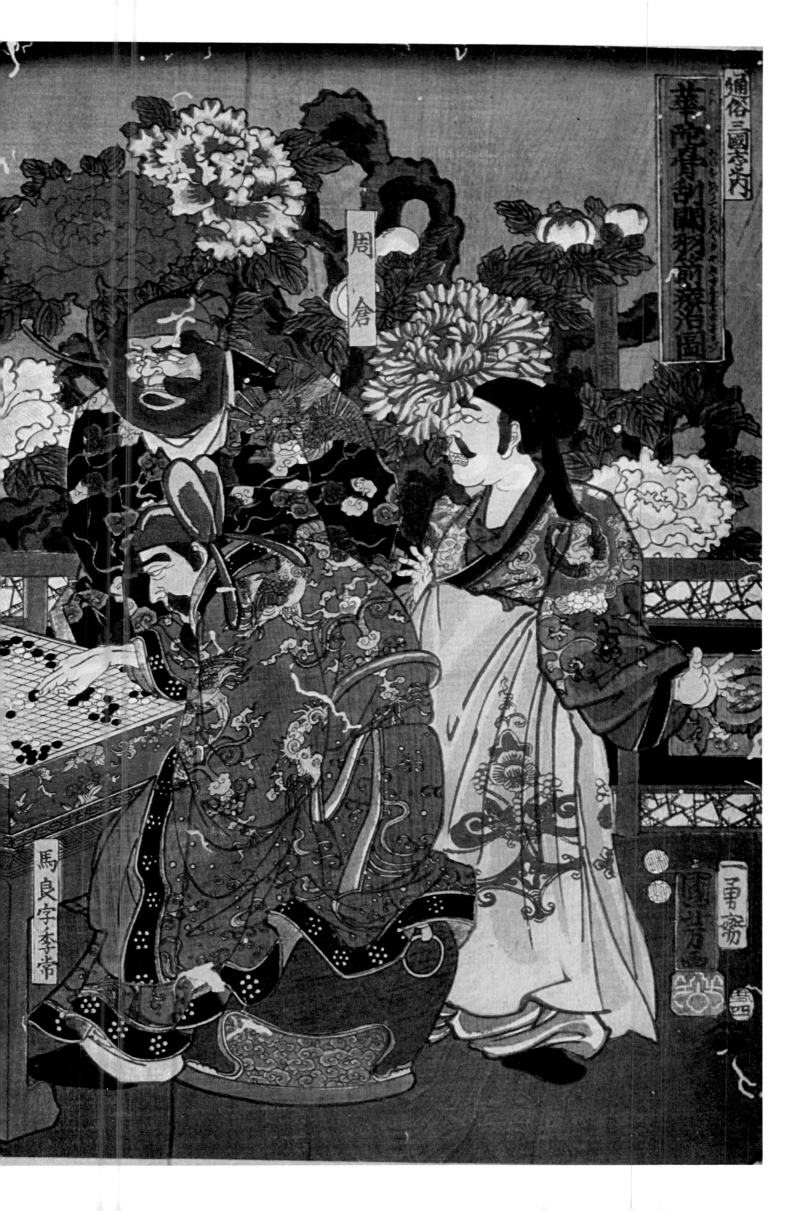

華佗書割開羽前療治圖

通俗三國志之内

周倉

馬良字季常

國芳画

CONTENTS

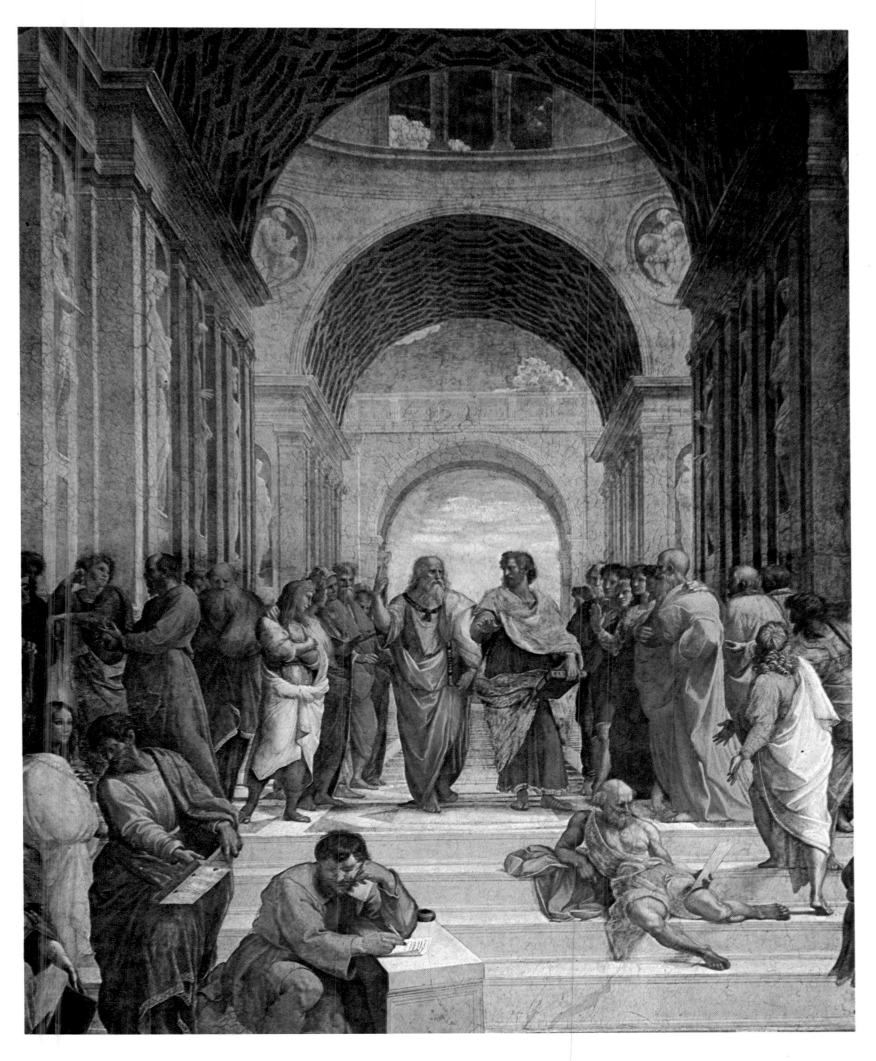

564 (detail) *Raphael's fresco* The School of Athens (*1510–11*) *was painted in response to the remarkable intellectual and artistic ferment in Renaissance Italy.*

Stanza della Segnatura, Vatican Palace, Rome

EARLY TYPES
OF MEDICINE

Prehistoric Medicine

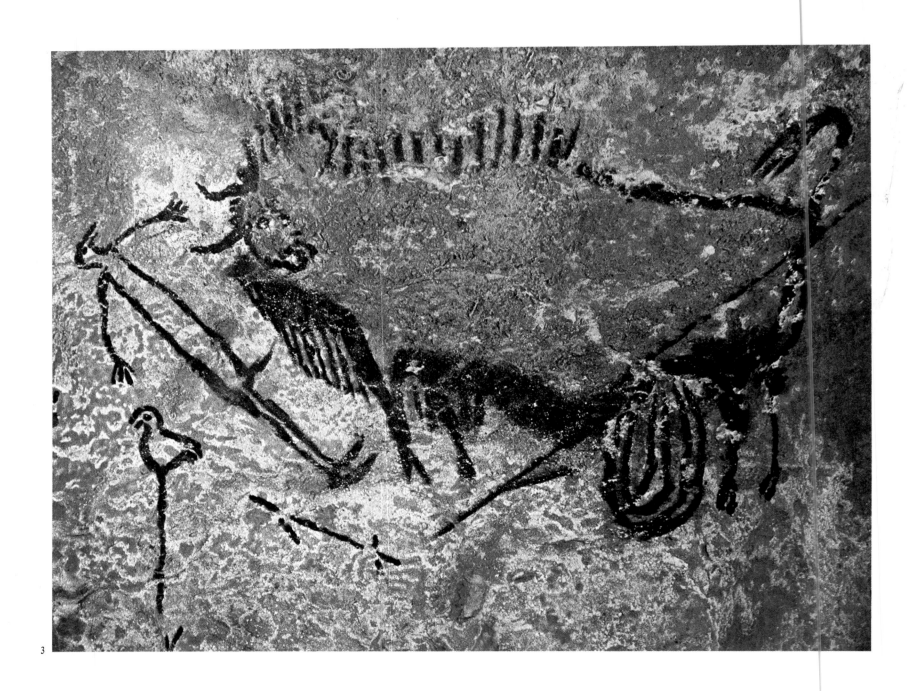

B EFORE there were humans on earth, there was disease. But were the diseases of early animals the same as those of evolving humans? And how did early humans treat their illnesses? For possible clues one must search among the surviving prehistoric skeletons and artifacts.

Studies of animal fossils have shown that prehistoric creatures were subject to manifold diseases and injuries. Fractures seem to have been common, and while some healed with little deformity, others show effects of infection (osteomyelitis), poor apposition of the bony fragments, and extensive calluses (bone "scars" associated with healing). Possibly the earliest callus known is in the arm bone of a reptile of the Paleozoic Permian period. Inflammations of both the surface of bones (periostitis) and their inner substance (osteitis) have also been reported. Arthritis in dinosaurs and prehistoric bears was evidently so common that scholars have named it "cave gout."

Paleopathology, a term given wide circulation by Sir Marc Armand Ruffer in the nineteenth century, is the study of the abnormalities which can be demonstrated in the human and animal remains of ancient times. Investigations of human remnants from historic periods have uncovered many disease entities, for instance tuberculosis and parasitic infestation in the mummies of ancient Egypt, but what of the bony remains of humans from prehistory? Clear-cut abnormalities in their skeletons and teeth also testify to the prevalence of a number of pathologic conditions. In addition, some of the bone irregularities (decalcification, overgrowths, and thickenings) may represent secondary effects of general illnesses.

Questions are still unanswered concerning some types of illnesses. For example, although Egyptian mummies show characteristics of tubercular disease of the spine, the same kind of infection has rarely been found in Neolithic bones. Nor is it yet incontrovertibly determined whether certain pathologic changes in ancient bones recovered in the Americas are attributable to pre-Columbian syphilis or to a different spirochetal disease, or whether the bones belong to a later period than supposed. Bone wasting (osteomalacia) has been interpreted by some as a sign of poor nutrition, but true rickets appears to have been rare, probably because living outdoors most of the time would have been preventive. Even the specimens claimed to be rickets were uncovered only in northern climes.

Fossil teeth show signs of erosion, abscess, and pyorrhea. When the first specimens were discovered in the nineteenth and early twentieth centuries, the now-abandoned concept that focal infections of the teeth and tonsils were a cause of arthritis was prevalent. Paleopathologists therefore linked tooth infection with the arthritis seen in prehistoric skeletons. This habit of judging the past by tenets of the present has been with us through the centuries. Cavities (caries) were also a problem by late Paleolithic and certainly Neolithic times. They became a common disorder in ancient Egypt, especially in its later history.

When it comes to prehistoric diseases of the soft parts, except for inferences drawn from changes in the bones, clear-cut evidence is absent because of failure of the tissues to survive. No bodies or organs earlier than 4000 B.C. have been discovered. Microscopic imprints on rocks seem to indicate the presence of bacteria in prehistoric periods, but since even now the vast majority of the billions of microorganisms are not harmful we have no way of knowing whether these were pathogenic (disease producing).

In the mummies of early Egypt, arteriosclerosis, pneumonia, urinary infections, stones, and parasites have been identified, which may suggest that such conditions also prevailed in earlier unrecorded epochs. We do not know whether prehistoric man suffered arteriosclerosis, but its very presence—sometimes in advanced degree—in ancient Egyptian mummies may have bearing on our modern ideas concerning its causes. If early humans existed without strains similar to those of technically advanced civilization, then stress would have an unlikely relation to arteriosclerosis. It does appear, however, that man's illnesses, for the most part, have been mere continuations of the diseases and

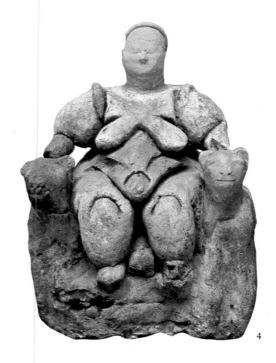

4

3 *In prehistoric scene (c. 15,000–10,000 B.C.) painted on cave wall at Lascaux, France, wounded bison, intestines spilling out, stands over ithyphallic figure, apparently dead. Interpretations of scene vary, but purpose was probably an appeal to supernatural forces rather than simple record of hunting accident.*

4 *Seated female figure (c. 6500–5700 B.C.), found in excavations of Çatal Hüyük in central Turkey, thought to be fertility goddess shown giving birth, one of earliest representations of delivery in this position. Archaeological Museum, Ankara*

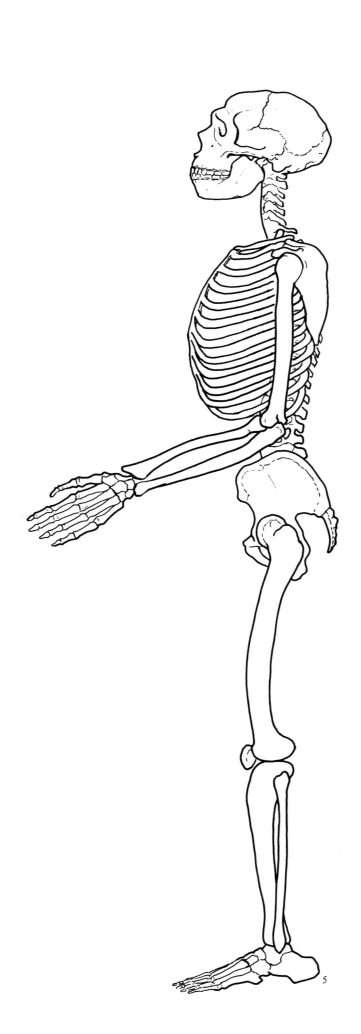

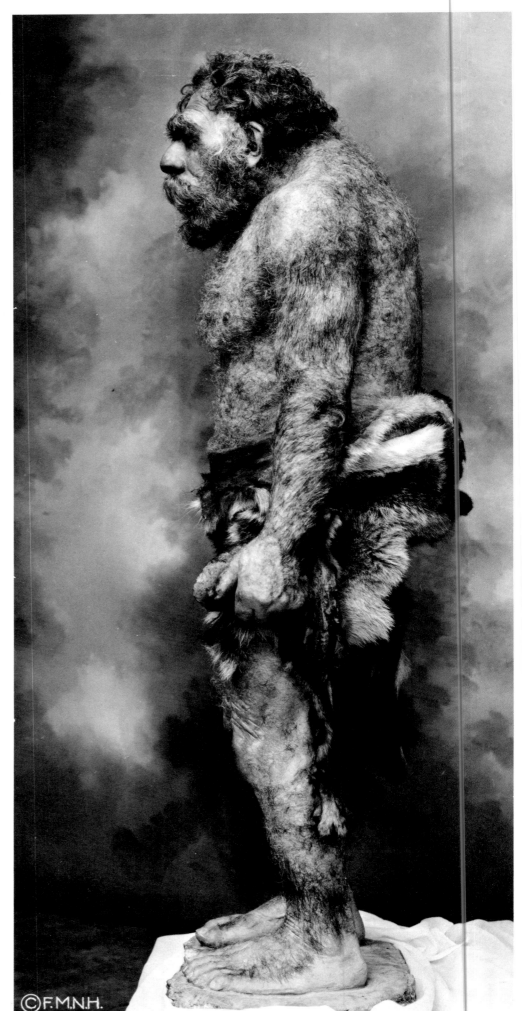

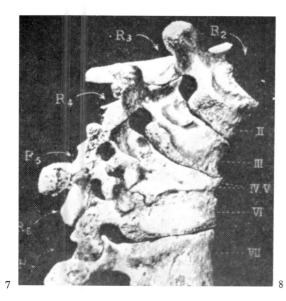
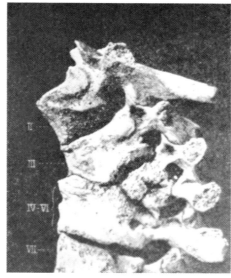

7

8

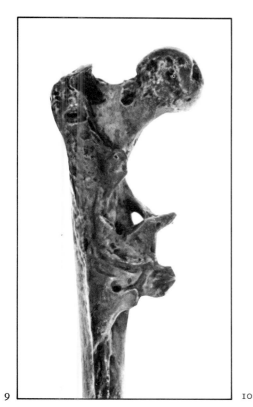
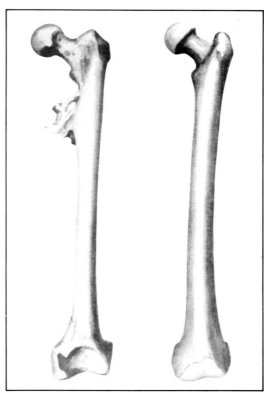

9

10

5, 6 *Neanderthal skeleton and lifelike reconstruction by Frederick Blaschke of early species of* Homo sapiens *active 40,000 to 70,000 years ago. First impressions of Neanderthal man were based on skeletal remains discovered in 1856, now considered those of man with advanced arthritis, which accounts for bent knees and rounded spine.*

7, 8 *Are these the lesions of tuberculosis on spine of Neolithic man, c. 7000–3000 B.C.? If so, they are probably the oldest example of bone tuberculosis.*

9, 10 *Bone tumor, or overgrowth after trauma, on femur (leg bone) of* Homo erectus, *earlier human species than* Homo sapiens. *Modern leg bone compared shows virtually identical size and shape despite intervening 250,000 years.*

11 *Fossilized water lily pollen (magnified 1900 times by electron microscope) of Pleistocene epoch, coterminous with first appearance of modern man, who might have suffered allergies from the beginning.*

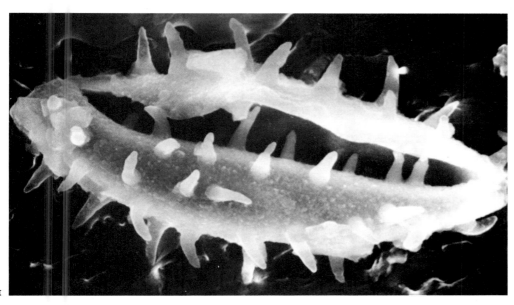

11

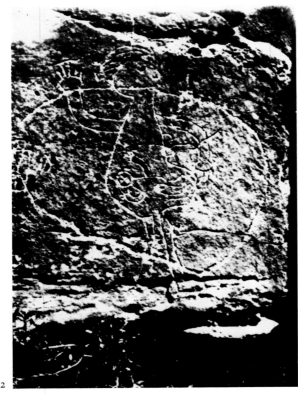

12

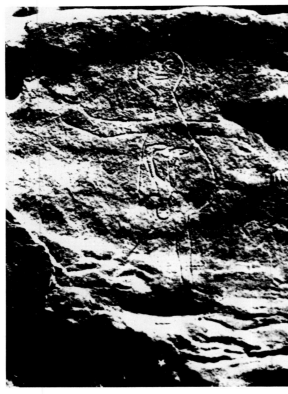

13

bodily mechanisms of the creatures who preceded or accompanied him.

What of the length and quality of life in prehistoric times? About 2600 B.C., the legendary "Yellow Emperor" of China is supposed to have said in the great *Canon of Medicine*, "I have heard that in ancient times the people lived to be over a hundred years, and yet they remained active and did not become decrepit in their activities." The emperor's rosy view of the distant past is not borne out by the findings. Bones from Paleolithic, Mesolithic, and Neolithic periods strongly suggest that a lifetime was much shorter than in more recent epochs, averaging approximately thirty to forty years.

In virtually all reported studies, men seemed to have lived longer than women, the common assumption being that pregnancy and childbirth were responsible for the difference. Skeletons of early women have been uncovered with fetuses wedged tightly in the pelvis, and also with newborns buried beside them. However, difficult labor was probably less common in the earliest millennia, the numbers of births per woman were much fewer than often assumed, and infection after delivery was probably infrequent. Furthermore, even after childbearing age women had shorter life expectancies than men of comparable age (the opposite of recent experience). A possible explanation for the shorter life spans of prehistoric women is that chronic malnutrition, starting in infancy and continuing through childhood, made women less resistant to illness. According to this idea, men and boys, as leaders, hunters, and warriors, were considerably better fed than women and girls who were the home laborers, crop cultivators, and childbearers.

How did early humans treat their illnesses? Some writers have surmised from the self-treatment of sick animals—licking wounds, delousing one other, and eating emetic grasses—that prehistoric man also employed similar care. In the first century of the Christian Era, Pliny repeated the tall tale about the hippopotamus which when ill would plunge its knee into a sharp reed to let out blood and heal itself (another example of applying the tenets of one's own time to other epochs—in this instance the idea that bloodletting was an effective medical treatment).

Was animal instinct a compelling force that enabled humans to find food, plants, substances, and procedures to nurture themselves? If so, it may have been the beginning of healing methods. The almost reflex rubbing of an injured part, using heat to relieve discomfort, and applying cold to deaden pain may all parallel the similar activities of animals who wallow in cool water and apply mud to irritated areas. Sucking skin that is pierced by insect stings and exerting pressure to stop bleeding possibly also could have been useful "medical" therapy performed by early man.

However, we also know that not all manipulations are beneficial. Nor were they necessarily well handled by prehistoric humans. For example, in noticing that menstruation relieved bodily tensions did prehistoric people thereby embark on the system of bloodletting that was to dominate healing practices for thousands of years? Or did phlebotomy (opening a vein) result from philosophical speculation rather than empiric observation?

We do not know whether *any* treatment was used by the earliest humans. Salutary outcome of sickness or injury does not necessarily mean that therapy was employed; many illnesses and wounds heal themselves. In one collection of prehistoric specimens, over half of the fractured bones seem to have healed with good results, but well-aligned healing of fractured bones of wild animals has also been observed. Furthermore, we have to guess at the knowledge of the body possessed by early humans. Cave pictures have received considerable attention and a variety of interpretations. For instance, the remarkable drawing in red ochre of a mammoth in the Pindal cave in Spain, presumably of the Paleolithic period, shows a leaf-shaped dark area where the heart should be. Whether this was meant to represent the ear, the heart, some other part, or was merely a decoration is not known. If it is truly the drawing of a heart it would be the first anatomical illustration.

22

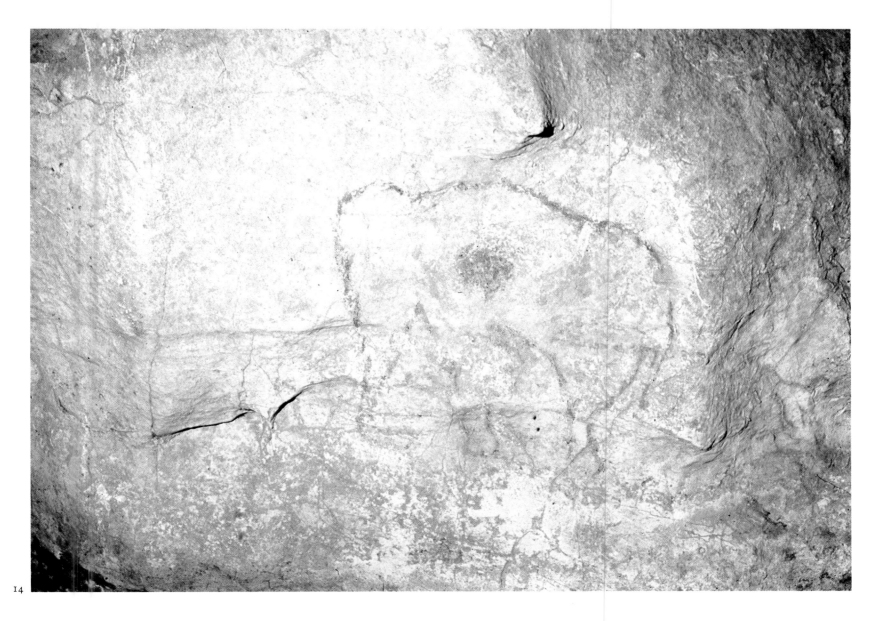

14

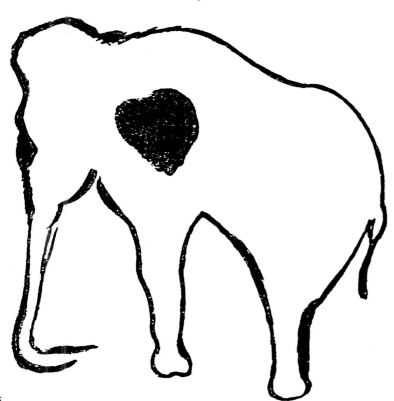

15

12, 13 *Rock-incised human figures in Spain showing pregnant woman carrying fetus in abdomen, which indicates some prehistoric knowledge of internal organs, and baby emerging from womb at birth.*

14, 15 *Paleolithic drawing of mammoth in El Pindal cave in Spain, with dark smudge at shoulder which may represent heart. Shown with contemporary redrawing, after Kühn, for clarification.*

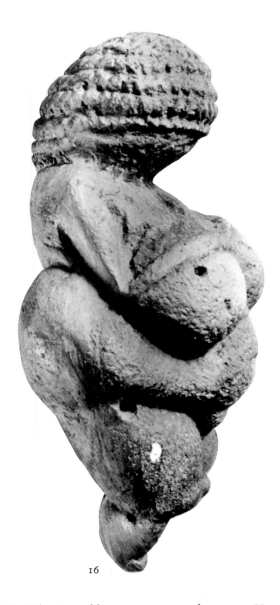

16

16 *Side view of limestone statuette known as Venus of Willendorf (c. 30,000–25,000 B.C.), considered to be fertility figure, a supernatural aid to fecundity and safe births. Naturhistorisches Museum, Vienna*

17 *Terra-cotta figure with red glaze from Cyprus thought to be fertility goddess (c. 3000–2500 B.C.). Color on figure may stand for blood (life?) and relate to prehistoric custom of painting deceased red at burial, perhaps in hopes of resurrection. The Louvre, Paris*

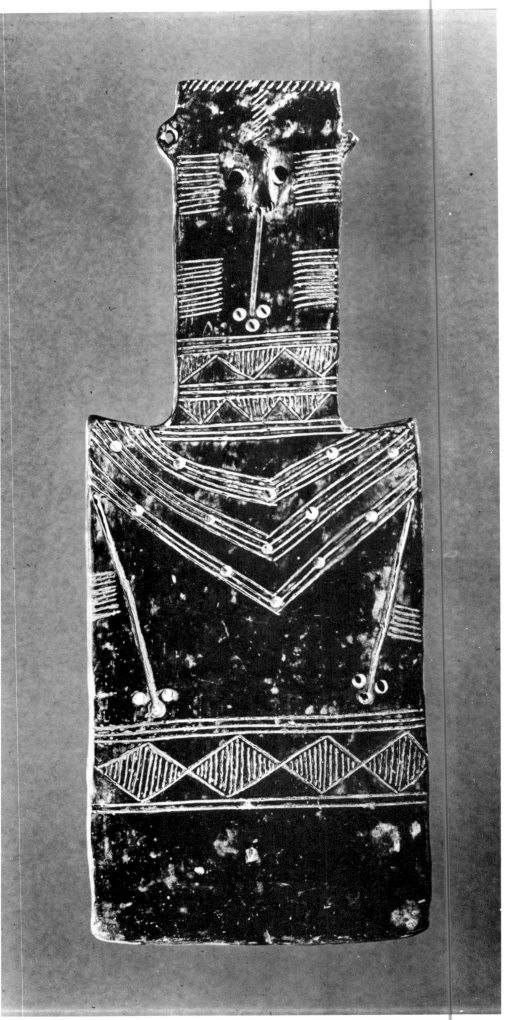

17

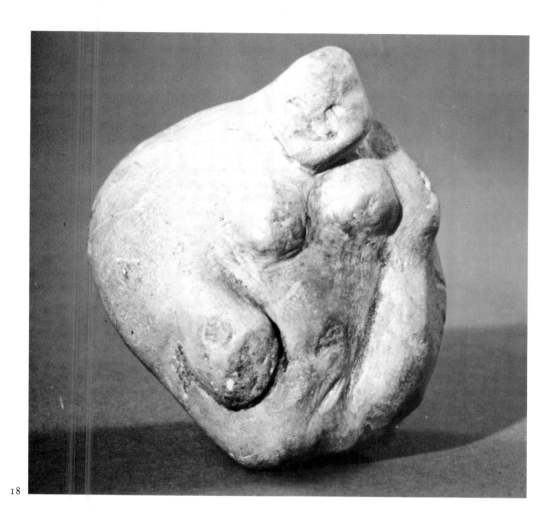

18 *Chalk figure of female from Neolithic Bronze Age (c. 2000–1800* B.C.*) found in pit at flint-mining site of Grime's Graves, Norfolk, England. British Museum, London*

19 *Reconstruction of prehistoric natural hot water baths showing Bronze Age tubings found at site of underground springs still used for hydrotherapy. St. Moritz, Switzerland*

18

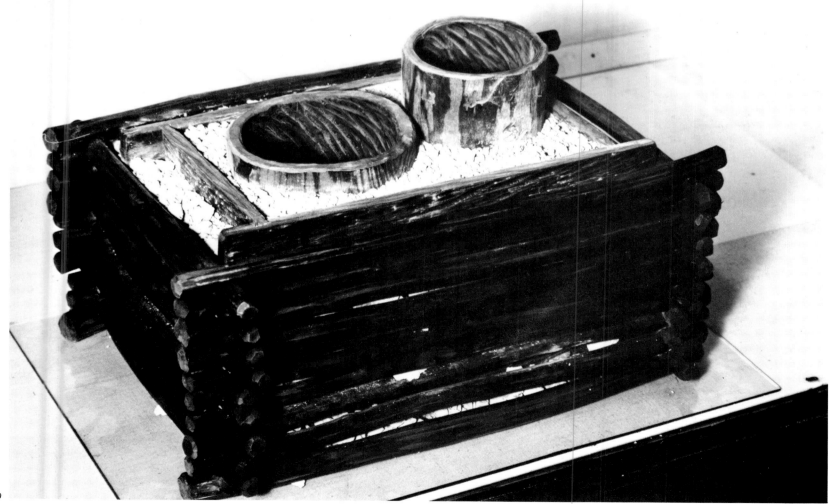

19

20, 21 *Mysterious, partly painted, partly engraved figure thought to represent shaman, or healing priest, in Les Trois Frères cave in France. Redrawing, after Breuil, shows complete effect.*

22 *Amber horse (c. 3000 B.C.), considered to be amulet with magical properties for warding off sickness and evil spirits. Museum für Vor- und Frühgeschichte, Berlin*

23 *Buffalo dancer in Rio Grande Pueblo ceremony shows continuity from prehistory of symbolic borrowing of animal power to heal sickness. Note similarity to prehistoric figure in Les Trois Frères cave.*

24 *Paleolithic shaman in animal mask shown performing ceremonial dance in engraving on fragment of reindeer rib, c. 30,000–27,000 B.C. Pin Hole Cave, Creswell Crags, Derbyshire. British Museum, London*

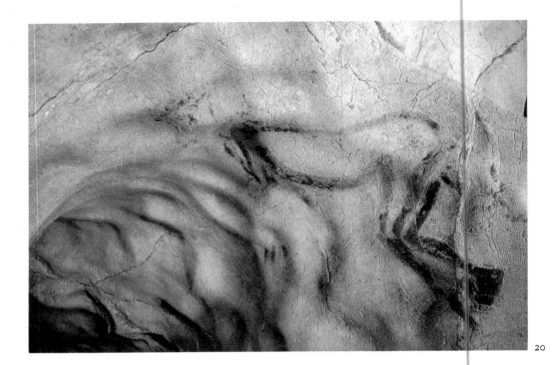

20

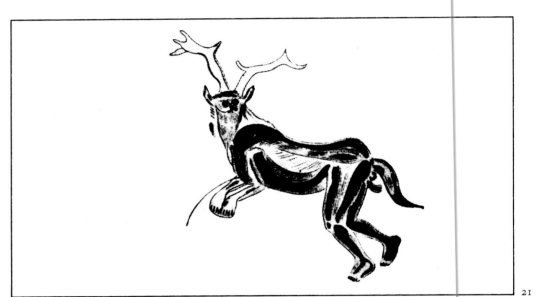

21

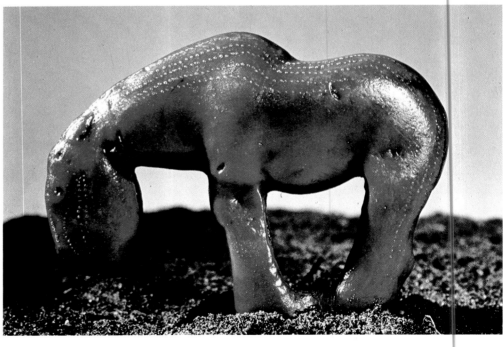

22

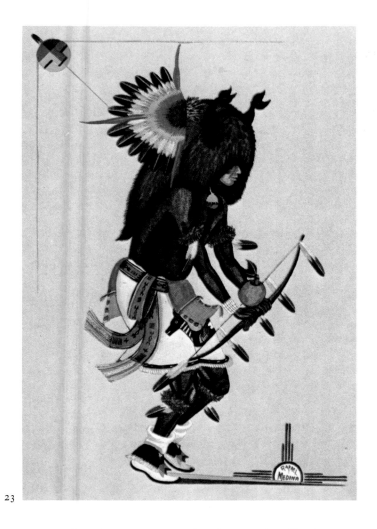

23

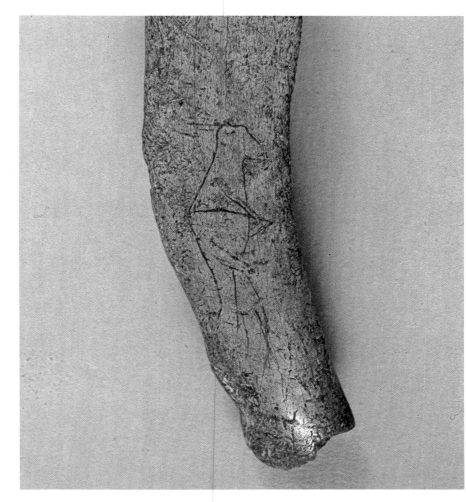

24

Did prehistoric people develop a cult of healing? A painting in the Trois Frères cave in France of an erect, possibly dancing figure with deer head or mask has been thought by some to represent the first shaman, or healing priest. Another Paleolithic fragment shows a reindeer stepping over a supine pregnant woman. Was this a ritual to transmit strength or was it a medical method to hasten labor?

In the Neolithic period (about 10,000–7,000 B.C.) humans apparently shifted from food-gathering to food-producing. One can assume that medicinal herbs were among the plants grown, but whether and when they were recognized to possess healing properties is not known. It is also possible that more secure shelter and more regularly available food led to fewer illnesses. With the use of tools Neolithic men and women became craftsmen. They may also have used implements for surgical purposes since examples of trepanation (removal of a segment of bone from the skull) dating to the Neolithic period have been discovered in France. Signs that the skull wound was healing indicate that a fair proportion survived the operation. However, each of many possible reasons for the procedure has had its advocates. That it may have been a religious rite is suggested by its performance even sometimes on the dead and by use of the removed button of bone ("rondelle") as an amulet. It may have had a magico-medical purpose of letting out a demon, as has been observed in some primitive peoples. On the other hand, it could have been a treatment for fractures or a means of removing bone splinters. Indeed trepanation may have been employed at different times for all of the above reasons.

Although the knowledge of prehistory is considerable from fossils, paleontology, physical anthropology, paleopathology, sculpture, and cave art, the answers to many of our questions are still conjectural. Folklore, known medical practices of primitive peoples, and the archaeological and literary evidences of ancient civilizations may well give additional indications of what preceded them, but this information can also be misleading since primitive societies and ancient cultures themselves have often undergone change through the centuries.

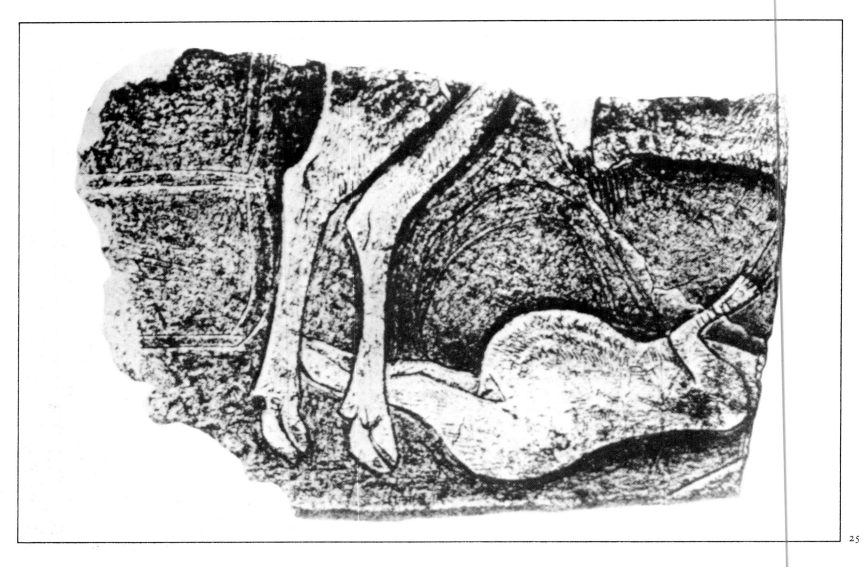

25

25 *Pregnant woman shown beneath reindeer in Paleolithic carving on reindeer bone, which may indicate a symbolic transference of strength to woman or unborn child.*

26 *Trephined skull of Neolithic period that shows healed wound edges indicating recovery from operation whose purpose, whether medical or magical, remains unknown. Nationalmuseet, Copenhagen*

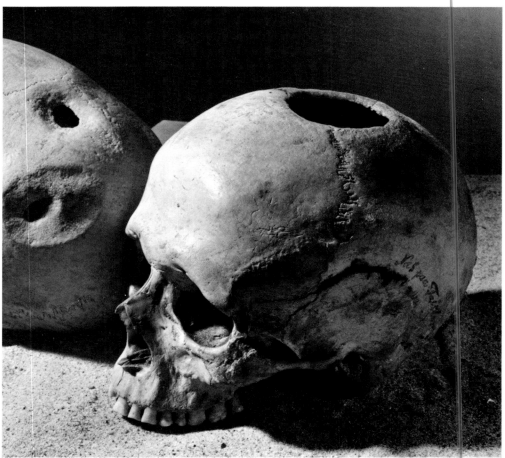

26

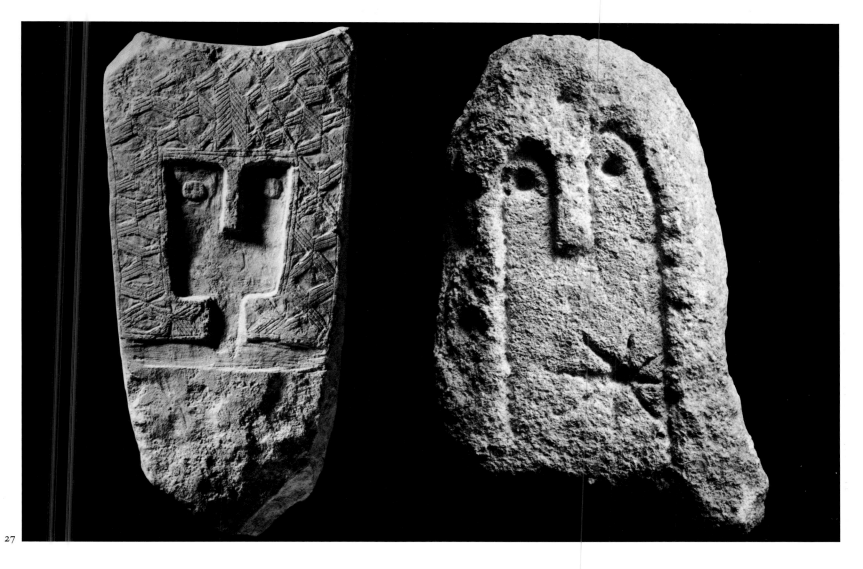

27

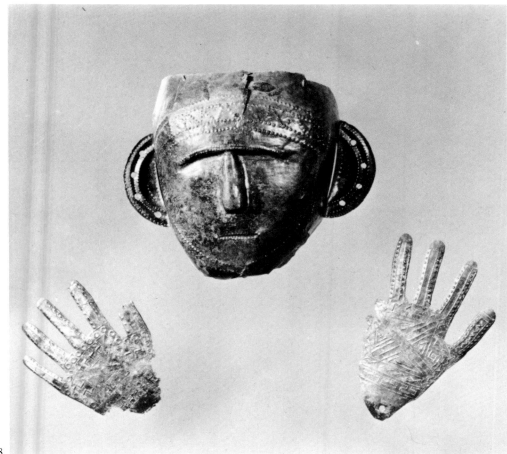

28

27 *Neolithic menhirs which seem to have had funerary or religious purposes and may show likenesses of the dead or represent gods. Left, from Rocher-des-Dômes, Avignon. Right, from Lauris, Vaucluse. Musée Calvet, Avignon*

28 *Bronze Age mask and hands made of bronze formerly affixed to container of ashes and thought to be a likeness of the deceased. Steiermärkisches Landesmuseum Joanneum, Graz, Austria*

Primitive Medicine

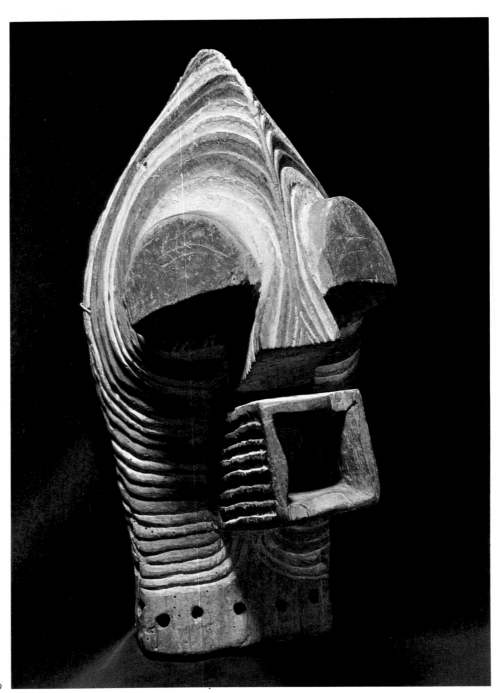

29

T HE medical ideas and practices among primitive cultures of today show considerable variety, differing in accord with geography and a society's historical heritage. Yet there are similarities which seem to be common to most primitive societies, and these may offer clues about the nature of medicine before recorded history.

HEALTH AND DISEASE

Judging from what we know of present-day primitive cultures, religion, magic, and medical treatment were seen in prehistory as inseparable from each other. The supernatural world was immanent in all things, affecting one's health, livelihood, and social activities, but not all illnesses were thought to be religiously or magically generated. Primitive man apparently often distinguished between ordinary conditions (such as old age, coughs, colds, and fatigue) and illnesses caused by spirits and evil forces that required the special services of a medicine man, shaman, or witch doctor.

The primitive patient and healer, believing in and seeking supernatural origins for most happenings, including sickness, were psychologically prepared for the effectiveness of magic. Illness could result, for instance, from the projection of an evil force or foreign object into a person by magic or sorcery. Even at a distance an effigy (or a hair or discharge from the body) could be manipulated by certain people to make the victim sicken or die. Remnants of these ancient superstitions are still with us in voodoo and the symbolic burning of someone in effigy. In some societies there were both good and bad spirits; in others, spirits were benign when pleased, harmful when offended.

Also, the dead often lingered in spirit form, trying to take over the bodies of the living. Some primitive funeral ceremonies were based on diverting the spirit of the departed from its intentions by appeasement with offerings or by preventing the spirit from recognizing members of the family. On the other hand, in addition to the risk of being possessed by a spirit, there was a danger of losing one's own soul.

A sick or disabled person was regarded in different ways by different peoples. Among the Cherokees and Navahos the ill were treated with kindness, the crippled and deformed with acceptance. In tribes faced with famine, suicide by the aged was often an accepted means of removing the burden of their dependence. The Eskimos set their old folks out unsheltered on the ice when food supplies were low. In some primitive groups the disabled were killed and eaten to preserve their life force for the tribe. Among the North American Indians, those who recovered from serious illness were looked upon with awe as possessed of unusual powers.

As for the mentally ill, primitive societies have shown the same variety of attitudes as advanced cultures. To some a deranged individual might appear to harbor an evil spirit and was therefore to be shunned, maltreated, or killed; to others the spiritual forces inside the person were worthy of respect. Among the Eskimos and Siberian peoples, psychotic behavior might signify the qualifications for becoming a shaman, who was chosen, or chose himself, just because of psychic experiences.

THE PRACTITIONERS

At the core of ministering to the sick was a central figure. We know him as medicine man among the North American Indians, shaman (the word is Tungusic) among the Eskimos and Siberian groups, and as witch doctor in the Congo. We tend to use the names interchangeably, although there are differences. Sometimes this healer was the sole practitioner in a tribe or clan. In larger groups there might be a number of them, even organized into a secret society. They all had certain characteristics in common. The healer was accorded a high place socially and politically, and he was considered learned in tribal lore and traditions.

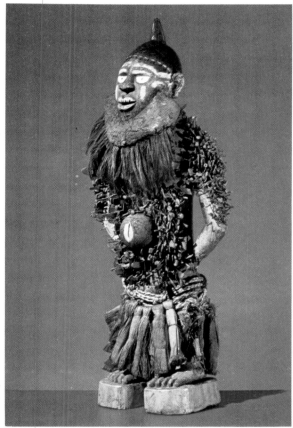

30

29 *Painted and carved wood* kifwebe *mask sometimes worn by Congo witch doctors in dances to rid Basonge villages of sickness. Collection Kamer, Cannes*

30 *Bakongo nail fetish used in Congo for either aggressive or protective magic, as directed by witch doctor. A nail is driven into figure each time its powers are called on. Field Museum of Natural History, Chicago*

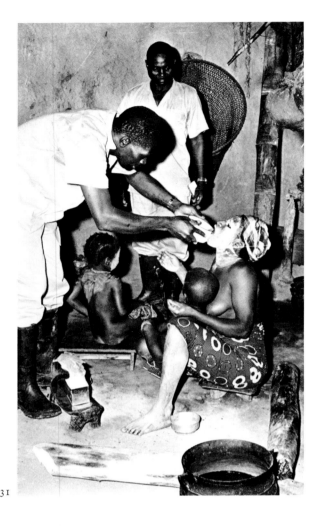

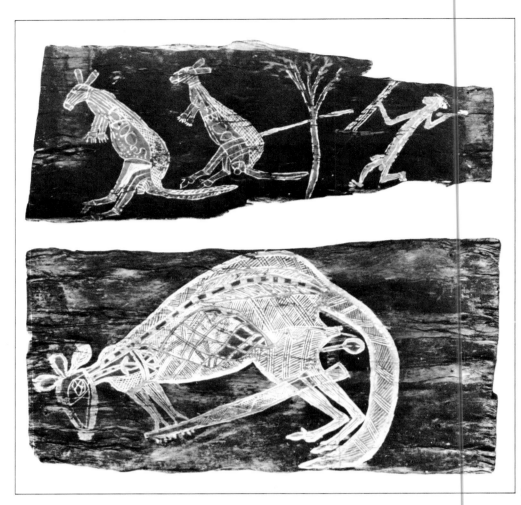

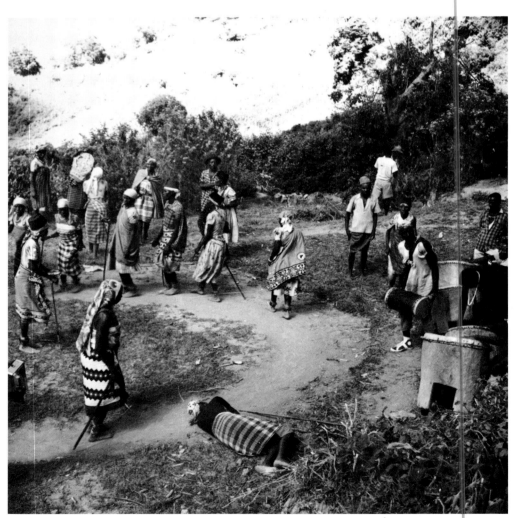

31 To chase away evil spirits causing illness, West African woman and daughter have had their faces whitewashed. However, they also are given antimalarial medication, thus combining magical and empirical remedies typical of primitive medicine.

32 Bark paintings from Oenpelli, western Arnhemland, Australia, showing kangaroos in so-called X-ray style, which indicates some anatomical interest and knowledge among primitive hunter-culture peoples.

33 African medicine men sometimes treat mental illness by causing patients to dance to rapid drumming, eventually inducing a state of trance characterized by automatic actions and hysterical convulsions, which is often followed by a condition of calm and relaxation. World Health Organization

A man's entrance into this calling might follow a recurring dream, a strong sense of mission, or an overt demonstration of unusual psychic power. Apprenticeship to an experienced doctor was common, and rituals and trials often accompanied his training. Women could also follow this special career, and in many primitive societies they were fully accepted as healers and sorcerers.

In virtually none of the primitive societies was entrance into this vocation taken lightly. Among the American Indians and also in the African Congo, a doctor could amass wealth but was vulnerable to attack if his medicine was "bad"; that is, if he did not utilize all the accepted methods. The outcome did not always have to be successful, but the techniques were expected to be above reproach. This resembles our contemporary legal strictures requiring medical procedures to conform to the standards of the community.

Although curing the sick was an important activity, the primitive healer was also responsible for protecting his people against bad weather, poor harvest, loss of flocks, or almost any catastrophe, and all religious ceremonies were under his charge. In the Congo, there were special witch doctors for virtually every ailment and every event. There were similar specializations among the Amerindians. For instance, the Arizona Indians had a specialist for the weather, for sicknesses, for injuries, and for snakebite. For illnesses not requiring religious rites, herbalists—male or female—were usually consulted, but chants and prayers accompanied the administration of drugs. Among the Ural-Altaic communities the supernatural duties of a shaman might be divided among a communicator with the spirits, a soothsayer foretelling events, and a sorcerer to cast magical spells.

The healer required special accessories. The shaman of Siberia had his drum, a distinctive hat, sometimes a mask, and a voluminous coat containing many magical and symbolic items. The North American medicine man carried a complex store of therapeutic and religious items in his medicine bag (which was sometimes a human scrotum): parts of animal and human bodies, plants, sticks, stones, and instruments such as a sucking tube.

The term "medicine" among the Indians of North America covered much more than just remedies for illness. Every venture had its "medicine": beneficial acts were "good medicine," unsuccessful efforts were "bad medicine." Every brave carried a medicine bag in which his good luck and the power of his spiritual force symbolically resided. Losing one's medicine bag was a catastrophe.

METHODS

Since illness among primitive peoples was caused by gods, spirits, and magic, the purpose of diagnosis was to determine the offense committed and the person or spirit administering the punishment. Was any taboo violated? Was any person wronged? Having taken the "history," a witch doctor might consult the gods—sometimes while in a trance—to discover which spirit or mortal was casting the spell. If the patient's soul were lost, had it wandered to some remote spot or did it inhabit someone else? Various means of divination were used: casting of bones, observing the reactions of animals to poison, moving beads to the chanted names of likely suspects. In some cultures, people thought responsible for casting a spell might be forced to undergo ordeals by poison, fire, or water to determine if they were guilty.

Treatment could be complicated, involving elaborate ceremonies, chants, mystical signs, charms, and fetishes. The African witch doctor might ensnare the offending spirit in a cockroach enticed into a basket trap by bits of food or blood. The Amerindian medicine man might spend days in dancing, shouting, and beating drums. The point of the healing rites was to drive out evil spirits, lure back a lost soul, or propitiate an offended god.

A special type of therapy indigenous to American Indians of the West was the sand painting. Elaborate, colored designs were constructed in the sand to provide a

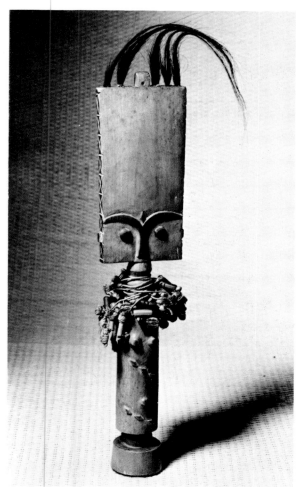

34

34 *Wooden doll with rectangular head carried by pregnant women of the Ashanti tribe in Ghana, who believe that appropriate doll will magically influence the sex of the unborn child. Nationalmuseet, Copenhagen*

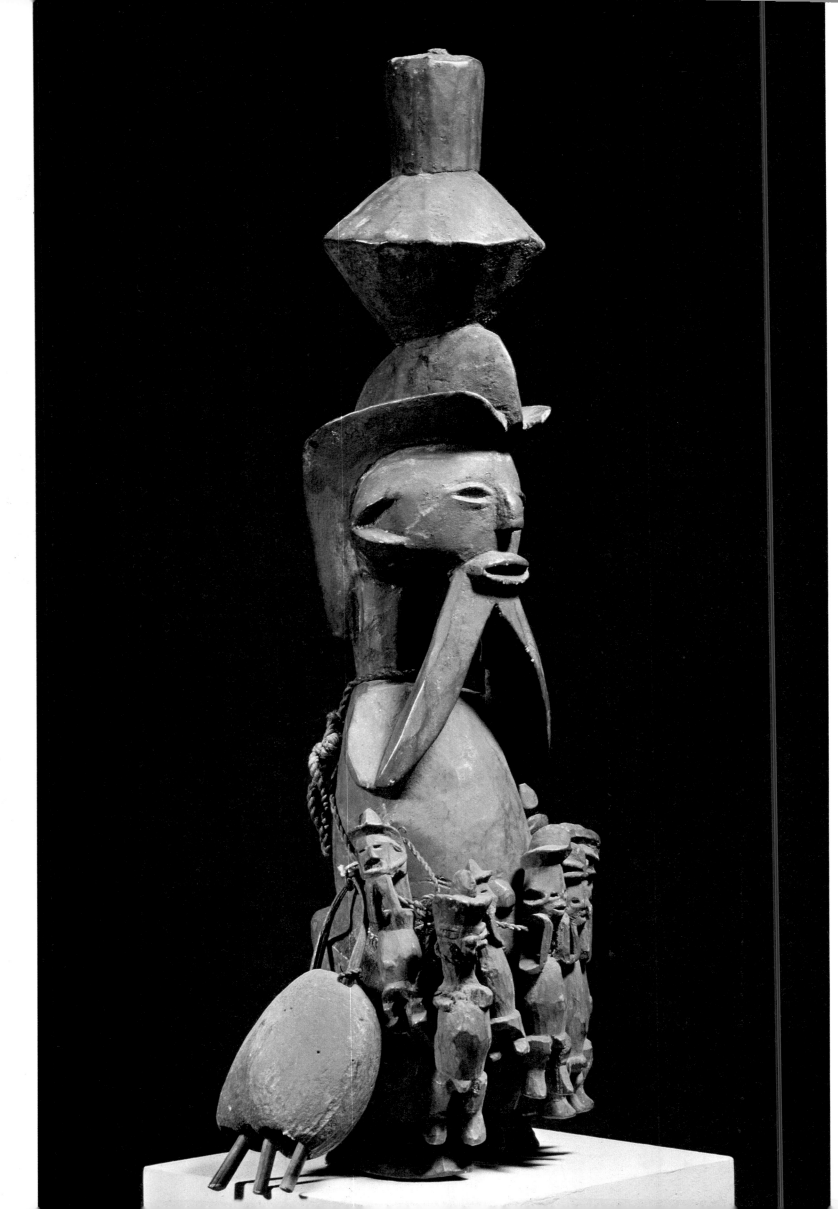

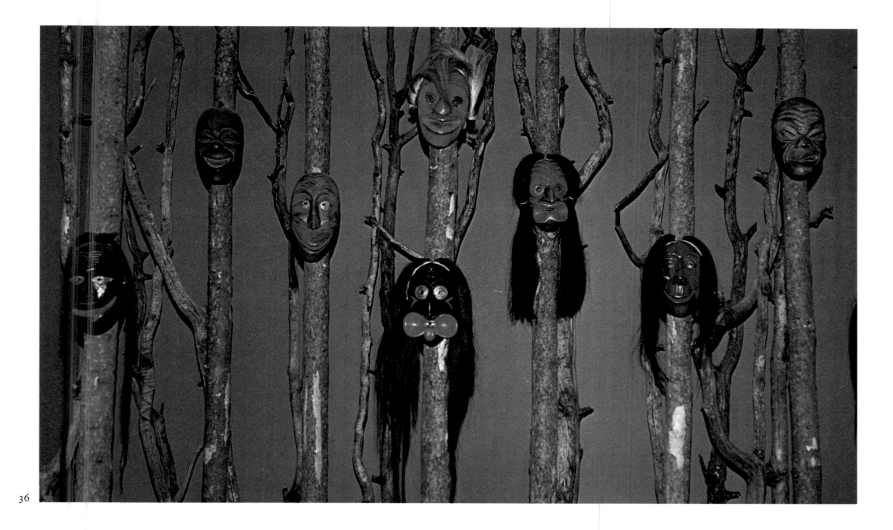

36

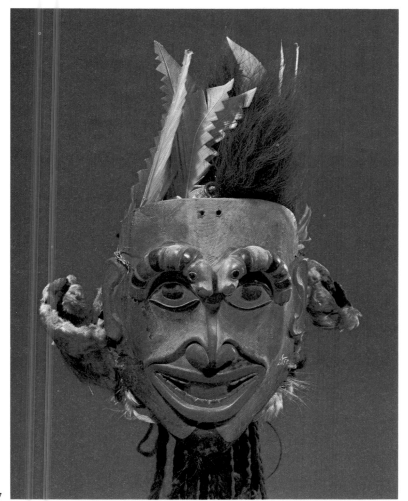

37

35 *Bahungana fetish figure from the Congo, with "medicine" bag and many miniature figures attached that contribute to its power. Museum für Völkerkunde, Berlin (Dahlem)*

36 *Masks worn by members of Iroquois False Face society to visit sick friends. Masks represent cheerful spirits invoked to aid patient's recovery, much as might be done by modern self-help groups. Denver Art Museum*

37 *Tlingit shaman's crown made of human hair, feathers, bird skin, blue jay feathers, and bearskin collected by George Emmons at Klukwan, Alaska. American Museum of Natural History, New York*

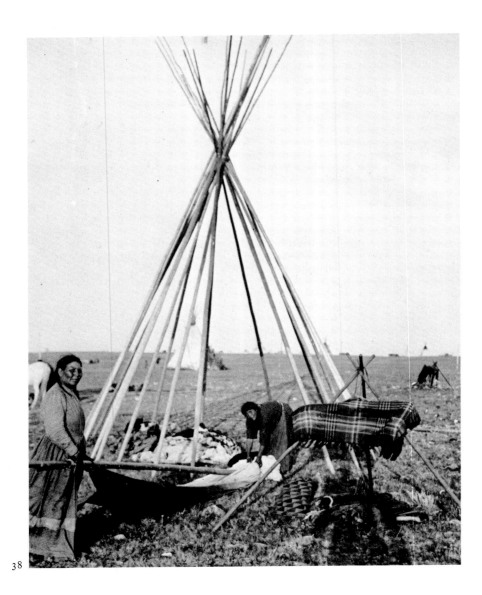

38

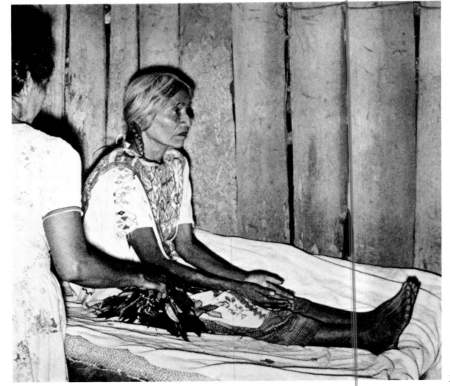

39

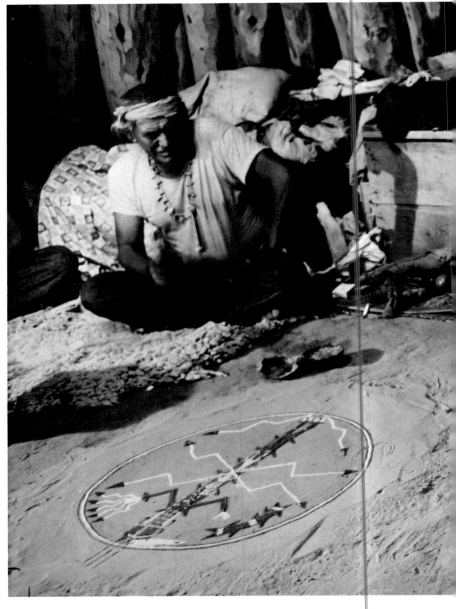

41

38 *Before erecting tepee, these American Indian women place medicine bundle, containing owner's good fortune and spiritual power, on stick tripod to placate or ward off evil spirits. Montana Historical Society, Helena*

39, 40 *Mexican medicine woman treats patient by "cleansing" her, passing medicinal leaves over her body; then, covering patient with plantain leaves, she chants incantations and prayers. Museo Nacional de Antropología, Mexico*

41 *Interior of Navajo hogan in Arizona, showing sand painting ritual being performed to aid sick child. American Museum of Natural History, New York*

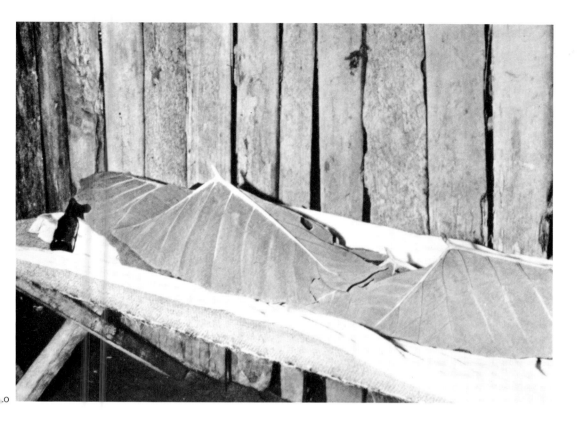

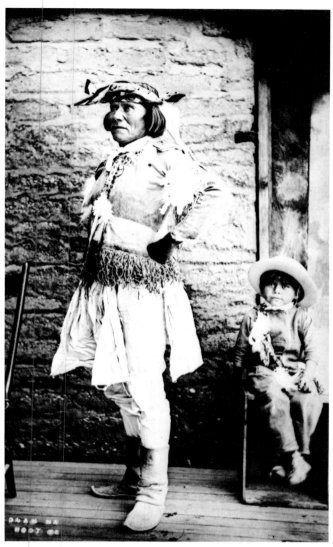

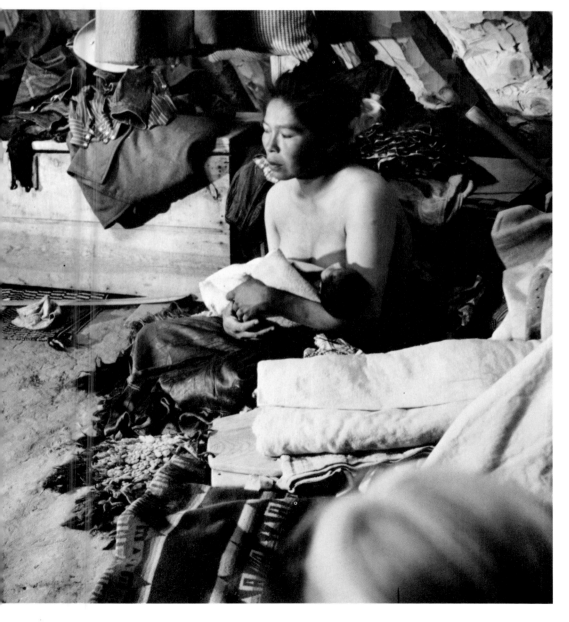

42 *Clan-na-hoot-te, an Apache tribal doctor photographed in 1884. Medicine men often had numerous accouterments in common: drums, rattles, feathered wands, sucking tubes, and necklaces of animal claws and human bones. Special Collections, University of Arizona Library, Tucson*

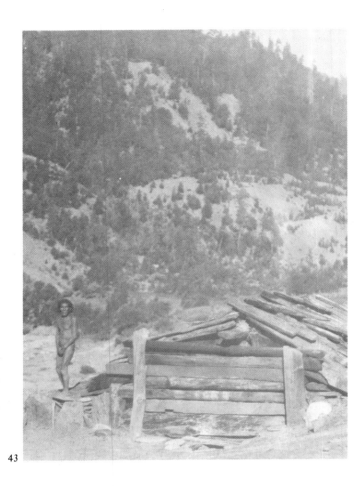

43

43 *Man of the Karok tribe surprised while leaving tribal sweat lodge, where men gather periodically for heat treatment thought to maintain health and cure illness. Photographed along the Klamath River in California or Oregon, 1894. National Anthropological Archives, Smithsonian Institution, Washington, D.C.*

44 *During Bakongo circumcision rites de passage, Zombo youths live for months isolated in lodges, from which they intermittently venture out in masks to frighten women into giving them food and money.*

45 *Mexican female witch doctor "smokes" patient and invokes powers of pagan and Christian divinities. She then sucks out evil from patient's head and cleanses body by passing egg or black hen over it. Museo Nacional de Antropología, Mexico*

46 *Bilbo, or American Indian medicine man, displays offending object supposedly extracted from body of sick person, thus convincing him and relatives of his recovery. National Library of Medicine, Bethesda*

medium through which the spirits could act to cure a sick person. The paintings were begun at sundown and had to be destroyed by the next nightfall lest this powerful medicine cause harm rather than good.

Sometimes a more direct attack was mounted, as for example by sucking, cupping, bleeding, fumigating, and using steam baths. Among American Indians the practice of appearing to suck out an offending object from a patient's ear, scalp, or other part was common, but it is probable that removing the foreign object was to the medicine man as much a symbolic act as it was deception.

There was also considerable rational empiricism in the magical methods. Religious rituals were frequently accompanied by the secular manipulations of massage, poultices, and drug lore, but the explanation for their use may have been supernatural. The American Indians had an especially rich knowledge of medicinal herbs. Some drugs were used for magical purposes because they suggested some aspect of the disease: yellow plants for jaundice, hairy plants for baldness, thistles for sore throat. However, one can compile a huge list of plant decoctions which were empirically effective for specific ailments. Medicinal plants seem to have been well understood by medicine men who used them according to their pharmacologic action: antifebrile, laxative, emetic, antispasmodic, diuretic, local analgesic, respiratory-soothing, pain-relieving, sedative, stimulating. Hallucinatory drugs were favorably known in many primitive societies, and the Omaha, Kiowa, and Fox tribes of the American West even organized societies of peyote (mescal) button devotees. Other plant substances such as jimsonweed produced the mental state suitable for certain ceremonies of the Mariposa Indians.

Surgery

Surgery consisted principally of treatment for wounds and injuries to the bones. Among the peoples who applied salves and other substances to open wounds, sealing them off and preventing drainage, it is likely that infection was common. On the other hand, some primitives took pains to keep wounds protected and dry. When sewing up lacerations with strips of tendon and needles of bone, some Amerindian tribes (the Dakotas, for instance) placed a strip of bark between the wound edges which probably permitted drainage and promoted healing from the inside out.

Hemorrhage was controlled by pressure, tourniquet, cautery, and styptic plant substances, for ligature of blood vessels was apparently unknown. Although amputations were performed, they seem to have been mainly ritualistic. Removal of spears and arrows was sometimes accomplished with great skill. Small abscesses were drained, and the tribes of the Great Lakes region are said to have opened abscesses of the chest cavity.

The treatment of fractures among the American Indians was sophisticated in some tribes. They fashioned splints of wood and casts of hardened hides, with openings to permit further treatment of compound fractures where bone protruded through the skin. Reduction of dislocations was also practiced. Surgical procedures were not always performed by the medicine man, for there were often others skilled in this kind of work.

During surgery, drugs were used to deaden the senses or to relieve severe pain from a wound. In Central Africa a beverage which may have been alcoholic was used to lessen consciousness. Before some tribal ceremonies, a performer would smear his skin with plant substances which numbed it and permitted him to bear intense heat and the pain of sharp instruments.

Trepanation was practiced in many ancient primitive societies, as it had been in prehistoric times, and in recent primitive cultures the procedure seems to have been ritualistic or a way of letting out spirits. Whether there was also an earlier more pragmatic medical use in treating skull injuries, as some have suggested, is not known.

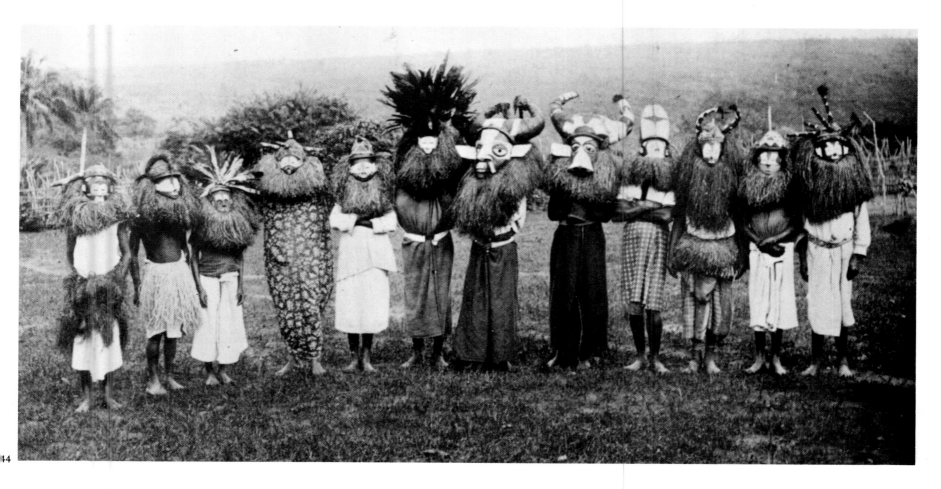

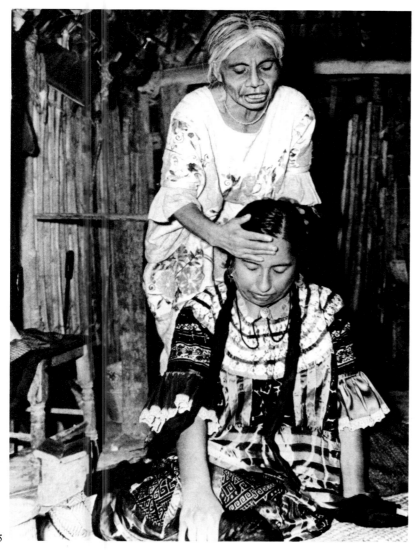

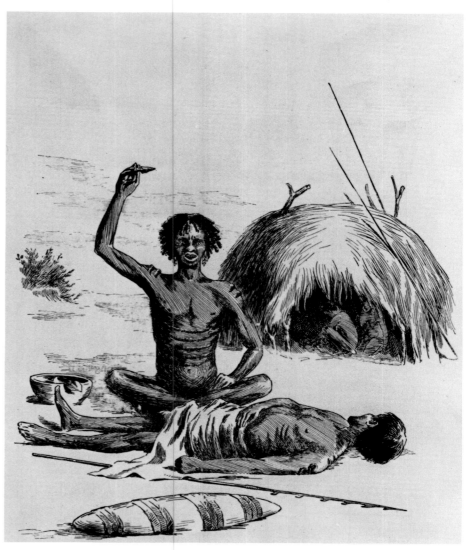

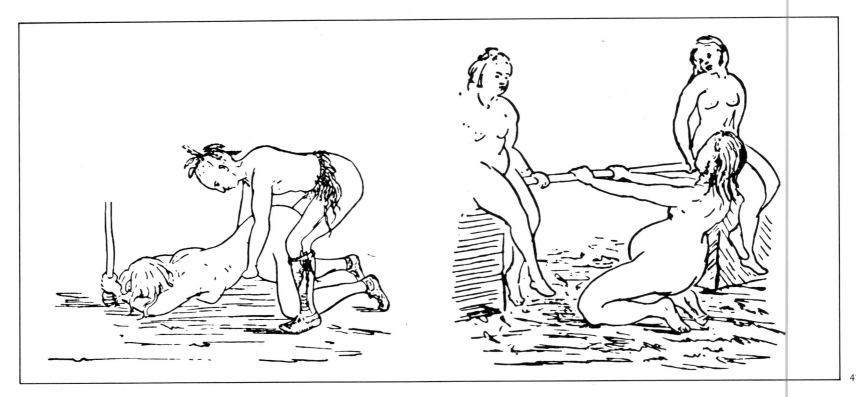

47 *Kutenai Indian woman, on knees and elbows, being helped to give birth by outside pressure on uterus. Chippewa Indian woman shown in labor in kneeling position.*

48, 49 *The Ibibio* ekpo *society owns sickness masks which portray spirits held responsible for certain illnesses such as leprosy and gangosa, the consequences of which are shown with great realism in mask on left with truncated nose, probably due to leprosy (Museum voor Land- en Volkenkunde, Rotterdam), and on right, illustrating that gangosa destroys mainly lower parts of the nose. Collection Dr. M. Kofler, Riehen/Basel*

50 *Douala statuette from Cameroon showing self-administered enema, used to instill medicines and sometimes hallucinogenic agents as well as to evacuate the bowels. Musée de l'Homme, Paris*

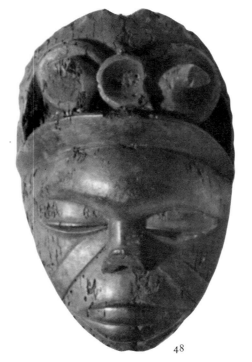

48

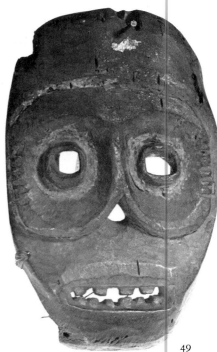

49

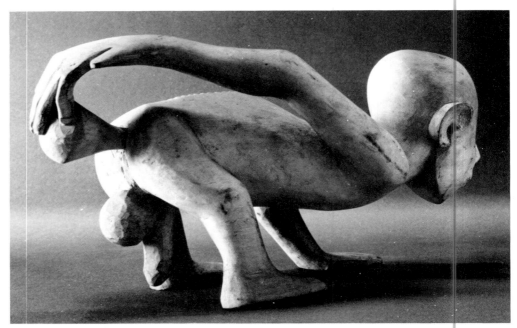

50

Obstetrics was in the hands of women. Attitudes varied with the group and its environment, but most nomadic peoples seem to have had less concern for pregnant women than the more settled groups. In many tribes of North America the afterbirth (placenta) was expelled by massage (the Credé maneuver practiced in modern hospitals today). Among some peoples, women returned to work almost immediately after delivery; among others, days or even weeks were spent in recuperating. Certain groups practiced couvade, a custom whereby the father takes to bed as if bearing the child and goes through ritual acts which presumably draw away evil spirits that might harm the mother and baby.

PUBLIC HEALTH AND HYGIENE

Apparently primitive societies were subject to many of the same diseases which afflict humans today if we are to judge by the multiplicity of ailments under the care of specialized shamans, including stomach upsets, diarrheal diseases, respiratory illnesses, rheumatic ailments, and menstrual disorders. However, some diseases were definitely introduced later by advanced civilizations. For instance, the virtual absence of immunity of American Indians to smallpox and yellow fever suggests that these illnesses were not indigenous. On the other hand, sleeping-sickness among Africans was dealt with often by witch doctors and was probably an affliction of long standing. Unsettled questions still remain on the origins of some epidemic scourges among the primitive communities such as syphilis and tuberculosis.

There were methods of preventing disease other than ceremonial and religious among some primitives, but the time of their introduction is unknown. Long before the colonial period in Africa, some tribes had practiced a type of protection against smallpox by variolation (inserting fluid from smallpox blisters under the skin). This was aimed at producing a mild form of the disease which would save the person from severe illness, for it was recognized that one never acquired it a second time. In some parts of Asia smallpox scabs in water had been pricked into the skin since ancient times, and the Chinese were known to blow powdered scabs into the nostrils. Whether these methods were the heritage of prehistory has not been determined.

In some respects the ill or wounded primitive may have been better off than the sick of a more advanced civilization since he was often isolated in a separate hut or lodge with less chance of contracting (or transmitting) infections. In contrast one can cite the frequent contagions in medieval hospitals and the terrible wound gangrenes in the poorly ordered hospitals of the American Civil War.

THE HERITAGE OF PRIMITIVE MAN

In developing ways of coping with the problems and afflictions of life, primitive man arrived at some solutions which have continued to be effective into modern times. By trial and error he found plant and mineral substances which even today are used to alleviate specific complaints. Primitive man also observed that some dread diseases never struck a person twice and worked out ways of purposely contracting a mild case rather than risk the full-blown effects. He recognized that excessive bleeding could be stopped by applying extreme heat to a wound, but he also believed that releasing moderate amounts of blood by opening a vein improved certain conditions.

Of course many of his most favored techniques had no rational or pharmacological basis, but he certainly recognized the psychological benefits to the sick of a healer's even appearing to do something effective, that under certain conditions the body seems better able to cure itself.

We do not know in what remote period primitive man first decided to invest the healing arts entirely in a specialist, but by the time mankind had reached the stage of "civilization" the doctor was already in practice.

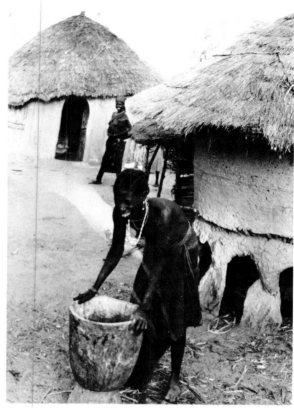

51

51 *Among primitives, some everyday and ritual practices were unsanitary, but others were protective, such as burying excrement to prevent bewitchment and keeping streams clean to avoid offending river gods. World Health Organization*

52 *Wooden pattens worn in the Nilotic Sudan as protection against guinea worm were pragmatic hygienic measure developed by primitive people to supplement magical methods of maintaining health. Wellcome Institute for the History of Medicine, London*

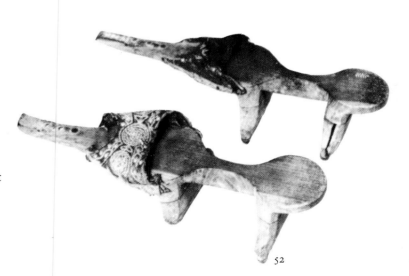

52

Medicine in the
Pre-Columbian Americas

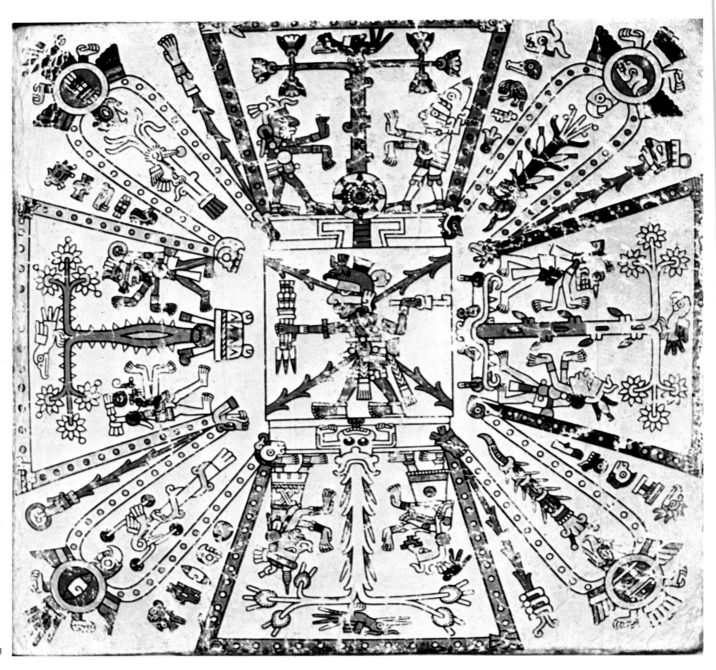

53

WHEN the *conquistador* Hernán Cortés and his followers crossed the Gulf of Mexico for the first time in the year 1519, they expected to find primitive natives like those encountered in the Caribbean islands to the east. Instead, they found the Aztecs, rulers of the greatest empire in the New World, with advanced forms of government, planned cities, engineering and architectural skills, a system of writing and recording history through pictograms, a developed agriculture, and a sophisticated understanding of mathematics and other sciences, including medicine. The Spaniards' astonishment was further compounded when they first saw and later conquered the Aztecs' capital Tenochtitlan (present-day Mexico City), which rivaled the capitals of Europe.

To the south, another people, the Mayans, were settled in the Yucatán peninsula, Guatemala, and Honduras. Although in decline for centuries (having already abandoned some of their cities), the Mayans exhibited a cultural and scientific sophistication whose equal was only rarely found in the Old World. Even further south, in the Andes, was the extensive empire of the Incas.

The civilizations of the New World which so astonished the Europeans were, at that time, experiencing the final waves in a history that extended back thousands of years. Besides the three major civilizations mentioned, many other tribes, some quite advanced, others seminomadic hunters, had also existed.

About thirty-five hundred years ago, in the humid jungles of Tabasco and Veracruz, the Olmecs, a sensitive, brilliant people, began a civilization which was to define much of the cultural values of all the peoples of Mesoamerica. At about the height of their splendor, however, the Olmecs suddenly disappeared for reasons unclear even today. Fifteen hundred years ago the Maya achieved impressive advances in art and science. Their calendar was more accurate than many formerly used in the Old World, and they were able to predict with uncanny accuracy eclipses and even the movements of the planets.

About the year A.D. 1000, the people called Toltecs established their empire in central and southern Mexico, which was perhaps the first politico-military state in the New World. Several hundred years later, the hitherto semibarbarian and culturally insignificant Aztecs migrated into the area and within a century had established complete dominance. Like the Toltecs before them, they adopted many of their predecessors' cultural qualities, which derived ultimately from the Olmecs. In the coastal regions of Peru, centuries before the birth of Christ, organized communities with rich cultural histories already existed, and, in the Bolivian Andes, the ruins of Tiohuanaco tell of a past splendor whose era we cannot precisely fix.

The Aztecs and other tribes believed that before the appearance of man a race of giants or gods had sacrificed themselves for the maintenance of the sun and that it was necessary for man to continue this practice. Blood was thought to sustain the sun, and elaborate sacrificial altars were constructed where, with sharp obsidian knives, priests tore beating hearts from living human beings! A large number of people throughout Mesoamerica were sacrificed in this way, and, to maintain an adequate supply for sacrifice, local wars often had the express purpose of providing victims. The Spaniards cited this abhorrent practice to justify the forced conversion to Christianity and subjugation of native populations.

An unfortunate side effect of Spanish rejection of some aspects of native culture (because they were "works of the devil" or "magic") was the destruction of the vast majority of local records, including the history and literature of many societies. Hence, our reconstruction of pre-Columbian life depends in large part on the chronicles of the Spaniards themselves (both *conquistadores* and missionaries) or of natives converted by them. Fortunately, the intense fascination of the conquerors with the conquered led to a rich and extensive reporting, colored only by religious and philosophical differences.

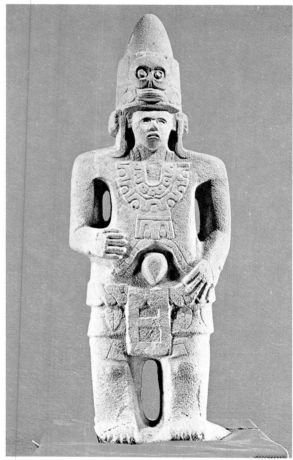

54

53 *The need to see a pattern in a mysterious universe is as old as the human race. Mixtec map of the Five World Regions identifies four past worlds at cardinal points and present earth in center, each represented by god who directs the history. From Mayer Fejervary Codex, A.D. 1000–1500. Merseyside County Museums, Liverpool*

54 *Figure from El Naranjo, Central Veracruz, with exposed heart in place of navel, mythical location for center of world as well as human life. Museo Nacional de Antropología, Mexico*

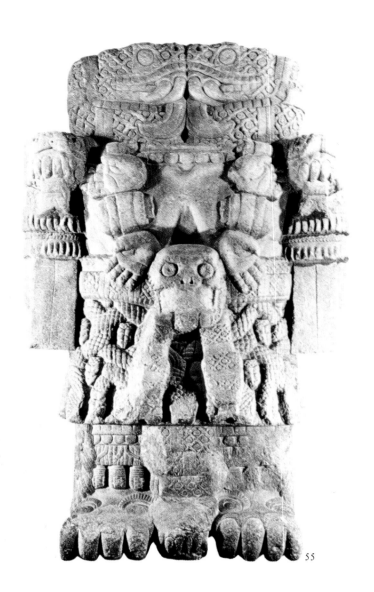

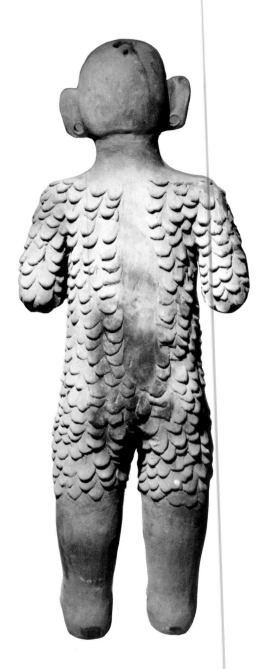

55 *Supreme Aztec goddess Coatlicue*

56 *Eagle devouring a human heart on painted terra-cotta relief from Central Mexican Highlands. Gift of Frederick E. Church, 1893, Metropolitan Museum of Art, New York*

57 *Large reddish-clay figure of priest shown clad in human skin of flayed sacrifice to the god Xipe Totec. Early classic period, Veracruz. Collection Stendahl, California*

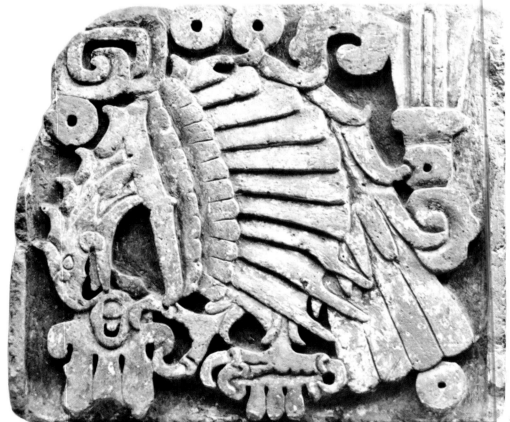

44

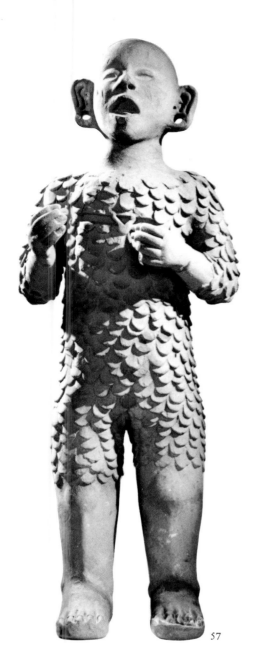

57

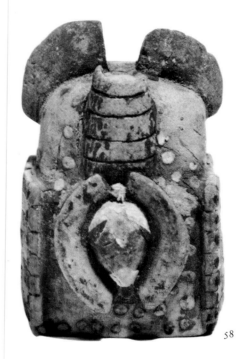

58

58 *Wooden box in form of jaguar. Back shows simplified representation of heart, lungs, and bronchi. Nazca culture, Tiahuanaco, c. 900–700 B.C. Staatliches Museum für Völkerkunde, Munich*

59 *Nayarit funeral procession modeled in brown clay with red and white paint. Corpse is carried on shoulders of attendants, and procession is led by servants carrying plates of food offerings on their heads. Collection Dr. and Mrs. George C. Kennedy, Los Angeles*

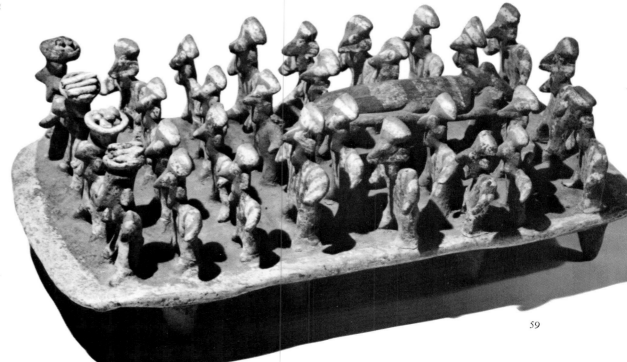

59

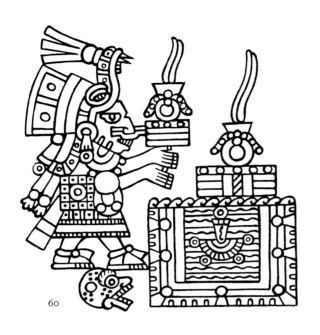

60

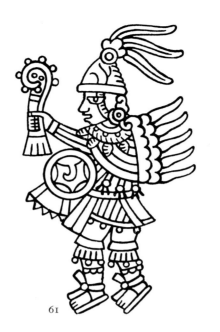

61

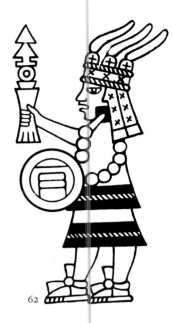

62

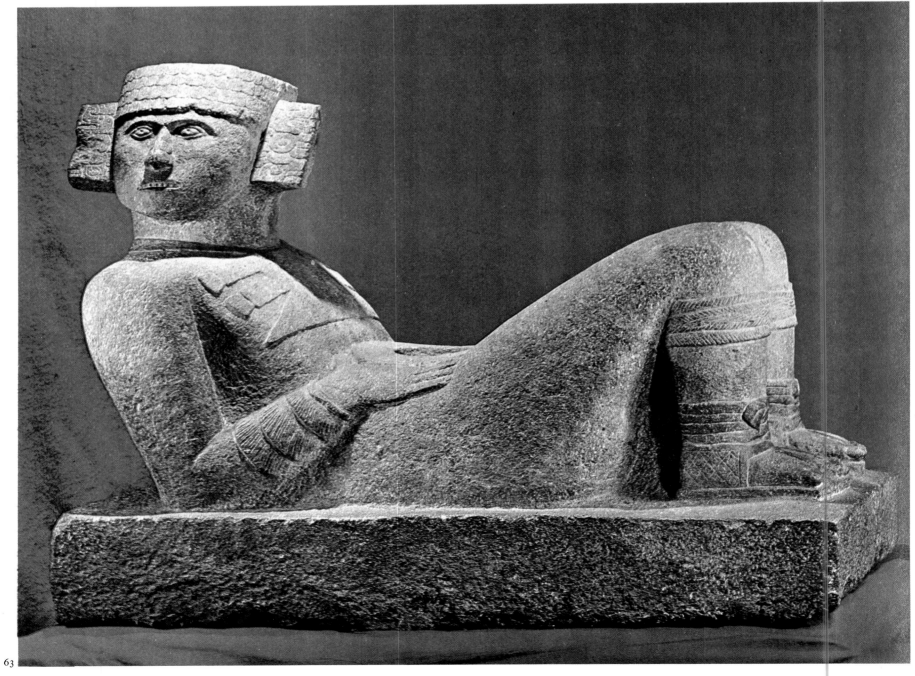

63

Attitudes toward Disease

The pre-Columbian cultures maintained an intricate blending of religion, magic, and science to combat sickness, similar to the medicine of primitive societies: religion because certain gods were responsible for diseases whereas others would protect their devotees; magic since many diseases thought to be caused through enchantment by enemies or rivals had to be cured through magic; science in that plants, minerals, and medical procedures were used whose value is accepted to this day. Without doubt, however, magic and religion were more important than science.

Disease represented a loss of balance between favorable and unfavorable influences. It was important to determine the responsible force in order to placate or expel it. For the pre-Columbian native, nothing was natural, not even death; a supernatural power toyed with mankind, as in other ancient civilizations. Causation was inevitably otherworldly, but the origin and development of disease would vary according to the circumstances.

The decline of Mayan society might have had some connection to the persistence of endemic, contagious disease, most probably yellow fever, or "black vomit," as it was characterized by the Maya in their pictograms and by the Spanish conquerors. It is possible that this disease was responsible in part for the Mayan exodus from their homes and temples, their abandonment of magnificent cities later covered over for centuries by the jungle.

Medicine and its Practitioners

In most societies of Mesoamerica, primitive medical practices coexisted with sophisticated concepts and procedures. As in the primitive medicine of less advanced civilizations, magical practices (the invocation of spirits or influences) were mingled with procedures shown by experience to be effective, procedures employed largely in response to an immediate need, such as a wound, an injury, or severe pain.

As in most primitive societies, the roles of doctor, witch doctor, and priest were commonly united in the same person. In the Americas, the witch doctor relied heavily upon ceremonial clothing and ritual gestures as he would kneel beside the sick person, rub the diseased part, and then attempt to suck out the cause of disease. In front of relatives and friends gathered around the sick person, the witch doctor with grotesque gesturing, would regurgitate arrowheads, small toads, and other strange things to which the disease had been attributed (as did the Amerindian medicine man and the Congo witch doctor).

Another kind of healer-priest was the Old World shaman, characterized by his use of trances. In the New World, shamanism was widespread throughout the continents, but its presence was especially strong in both the extreme north and south (in Chile, for instance), and that is cited as supporting the theory that the original inhabitants of the Americas came from Asia.

Another characteristic of these practitioners was the separation they made between magical practices (which they, in general, retained for themselves) and simple surgical procedures (which were commonly entrusted to lesser personages). The witch doctor set himself apart from the general population, and his clothing and way of life distinguished him. Not only did his embellishments signify distinction and superiority over other members of the group, but they were intended to produce a terrifying aspect which would impress and frighten demons.

Even though all these characteristics of the healer-priest seem to have been common to the various pre-Columbian populations, his different attributes were adapted to the social organization of each group. Among the Maya, who possessed a theocracy, the art of healing was entrusted to the *hemenes*, priests who were organized into a true medical society whose knowledge was thought to be inherited

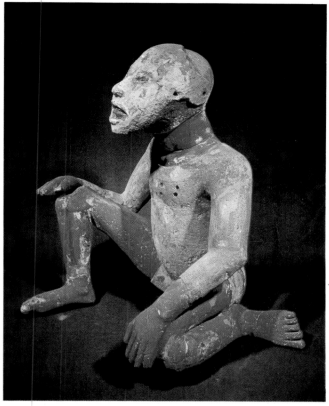

64

60 *Tlazolteotl (also Toci and Tetehuinan), goddess of medicine men. Old Codex*

61 *Quetzalcoatl, god of fertility and life. Old Codex*

62 *Tzapotlatenan, goddess of drugs. Old Codex*

63 *Mayan sculpture Chac-mool from Chichén Itzá placed at entrance of temples in Toltec period. Receptacle on stomach is for offerings, usually fresh blood or pulsating hearts. Museo Nacional de Antropología, Mexico*

64 *Painted Tula statue from Hidalgo, c. 1000–1168, representing sacrifice to Xipe Totec, "our lord the flayed one." Collection Mr. and Mrs. Robert Rowan, Pasadena, California*

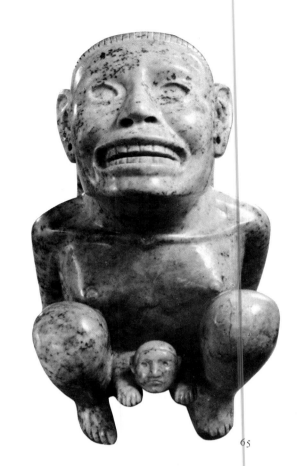
65

65 *Aztec goddess Tlazolteotl, carved in aplite speckled with garnets, in the act of childbirth. The Robert Bliss Collection of Pre–Columbian Art. Dumbarton Oaks, Washington, D.C.*

66 *Aztec temascal, or steam bath, was headquarters for massage specialists, who treated rheumatism, paralysis, and neuralgia. Biblioteca Nazionale Centrale, Florence*

67 *Brown clay Nayarit figures, with yellow, red, and black paint added, may represent sick person with attendant. Collection Stendahl, California*

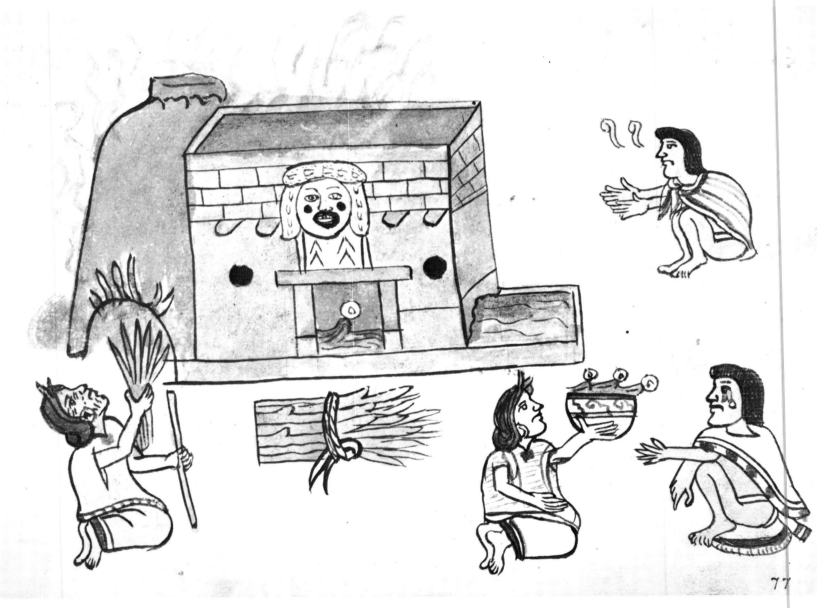
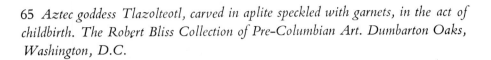

77

66

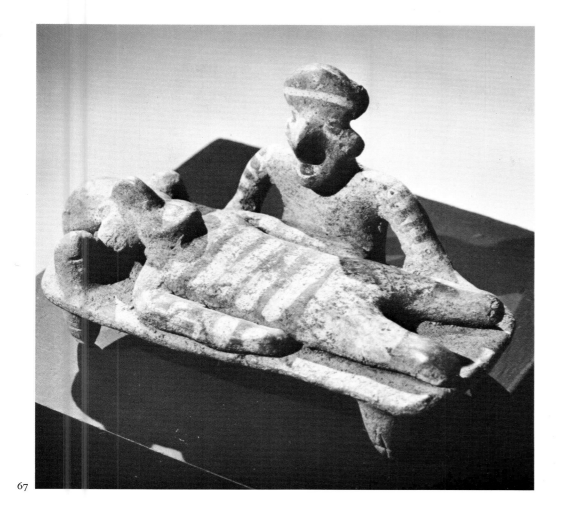

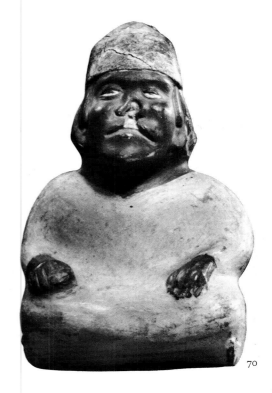

67

70

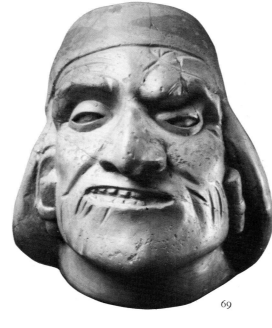

69

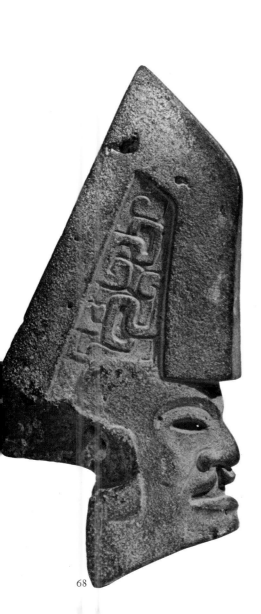

68

68 *Tajin culture head with harelip, from Veracruz. Staatliches Museum für Völkerkunde, Munich*

69 *Face which seems to show paralysis on one side, usually the result of stroke. Museum für Völkerkunde, Berlin (Dahlem)*

70 *Figure shown with what may have been leprosy, or mutilation administered as punishment. Museum für Völkerkunde, Berlin (Dahlem)*

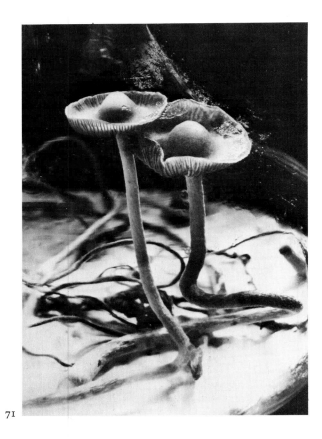

71

from the gods. In addition, there were *hechiceros* of lesser status who did not form part of the priestly caste and were responsible for the practice of bleeding, treating wounds, opening abscesses, and reducing and treating fractures.

Among the Aztecs, the medical profession acquired a hereditary character. It was a father's duty to entrust the knowledge of medical functions to his son; nevertheless, the son was not permitted to practice while his father was alive. Healers were divided into a series of specialties. The most common was the healing with herbs and by means of external manipulations done by the *tictl*, who combined with invocations and magical gestures some knowledge of the human body and the properties of plants and minerals. In addition to this specialist (which we might call clinical healer), others were entrusted with the tasks of pulling teeth, attending births, and setting fractures. The high quality of medical care by Aztec physicians was reflected in the *conquistadores'* common preference for them over their own physicians trained in Europe. Philip II sent one of his doctors, Francisco Hernandez, to Mexico to study the native medicine and put together a catalog of medicinal plants.

The treatment of disease is in large part dependent upon the concept of causation: if a disease is believed to be magically or supernaturally derived, then curative procedures will be likewise of a magical nature. On the other hand, when drugs and medical procedures are thought to be effective, an empirical medicine will result which will incorporate them. The healer-priest of the Americas combined both types of treatment. Therapy was based upon herbs, mineral substances, animal products, and simple procedures, like bleeding, enemas, and plasters, but also on religio-magical endeavors such as ritual dances and offerings.

MEDICATIONS

In Mexico, the climate favored the growth of many species of plants which were of great importance to Aztec doctors. Many years before Europeans cultivated them, Montezuma maintained a royal nursery of medicinal plants which supplied medications to the rest of the kingdom. Among these were narcotics, numerous medicines for diarrhea, drugs to induce abortion, and salves for skin diseases. But above all, the Aztecs preferred drugs which induced purging, vomiting, or sweating to expel bad spirits.

The Incas employed many plant remedies, especially quinine derived from cinchona bark, which was effective in the treatment of malarial fevers, and the coca leaf (containing cocaine), which was used both to calm and stimulate. Other common plant-derived drugs were atropine, ipecacuana, curare, theophyllin, and many another medicine which appears in today's pharmacopeia.

Plants whose principal active components caused profound psychic effects fulfilled an important function in the religious ceremonies as well as in medical practices. The three basic plants used were peyotl, a type of cactus, teonancatl, a variety of fungus, and ololiuqui, a type of vine; their active substances were mescaline, psilocybin, and psylocine. Among these plants, we should also include the chamico, which has an atropinic effect and had widespread use in Chile.

SURGERY

Surgical procedures were highly developed among some of the pre-Columbian peoples. Wounds were cleaned and closed with astringent vegetable concoctions or egg substances of divers birds and then covered with feathers or bandages made of skin. Common bleeding was controlled by placing masticated herbs over the wounds. In addition, the ancient Peruvians stanched scalp bleeding by wrapping a large cord with a type of gauze around the head several times at the base of the skull, like a tourniquet, until sufficient pressure stopped the bleeding. Among both the Incas and other pre-Columbian peoples, the surgeon was often a separate

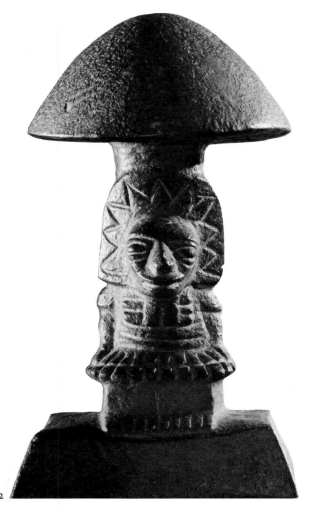

72

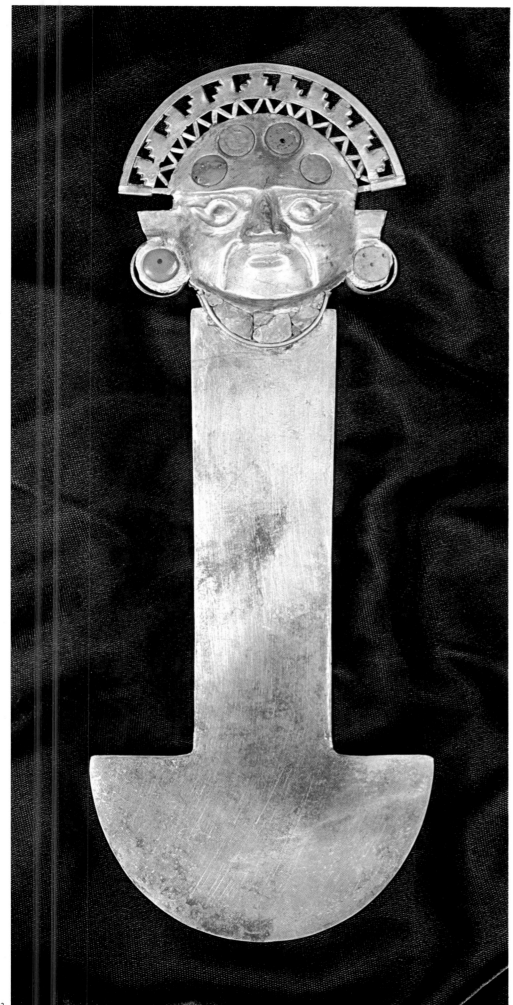

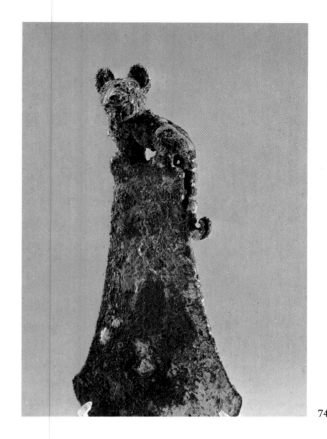

74

71 *So-called "magic" mushroom* Psilocybe mexicana Heim, *with active ingredients which induce hallucinations. Archives Sandoz, Basel*

72 *Mayan stone god of classical period, 300–700, in form of mushroom. Archives Sandoz, Basel*

73 *Tumi knife of a type used for trepanation. Middle Chimu, 1200–1460. Private collection*

74 *Cast copper knife, with traces of shell and stone inlay, of Mochica period, 300 B.C.–A.D. 500. Private collection*

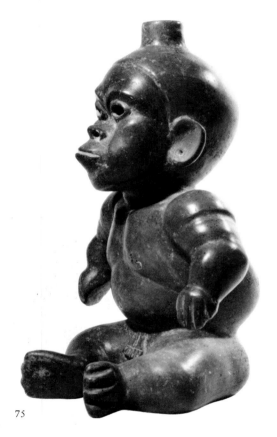

75

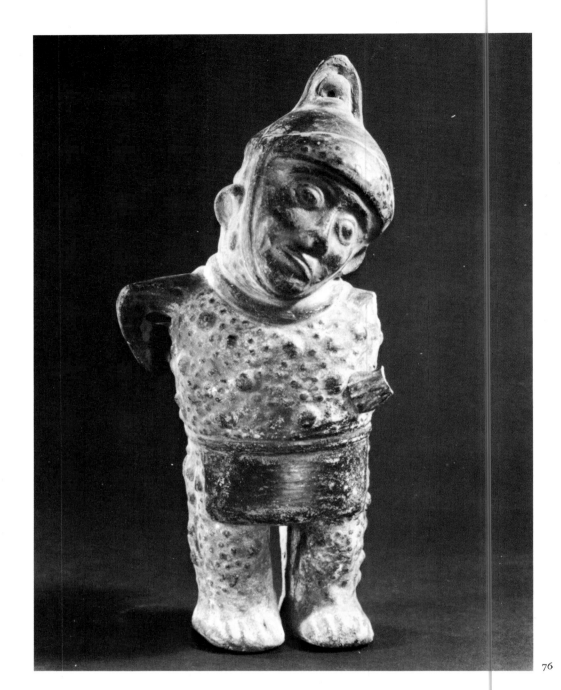

76

75 *Burnished red clay figure of hunchback, from Colima. Collection Samuel Dubiner, Tel Aviv*

76 *Mochica ceramic figure of naked man covered with bumps, probably representing verruca, a common Peruvian disease. Museum für Völkerkunde, Berlin (Dahlem)*

77 *Colima figure of reddish brown clay probably showing effects of elephantiasis, one of wide range of ailments so depicted. Collection Jacques Sarlie, New York*

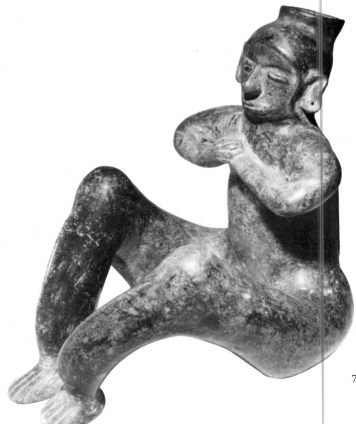

77

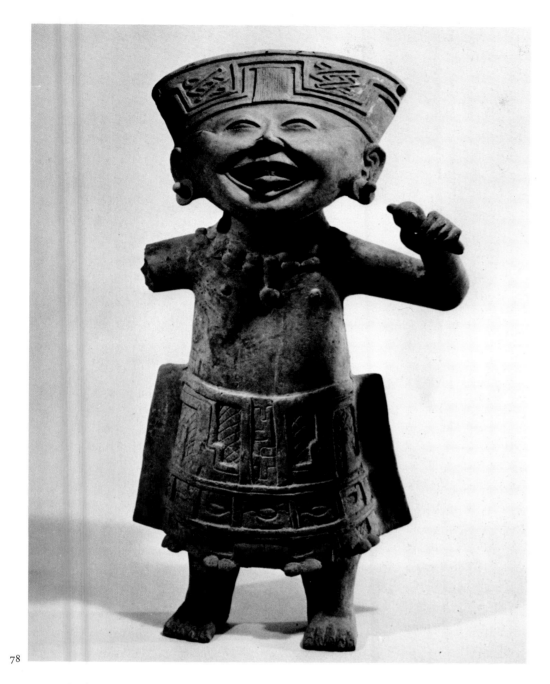

78

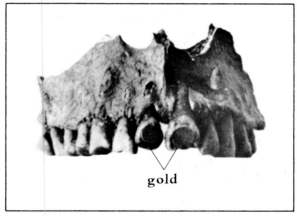

gold

79

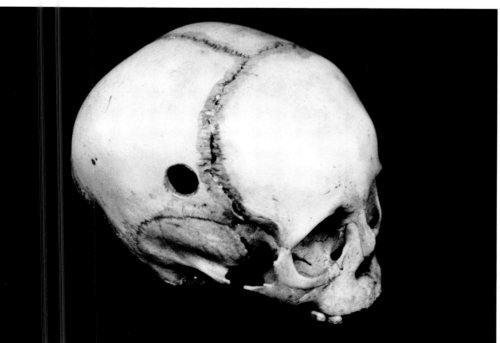

80

78 *Laughing face figurine of buff clay, holding rattle, of late classic period, from Veracruz. Collection Mr. and Mrs. Ellsworth La Boyteaux, Orinda, California*

79 *Fragment of ancient skull with gold-inlaid teeth excavated at Atacames site, Esmeraldes Province, Ecuador. Museum of the American Indian, Heye Foundation, New York*

80 *Skull found in Peru showing evidence of trepanation. Department of History of Medicine, University of Kansas, Lawrence*

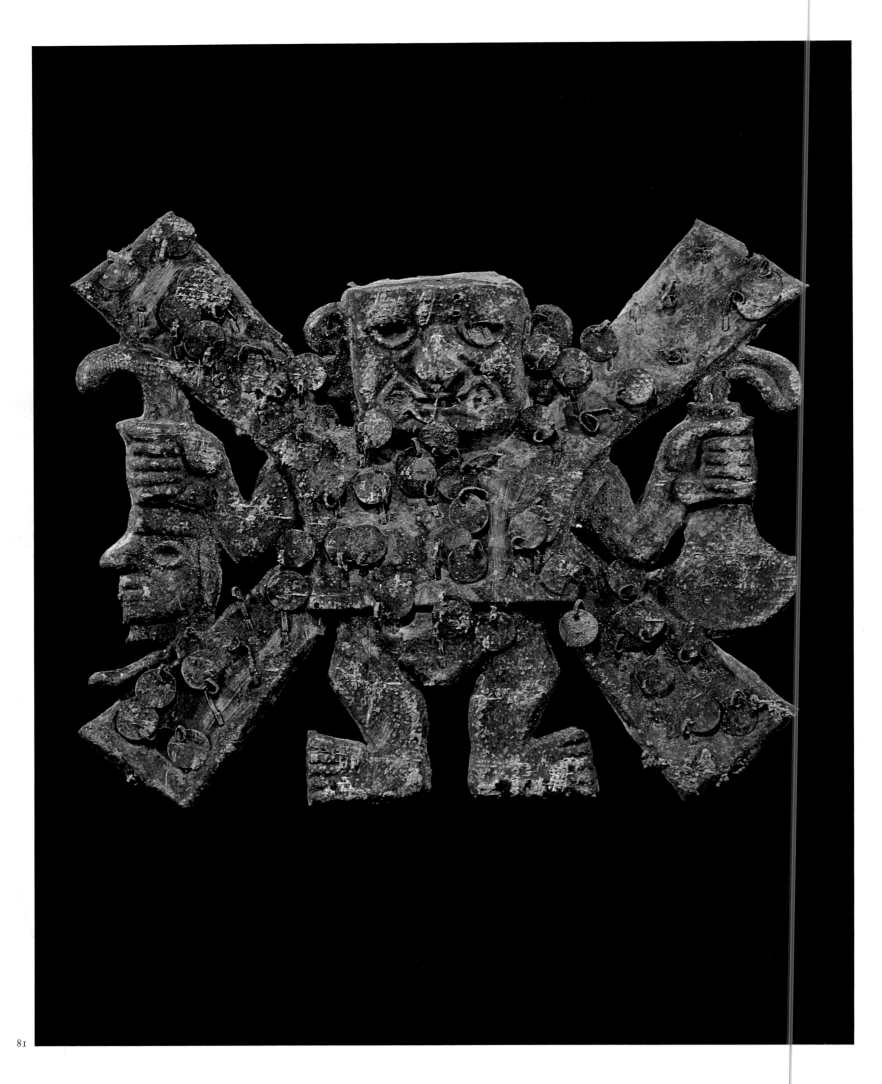

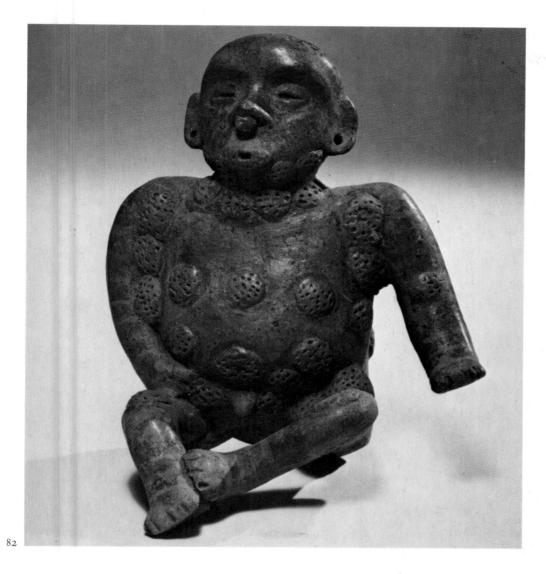

82

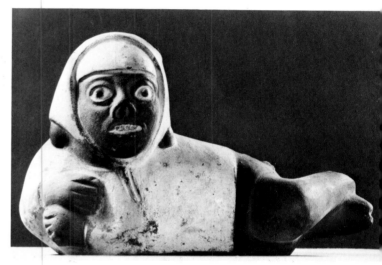

83

practitioner who looked after wounds and performed bloodletting and other lesser surgical practices. He also accomplished the astonishing feat of trepanning the human skull. Many skulls, some with several trepanations in different stages of healing (which indicates survival), have been found and testify to the skill of this practice. Here, too, it is not known what the purpose was.

PUBLIC HEALTH

The Aztecs formed an empire which was startling to the *conquistadores* not only for its material and cultural splendor but also for its cruelty and lack of concern for human life. Violence was a principal cause of death among the Aztecs, whether in war or upon the sacrificial altars. Nevertheless, the Spaniards were also astonished by the sophisticated means of maintaining public health in the fabulous Aztec capital Tenochtitlan. A system of drainage provided adequate disposal of wastes, and in each street (as we are told by the *conquistador* Bernal Diaz) there were public latrines which allowed personal privacy. Refuse was carefully collected and buried outside the city limits, and cleaning the streets was the responsibility of each district. Thus, at the beginning of the sixteenth century, Tenochtitlan was not only a prosperous city but also a healthy one. In none of the numerous Aztec codices were epidemics described. The first one to devastate the city, smallpox, occurred after the arrival of the Spaniards. (The venerable question of whether syphilis was exported to Europe from the New World by the returning sailors of Columbus or whether it was always endemic in Europe and Asia before its epidemic spread remains unsettled.)

The cultures of the pre-Columbian Americas had medical practices closely resembling those of primitive societies; yet their civilizations were highly developed in many other respects.

81 *Silvered-copper repoussé plaque showing Mochica dignitary holding trophy head and ceremonial knife, 300 B.C.–A.D. 300. Private collection*

82 *Brown clay Nayarit figure of man with pustules on body which may represent syphilis. Collection Dr. and Mrs. William F. Kaiser, Berkeley, California*

83 *Man shown with both feet amputated. Museum für Völkerkunde, Berlin (Dahlem)*

ANCIENT CIVILIZATIONS

Mesopotamia

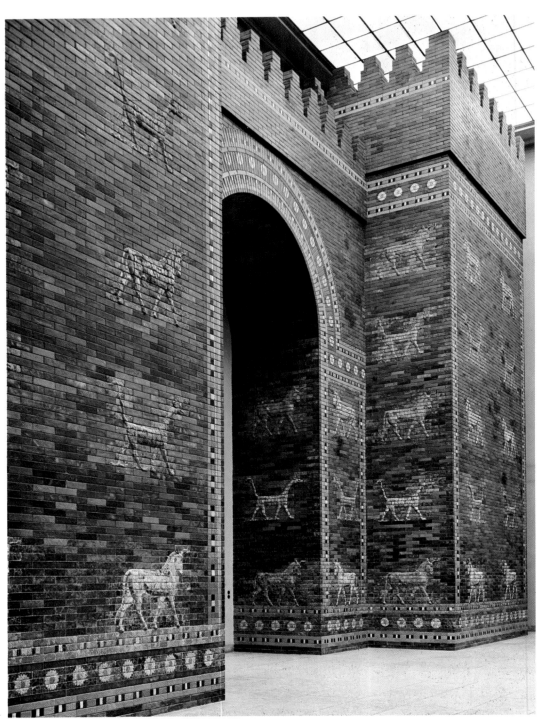

THE ancient region of southwest Asia known as Mesopotamia is literally "between rivers": the Tigris and Euphrates, which have their headwaters in the mountains of Asia Minor and ultimately merge as they flow into the Persian Gulf, nearly a thousand miles to the east. This fertile land, tilled for ten thousand years, also has been called the Cradle of Civilization. Here, about five thousand years ago, man first attempted to develop a system of writing, and here the first cities in the world were built.

In the course of the fourth millennium B.C., city-states developed in southern Mesopotamia that were dominated by temples whose priests represented the cities' patron deities. The most prominent of the city-states was Sumer, which gave its language to the area and became the first great civilization of mankind. About 2340 B.C., Sargon the Great (c. 2360–2305 B.C.) united the city-states in the south and founded the Akkadian dynasty, the world's first empire.

The next major civilization was centered on Babylon, and the most famous ruler of the Old Babylonian dynasty was Hammurabi (r. 1728–1686 B.C.), whose code of laws is the most prominent work of the period. Many thousands of inscribed clay tablets from this era still exist and make it one of the best-known cultures of Near Eastern antiquity.

The civilizations of Mesopotamia exerted powerful influences on their neighbors not only in their own time but also in subsequent centuries. Hebrew, Greek, Christian, and Islamic cultures owe many debts to ancient Mesopotamia. Some of the most famous early Bible stories have precursors in venerable Sumerian legend. The story of the Flood and Noah's Ark is lent credence by the discovery of ancient Nineveh beneath eleven feet of silt, and the description of the Tower of Babel in the Bible seems to fit the ziggurat temple-form of early Sumerian city-states. Perhaps Mesopotamia's most important contribution to the world was the introduction of a writing system, attributed to the Sumerians of about 3000 B.C. Although the Sumerian language itself did not long survive, the writing, called cuneiform, was adapted to Akkadian and its Babylonian dialect and was used to preserve the records and literature of Mesopotamia on clay tablets. Found by the thousands among the ruins of Babylon, Mari, and Nineveh, many of these tablets list representative plants, animals, and implements and provide a rudimentary zoological and botanical survey of the area. Others list the dynasties of rulers and major events which have enabled historians to work out a satisfactory chronology for the era.

Many other innovations came from the region of Mesopotamia: metallurgy, the wheel, the arch, clock dials, and uniform weights and measures. The sexagesimal system from which we derive our sixty-minute hour had its origins in Babylonian mathematics. The Chaldeans, a late Babylonian people, under Nebuchadnezzar developed extensive information on astronomy as well as concepts of astrology which were used in the medicine of Greco-Roman, Arabic, and medieval times. The earliest known regulations of the practice of medicine were found in the Code of Hammurabi (c. 1700 B.C.).

IDEAS ABOUT DISEASES

Although the various Mesopotamian cultures had their differences, there was a certain basic agreement on cosmology. As among their primitive forebears, illness was a curse, a punishment by the gods which could be visited on the family and descendants as well as on the sinner who had knowingly or inadvertently violated a moral code. However, there was probably some realization of nonspiritual causes for illness since physicians were admonished, for ethical reasons, to avoid continuing treatment for hopeless cases.

There was a pantheon of numerous deities, some of them patrons of the local region or city-state. For the most part, the chief early Sumerian gods remained supreme throughout the era, either unchanged or mingled with the Semitic gods

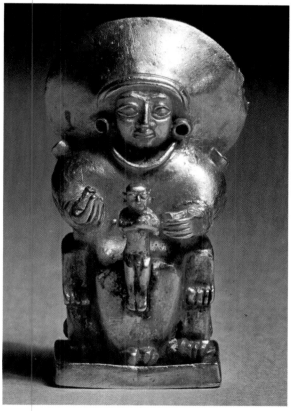

85

84 One of eight monumental gates (this one restored) to the Babylon of Nebuchadnezzar II, c. 575 B.C., dedicated to fertility deity Ishtar, most widely invoked goddess in religion of Babylonia and Assyria. Staatliche Museen, Berlin

85 Gold figure of Mesopotamian mother and child, c. 1400–1200 B.C., probably a fertility image. Collection Norbert Schimmel, New York

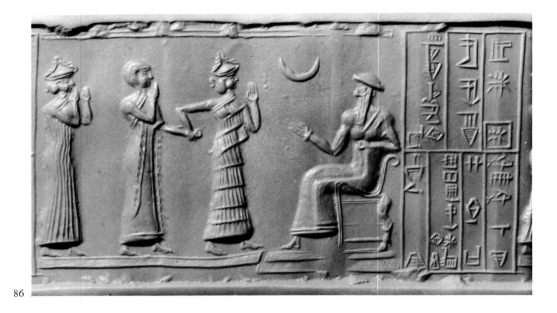

86

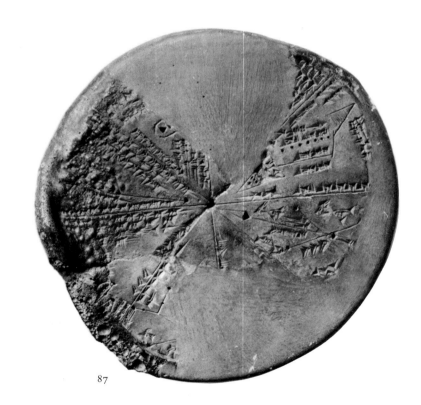

87

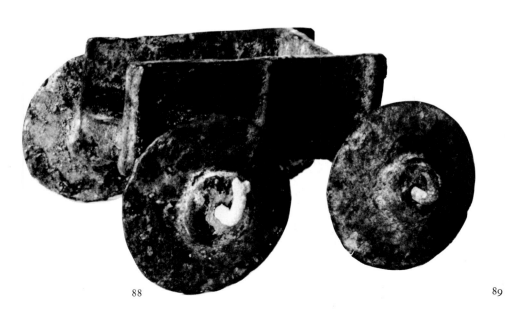

88

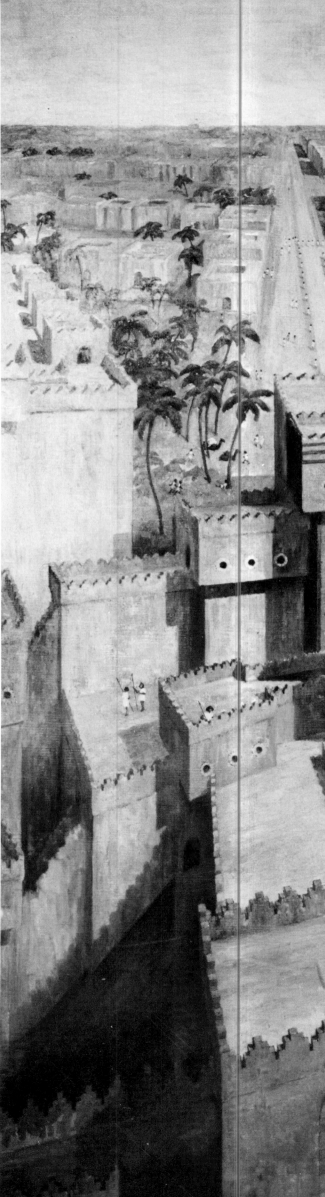

89

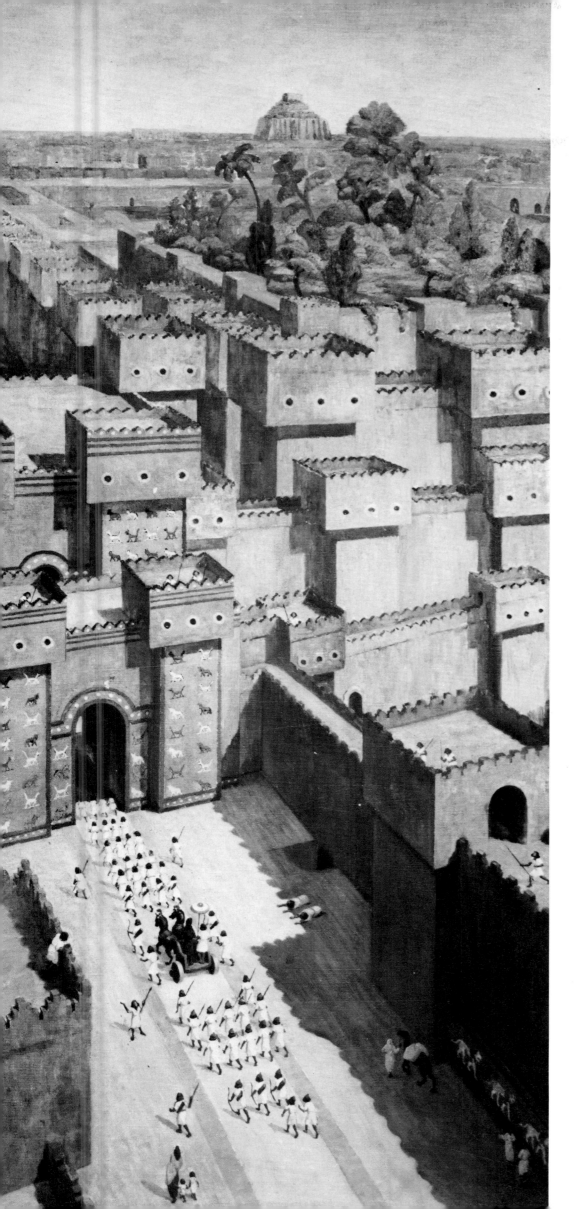

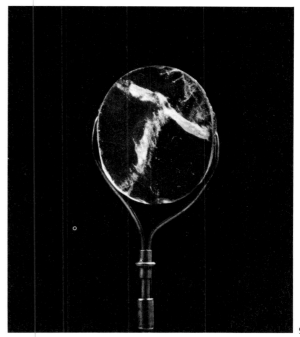

90

86 *Rolled-out impression of Sumerian cylinder seal, c. 2000* B.C., *probably developed to identify property in commercial trade. Text reads: "Ur–Nusku, son of Kaka, a merchant." British Museum, London*

87 *Assyrian astrolabe found at Nineveh, 7th century* B.C., *used to locate celestial bodies in calculating astrological influences on events and treatment. British Museum, London*

88 *Assyrian cart model (restored) of 3d millennium* B.C., *indicating early use of wheel, apparently a Mesopotamian innovation. Medelhavsmuseet, Stockholm*

89 *Artist's reconstruction of Babylon at time of Nebuchadnezzar II, showing Ishtar Gate through which New Year's procession carried images of gods, notably Marduk, a high healing god, and Shamash, the sun god. Oriental Institute, University of Chicago*

90 *Polished crystal, excavated at Nineveh, that may have been used as lens, considering high state of Mesopotamian science. British Museum, London*

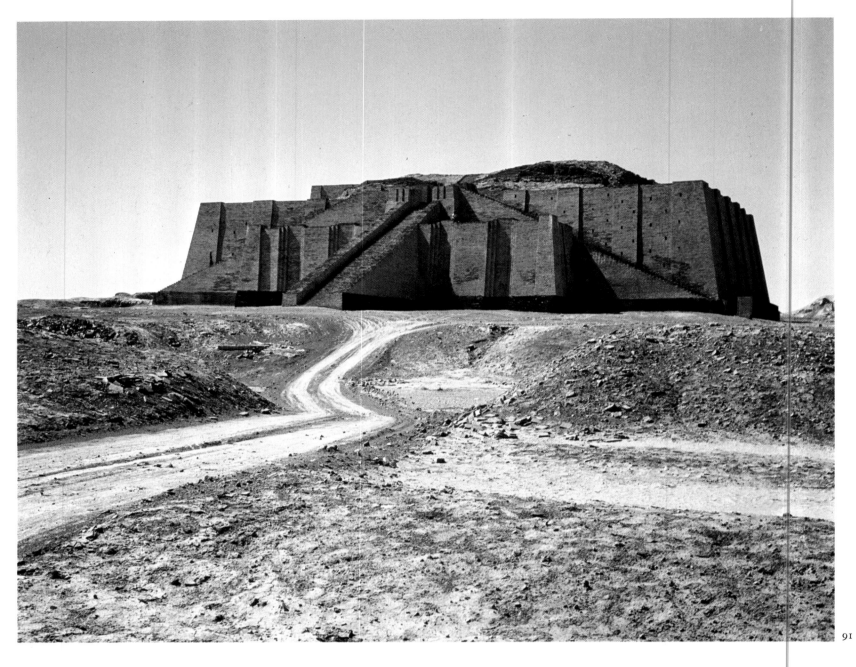

91

91 *Ziggurat of Ur, c. 2100* B.C., *Sumerian temple form surmounting brickwork mound, which possibly contributed to Biblical account of Tower of Babel*

92 *Fragment of clay tablet from Uruk, c. 3200* B.C., *one of earliest cuneiform documents found in Mesopotamia, where writing apparently began. Iraq Museum, Baghdad*

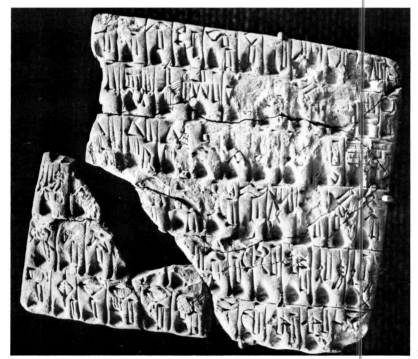

92

of later times. The three principal deities of Sumer were Anu, Enlil, and Enki. Enlil had a son, Ninib, who was a healing god. An important Babylonian god was Ea, Lord of Water and the first great cosmic ancestor of physicians, whose son Marduk became the most influential god in Babylonian worship. Marduk was the father of Nabu, who ruled over all science, including medicine, and to whom a temple was erected where a medical school developed. It is worth noting that one healing god, Ningishzida, has been pictured with a double-headed snake as his emblem, an indication of how long the snake has been a medical symbol. Indeed, in the early Sumerian epic of Gilgamesh, the search for the secret of immortality was thwarted when a snake stole and ate the plant of everlasting life. The snake immediately shed its skin and appeared rejuvenated, which qualified it as a symbol of regeneration and the cure of illness.

There were also evil demons who filled the spirit world. Each brought a different disease: Nergal gave fever, Ashakku debilitating consumption, Tiu headache, Namtaru throat ailments. Especially feared were the Evil Seven who wandered about afflicting the unwary. Because of them, physicians did not treat patients on the days of an illness divisible by seven.

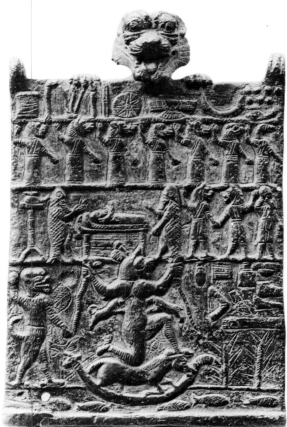

METHODOLOGY

Mesopotamian doctors depended on divination to uncover the sin committed by a sick person and to learn the expiation demanded by the gods, but they also observed a patient's symptoms to estimate their seriousness. One method of divination particularly associated with Mesopotamian medicine was hepatoscopy (detailed examination of the liver, and other entrails, of sacrificed animals). Although the Mesopotamians seem to have had no overall idea of anatomy, they regarded the liver as the seat of life since it appeared to be the collecting point for blood. Clay models of livers have been found with markings that probably were used to instruct neophytes in the art of divination or to guide the priest himself.

Recitations, ceremonies, prayers, and sacrifices were common religious means of beseeching the gods for a cure; however, along with these a veritable pharmacopoeia of drugs was used regularly in the treatment of disease. In addition to clay tablets which report illnesses with their symptoms and diagnosis, prognosis, and treatment, others were found that list drugs and their appropriate uses. Hundreds of plants, minerals, and animal substances were the therapeutic agents. They were given by mouth in compositions, applied as salves and fomentations, blown into orifices, inhaled as vapors and fumigations, and inserted as suppositories and enemas. Oil was apparently the principal balm for open wounds, probably preventing the adherence of overlying dressings. The medications were administered according to rituals, the time of the day, and the positions of constellations.

No cuneiform tablets devoted exclusively to surgery have survived, but since virtually all of the medical rules in the Code of Hammurabi concerned the outcome of operations, we can be certain that surgical practices were common. Wounds, abscesses (especially of the eye), broken bones, sprained tendons, and brand marks of slaves were all clearly in the province of surgery. Furthermore, references to bronze lancets in the Code and elsewhere indicate the use of instruments in surgical operations, and there have been a few isolated archaeological recoveries of knives. A possible trephine has also been unearthed, but no examples of trepanned skulls have yet been found in the land "between rivers." However, they have been uncovered in nearby Judea, which got its medical knowledge from Mesopotamia.

PRACTITIONERS

Medical practice appears to have been in the hands of three types of priests, only one of which was concerned exclusively with sick people. The *baru* as a diviner

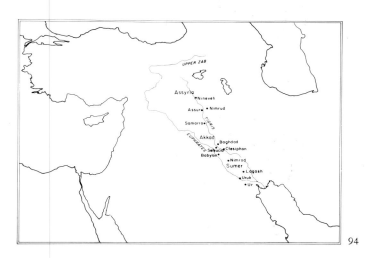

93 *Assyrian bronze amulet showing exorcism, with sick person in center, priests in fish guise symbolizing Ea, great god of water, and female demon Labartu about to depart on boat, possibly to flee exorcism. The Louvre, Paris*

94 *Map of Mesopotamia*

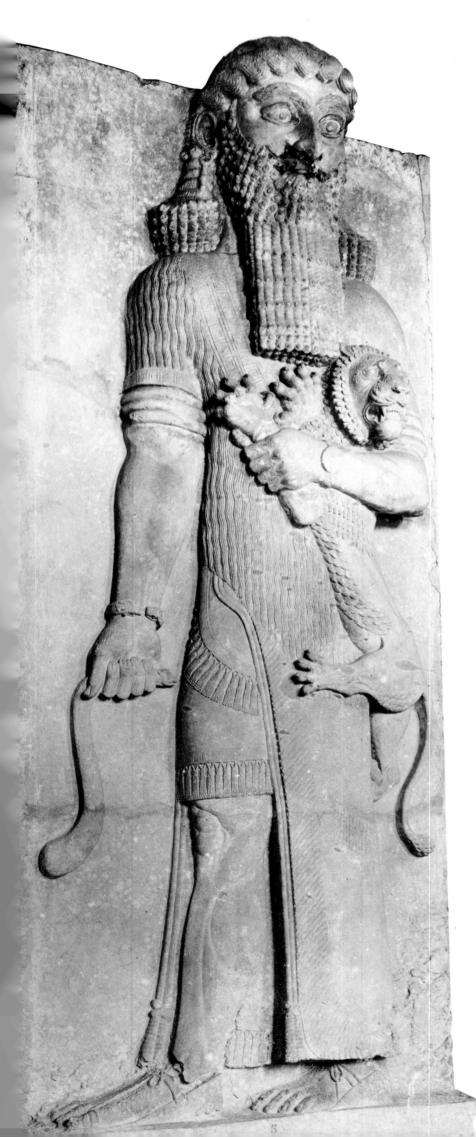

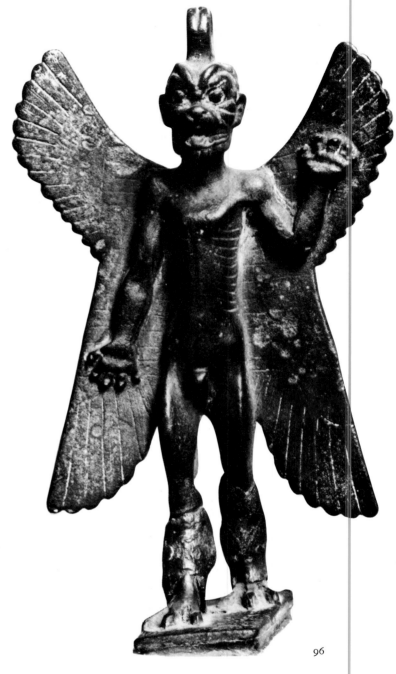

96

95 *Alabaster sculpture from Khorsabad thought to represent Gilgamesh, hero of Mesopotamian epic, recorded on clay tablets earlier than 2000 B.C., containing Babylonian account of Biblical Flood: The Louvre, Paris*

96 *Bronze figurine of dreaded sickness demon Pazuzu, c. 1000–500 B.C. The Louvre, Paris*

97 *Oldest known medical handbook, c. 2200 B.C. Sumerian physician's collection of empiric prescriptions, an indication that medical treatment was not always religious or magical. University Museum, Philadelphia*

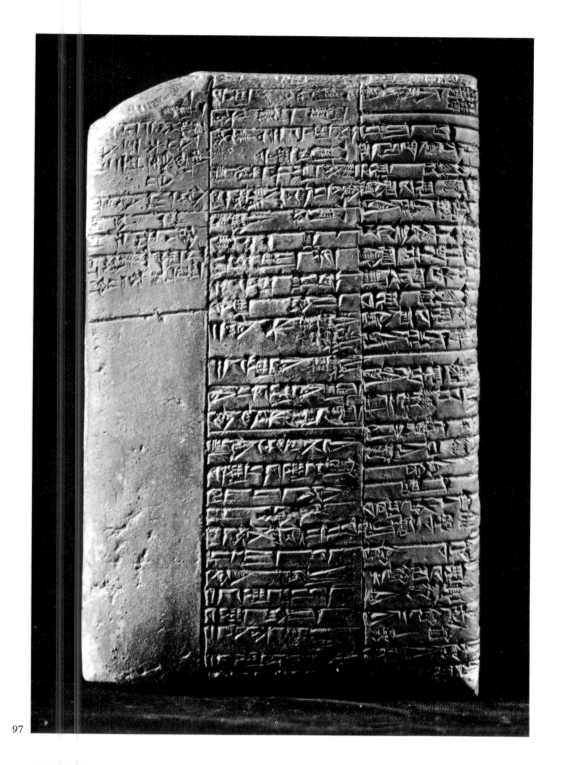

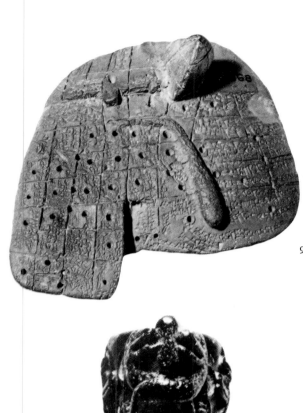

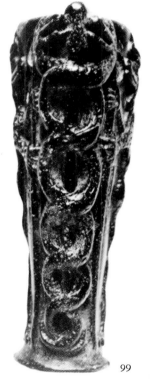

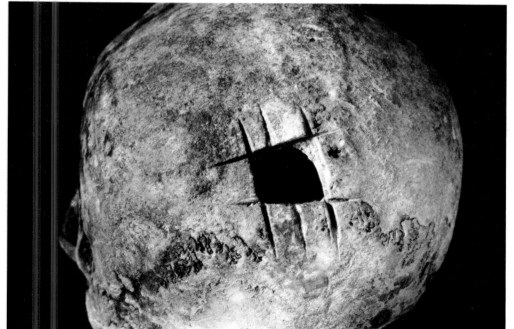

98 Inscribed Babylonian clay model of sheep's liver, 19th–18th century B.C., used as reference in divination and prognosis of illness while examining liver of sacrificed animal. British Museum, London

99 Dark green soapstone ceremonial beaker, c. 2000 B.C., dedicated to Ningishzida, god of healing, whose symbol, thought to have been intertwined snakes, is seen here in earliest representation. The Louvre, Paris

100 Trephined skull found in excavations at the ancient Judean city of Lachish. Institute of Archaeology, University of London

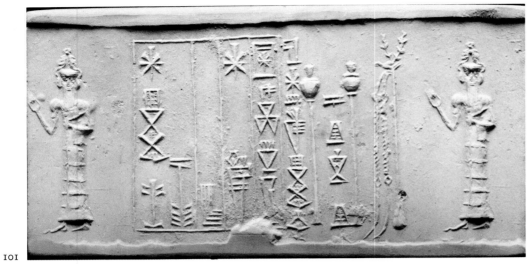

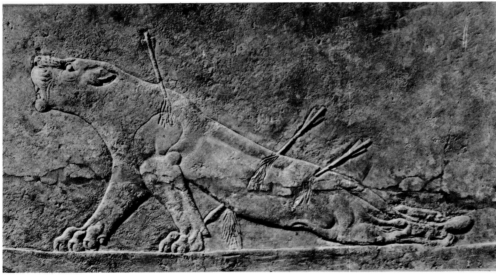

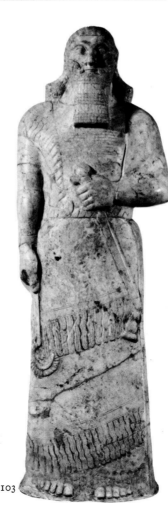

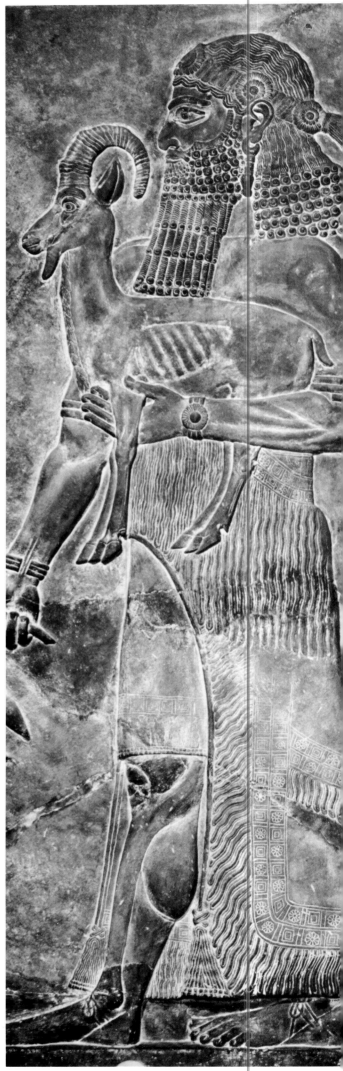

101 *Impression of Dr. Urlugaledina's cylinder seal,*
c. 2000 B.C., *found at Lagash. Text reads: "O god*
Edinmugi, vizier of the god Gir, who attends
mother animals when they drop their young!
Urlugaledina the doctor is your servant." The
Louvre, Paris

102 *Wounded lioness from alabaster relief "The*
Great Hunt" in palace of Ashurbanipal II at
Nineveh, 7th century B.C., *showing paralysis of*
extremities from spinal injury. British Museum,
London

103 *Statue of Ashurbanipal II, 7th century* B.C.,
whose excavated library of clay tablets is chief source
of knowledge about ancient Mesopotamian
civilization. British Museum, London

104 *Assyrian alabaster relief, 8th century* B.C.,
showing priests, one carrying opium poppies,
preparing to sacrifice gazelle to gods. The Louvre,
Paris

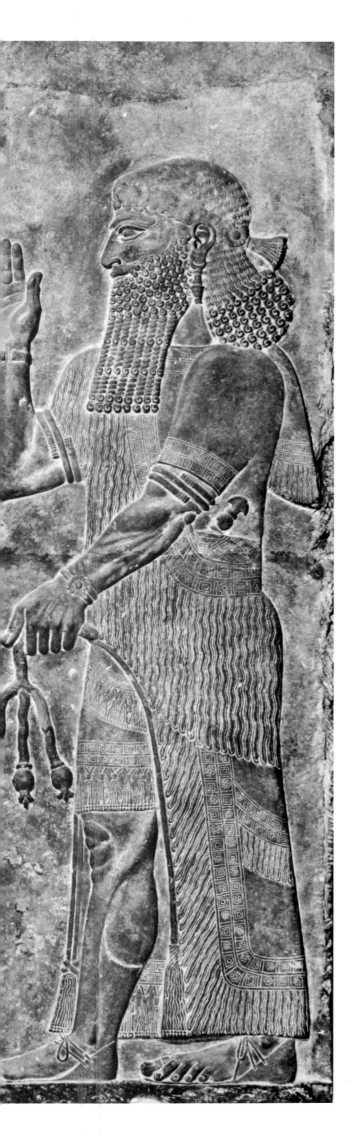

dealt with diagnosis and prognosis, but not only of illness. He also had to discover the causes and probable outcome of many other kinds of catastrophe. The *ashipu*, as an exorcist who drove out evil demons, was called on to rid a house, a farm, an area, and also sick people of occupying spirits. The *asu* apparently acted principally as a physician, employing charms and divination but also drugs and operations. The name of Biblical king Asa (Asa-El), "healer of God," may have derived from the Babylonian *asu*.

The healing priests received their education in schools that were associated with the temples. The source of their learning, in addition to practical instruction, was the large number of texts available in the form of clay tablets. By the seventh century B.C., for instance, the library of Ashurbanipal contained over twenty thousand tablets, which were only discovered about a hundred and fifty years ago at the site of ancient Nineveh. They are still the most extensive source of knowledge about Mesopotamian society, including medicine, but recently tablets have been unearthed that date back to Sumerian times.

The priest-physician ministered mainly to the court, nobility, and upper classes, but apparently there were also barbers who performed some surgical procedures and did the branding of slaves. They also treated tooth disorders and did extractions. Veterinary practice may have been handled by either the low-class barber or the upper-class *asu*, but whether there were exclusive healers for animals, "doctors of oxen or asses," is not known.

Medical practice, as well as other professional activity, was evidently regulated by well-defined laws. The Code of Hammurabi devotes ten short statements out of the 282 provisions to the fees due medical practitioners and their punishments for failure.

> If a doctor has treated a freeman with a metal knife for a severe wound, and has cured the freeman, or has opened a freeman's tumor with a metal knife, and cured a freeman's eye, then he shall receive ten shekels of silver.
>
> If the son of a plebeian, he shall receive five shekels of silver.
>
> If a man's slave, the owner of the slave shall give two shekels of silver to the doctor.
>
> If a doctor has treated a man with a metal knife for a severe wound, and has caused the man to die, or has opened a man's tumor with a metal knife and destroyed the man's eye, his hands shall be cut off.
>
> If a doctor has treated the slave of a plebeian with a metal knife for a severe wound and caused him to die, he shall render slave for slave.
>
> If he has opened his tumor with a metal knife and destroyed his eye, he shall pay half his price in silver.
>
> If a doctor has healed a freeman's broken bone or has restored diseased flesh, the patient shall give the doctor five shekels of silver.
>
> If he be the son of a plebeian, he shall give three shekels of silver.
>
> If a man's slave, the owner of the slave shall give two shekels of silver to the doctor.
>
> If a doctor of oxen or asses has treated either ox or ass for a severe wound, and cured it, the owner of the ox or ass shall give to the doctor one sixth of a shekel of silver as his fee.

Although estimating relative monetary values in modern terms is difficult, one should compare the fees in the Code with the five shekels of silver yearly rent for a middle-class dwelling or the one-fiftieth of a silver shekel daily pay for an ordinary craftsman, which indicates a generally high schedule of medical fees. The severe punishments for a physician's failures listed in the Code (such as cutting off the hands) should be matched against the punishments (which could include execution) meted out for the failures of other professionals and the transgressions of any person against another.

If a man has destroyed the eye of a patrician, his own eye shall be destroyed.

If a man has knocked out the teeth of a man of the same rank, his own teeth shall be knocked out.

If he has knocked out the teeth of a plebeian, he shall pay one-third of a mina of silver.

One may wonder whether under risk of such stringent penalties any practitioner could have had the nerve to perform an operation, but it may well be that the Code was not enforced to the letter. Indeed, earlier Sumerian writings recently discovered indicate that punishments were less severe than called for by the later Code.

One fact seems clear. Whatever may have been the restrictions and regulations, a goodly number of healers—whether priests or barbers—practiced medicine and surgery throughout the history of Mesopotamia. It is therefore difficult to account for the statement of the Greek historian Herodotus (fifth century B.C.) that: "They have no physicians, but when a man is ill they lay him in the public square, and the passersby come up to him, and if they have ever had his disease themselves or have known any one who has suffered from it, they give him advice, recommending him to do whatever they found good in their own case, or in the case known to them. And no one is allowed to pass the sick man in silence without asking him what his ailment is."

PUBLIC HEALTH AND HYGIENE

From the numerous instructions on clay tablets recommending religious and empiric methods of treatment, one can infer that the physician was called upon to treat a large number of ailments. They were not grouped together as disease entities, as they are today, but were listed and classified according to the location of the symptoms. For instance, in the head there were aches, eye and ear pains and swellings, and tooth abscesses. Chest problems were cough, pain, and the spitting of blood. Cramps, vomiting, and diarrhea were illnesses of the abdomen.

Epidemics must have occurred often; the many wars and invasions were likely events to foster pestilence. Certainly plagues of some kind were reported in the cuneiform tablets of the eighth century B.C., and fevers, probably of varying causes, were mentioned frequently in the medical texts. The shaking chills which Alexander the Great suffered in his last illness while campaigning in Mesopotamia in the fourth century B.C. may have been due to malaria.

A sick person of any rank was in a special category and was excused from work and even from service to the king. On the other hand, since disease was caused by spirits having possessed the body, the afflicted person was shunned as much as possible to avoid transference of the offending demon. This relative isolation was hygienically beneficial to the community although its purpose was based on religio-magical reasoning. The taboo against touching the sick was carried over into Hebrew culture, where it became a key factor in a system of public hygiene—just one further example of Mesopotamia's long-lasting influence on contemporary and later cultures.

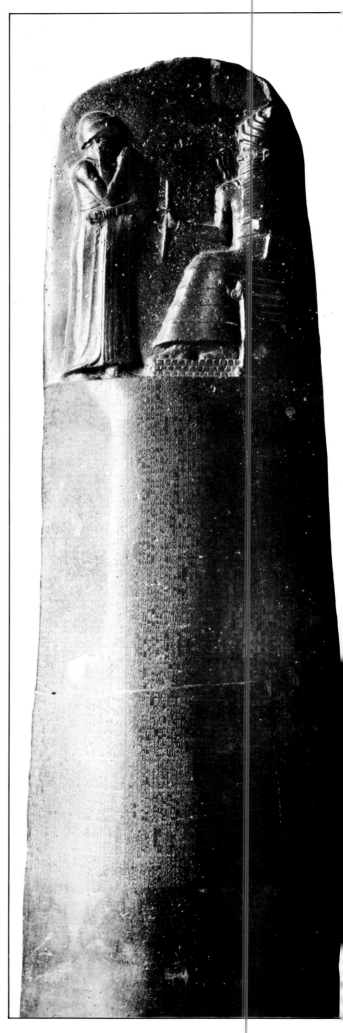

105

68

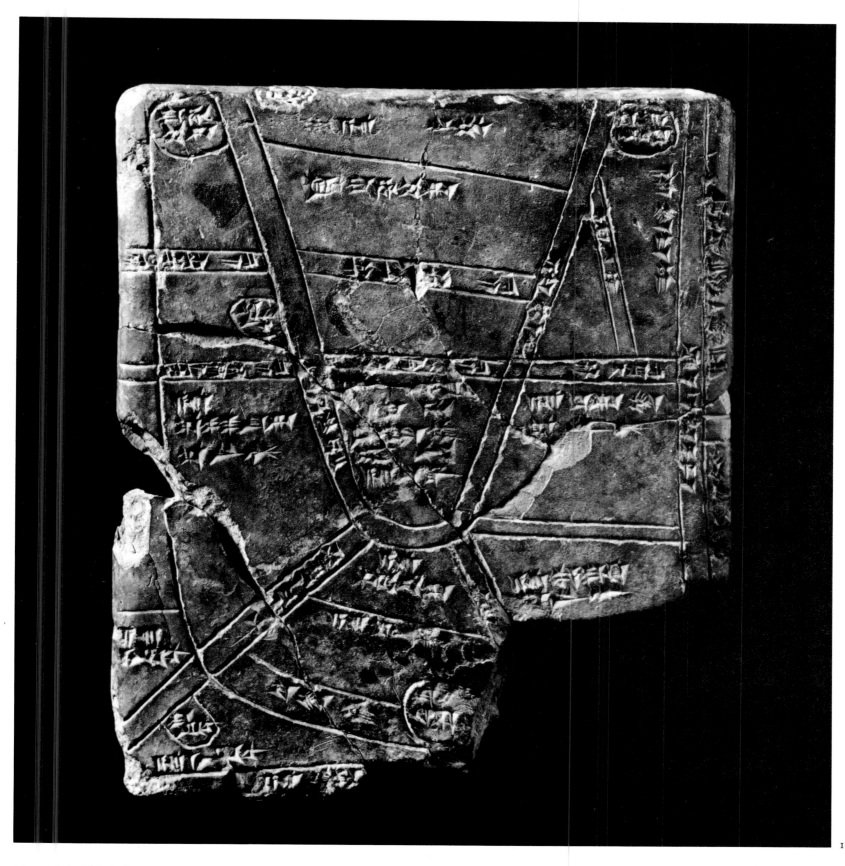

105 *Polished black diorite stele, c. 1792–1750*
B.C., *found near Susa, with Code of Hammurabi*
inscribed and bas-relief at top showing king receiving
laws from sun god Shamash. The Louvre, Paris

106 *Clay tablet map, c. 1300 B.C., showing*
irrigation system on royal estate near Nippur and
surrounding villages marked by circles. University
Museum, Philadelphia

Ancient Hebrew Medicine

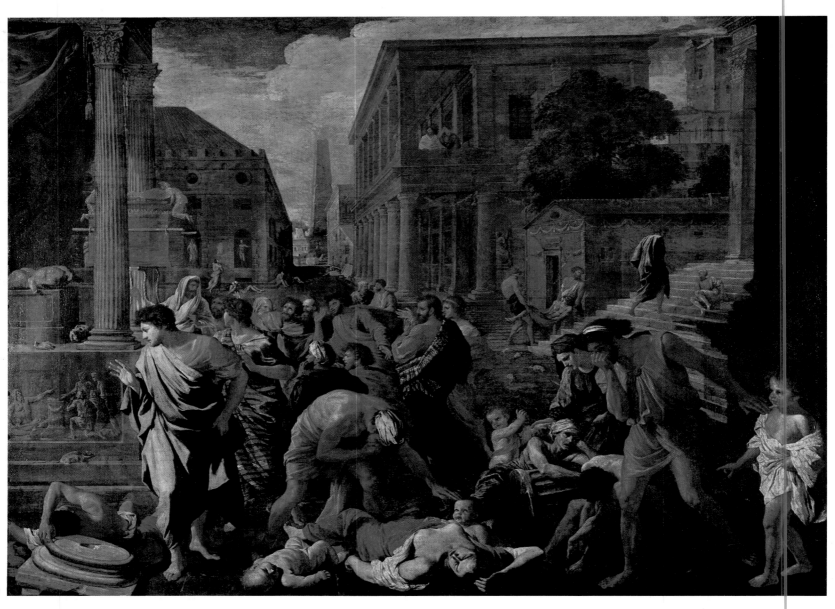

THE Biblical Hebrews may have inherited a number of their beliefs from ancient Mesopotamian cultures, among them a conviction that disease was divine punishment and therefore a mark of sin. This belief was passed on as a basic concept to Christian medieval Europe. Assyro-Babylonian taboos against close proximity to the sick were also continued by the Hebrews in their isolation of the unclean, who, in addition to the diseased, included the dead, a potential source of soul transference among the Mesopotamian peoples.

Hebrew reliance on strict codes which controlled virtually all behavior was another Mesopotamian characteristic. Furthermore, the assignment of the Sabbath as a day of rest, observed by orthodox Jews even today, matches the severe Assyrian restriction of activities on the seventh day of the week, when the king engaged in no official business and physicians were not even permitted to treat the sick.

There were, however, important differences between Hebrew and Assyro-Babylonian concepts. For instance, the Biblical Hebrews, although they believed in supernatural causation of disease, did not envision the world as filled with demons and spirits. (Many centuries later, however, in medieval times, Jewish folk superstition did subscribe to cabalistic views on possession by spirits.) To the ancient Hebrew it was essentially Jehovah, God Himself, who was to be placated as the giver and taker of health. In the same vein, contamination was not a matter of evil spirits having passed from the sick to the well but a sign of one's spiritual impurity from having violated the prohibition against touching the unclean, the sick person being punished by God. Hygienic laws were to be obeyed for religious and disciplinary rather than medical reasons. These regulations reached into virtually every activity: isolation of the sick, time and location of burial, frequency of sexual intercourse, washing before meals, bathing after coitus and menstruation, slaughtering of animals, and preparation of food.

Much has been made of a presumably medical basis for the food prohibitions in Jewish tradition, but there may be other explanations. One recent suggestion is that the taboo against pigs was originally related to their competition with humans for water and grain (scarce commodities in a barren land), in contrast to cattle and sheep which consume relatively little water and graze on forage inedible to man. Since transmissible parasitic diseases and infestations such as tapeworm are also found in sheep and cows, singling out trichinosis in pigs would not be wholly logical. However, to discourage the raising of swine so as to conserve water and grain resources for human consumption, a strict religious taboo may have been necessary—considering man's nearly universal agreement on the delectableness of pork. Medical observations may indeed have been at the core of hygienic codes, but the Biblical listing of seemingly unrelated creatures prohibited as food is difficult to associate with purposes entirely hygienic.

Plagues and epidemics were mentioned often in the Bible, with special attention given to leprosy, which was feared and isolated, but, as among the Assyro-Babylonians, many skin diseases considered to be leprosy probably were not. There were, however, references to many other types of illnesses and symptoms in the Bible.

Physicians were drawn from the priestly tribe of Levites and were prohibited from practicing if deficient in vision; nor was examination permitted at twilight, on cloudy days, or in a dim room. Some passages in the Bible suggest that physicians were held in high esteem. "When thou feelest sick call upon God and bring the physician, for the prudent man scorneth not the remedies of the earth." However, other statements in the Bible suggest that admiration was mixed at times with mockery. "In his disease he sought not the Lord but went to the Physicians. And Asa slept with his fathers."

Hebrew medical practices were much like those of the peoples among whom they lived. A number of medications were mentioned in the Bible, such as mandrake, balsams, gums, spices, oils, and possibly narcotics, but the relatively limited list of drugs recorded is remarkable when one considers the abundant

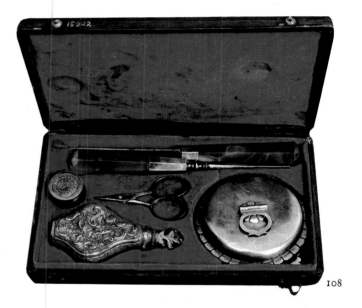

108

107 The Plague at Ashdod, *depiction by Nicolas Poussin of Biblical plague, c. 1030 B.C., described in First Samuel as divinely visited upon Philistines for seizing Hebrews' Ark of the Covenant. Details of story point to plague as bubonic and implicate rats. The Louvre, Paris*

108 *Case of silver-mounted instruments used in performing the Hebrew rite of circumcision. Inscribed in silver box, "Hollandia 1801." Wellcome Institute for the History of Medicine, London*

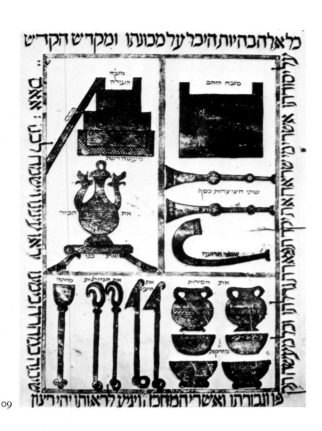

109

109 *Illustration in Hebraic Bible, dated 1299, done in Perpignon by Saloman, son of Raphael, showing Jewish ceremonial paraphernalia, including circumcision knives and sacrificial vessels. Ms. Hebrew No. 7, Bibliothèque Nationale, Paris*

110 *Illumination by Fouquet in medieval edition, 1420–81, of Antiquities of the Jews by Flavius Josephus, showing Roman general Pompey in Temple of Jerusalem, B.C. 63, at time of its conquest which placed the Jews under Roman rule. Ms. Français 247, f. 293, Bibliothèque Nationale, Paris*

materia medica of Mesopotamian and Egyptian physicians. There was little reference to surgery in the Bible except for ritual circumcision, and that may have come from the Egyptians. Midwives were spoken of, but their ministrations seem not to have extended beyond comforting and attendance.

Although Biblical information on medicine is relatively limited, a rich collection of medical lore is found in the later Talmud, the authoritative collection of Jewish tradition. There are two Talmuds, the Jerusalem and the much longer Babylonian, both written over the same period (second to sixth century A.D.). The Temple of Solomon in Jerusalem was destroyed for the first time by the Babylonians in 586 B.C., and this marked the beginning of the Babylonian captivity of the Jews. In the first century A.D. Jerusalem was sacked again, this time by the Romans. After each of these catastrophes, Jews scattered over many lands and established schools for preserving their learned and religious traditions; the Talmud became the bedrock on which Jewish education rested. Although the Talmudic medical writings demonstrated remarkable insights and observations, they reflected as much the attitudes and methods of the various peoples among whom the Jews lived over the centuries as they did their own Biblical inheritance. For instance, the Talmudists relied on the humoral theories of the Greeks, which attributed disease to the imbalance of the four humors of the body: phlegm, blood, yellow bile, and black bile. Similarly, they followed Greek philosophers in specifying the four elements of the universe as air, fire, earth, and water.

Since Jews were among the many races and nationalities that flocked into the great center of Greek learning at Alexandria in the fourth century B.C., they followed the teachings there on anatomy and physiology, as well as on diet, massage, and drugs. The many medical sects numbered among them Jews whose writings found their way into the Talmudic commentaries. Although dead bodies were avoided as unclean, Jews evidently performed occasional human dissections, for Rabbi Ishmael in the first century A.D. is said to have boiled and then studied the body of a prostitute. However, most of the anatomical information in the Talmud came from Alexandrian human dissections and from examination of animals to determine whether they were free of abnormality and suitable as kosher food.

In terms of surgery, the Talmud discussed the means of reducing dislocations and the management of injuries to many organs. Sometimes detailed techniques were described, as, for instance, the methods for dealing with an imperforate anus whereby, after oiling and sunburning, a small incision would be made over the spot where the anus should have been. Of course, circumcision remained the "seal of the covenant" to be performed on all boys at a prescribed time after birth.

Although barbers and other uneducated healers might engage in the accepted practice of bloodletting and minor mechanical procedures, medicine was practiced by professionals called *rophe*, who seem to have participated in both medicine and surgery. The doctors who limited themselves entirely to surgical procedures were referred to as *uman*. There were probably also veterinary surgeons since one was mentioned in the Talmud by name.

The precepts and prohibitions of Biblical times on personal and public hygiene were continued in the Talmud. "Physical cleanliness is conducive to spiritual purity" (Avoda Zara in the Jerusalem Talmud). For instance, the leper continued to be regarded as unclean and his clothing was to be burned. A type of isolation outside the city for some of those with other sicknesses was also mentioned. The later Hebrews apparently recognized that certain diseases were transmissible through contaminated objects, and women, as in the Bible, were unclean and could not participate in religious or sexual activity until seven days after cessation of the menstrual flow. The restrictions on preparing food were maintained.

In much later times, during the Middle Ages, Jews were to be a repository of Greek and Roman learning. In the period of Islamic supremacy they acted as a bridge between the Muslim East and Christian West.

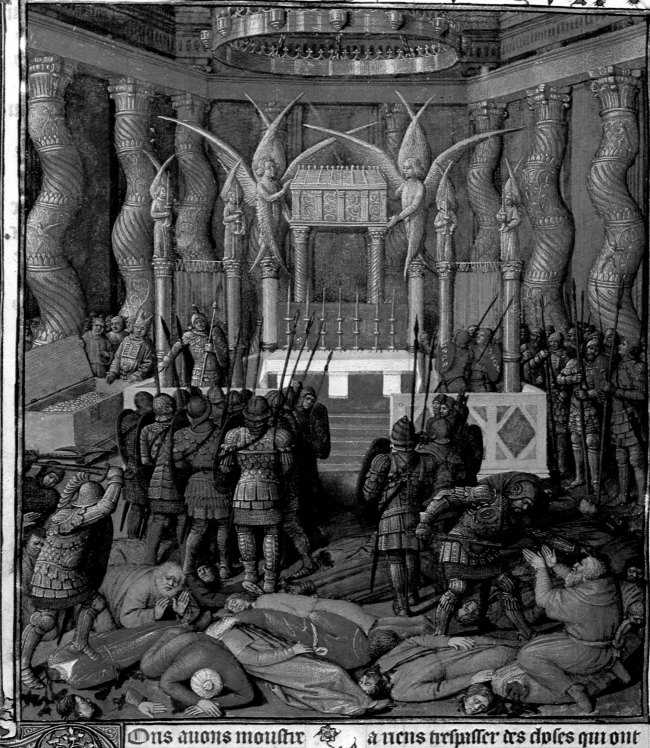

Ons auons moustre
au uolume de dauant
cestuy a la mort de la
royne alexandre. Oz
racomptons les choses qui sensuiuet
et ne tendons a nulle autre chose foz

a nous trespasser des choses qui ont
este faictes en puruoiant ala memo
yre de ceulx qui les liront. Car a
ceulx qui escripuent hystoires ou ra
comptent choses anciennes il conui
ent pour lancienete mettre ou faire

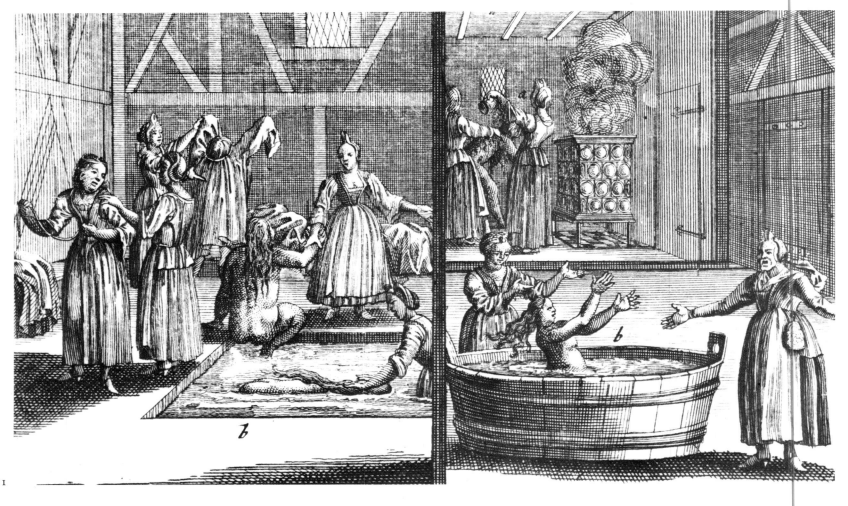

111

111 *Engraving of Jewish women in ritual bath from Kirchner's* Jewish Ceremony, *Nuremberg, 1726. Although Jewish hygienic precepts were followed for religious reasons, they contributed to development of preventive health measures. Österreicherische Nationalbibliothek, Vienna*

112 *Cabala scheme used by Jews in Middle Ages to conjure good results, including cure of illness, in contrast to virtual absence of magic and spells in medicine of Biblical Hebrews. Ms. 2406 Heb. 763, f. 35, Bibliothèque Nationale, Paris*

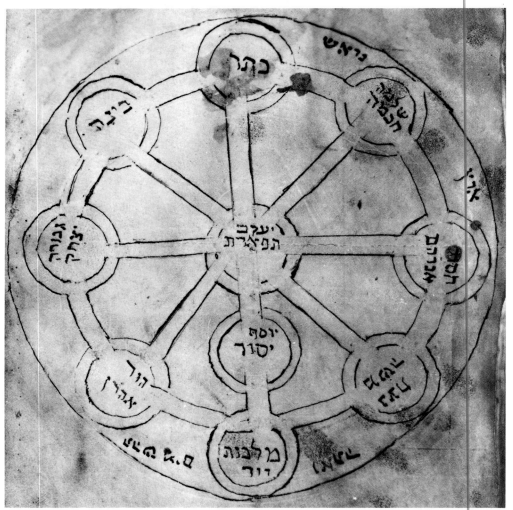

112

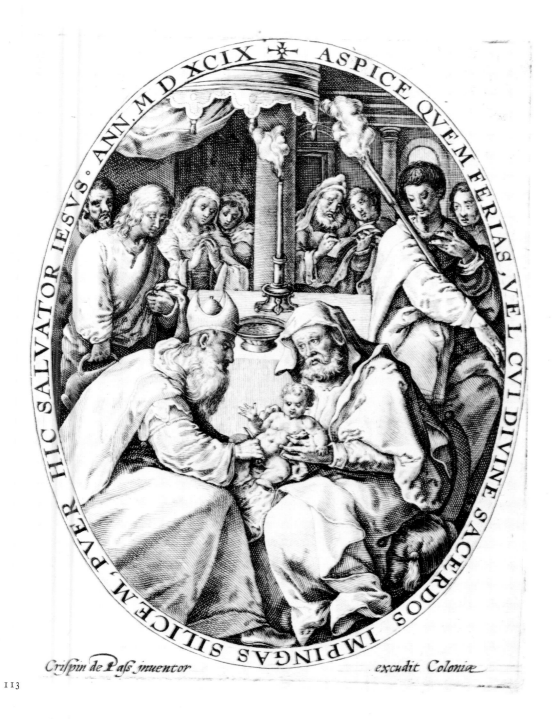

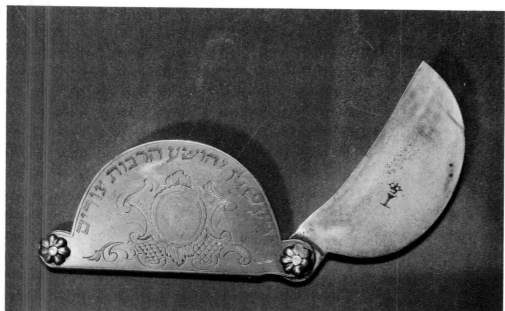

113 *Engraving by Crispin de Passe, 1599, showing circumcision, prescribed ritual among Jews of religious rather than medical significance, although considered hygienic measure by many physicians. Collection Charles M. Lea, Philadelphia Museum of Art*

114 *Eighteenth-century knife used in circumcisions. If two sons of same mother died of uncontrollable bleeding, subsequent offspring were not circumcised, indicating awareness of hereditary bleeding tendencies. Collection Putti, Istituto Rizzoli, Bologna*

Ancient Egypt

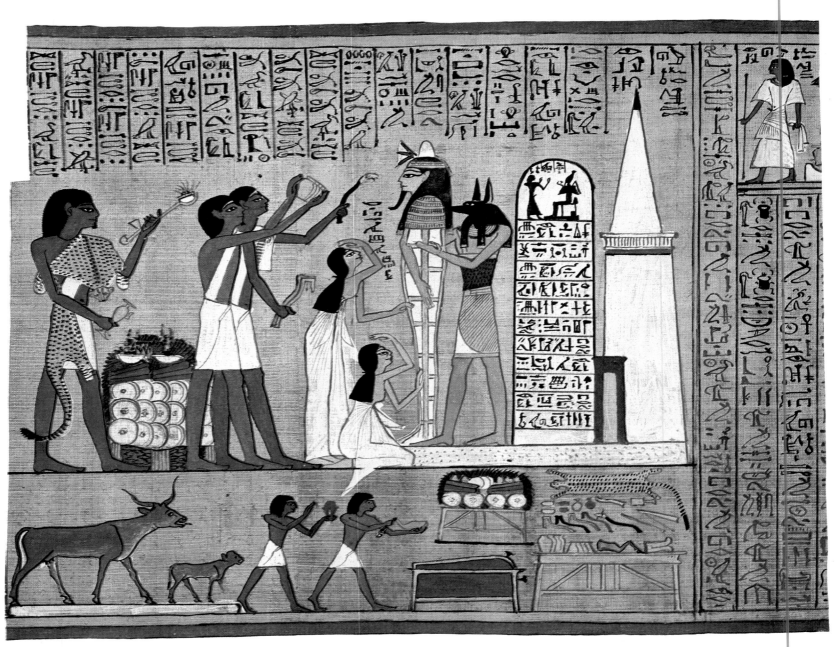

Until the seven known medical papyruses were discovered during the last century, our knowledge of ancient Egyptian medicine came principally from the writings of Greek and Roman commentators such as Homer, Herodotus, Hippocrates, Pliny, Diodorus, and Clemens. The writings of Egyptians themselves, though abundant on historic ruins, were virtually indecipherable until the Rosetta Stone was discovered in 1799 during Napoleon's conquest of Egypt. This basalt stela bore a tribute to Ptolemy V (196 B.C.) carved in hieroglyphics and repeated in demotic, or simplified, characters, and also in Greek, providing Jean-François Champollion necessary keys to decipher the language and open doors to a wider understanding of ancient Egypt.

Medical Documents

The oldest of the medical papyruses is the fragmentary Kahun Papyrus, which deals with veterinary medicine and women's diseases. The Edwin Smith Papyrus (of about the seventeenth century B.C.) is concerned with surgical matters, starting at the top of the head and working down—a type of medical organization often to be seen in subsequent texts in other countries—but the text stops abruptly at mid-chest. For the most part, this document is an empiric, secular, instructional system of practice, and evidently a copy of a much more ancient treatise. The Georg Ebers Papyrus, dating from the early sixteenth century, is the longest of the medical papyruses. An extensive medical therapeutic text covering many subjects, among them pharmacologic and mechanical means of treatment, it also contains many incantations and verbal charms.

The Hearst Papyrus (about the sixteenth century B.C.), the London (fourteenth century), the Berlin (early thirteenth century), and the Chester Beatty (late thirteenth century—dealing almost entirely with the treatment of diseases of the anus) may have been practical handbooks, whereas the Smith and Ebers papyruses may have been teaching materials. Part of the Ebers document is repeated in the Smith, and the Berlin Papyrus contains an entire treatise which also appears in the Ebers.

The oldest medical text extant anywhere is a cuneiform tablet from Mesopotamia. The most ancient known Egyptian medical writings date from a later period, but they refer back to texts far older. Most important among the more ancient treatises were: *Book on the Vessels of the Heart, The Physician's Secret: Knowledge of the Movement of the Heart and Knowledge of the Heart,* and *Collection on the Expelling of the Wehedu* (a toxic principle in the body).

In the second century A.D., the Christian writer Clemens of Alexandria spoke of forty-two sacred books the Egyptian god Thoth gave to humankind, said to contain the fountainhead of all knowledge. Thoth had by that time become incorporated into the Greek god Hermes as Hermes Trismegistos (or, "thrice great"), and the legendary collection was therefore called the "Hermetic Collection." Six of the Hermetic books were supposed to have been devoted to medicine, and Georg Ebers believed that his papyrus was the fourth medical book of the Collection.

Many mystical or fraudulent writings attributed to Hermetic origins kept appearing and reappearing in the centuries after Clemens. Secret processes and remedies became part of the medical folklore of the Mediterranean world, and the word "alchemy" may have come from the ancient name for Egypt: "Chem."

History

It is now believed that about 3000 B.C. the two kingdoms of Upper and Lower Egypt were united under King Menes, a ruler of the Southern Kingdom (Upper Egypt). Early in history, the ruling kings of Egypt were regarded as gods, but they retained human qualities, as did the cosmic gods. As sons of Ra, the sun-god, the

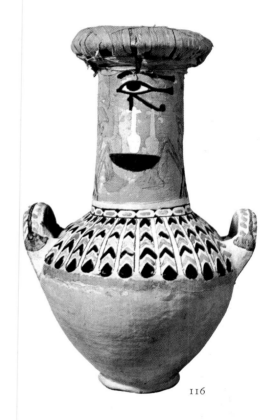

116

115 *Scene from XIXth-dynasty Theban Book of the Dead of Hunefer (c. 1300 B.C.) showing jackal-headed Anubis holding coffin containing embalmed body of Hunefer before weeping family and priests performing "Opening of the Mouth" ceremony, which prepares deceased for afterlife. British Museum, London*

116 *Clay vase with painted linen wrappings from XVIIIth-dynasty Tomb of Khai (c. 15th century B.C.) emblazoned with Eye of Horus sign, which may have been origin of prescription symbol ℞. Museo Egizio, Turin*

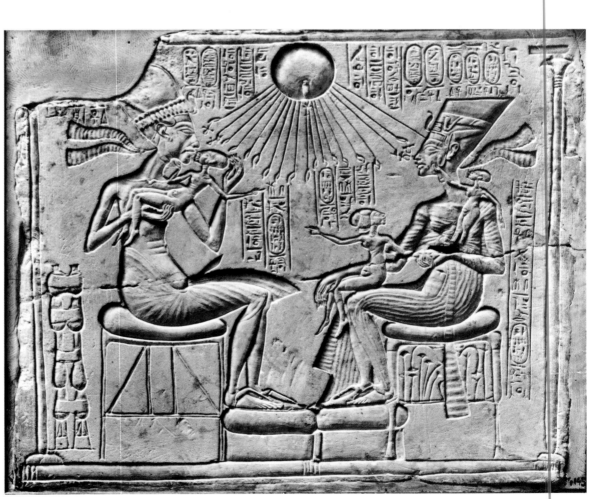

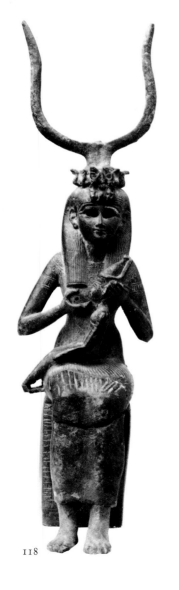

kings were both spiritual and temporal heads of state. Significant developments of this time were the Egyptian alphabet and the tools of writing: papyrus, reed pens, and ink.

The following period, about 2780–2200, is sometimes referred to as the Old Kingdom, and the great pyramids were probably constructed during this time. Over the next few centuries (Sixth to Eleventh dynasties), the strong central government weakened, but it was at least partially reestablished during the Eleventh and Twelfth dynasties, which marked the Middle Kingdom (2000–1750). This period has been called the "Classical Age" as an indication of its high intellectual emphasis, and medicine apparently held a prominent place in the pursuit of learning.

In the Thirteenth dynasty (1750–1580), Egypt was invaded by the Hyksos, a Semitic people from Lower (Northern) Egypt, who held sway for about two hundred years and merged many of their gods and customs into Egyptian culture. Gradually the Hyksos overlordship was destroyed, but the struggle resulted in the establishment of a military state in the Eighteenth dynasty, under Ahmose and then Amenhotep I, which ushered in the period of the New Empire (1580–1350 B.C.). During this time, the extraordinary Queen Hatshepsut became the first woman ruler of all Egypt and extended the influence and power of her country. It was not uncommon later for queens to rule Egypt, but even as consorts of the pharaoh they wielded important political power. Whether there were actually women physicians, as has been deduced from philological evidence of a feminine form of the Egyptian word for physician, is not yet fully established.

It was also during this age that Pharaoh Amenhotep IV moved away from worship of the state god Amen and favored the developing cult of the sun-god Aten. He left Thebes to establish a new capital, Akhetaten (horizon of Aten), dedicated to the worship of this one god, and changed his name to Akhenaten (of service to Aten) in tribute. After Akhenaten's death, his son-in-law and successor, Tutankhaten, returned the court to Thebes, restored the god Amen to supremacy, and changed his name to Tutankhamen. The discovery in November, 1922, of this ruler's intact tomb, sealed for more than 2,000 years, was a major contribution to Egyptology.

After Tutankhamen, power shifted back to a dynasty of Hyksos derivation. The story of the enslavement of the Hebrews probably dates from this period in the thirteenth century B.C., and Ramses II, builder of the great temple of Abu Simbel, may have been pharaoh during the Exodus. Another pharaoh of Biblical times was Merneptah. The Royal College of Physicians in examining his mummy found that he had died in old age with bald head, obese abdomen, and an arteriosclerotic aorta (the main artery of the body).

Over subsequent centuries, as pharaonic power waned, the country successively fell under the hegemony of Libya, Ethiopia, Assyria, and finally Persia, when Egypt became a satrapy of that empire. In 323 B.C. Alexander the Great, the Macedonian Greek conqueror, defeated Persia and set his general Ptolemy on the throne as king of Egypt. (The famous Cleopatra VII of Roman times was the last of this Greek Ptolemaic dynasty.) Alexandria, the city in Egypt founded by Alexander, became the medical and intellectual capital of the Mediterranean world.

THE GODS

All deities were associated with some aspect of health or illness. Many began as local divinities, later to be taken up by the whole kingdom as cosmic gods. Others were melded into some other deity. Ra, the sun-god, held the highest place in the pantheon. Isis, a sort of primal earth-mother, was worshiped as a healing goddess. Her cult persisted for many centuries, and temples dedicated to her healing powers were still being established at the time temples to Asclepios began to appear in the Greek world. A brother of Isis was Osiris, a personification of the Nile, who was dismembered by another brother, Seth. Isis lay upon her brother Osiris,

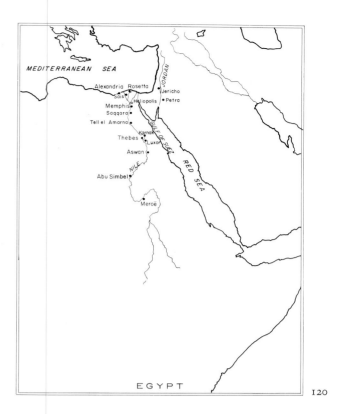

117 *Section of medical papyrus (c. 1550 B.C.), one of seven extant, discovered by Georg Ebers at Thebes in 1872. Contains recipes, treatments, and both magical and religious incantations. Universitätsbibliothek der Karl-Marx-Universität, Leipzig*

118 *Figure of the healing goddess Isis, sister and wife of Osiris, personification of the Nile, and mother of Horus, god of light. The Louvre, Paris*

119 *Akhenaten, seated with Queen Nefertiti, on limestone relief (c. 1360 B.C.) from Tell el Amarna, holding daughter under life-giving rays of sun-god Aten, whom Akhenaten had elevated over Amen as chief god of Egypt. Egyptian Museum, Cairo*

120 *Map of Egypt*

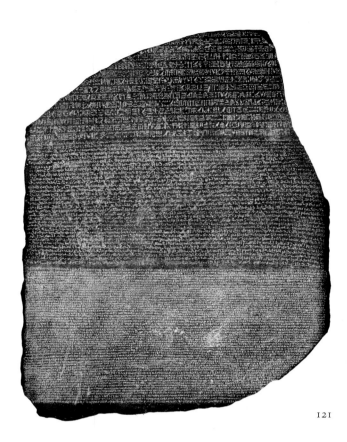

121

121 *Basalt fragment called the Rosetta Stone (c. 196 B.C.) for place of discovery during Napoleon's Egyptian campaign in 1799. Comparison of text in hieroglyphic, demotic, and Greek scripts led to decipherment of ancient Egyptian writing. British Museum, London*

122 *Gold statue of Amen, local deity of Thebes elevated to ruling god of Egyptian pharaohs, whose temple priests included healers. Metropolitan Museum of Art, New York*

123 *Solid-gold mask, inlaid with lapis lazuli and semiprecious stones, of inner coffin (c. 1360 B.C.) of Tutankhamen, pharaoh who renounced sun-god Aten and restored Amen to primacy among Egyptian gods. Egyptian Museum, Cairo*

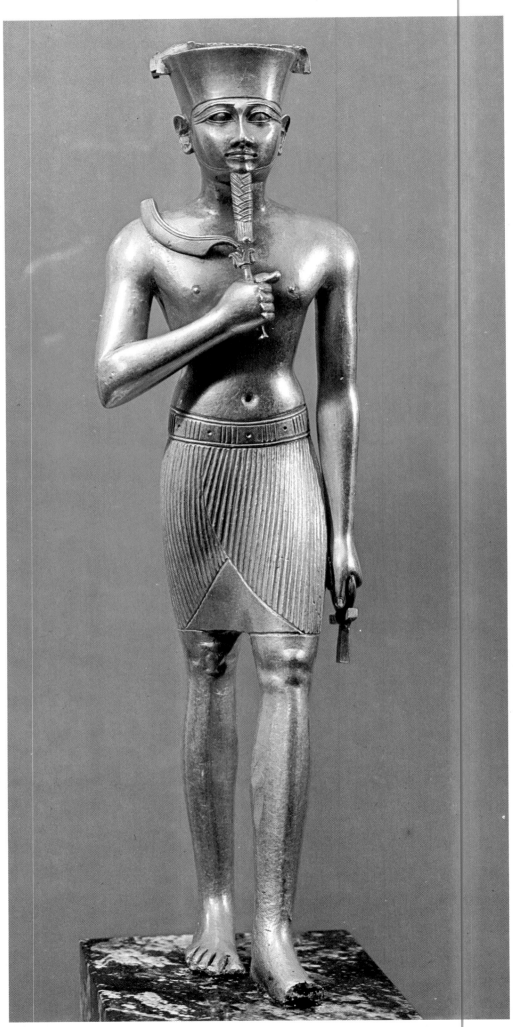

122

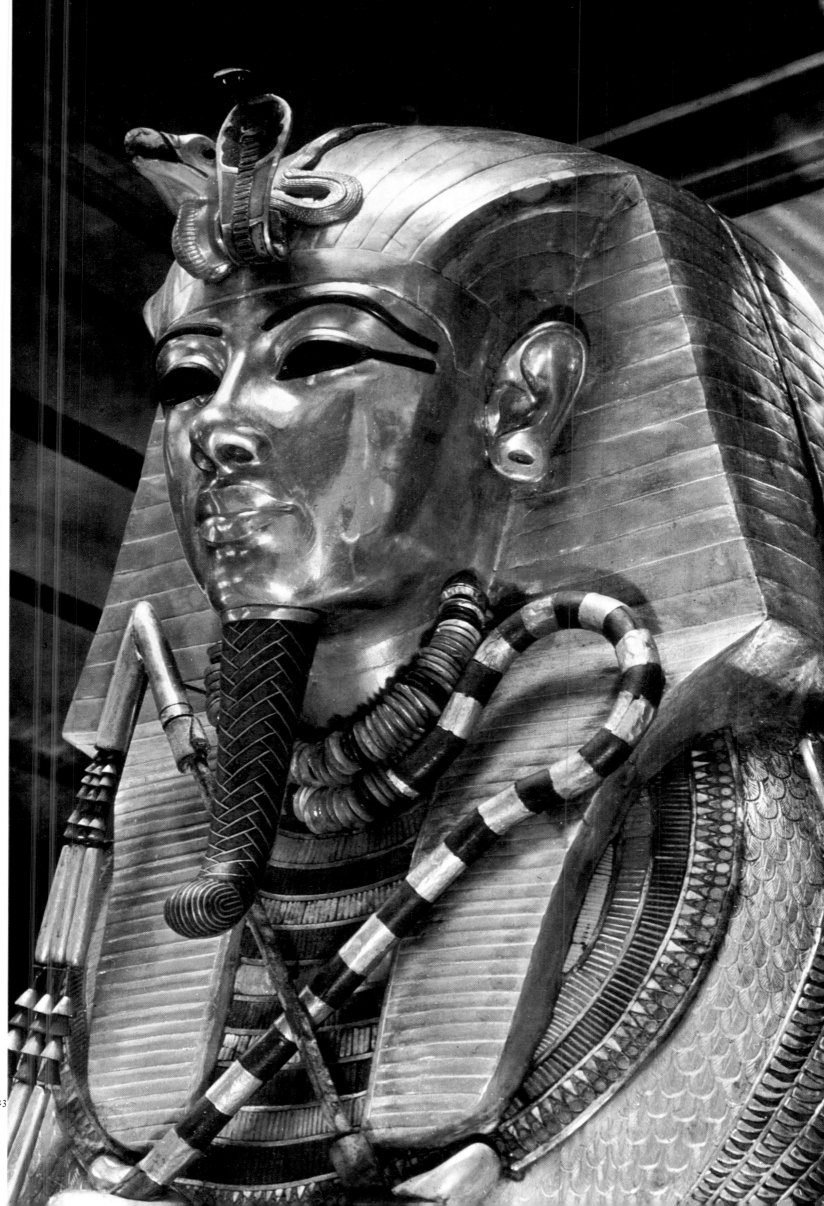

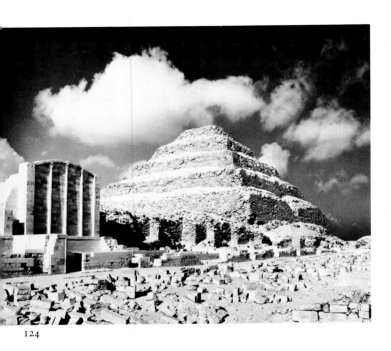

124 *Step pyramid at Saqqara (c. 2650 B.C.), tomb complex of IIId-dynasty King Zoser, said to have been built by Imhotep, who became deified as most famous Egyptian god of healing.*

125 *Falcon-headed Horus, guardian of health, shown making libation. The Louvre, Paris*

126 *Gold-painted wooden figure of Ptah, principal god of Memphis and patron of artisans and artists, later called father of Imhotep and a patron deity of physicians. From tomb of Tutankhamen, Metropolitan Museum of Art, New York*

127 *Seated statue of Imhotep (c. 2600 B.C.), vizier, scribe, poet, architect, and physician, who, as deified Egyptian healing divinity, was merged with Asclepios, Greek god of medicine, during Hellenic times as Asclepios-Imhoutes. The Louvre, Paris*

128 *(Overleaf) Opening scene of papyrus* Book of the Dead *of Khai (c. 1540 B.C.), showing Khai and his wife Merit paying obeisance to the god Osiris. Museo Egizio, Turin*

restored him, and also conceived her son Horus. The evil Seth, who together with his sister and consort Nephthys was a prime bringer of disease to humans, then destroyed the eye of Horus. Thoth, the source of all knowledge and physician to the gods, healed the eye. (Following divine example, Egyptian royal couples were often brother and sister. The custom of sibling marriage was also adopted at court, and eventually by the lower classes. By the second century A.D., it was estimated that two-thirds of the citizens of Arsinoe were offspring of sibling unions.)

Among other supernatural healers were Hathor, mistress of heaven and protector of women in childbirth; Bes and Thoëris, to whom pregnant women also prayed; Keket, who ensured fertility, and her ram-headed consort Khnum, who actually fashioned each child and created its *ka*, or spiritual projection. During Ptolemaic times, Serapis was a local deity who rivaled Asclepios among the populace of Egypt as god of healing.

The two most important healing divinities were Thoth, physician to the gods, and Imhotep, whom Sir William Osler called "the first figure of a physician to stand out clearly from the mists of antiquity." Thoth became a patron god both of physicians (as the source of medical knowledge) and of scribes (as the inventor of writing).

The other important god of healing, Imhotep, began as a historic personage in the Pyramid Age (about 2600 B.C.) as a many talented genius: vizier to the pharaoh, architect (he is said to have built the step pyramid at Saqqara), poet, scribe, and apparently also physician although no writings or teachings have been ascribed to him. By the sixth century B.C. he had displaced Thoth as the chief healing god of Egypt and been given a divine father, the god Ptah. In time the Greek Asclepios and the Egyptian Imhotep were combined as Asclepios-Imhoutes.

DEATH AND AFTERWARDS

The attitude toward death is a key to much of ancient Egypt's civilization and contains many paradoxes. Life was a preparation for afterlife; yet life was lived to the fullest—at least among royalty and the rich. Burial practices were a paean to life after death—which was to be a new existence, a joyful experience. Nevertheless, the dead were mourned openly and elaborately, even at times with self-flagellation. Embalmers often removed the internal organs of the dead body and left only a shell, yet this preserved remnant was important to spiritual reawakening in the hereafter. The living body was the abode of a divine spark which left after death to become a ghost or demon, but the soul (*ka*), a sort of spiritual double of the person, remained forever in the embalmed body. An important ritual called "the opening of the mouth" was often depicted in the *Book of the Dead,* a guidebook to the afterlife and regulator of all funerary practices. Presumably it readied the body for receiving the life force necessary for future resurrection.

EMBALMING

The extent of embalming was determined by the status of the deceased and the money to be spent. The most elaborate procedure called for, among other things, four stone canopic jars in which to preserve the extracted liver, lungs, stomach, and intestines. To ensure that these organs would function for eternity, the covers of the jars were carved to represent the four sons of Horus: Dutamutef the jackal-headed, Kebehsenuef the falcon-headed, Imsety the human-headed, and Hapi the ape-headed. The cranial contents were removed through the nostrils with hooks, and the skull and abdominal cavity were then washed out with spices. The body was soaked for seventy days in natron (a mixture of clay and salts of carbonate, sulfate, and chloride) and then thoroughly washed. Finally, the corpse was coated with gums and wrapped in long strips of fine linen. Less costly embalming included only some of the preparations, and the poor were simply buried in the sand.

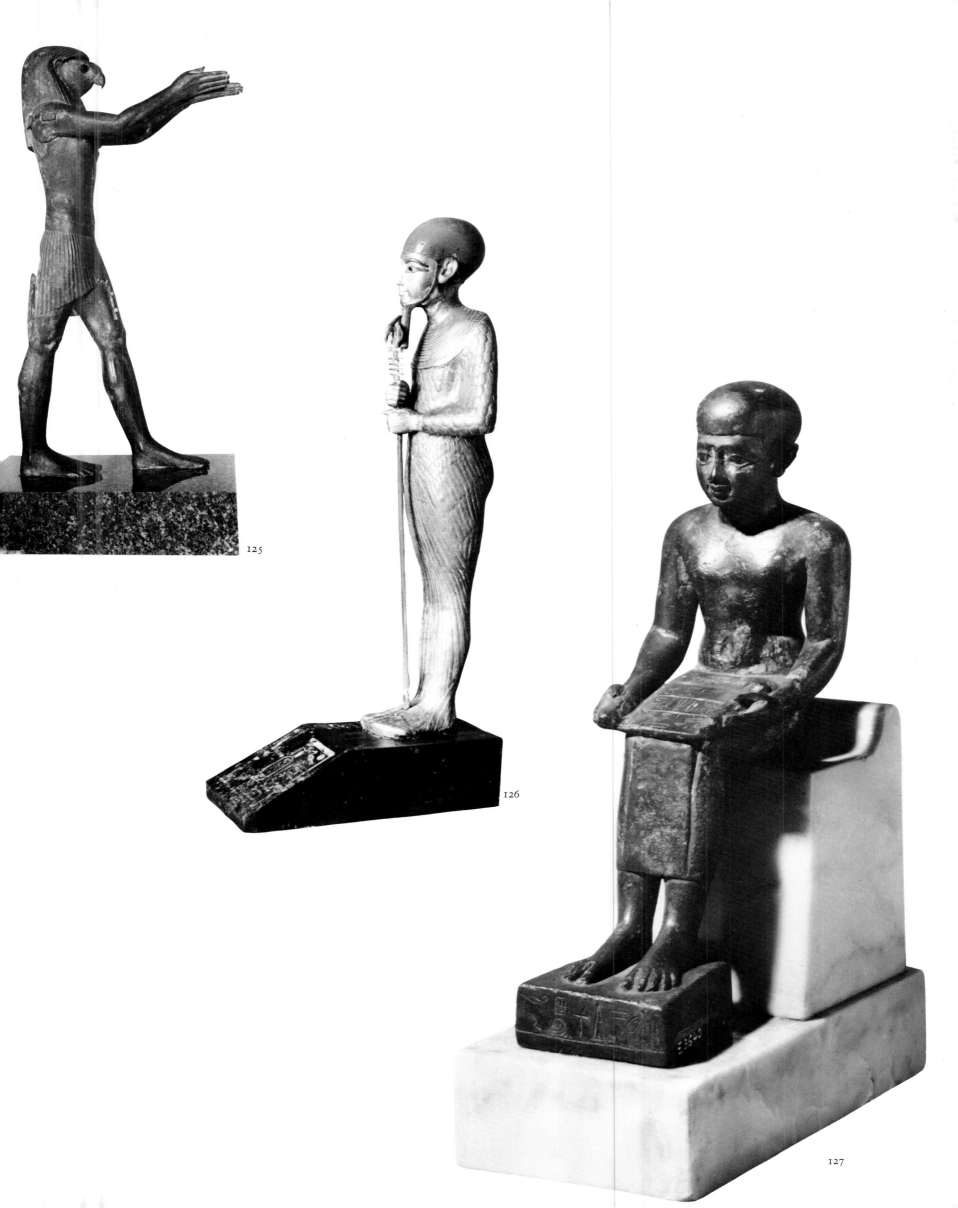

125

126

127

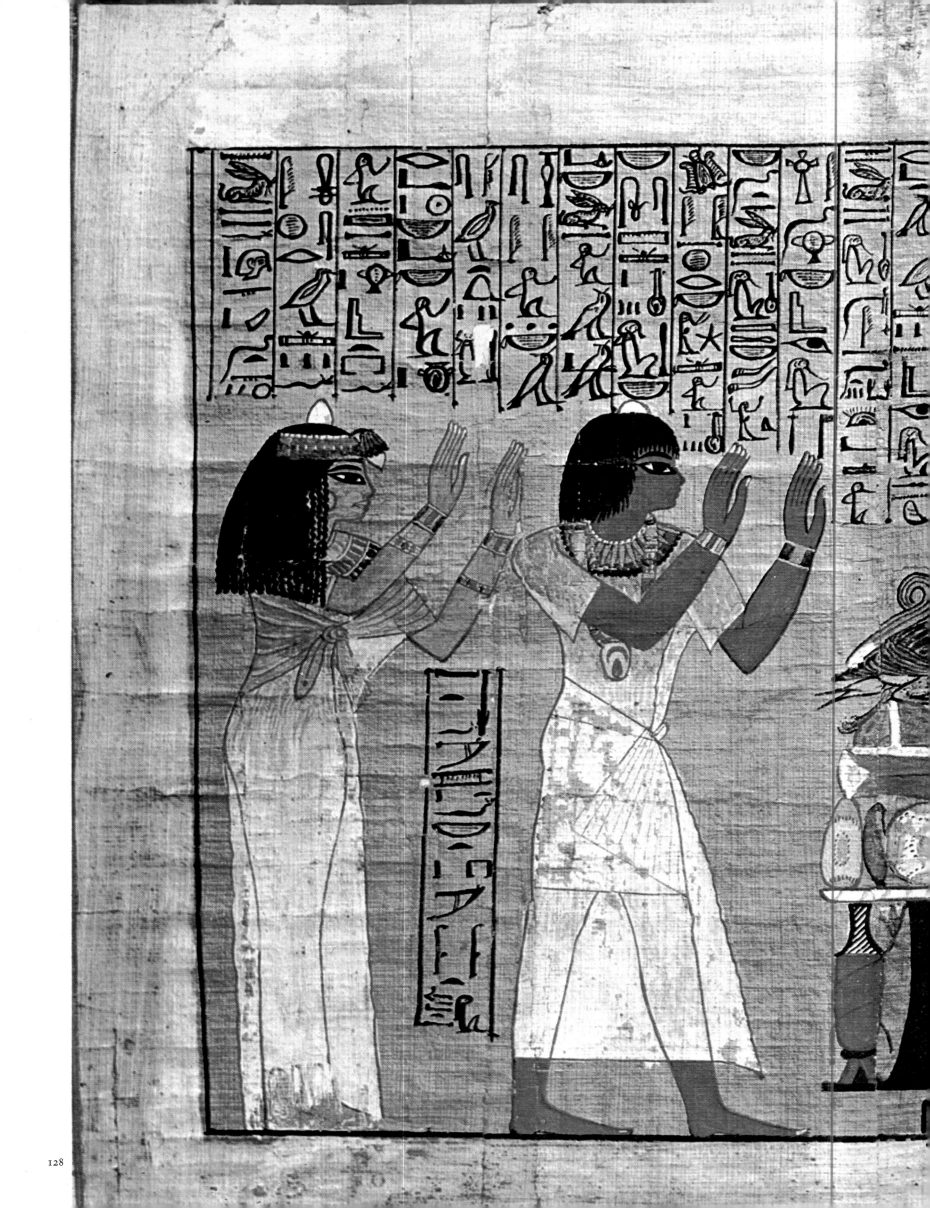

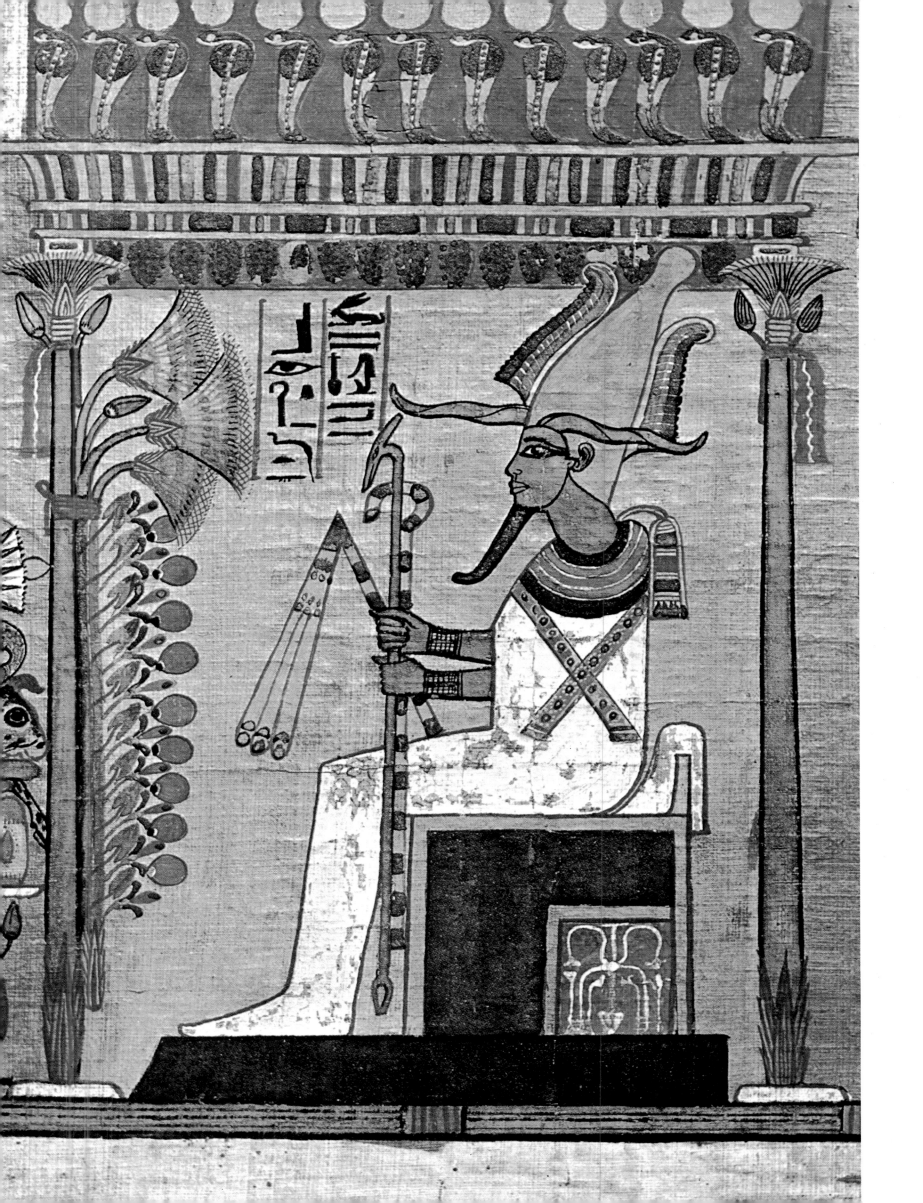

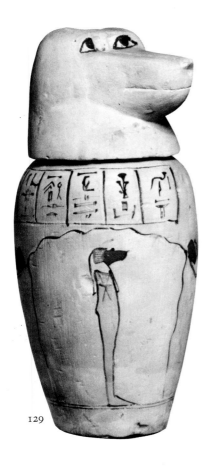

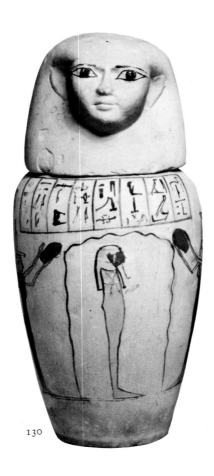

129   130

129, 130, 133, 134 *Set of four canopic jars used to preserve liver, lungs, stomach,
and intestines extracted from deceased during embalming. Lids represent four sons of
god Horus, who protect remains in eternity. Walters Art Gallery, Baltimore*

131, 132 *One of four miniature gold coffins (c. 1360 B.C.), inlaid with carnelian
and glass, used to house preserved viscera of XVIIIth-dynasty King Tutankhamen.
Metropolitan Museum of Art, New York*

135 *Bronze coffin of embalmed sacred cat (c. 940–664 B.C.) illustrating Egyptian
regard for animals, in whose guise their gods often took form. Collection Norbert
Schimmel, New York*

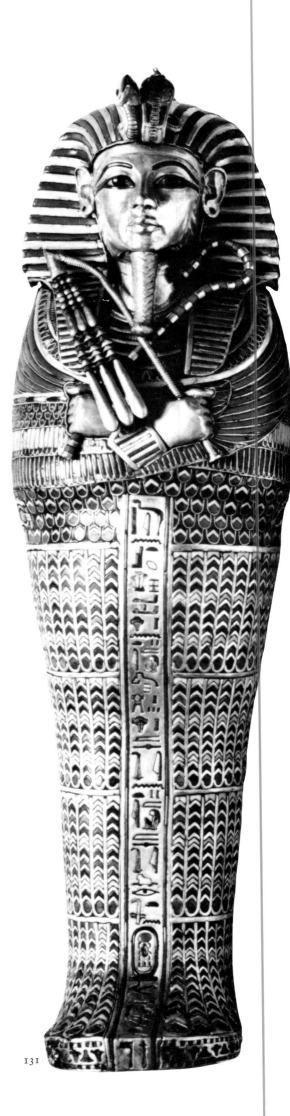

131

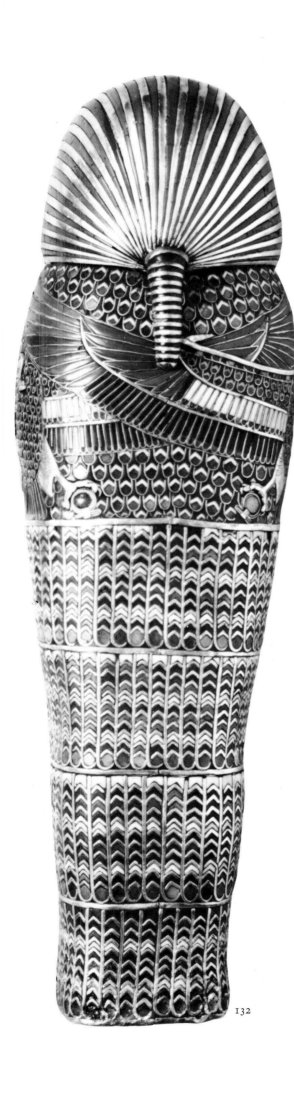

132

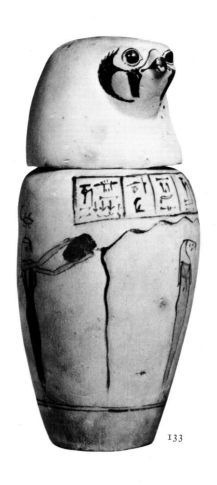

133

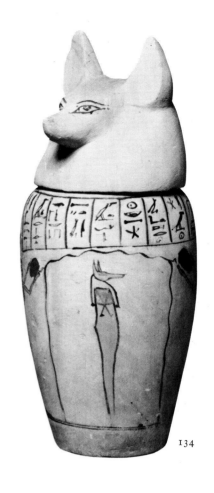

134

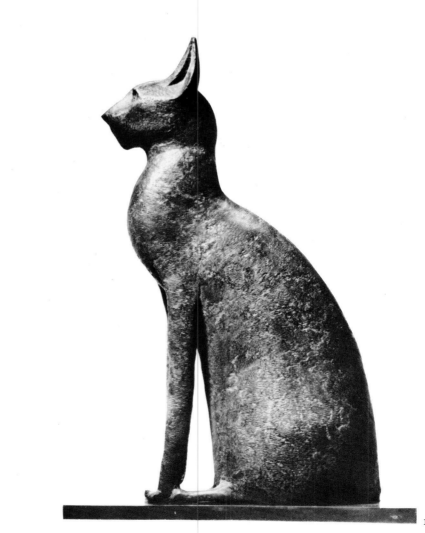

135

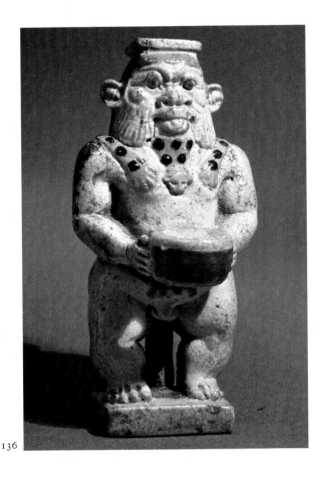

136

136 *Cosmetic* kohl *container of cream-colored faience (c. 1320–1280* B.C.*) in form of Bes, god of household and pregnancy, as attendant. Collection Norbert Schimmel, New York*

137 *Fragment of sycamore wood coffin lid of Djed-Thoth-Ef-'Onch (4th century* B.C.*) with inlaid colored enamel hieroglyphics giving deceased's name and portion of* Book of the Dead. *Collection Drovetti, Museo Egizio, Turin*

138 *Scene from* Book of the Dead *(c. 1250* B.C.*) where heart of scribe Ani is weighed in scales against feather symbolizing Truth by jackal-headed Anubis in final judgment. Monster Amit waits to devour heart found wanting. British Museum, London*

139 *Gilded wooden coffin of ibis, with head and feet cast in silver, of Ptolemaic period. Ibis was representative figure of god Thoth, source of all knowledge and physician to the gods. Charles Edwin Wilbour Fund, Brooklyn Museum*

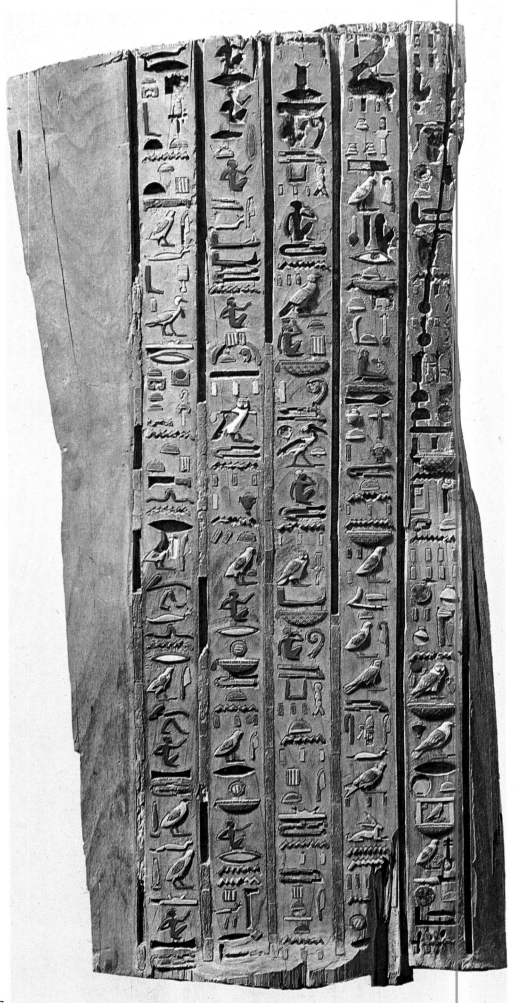

137

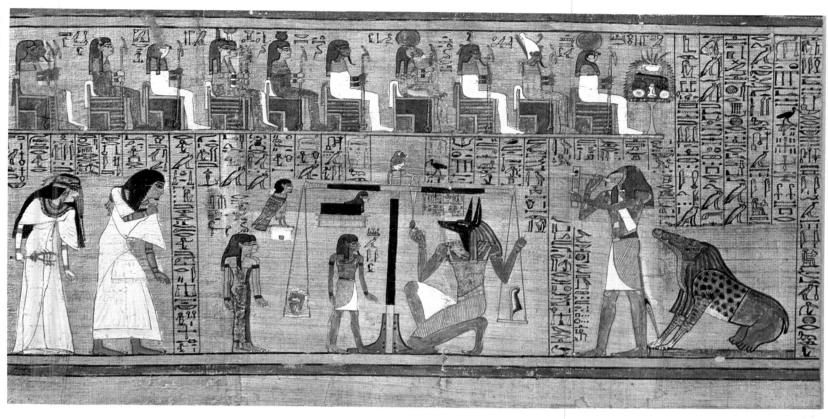

138

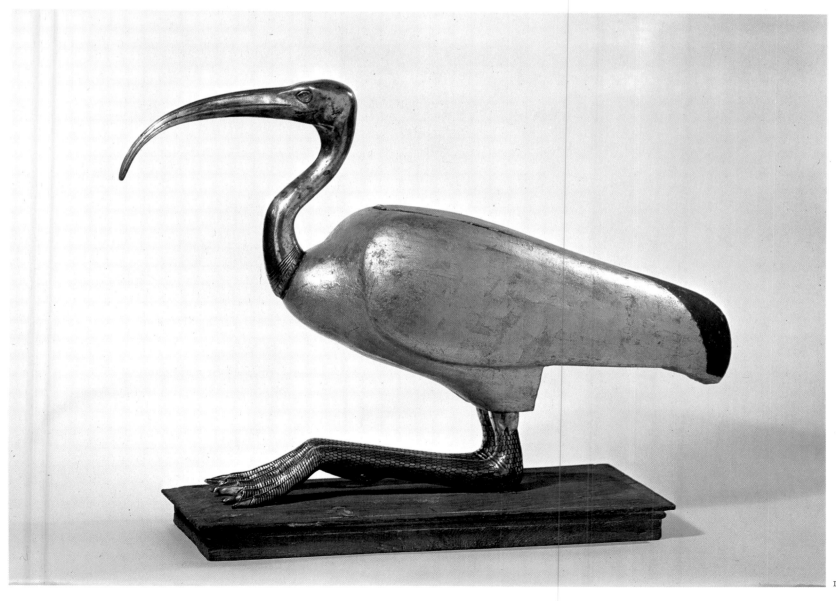

139

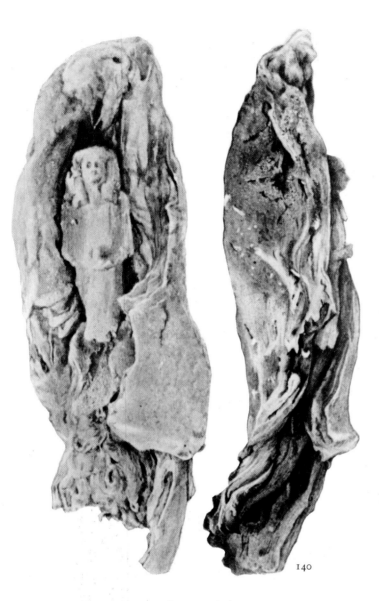

140 *Drawings of mummy's liver containing statuette of human-headed deity Imsety, son of Horus, placed there by embalmer to guard remains. New York Academy of Medicine*

ANATOMY AND PHYSIOLOGY

Despite the continual exposure of internal organs by embalmers, information on anatomy and physiology was sketchy and closely linked with theology. The listing of organs of the body was a religious recital of those belonging to the great god Ra, and each body part also had a special deity as protector. This projection of the human body into the cosmic scheme continued to be a universal medical and philosophical concept, especially emphasized in Europe during the Middle Ages.

A similar linkage of internal human functioning to the functioning of the outside world may have prompted the Egyptians to view the anatomical and physiological makeup of the body as a system of channels (*metu*) similar to the network of canals which spread throughout their land. The heart was at the center of the system, the station where the *metu* delivered and received. The pulsation of the heart was known, and the propagation of its beats throughout the body was perceived, for as the Smith Papyrus states: "Its pulsation is in every vessel of every member." Air came in through the nose (but also the ears), entered the channels, was delivered to the heart, and from there was sent to all parts of the body. However, the *metu* also carried blood, urine, tears, sperm, and feces. Around the anus, the channels coalesced into a sort of collecting system where the contents of the rectum could enter the network; however, they became the main cause of disease if allowed to build up. Hence, the intestinal contents were cleaned out regularly by emetics, purges, and enemas, and the anus became a prime target of medical treatment. Most medical therapies were directed toward the *metu*: to calm if irritated; to soften when too firm; to stimulate if sluggish; to cool when hot; to deflate if swollen; to relieve when painful.

The importance of the brain was well appreciated, and the Smith Papyrus spoke of a sensation of throbbing and fluttering beneath fingers palpating the surface of an injury-exposed living brain. The Papyrus also spoke of the effects on motor functions of brain injury; the results were seen to be different depending on which side was injured. Other organs were also mentioned and even described in the various medical papyruses, but the Egyptians misunderstood or misinterpreted much of what they saw.

PUBLIC HEALTH

Herodotus called the Egyptians the "healthiest of all men." Whether this remark was based on a general impression or on secondhand information similar to his erroneous conclusions regarding the absence of doctors among the Babylonians is not known. However, a sweeping statement with the opposite conclusion was made by Pliny five hundred years later, when he referred to Egypt as "the motherland of diseases."

The ancient Egyptians paid much attention to cleanliness of body and home, probably to a great extent for religious reasons. Among all economic and social classes washing was practiced every morning, evening, and before each meal, but since soap had not yet been invented a type of alkali was used. The purgings, vomitings, and enematizing which ancient Egyptians engaged in each month were also a sort of symbolic internal cleansing as well as a method of ridding the channels (*metu*) of dangerous intestinal contents.

The water of the Nile was thought to be of great purity and salutary effect, and its supply was usually abundant. An elaborate system of dams, basins, and canals fulfilled all agricultural needs. For the most part this network was effective, but Egypt was still dependent on the periodic rise and fall of its great river for the fertility of its land and the orderly flow of water through its sluices and reservoirs. It is doubtful that in ancient Egypt refuse was dumped into the river as it was in Greek, Roman, and Muslim times—when the Nile became a veritable cesspool. However, many canals, pools, and puddles always were suited to breeding insects.

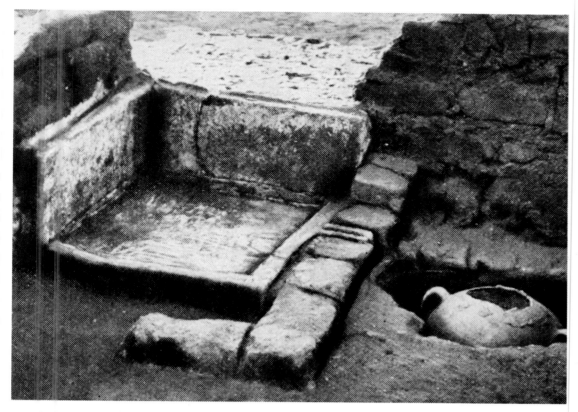

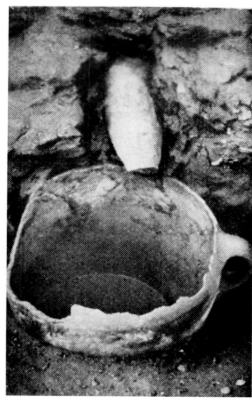

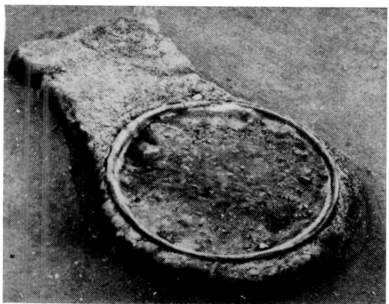

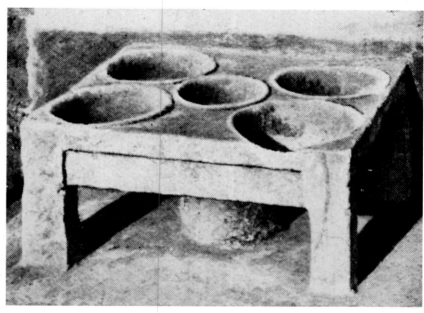

141 *Sanitary facilities in excavated house of noble-man Nekht at Akhetaten, city built by Akhenaten about 1360 B.C., dedicated to monotheistic worship of Aten. New York Academy of Medicine*

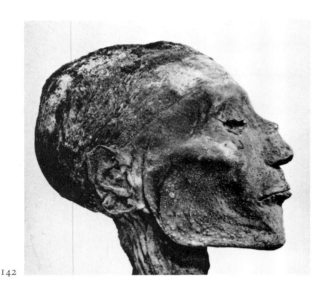

142 *Mummified head of the Pharaoh Ramses V, 1160 B.C., showing lesions thought to be those of smallpox. World Health Organization, Geneva*

Herodotus spoke of the need to find high ground or towers for sleeping places to avoid clouds of gnats.

DISEASES

A number of diseases can be reasonably well identified from descriptive reports in papyruses, pictorial representations, inscriptions, mummies, and contemporary accounts. Diseases resulting from water and food contamination, notably intestinal ailments, were evidently common and disabling, and parasitic infestations, especially by the schistosome and other worms, also have been discovered in mummies. Although malaria appears not to have been quite as common nor as severe as in Mesopotamia, India, and Greece, fevers of all kinds were a problem.

Diseases of the eye were frequent and included infections such as trachoma (which is still common in Egypt), night blindness, cataract, and distortions of the eyelids. Arteriosclerosis was surely a disease of the ancient Egyptian judging by pathologic findings in mummies, and epidemic diseases such as smallpox and plague were probably as much a scourge then as they were later. The vertebrae of mummies often suggest the late effects of Pott's disease (a tubercular infection).

Some ailments described in the writings resemble gonorrhea, but at present no obvious instances of syphilitic infections of the bones or soft parts have been proved. Leprosy may well have been present, but as in virtually all ancient civilizations it was probably often confused with other skin conditions. Acute illnesses were certainly well known even though their precise nature is difficult for us to reconstruct, but penumonia and appendicitis clearly may be inferred from some of the information available. Certainly the muscle wasting of poliomyelitis can be recognized in a few temple reliefs.

Arthritis, gout, and kidney and bladder stones were probably frequent, and tumors of the ovaries and of bone have been identified. The occurrence of cirrhosis of the liver is also generally accepted. The reported large consumption of beer and wine may have been a causative factor.

DIAGNOSIS

Egyptian methods of diagnosis used information from the patient, but the actual taking of a detailed history had not yet developed. Nevertheless, examination was complex and included probing of wounds with the fingers and study of the sputum, urine, feces, and other bodily emanations. Inasmuch as the pulse was recognized as transmitted by the heart, it was carefully checked in different parts of the body.

The papyruses contain many astute observations from which a reconstruction of some disease entities can be surmised. For example, hernias were clearly noted: "When you judge a swelling on the surface of a belly . . . what comes out . . . caused by coughing." References to bloody urine may call to mind cystitis (bladder inflammation), stones, or parasites. Indeed, infestations with worms of different types must have been as common then as they are now—to judge from the findings in mummies with organs intact.

Combinations of symptoms were occasionally grouped together, but for the most part the symptom *was* the disease: cough, fever, swelling, skin rash—each was an ailment itself. Inflammation as "disease" was recognizably described as follows in the medical texts: "It means that the wound which is in his breast is sluggish, without closing up; high fever comes forth from it, its two lips are red, and its mouth is open." Medical classifications, therefore, tended to be of symptoms rather than diseases.

PROGNOSIS

Although the Egyptian healers did not state a prognosis specifically, they did make

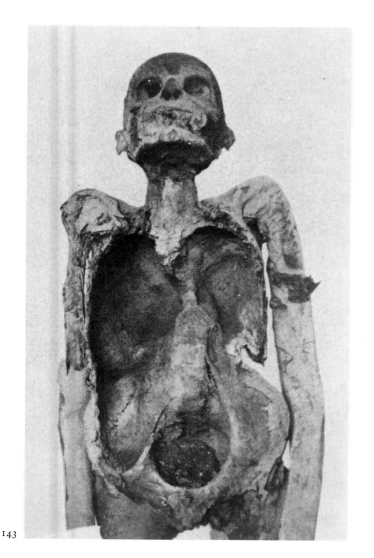

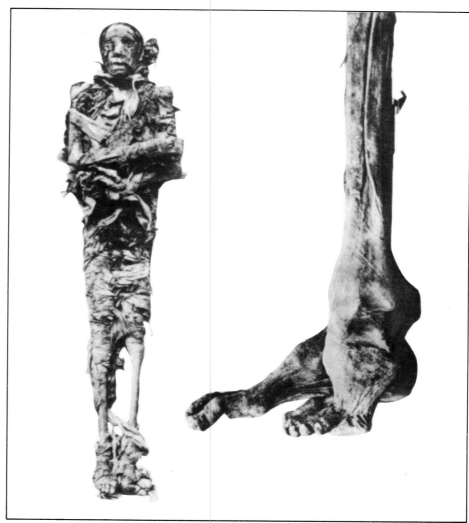

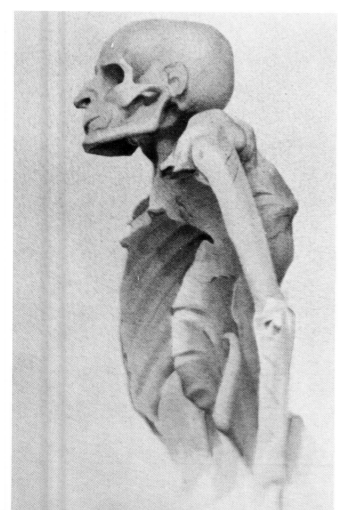

143, 144 *Mummy of priest of Amen (c. 1000 B.C.), with profile view showing protrusion of spine common to Pott's disease (tuberculosis of spine) and frontal view showing huge psoas abscess into which tubercular lesion drained. New York Academy of Medicine*

145 *Mummy and congenital clubfoot of XIXth-dynasty Pharaoh Siphtah (c. 1300 B.C.). Egyptian Museum, Cairo*

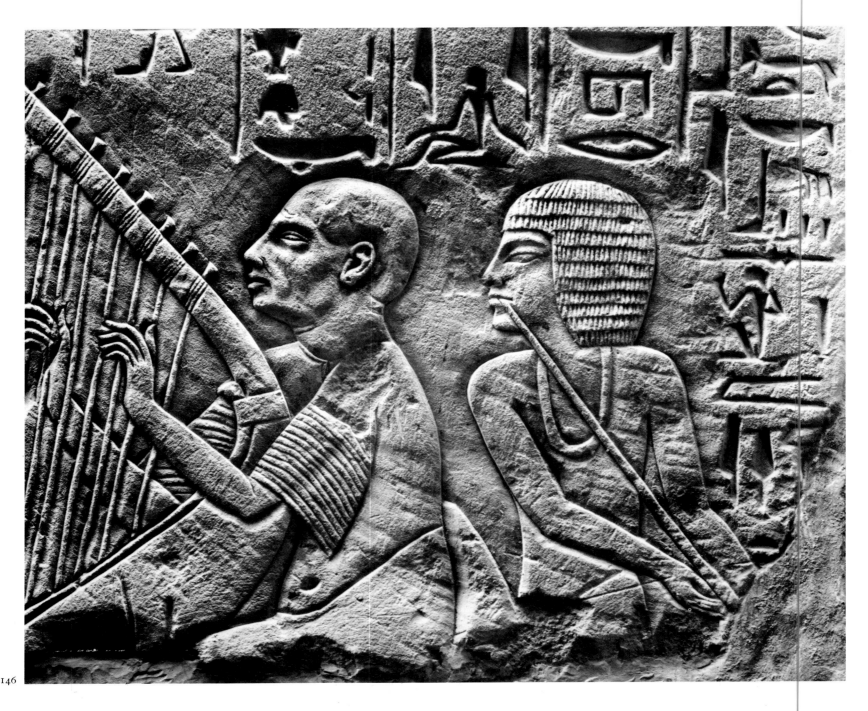

146

146 *Relief of blind harper from tomb of Patenemhab (c. 1552–1306 B.C.), Saqqara, indica-tive of long history of pervasive blindness in Egypt. Rijksmuseum van Oudheden, Leiden*

147 *Translation of hieroglyphs from* Precepts of Ani (c. 1500 B.C.) *advising moderation in drink, as well as avoidance of excess in other things. World Health Organization*

148 *XVIIIth-dynasty stele (1580–1350 B.C.) showing young man leaning on staff with withered leg characteristic of polio. Collection Carlsberg Glyptothek, Copenhagen*

Make not   thyself helpless   in drinking in the

beer shop.   For will not   the words   of [thy] report repeated

slip out from { thy mouth } without { thy knowing } { that thou hast uttered them ? }

Falling down   thy limbs   will be broken,   [and]

no one will   give thee { a hand [to help] thee up }   as for thy

companions in the   swilling of beer,   they will get up

and say, " Outside with   this   drunkard."

147

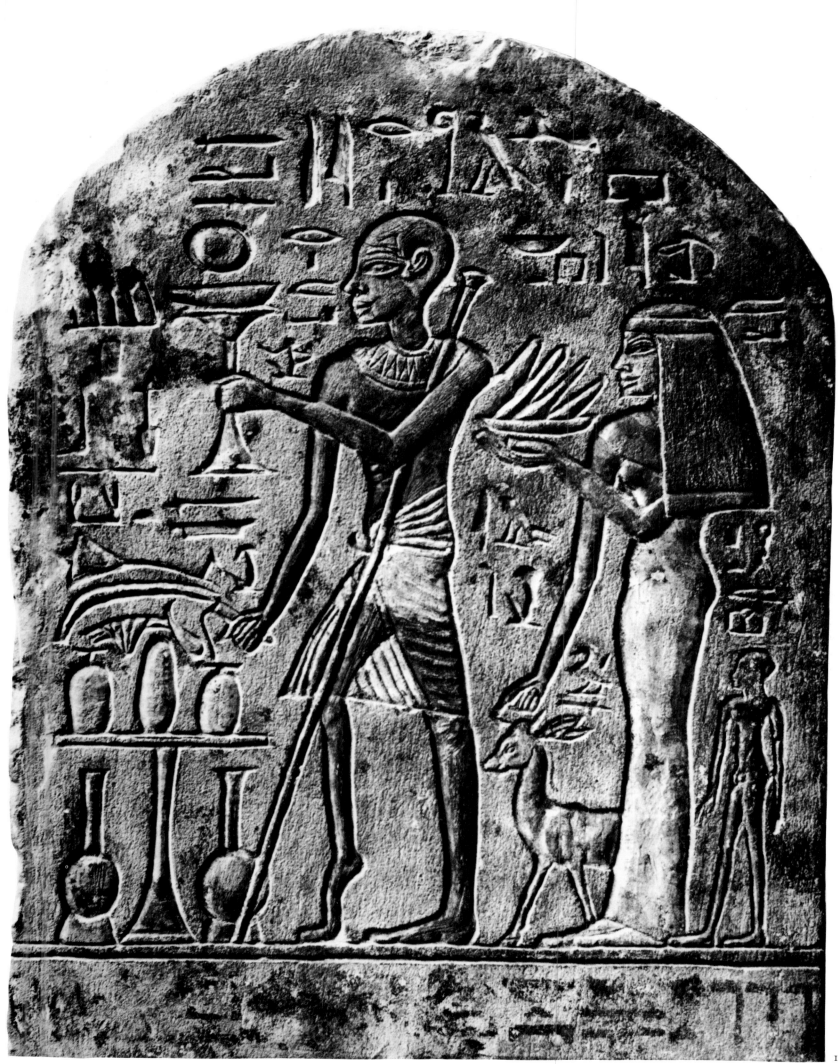

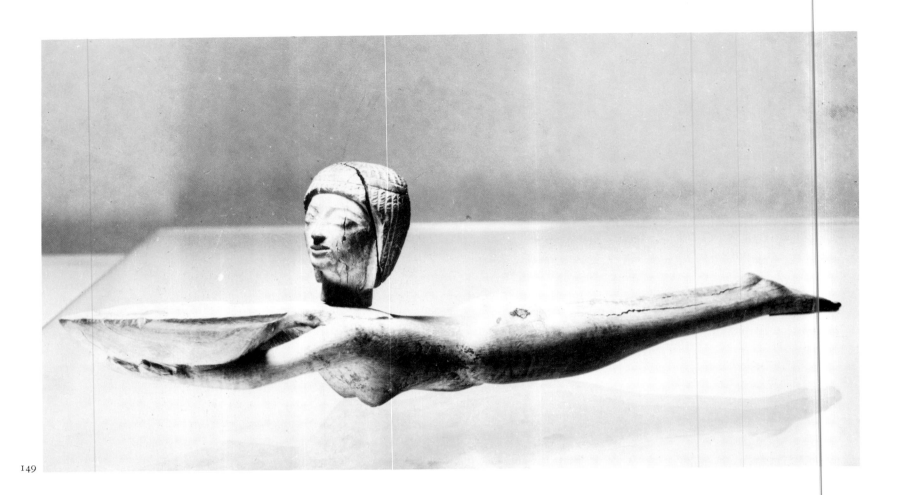

149

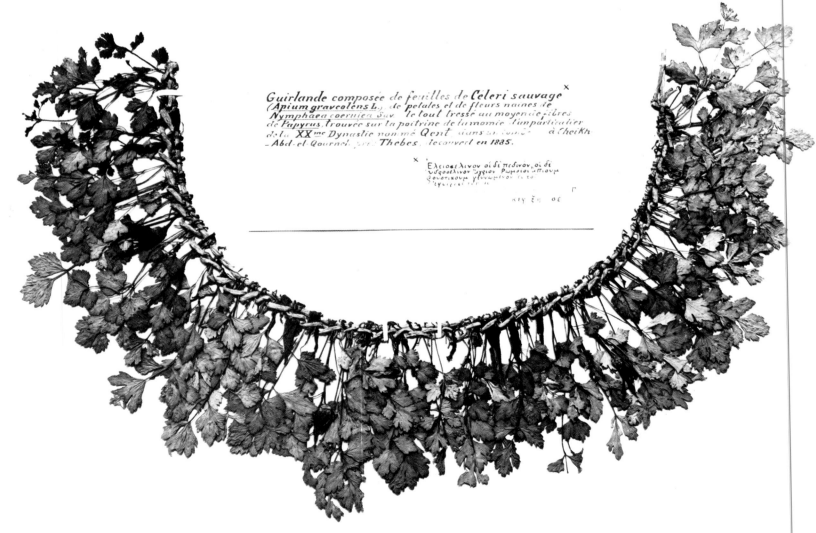

Guirlande composée de feuilles de **Celeri sauvage**
(**Apium graveolens** L.) de pétales et de fleurs naines de
Nymphaea coerulea Sav le tout tressé au moyen de fibres
de Papyrus, trouvée sur la poitrine de la momie d'un particulier
de la **XX**ᵐᵉ Dynastie nommé **Qent** dans son tombe à Cheikh
Abd-el-Qournah près **Thèbes**, découvert en 1885.

Ελκιοσελινον οι δι πεδινον, οι δι
υδροσελινον εγχιον Phμxιοι αττικια
φονατκουμ ετνναμενον εςτο
δεγειφρεται κη

κιγ ξη οε

150

decisions on whether to "contend with," or to avoid treating—which implied estimation of the future course of a sickness. A very serious illness which had even a chance of responding favorably the physician agreed to contend with, but conditions thought hopeless were denied treatment. This attitude of withholding medical ministrations to the incurable was a recurring theme throughout history, frequent especially in Greek times. The basis may well have been pragmatism or insensitivity, but honesty may also have underlain the decision.

TREATMENT

In treatment itself, religio-magical gestures played a vital role. Accompanying the administration of drugs and mechanical procedures were incantations to drive out demons and supplications to the gods for protection from evil spirits. Amulets could ward off illnesses of most kinds, but serious mental disease required the exorcism of demons, often calling for the use of excrement. For snakebite, rituals were virtually the only therapy—in marked contrast to the management of snakebite in India, where sound, rational medical principles were combined with the supernatural. Nevertheless, in most other healing activities the Egyptians combined their religious rituals with an exceptional and varied array of vegetable, mineral, and animal drugs.

MEDICATION

Their pharmacopoeia was vast. A great many of the medications and plants that later found their way into the herbals of Dioscorides, Galen, and Pliny, and also into the Hebraic, Syriac, Arabic, and Persian armamentarium came from Egyptian sources. But the Egyptians also imported substances from abroad: saffron and sage from Crete; cinnamon from China; perfumes and spices from Arabia and Abyssinia; sandalwood, gums, and antimony.

They administered medications in many forms—as pills, cakes, suppositories, ointments, drops, gargles, fumigations, and baths. Even enemas were a popular route for the introduction of drugs as well as a means of evacuating the bowels. (Incidentally, the ibis, symbol of the god Thoth, was supposed to have originated the enema by inserting its long beak into its own anus.) The liquid vehicles were water, milk, beer, and wine, each sweetened with honey, and the ingredients were expected to remedy a variety of problems, not just illness: recolor gray hair; restore thinning hair; beautify; clean house; create pleasant odors; and control flies and other insects.

Egyptian physicians made use of a wide variety of medicinal plants, but the most numerous remedies were purgatives and emetics. The cathartic oil of the castor plant was used both as an internal drug and as a medication for wounds and irritated areas. Products from the opium poppy may have come into use in Egypt relatively late, but some scholars believe the plant was a therapeutic drug in the second millennium B.C. Substances such as hyoscyamus and scopolamine (an ingredient of "twilight sleep" in recent obstetrical practice), which are both related to mandragora from the mandrake plant, probably also were employed, but the time of their introduction is not established. Some of the vegetable decoctions may well have had antiseptic action. The "rotten bread" prescribed in several formulas might have been effective on wounds because of the presence of antibacterial molds (just as penicillium mold is used today).

Minerals and metals in the Egyptian pharmacopoeia included antimony, copper, salt, alum, carbon from charred wood, and possibly also iron from meteorites. The paints used for beautifying a woman's eyes were probably high in antimony, which became an important pharmacologic substance in the Renaissance and after. Black eyelid linings apparently were produced by a composition of antimony or lead. (Many centuries later in Arabic times finely

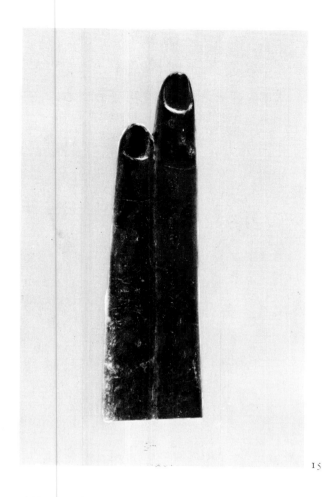

151

149 *Wooden cosmetic container used by women in reign of Amenhotep III (c. 1400–1360 B.C.) in perfuming their bodies and painting lips and eyes. Collection Norbert Schimmel, New York*

150 *Necklace made of wild celery leaves and papyrus found on mummy in tomb (c. 1181–1075 B.C.) near Thebes. Ancient Egyptians were considered very knowledgeable about plants and herbs and their medicinal uses. Egyptian Museum, Cairo*

151 *Limestone two-finger amulet to ward off disease, used in addition to religious and secular healing practices. Collection Norbert Schimmel, New York*

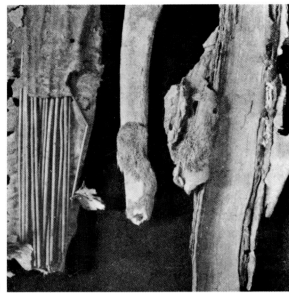

152

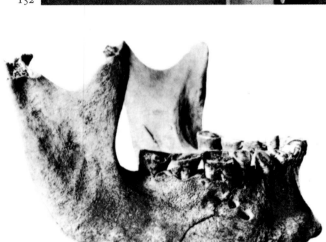

153

powdered antimony came to be called *al-kohl*. In the sixteenth century Paracelsus applied this term to the subtle spirit in wine, *alcohol*.) The green color in eye makeup probably came from copper salts. These natural substances are inherently antiseptic, but whether they were effective inadvertently in preventing or treating the eye infections common in Egypt cannot be ascertained. Yet it is of more than passing interest that copper preparations are the main agents of the present century against trachoma, a blinding infection very common in Egypt.

MECHANICAL TREATMENT

Most mechanical methods of treatment involved application of cold, heat, and dressings. Bloodletting by scarifying and puncturing the skin and by attaching leeches apparently also was a regular practice. Surgery was directed principally to the management of wounds and fractures, for which molded splints of bark and cloth steeped in resins may have provided comfortable fixation. Hemorrhage was controlled by pressure, sometimes with the addition of slabs of fresh meat, the muscle juices of which may have acted as styptics.

SURGERY

The surgical use of the knife, except for circumcision (common among all classes of Egyptians), is barely discussed in the few surviving medical papyruses, but there were several kinds of blades: stone, metal, and papyrus reed. The openings cut by embalmers in their work were stitched closed in at least some instances, and it is possible that stitching was used similarly by doctors. Trepanation, though widespread among early cultures, appears not to have been a prominent part of ancient Egyptian surgical practice. Cauterization, however, was clearly indicated for the removal of surface tumors and cysts. The fire-drill—a heated sharp utensil— is mentioned as a surgical tool, and in a textual reference to upgrading a medical school there is evidence that other instruments were available. We have learned that, among lesser surgical aids, the Egyptians made a type of adhesive tape by impregnating gums into linen strips used to pull gaping wounds together. Although some botanical and mineral concoctions used in treating wounds were in all likelihood antiseptic, many plant and animal substances were probably harmful in that they produced contamination and sealed off open drainage.

DENTISTRY

Tooth ailments must have been frequent and distressing. The earliest human remains show cases of severe wearing down of the teeth, even to the point of exposing the pulp—but with virtually no cavities. The evidence of cavities and abscesses in less ancient mummies has been interpreted to be a result of the eating of more refined, softer foods. But it is also possible that climatic, geological, and cultural changes altered the presence of cavity-preventing minerals in the diet.

Some mummies show evidences of severe infections, cavities, and loose teeth, but also teeth that were wired together and artificial prostheses. (Nefer-ir-etes, who lived about 2600 B.C., was mentioned as a maker of teeth). Possibly the fire-drill was inserted to drain abscesses, but the treatment of most infections of the teeth consisted of applying medications aimed at drawing out the "worms." This idea of worms as a cause of tooth disease was also prominent in Mesopotamia, and continued in Western medicine throughout the Middle Ages and even into recent centuries.

FEMALE DISORDERS

Women's diseases occupy a fair proportion of the medical writings. Healing substances were introduced into the vagina by tampons and also by fumigation, a

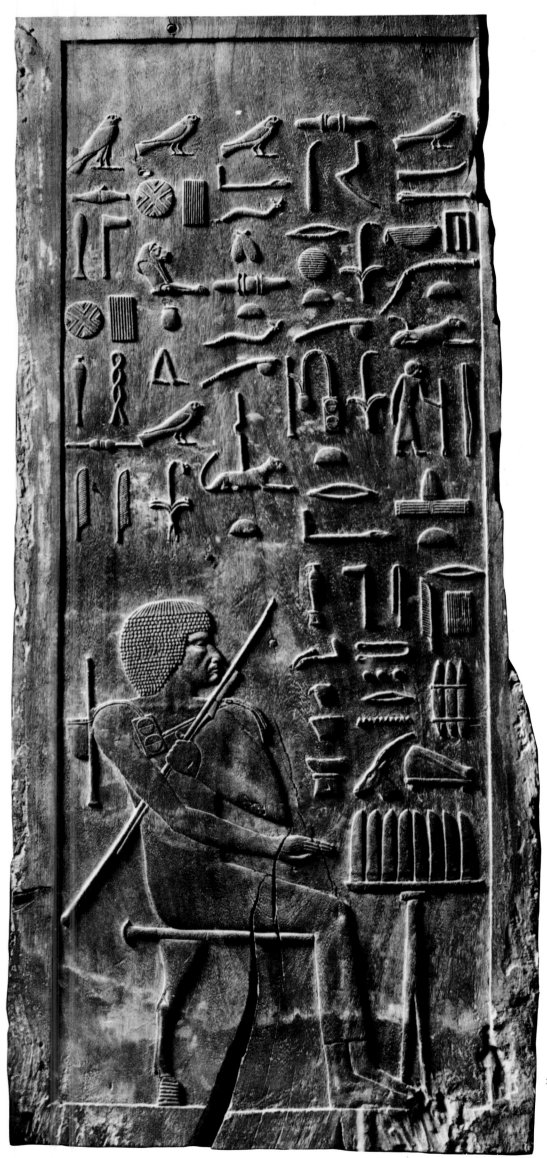

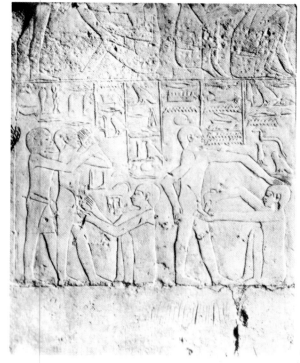

152 *Splints of palm fiber and reed bundles used about 2500 B.C. to immobilize injured limbs. British Library, London*

153 *Excavated jawbone from Old Kingdom period showing evidence of ancient operation: two holes bored in it to drain abscess. Peabody Museum, Harvard University, Cambridge*

154 *Wood panel from tomb at Saqqara of Hesi-Re, earliest known dentist (c. 3000 B.C.), showing his title, Chief of the Toothers and of the Physicians.*

155 *VIth-dynasty relief (c. 2200 B.C.) from Saqqara showing circumcision in progress. From cast in possession of Wellcome Institute for the History of Medicine, London*

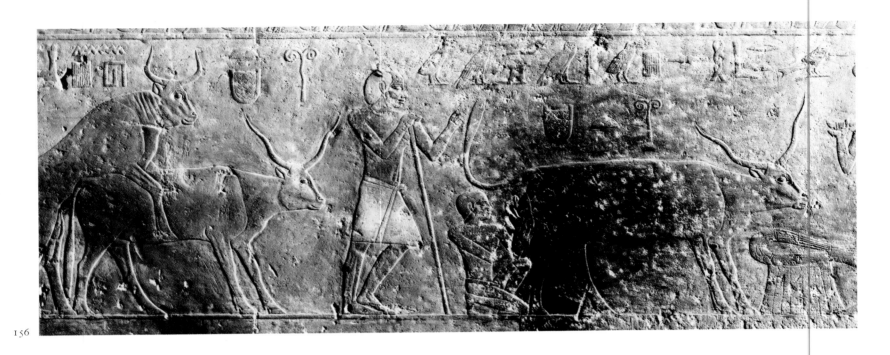

156

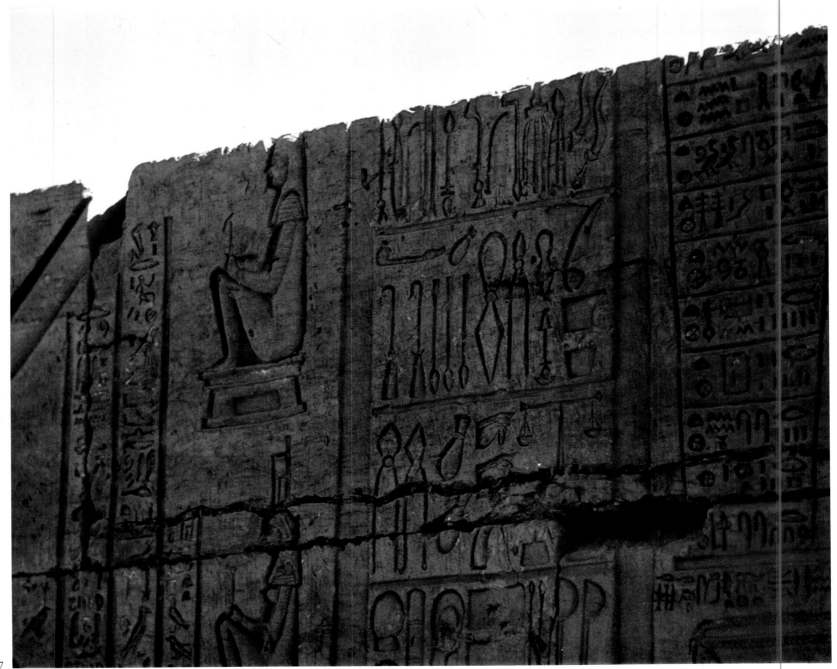

157

technique whereby a woman straddled hot stones on which a medicated solution was poured to produce vapors that could enter her vagina.

An exceptional method was offered for diagnosing pregnancy. A woman would urinate over a mixture of wheat and barley seeds combined with dates and sand. If any grains later sprouted, the woman was sure to give birth. If only wheat grew, the child would be a boy; if only the barley, a girl. This fanciful-sounding ritual may have had some success because of the hormonal content of urine, a factor in contemporary urine examination for pregnancy. Of course, fantastic and magical means of diagnosing pregnancy were also followed by the Egyptians.

Although contraceptive methods were described in the medical papyruses, fertility was most desirable. In addition to prayers and offerings to fertility deities, an infertile woman might have symbolic intercourse with a bull to open the pathway to conception. The necessary contribution of semen to fecundation was appreciated, but the understanding of sexual physiology was minimal. The people, and probably physicians as well, believed that impregnation could occur through the mouth as well as the vagina. Dung, honey, and a carbonate salt made up one contraceptive combination. Vaginal insertion of acacia leaf-tips was another method, and that plant has been found to produce lactic acid—a common ingredient of modern vaginal douches.

THE PRACTITIONERS

The reputation of medical practitioners was consistently high throughout Egypt and the rest of the Mediterranean world. Egyptian physicians were often called to treat members of the ruling classes in other countries and were mentioned frequently in court records of Persia and Palestine. However, they did not always emerge as superior practitioners. The Greek Democedes, who lived about 500 B.C., for instance, cured the ankle of the Persian monarch Darius and the breast of his daughter while Egyptian physicians stood by unable to help.

Although the Egyptian healer was a person of standing, he was not beyond reach of malpractice suits. He was warned to use only the methods promulgated in authoritarian ancient treatises, for then, even if the results were poor, he would be above reproach. This rigidity was a deterrent to following one's own observations, and woe to the doctor who deviated!

Altogether, the names of several hundred physicians can be gleaned from the writings, references, and inscriptions extant. Among them was Iry, called "Keeper of the King's Rectum," a court physician who, about 2500 B.C., attended to diseases of the eye and belly as well as the anus. Hawi was an Old Kingdom healer of the teeth and anus. This seemingly bizarre combination actually makes embryological sense, for the mouth (stomadeum) and the anus (proctodeum) are derived from the same types of tissue systems. The high position of Hesi-Re, a tooth specialist, as Chief of the Court College of Physicians suggests the repute and respect given to doctors concerned with teeth.

Herodotus, in the fifth century B.C., wrote this of the Egyptians: "Medicine with them is distributed in the following way: every physician is for one disease and not for several, and the whole country is full of physicians of the eyes; others of the head; others of the teeth; others of the belly, and others of obscure diseases." Yet specialization is not necessarily evidence of an advanced system of medicine. The Hermetic Collection of writings was apparently so large that to learn all would have been a gigantic task; thus there may well have been considerable incentive for concentrating on a limited area of knowledge.

The standards of training and of practice seem to have been set by the pharaoh's physician, who stood at the apex of the hierarchy. Beneath him were the palace physicians, among whom one may have been the supervisor of physicians. The others were inspectors of physicians, a group of lesser chief physicians, and a lower order of physicians comprising the great bulk of practitioners. There were

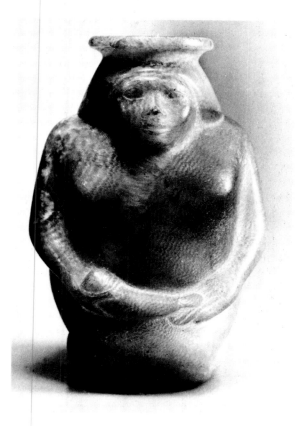

158

156 *Bas-relief from Saqqara showing cow giving birth, with human assistance, while (at left), bull mounts another cow, indicative of early understanding of role of semen in fecundation. The Louvre, Paris*

157 *Wall of Twin Temple of Kom Ombro on Nile showing surgical instruments, queen in labor, and obstetric chair, where woman delivers in semi-sitting position, a common posture for thousands of years.*

158 *Alabaster vessel (c. 1300 B.C.) in form of seated female, used by pregnant women for magical or medical ointments to rub on their bodies. Collection Norbert Schimmel, New York*

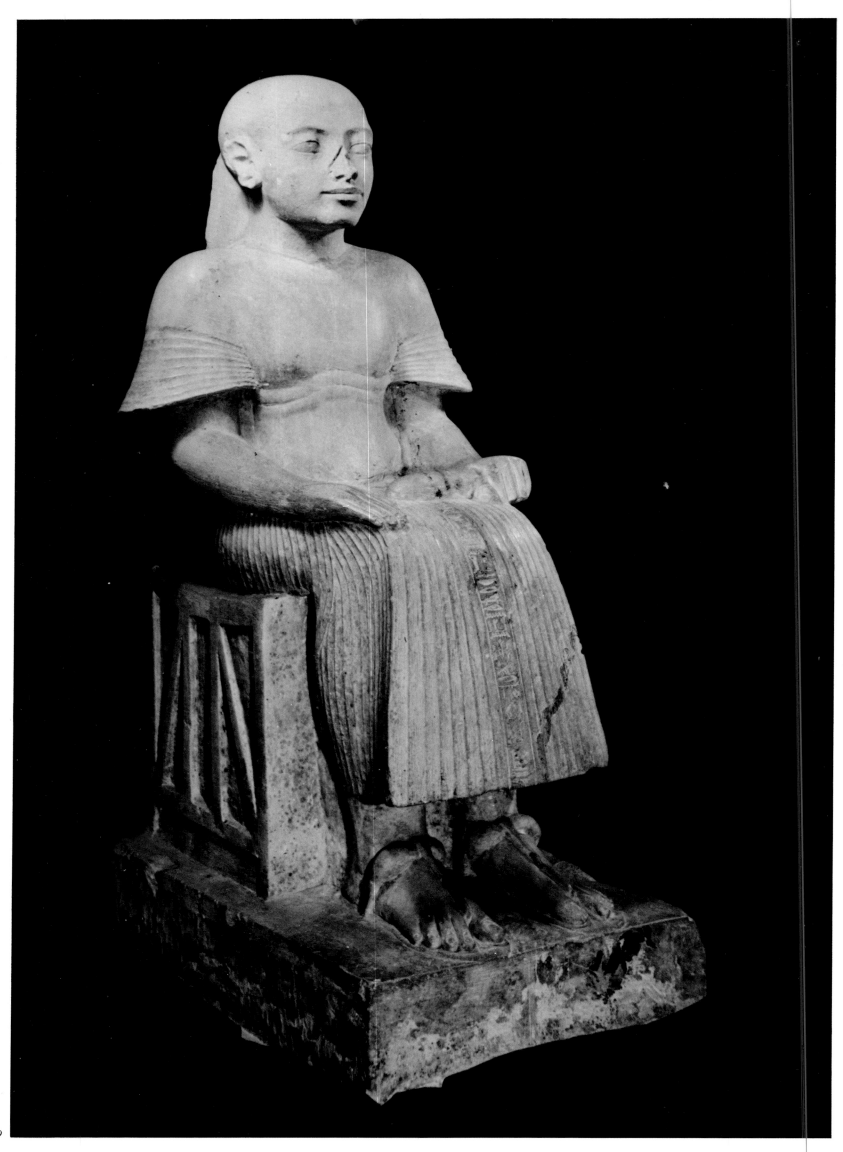

also physicians who took care of workmen and a special cadre of doctors for miners; these healers may have been salaried. (Herishef-nekhet, about 2000 B.C., was a chief physician who served at a quarry. Metm was termed a "physician of serfs.") Temple physicians, possibly of lower social standing, were available to all and visited patients' homes as well. Army doctors accompanied military expeditions and gave service to soldiers in the barracks.

Special schools for training physicians were attached to temples. User-hor-resinet, the chief physician at the time of the Persian hegemony, was sent to improve a medical school and boasted that he had selected no students from the poor, which suggests that medical students were not always from the upper classes. Whether they were educated as scribes as well as healers is not clear. However, Iwty in the New Kingdom was described as a royal scribe and chief of physicians.

An apprenticeship of some kind must have been a part of the schooling for surgery, but it is not clear whether surgery was a highly reputed specialty, a province of all physicians, or a separate but lower form of practice; perhaps its status varied with the period in history. However, since the Ebers Papyrus and the Smith Papyrus both deal with surgical matters, one may infer that physicians were expected to have knowledge of all types of medicine.

In the absence of a monetary system (gold as a medium of exchange was introduced only in the New Kingdom), physicians were usually paid with goods or services. Generally they were well rewarded. In the temple, however, physicians probably were salaried, ministering to the populace without fee. Whether paid with fees or salaries, physicians charged for dispensing medications. Although they may have obtained basic plants and drugs from various sources, they seem to have prepared their own medicines. Even the above-mentioned Iwty was said to have mixed his own salves.

Since the texts on which all medical lore depended were thought to have been given by the gods, particularly by Thoth, the writings were both divinely based and secret—a sacred trust of the healers. For instance, the book referred to in the Ebers Papyrus which described the functions of the heart was pointedly called *The Physician's Secret*. The Egyptian physician therefore, whether a priest or a specially chosen layman, was considered to possess divine knowledge and have special access to the deities and demons. Some of this tendency to ascribe possession of unimpartable information to professionals of the healing art has continued to permeate medical practice in all countries throughout the many intervening millennia. This divine self-image has had effects both beneficial and detrimental. The devotion, ethics, and skill which characterize elitism at its best are a benefit to the sick, so that even mediocre personalities can be exceptional physicians in the special context of treating. On the other hand the self-image of godliness can also breed arrogance, excessive secrecy, and unwillingness to recognize limitations.

159 *XIXth-dynasty physician Iwty shown seated with scroll on lap in pose reminiscent of representations of Imhotep, great god of medicine. Rijksmuseum van Oudheden, Leiden*

Ancient India

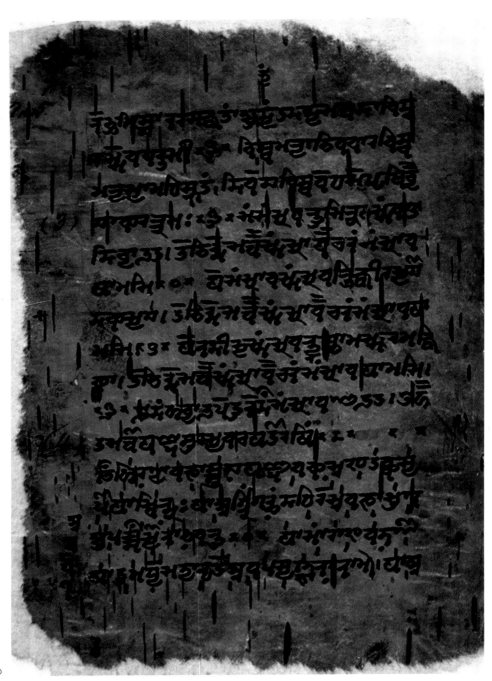

THE earliest culture in India of which we have archaeological evidence centered on Mohenjo-Daro and Harappa, chief cities of the Indus valley civilization, which flourished from about 2500 to 1500 B.C. An astonishing feature of this pre-Aryan urban culture was its advanced system of public sanitation. There were numerous wells, bathrooms, public baths, sewers, and chutes for collecting trash. Streets were laid out in regular fashion, and houses were well built and ventilated.

About 1500 B.C., an Aryan people invaded the Indus valley from the northwest and drove the earlier inhabitants down into the Indian subcontinent. These Aryan conquerors brought with them the basis for the subsequent religious and cultural development of India.

In the sixth century B.C., the Achaemenid Persian army of Darius I seized Gandhara and the Punjab region of northwest India, the easternmost extent of the Persian Empire. For a short time in the fourth century B.C., Alexander the Great, the Macedonian Greek leader, also occupied this northwest territory, but withdrew at the urging of his own army. Most of the rest of India was governed by the Maurya dynasty, which preserved the Aryan heritage. Asoka (273–232 B.C.), greatest of the Mauryan rulers, subsequently unified all of India except the southern tip. He was converted to Buddhism from the Hinduism of his ancestors and established it as the state religion.

Hinduism is one of the oldest living religions, having evolved over a period of four thousand years. Initially it was a synthesis of the ancient religion brought in by the Aryans and the religious traditions of the Indus valley civilization. The body of literature of the Aryans known as the Veda (Sanskrit for knowledge) is the oldest scripture of Hinduism. The foundations of traditional Indian healing, called Ayurvedic (knowledge of life) medicine, rested on these ancient teachings together with a number of commentaries and later writings by healers such as Charaka, Sushruta, and Vagbhata.

Indian medical practices were gradually dispersed all over Asia, including the southeast, Indonesia, Tibet, and Japan. Furthermore, the translation of the Ayurvedic literature into Persian and Arabic in the eleventh century A.D. led eventually to further spread of Indian medical lore into Europe as writings in Arabic became part of European culture in the Middle Ages.

It is noteworthy that Indian religion and mysticism would permit a system of secular medicine which engaged in sound, rational practices, even though not completely free of magical and religious associations. Initially, illness was thought to result from punishment by the gods for sinning, but as belief in reincarnation developed the transgression itself would lead to retribution by nature. Humans were continually reborn until their karma (sum of actions in one existence which determined destiny in the next) entitled them to nirvana, or merging with the cosmic spirit. The universe was considered an eternal cycle of creation, preservation, and destruction.

Although there was a complex Vedic pantheon, the deities were but parts of the eternal whole, for Brahman, the power and spirit of the cosmos, permeated everything in the universe. The principal Aryan divinities were Indra (god of weather and war), Varuna (all-seeing god of justice and cosmic order), Agni (god of fire and sacrifices), and Soma (personification of the hallucinatory plant—no longer identifiable—used in Aryan rituals). As the *Rig-Veda* stated:

> They call it Indra, Mithra, Varuna, and Agni,
> And also heavenly, beautiful Garutman;
> The real is one, though sages name it variously.

In classical Hinduism, Shiva was a powerful and fierce deity. His consort was Kali. Together they personified fertility, creativity, and good, as well as destruction and evil, but Shiva alone was the conqueror of death. Vishnu, preserver of the world, with his consort Lakshmi (goddess of life, beauty, and good fortune), was gentler but just as majestic and powerful. The gods were often interchangeable; for instance, Shiva was sometimes Rudra, who shot arrows to produce pain and

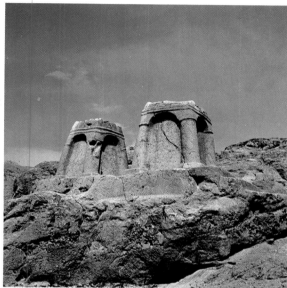

161

160 *Manuscript page from Atharva-Veda, earliest Indian text with much medical information, one of several Vedas (meaning "knowledge") of Aryan invaders, upon which Ayurvedic or traditional Indian medical practice was based, along with later commentaries by Charaka, Sushruta, and Vagbhata. Universitätsbibliothek, Tübingen*

161 *Twin fire altars at Naqsh-i-Rustam, Iran, near tomb of Darius I, whose vast Persian Empire also included Mesopotamia, Egypt, and northwest India in 6th century B.C. Fire was symbolic of Ahura Mazda, god of goodness and light in ancient Zoroastrian religion, still followed by Parsees in India.*

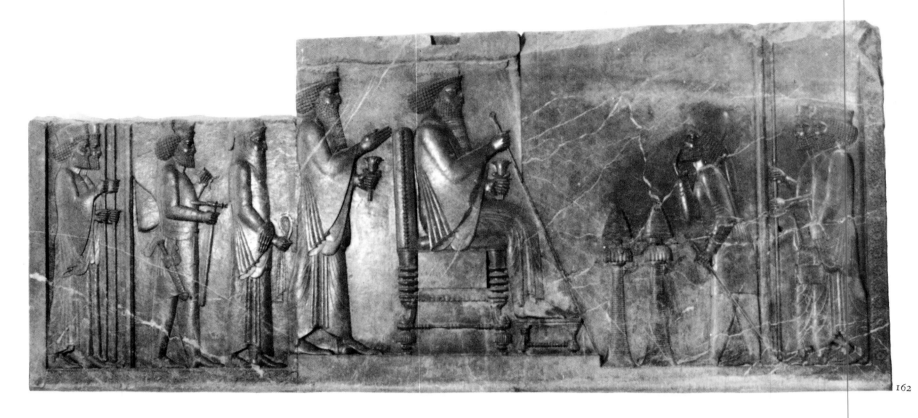

162 *Limestone relief (c. 490 B.C.) at Persepolis, Achaemenid imperial residence, showing Darius the Great seated on throne, with son Xerxes behind, giving audience to official. Rules governing medical practice in ancient Persia were laid down in* Vendidad.

163, 164 *Rock at Girnar near Junagarh, one of series inscribed with edicts of King Asoka (273–232 B.C.). Included are statements that Asoka erected hospitals for humans and for animals and supplied them with healing herbs.*

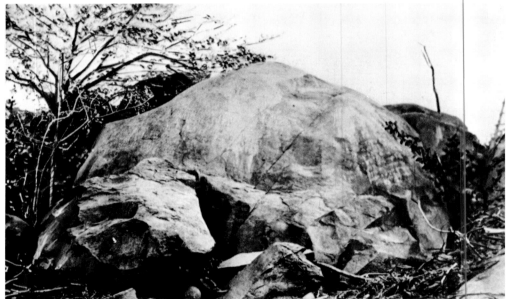

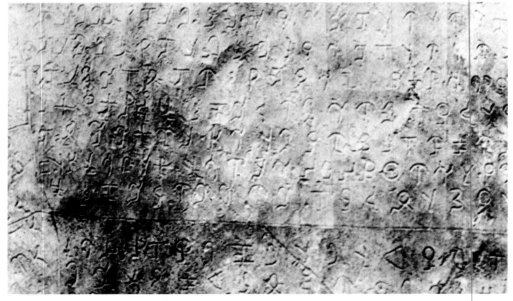

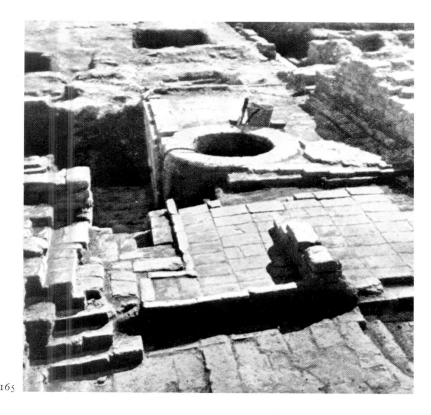

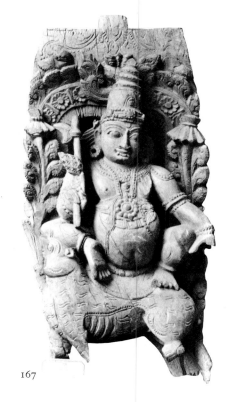

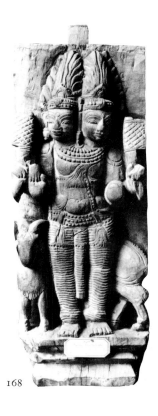

165

167   168

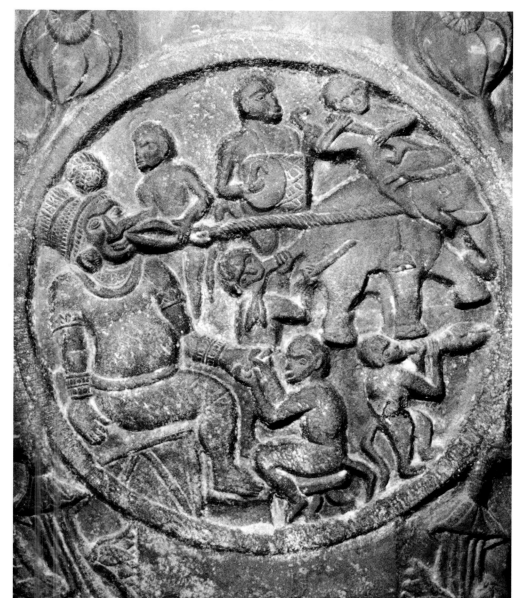

166

165 *Paved bathroom and brick well excavated in
ruins of Mohenjo-Daro (c. 3300 B.C.), in Indus
valley, indicative of advanced systems of sanitation
rivaling or surpassing contemporaneous cities in
Mesopotamia and Egypt.*

166 *Bas-relief from Bharut (2d century B.C.) showing giant having tooth extracted, fanciful presentation
of common-sense practice of removing diseased tooth.
Pragmatic medicine was closely intertwined with
mystical religious rituals. Indian Museum, Calcutta*

167 *Wooden relief of Indra, a principal god of the
Aryans, who was responsible for weather, war, and
bringing medicine to mankind. Musée Guimet, Paris*

168 *Agni, the Hindu god of fire, shown in wooden
relief, was appealed to in cases of fever. Indian physicians also relied on vast number of plant drugs.
Musée Guimet, Paris*

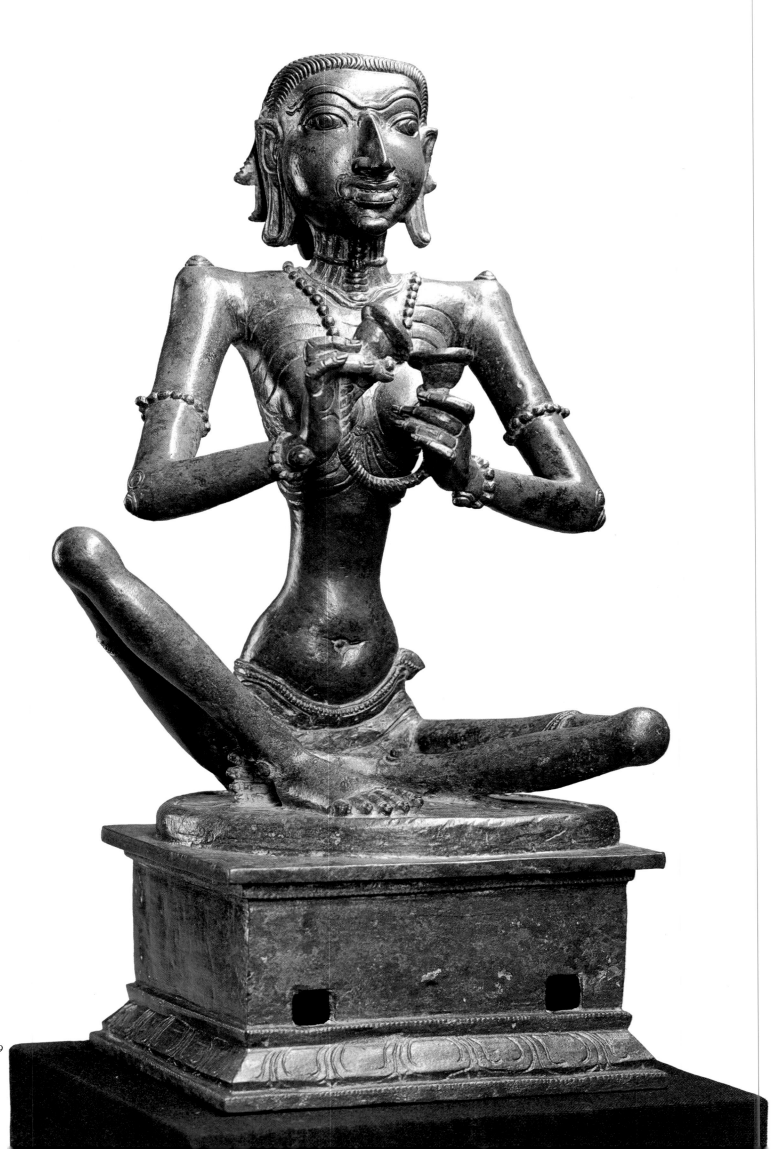

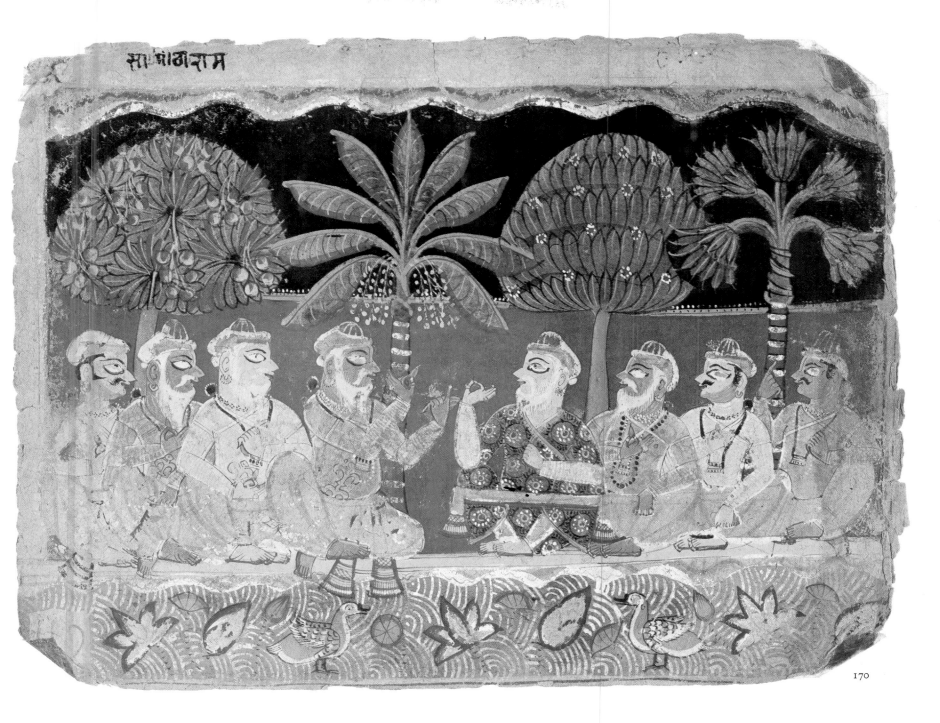

साधाबरास

170

169 *Twelfth-century* A.D. *copper figure showing devotee of Kali, goddess associated with disease, death, and destruction, who as Parvati was consort of Shiva, god of destruction and regeneration. William Rockhill Nelson Gallery and Atkins Museum of Fine Arts, Kansas City, Missouri*

170 *King Parikshit and the Rishis, from the* Bhagavata Purana *(1575), shown discussing the ancient epics on which religious and moral codes were based. Since Indian religions emphasized spiritual over material, development of rational, secular system of medicine was exceptional. Cleveland Museum of Art*

171 *Copper statue (c. 985–1016) of Hindu god Shiva, also identified with fierce Vedic god Rudra who caused pain by shooting arrows into victims, as did Greek deities Apollo and Artemis in bringing pestilence. Tanjore Museum, Madras*

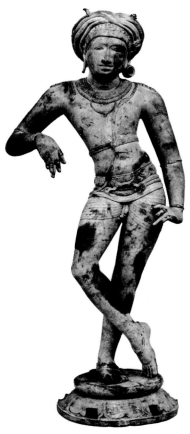

171

172 *Vishnu, among the greatest gods of Hinduism, shown in 14th-century copper figure as Krishna, one of his incarnations, a bulwark of good against evil. Nelson Gallery/Atkins Museum, Kansas City, Missouri*

173 *Dhanvantari, who became principal Hindu patron deity of medicine, seen hovering above Vishnu in bas-relief fragment (1113 B.C.) from Angkor Wat. Musée Guimet, Paris*

174 *Seventh-century A.D. relief from Mahamalla-puram showing mother goddess Devi in form of Durga slaying Bull Demon, typical of evil spirits afflicting man with illness, from whom deliverance was sought through agency of gods. Cleveland Museum of Art*

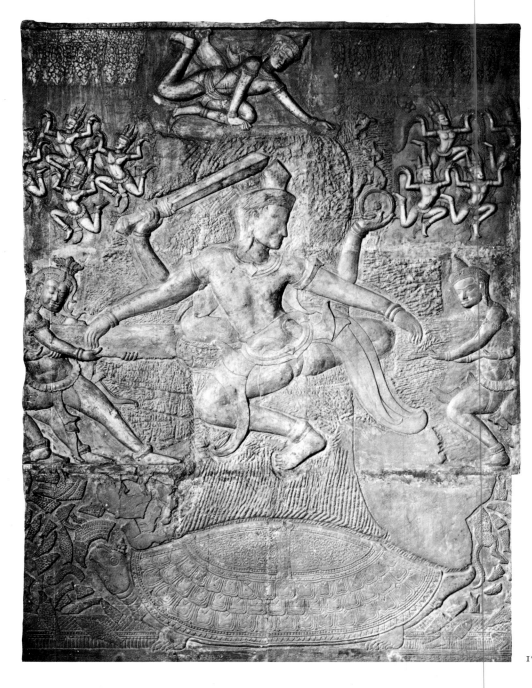

173

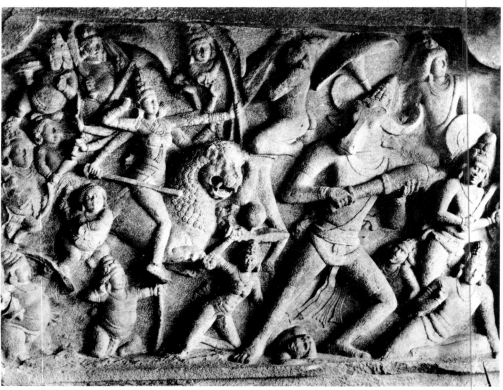

174

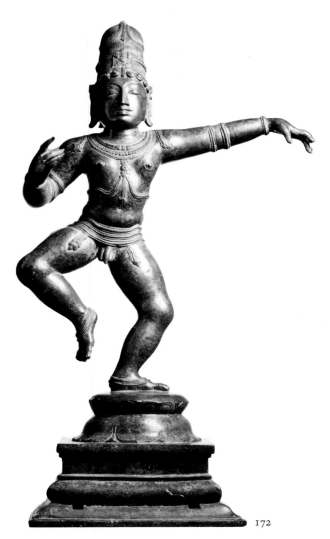

172

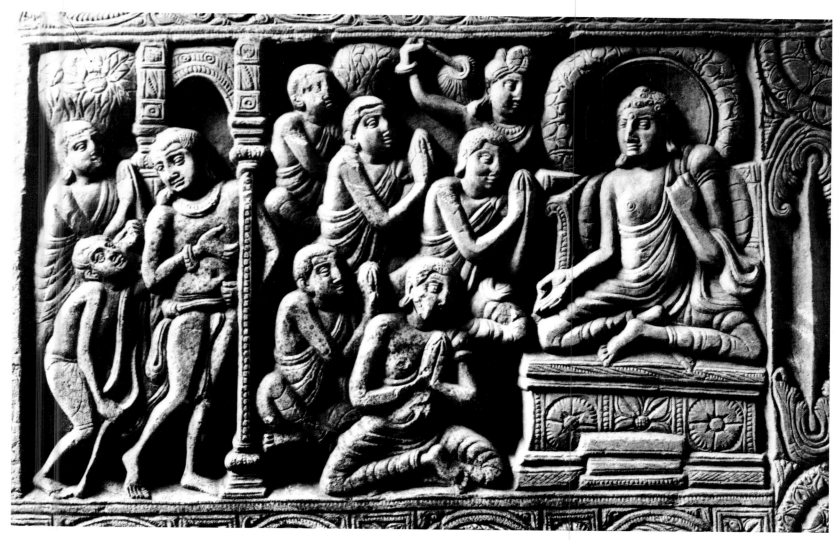

175 *Third-century* A.D. *relief showing Buddha teaching the "four noble truths" and the "eightfold path" to Nirvana, or eternal peace. King Asoka, a convert to Buddhism from Hinduism, aided spread of religion by sending missionaries to Ceylon and southern India. Musée Guimet, Paris*

176 *Manuscript page from* sutra sthana *section of Charaka Samhita, early Indian medical text. Among the influential writings on medicine, those of Charaka, Sushruta, and Vagbhata stand out, but estimates vary widely on their dating. Sanskrit Ms. Eggeling 2637: I.O.335, India Office Library, London*

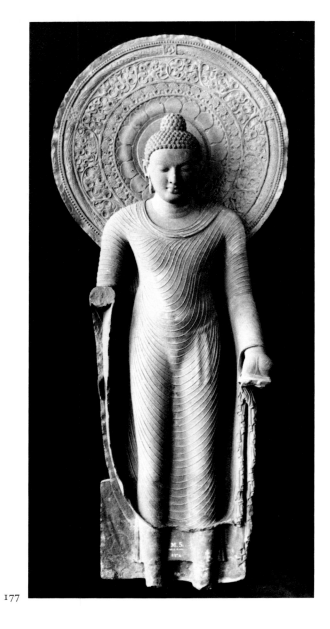

177

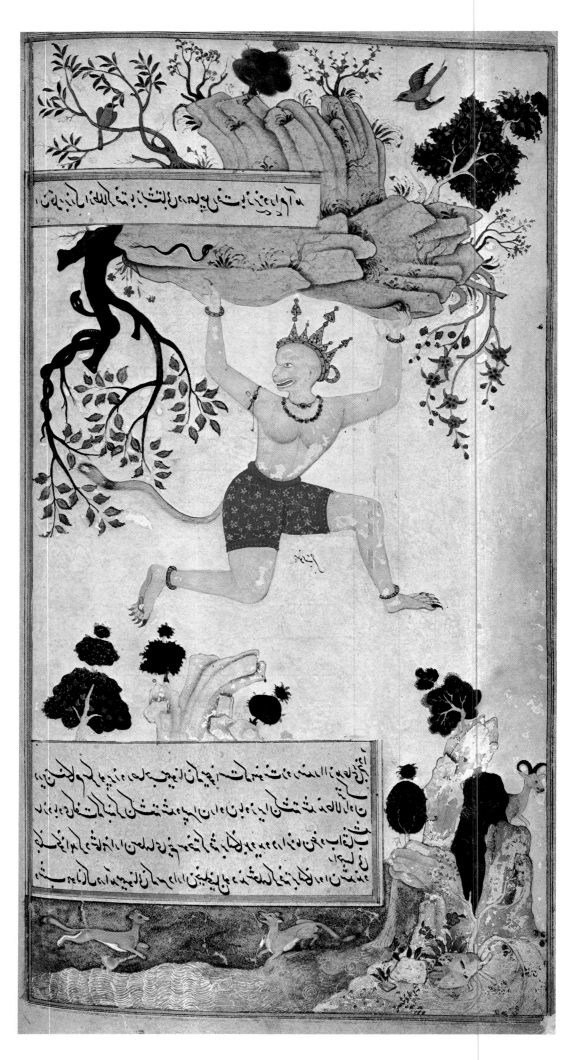

illness, as did Apollo in mythological Greece. Furthermore, the gods also took human incarnations, and thus Krishna and Rama were avatars of Vishnu on earth.

All of the gods affected health and illness, but Dhanvantari, one of the latest gods to appear, was most associated with medicine as its patron deity. He even appeared on earth as the king of Benares in one incarnation. In a legend Dhanvantari taught the sages the science of medicine. In another myth, it was Indra who imparted the secrets of life to the holy man Bharadvaja. His pupil Atreya, a great legendary physician, then transmitted this knowledge through the compilations of his disciples. Other medical gods were the twin Ashvins, who were patrons of eyesight and acted as doctors to the gods themselves.

The Vedas were the ancient hymns, prayers, and teachings of the Aryans, on which most of the religious and moral codes of India were based. The oldest, the *Rig-Veda*, as well as the *Yajur-Veda* and the *Sama-Veda*, were almost entirely religious. The *Atharva-Veda*, although also a collection of spells and incantations for the practice of magic, contained references to disease, injuries, fertility, sanity, and health.

Ayurvedic medicine was thus based on a vast literature which included not only the Vedas and their later commentaries (the *Brahmanas, Aranyakas,* and *Upanishads*) but also a body of medical writings by many contributors, of whom two stand out as the most influential: Charaka and Sushruta. Estimates have varied widely on their dates. Some have suggested the first century A.D. for Charaka and the fourth century for Sushruta, but there are also claims for more ancient times.

Inherent in Hinduism was the stratification of society into castes. Begun by the original Aryan invaders, the system later became more inflexibly structured by the doctrine of the Varna which divided all society into four distinct castes: Brahmins (priests and descendants of priests); Kshatriyas (warriors); Vaishyas (merchants, farmers, and artisans); and Shudras (the "untouchable" menial workers).

In the sixth century B.C. Buddhism arose chiefly as a reaction against the rigidity of Hindu teachings and the caste system. While retaining many of the Hindu rituals and gods, although they became less important, Buddhism preached through the "four noble truths" that suffering in life was due to the craving for bodily satisfactions from which one could be relieved only by doing away with desire. Nirvana, eternal peace, was achievable only by following the "eight-fold path." The taking of life in any form was strictly forbidden. Although for a time Buddhism gained ground rapidly and was carried to Ceylon, Tibet, and China, by the thirteenth century it had largely died out in India.

Many other sects and offshoots developed from Hinduism and Buddhism. For example, there was Yoga, a theistic philosophy which taught its devotees through exercise to suppress all activity of body, mind, and will so that the self would be liberated. Virtually all Indian religions emphasized the spiritual rather than the material, and so the development of a rational, secular system of diagnostic and therapeutic medicine was all the more remarkable.

METHODOLOGY

Methods of diagnosis included magical as well as rational approaches. Omens played an important role. The flight of birds, the sounds of nature, and many other observations were interpreted by the Indian physician as clues to the severity of the illness. Nevertheless, the patient was given intensive scrutiny, especially his sputum, urine, stool, and vomitus. Thus diabetes was detected by the sweet taste of a patient's urine. The pulse, classified into an elaborate system, was also an important diagnostic and prognostic tool.

The pharmacopoeia was voluminous. Some ancient remedies have only recently been added to Western medicine, but there may be many more useful drugs among those not yet studied. Charaka listed five hundred remedies and Sushruta over seven hundred vegetable medicines. The plant now called *Rauwolfia*

177 *Sandstone statue of Buddha, from Mathura (5th century* A.D.*), who in 6th century* B.C. *founded Buddhism, which forbade the taking of life, taught compassion for others, and in stressing charity stimulated hospital development. National Museum, New Delhi*

178 *Manuscript page (c. 1587–99) of epic* Ramayana *shows monkey general Hanuman bringing top of Himalayan mountain with healing herbs to restore life to killed and wounded in battle of monkeys and bears. Freer Gallery, Washington, D.C.*

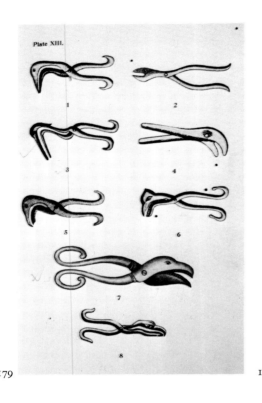

179

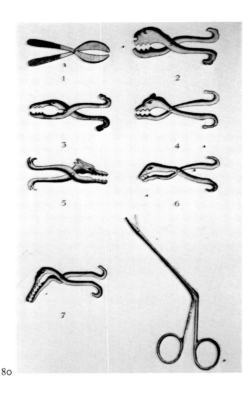

180

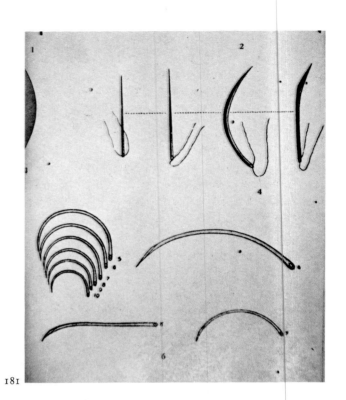

181

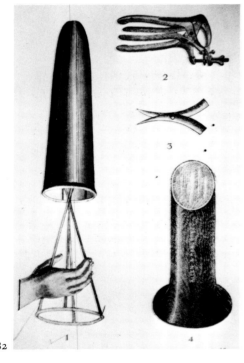

182

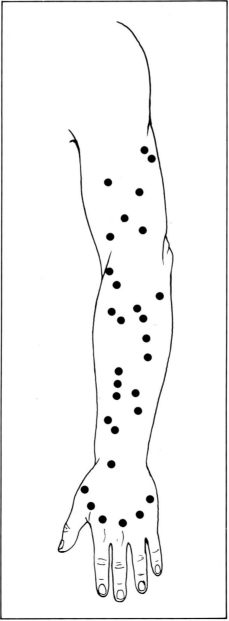

183

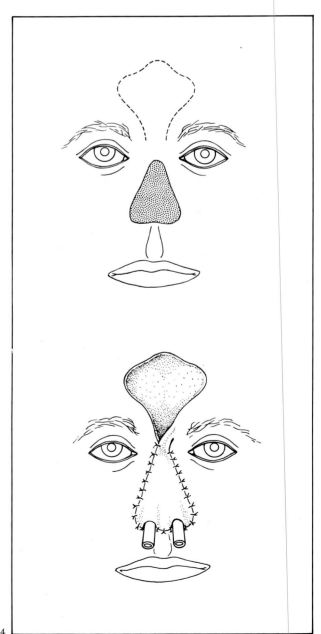

184

gaining exemption from taxes. The court doctor stood highest on the ladder, often acting for the ruler in passing on the entrance of a student into practice. The ruler's doctor was also an important political figure with considerable power and moral authority. He sat on the right hand of the sovereign during affairs of state. As in all times, doctors frequently exaggerated their own importance. Medical teachings pointed to the four foundations for cure: the physician, the patient, the medicine, and the nurse. Without the physician, said the teachers, the others were worthless.

The *Laws of Manu*—a body of rules for ritual and daily life compiled between 200 B.C. and A.D. 200—stated that physicians could be penalized for improper treatment. On the other hand, if the cured patient refused to pay, his property could be forfeited to the doctor. Ethically, Brahmin priests, friends, and the poor were supposed to be treated without charge. The finances of other patients were to determine the bills rendered. However, it is not certain how much medical attention was given the Shudras, the lowest caste, before Buddhism took their part.

The physician included both surgery and medicine in his practice. Sushruta wrote, "Only the union of medicine and surgery constitutes the complete doctor. The doctor who lacks knowledge of one of these branches is like a bird with only one wing."

As in primitive societies and other ancient civilizations women were midwives and the possessors of drug lore, but they were not considered fit for higher learning. Charaka and Sushruta rarely referred to women and then only in connection with the management of women's diseases and childbirth. A considerable amount of attention was given in the Vedic and medical writings to women, including their sexuality and illnesses. In all times a woman was supposed to be treated kindly. On the other hand, although the *Laws of Manu* forbade adultery for both men and women, extreme penalties for the transgression were prescribed only for the woman. Bearing and raising children and running the household were her functions. The *Laws of Manu* stated, "Wherever women are honored, the gods are satisfied, but when they are not honored, all pious acts become sterile."

The behavior of practitioners of the healing arts was expected to conform to the highest ideals of professional and personal life. Even the appearance, dress, speech, and manners, must be above reproach. Therefore the student who wished to be apprenticed to a high-caste teacher had to present evidence of good moral character, satisfactory parentage (descent from a physician was a great asset), and the same attributes which the ideal physician should possess.

The teacher and the student had a high sense of responsibility to each other, and only four to six apprentices were permitted to each teacher. During storms, festivals, or catastrophes, the pupil was excused from classes lest he be unable to concentrate. Instruction in theory consisted of reciting and memorizing the Ayur-vedic texts. Practical exercises included visiting the sick, collecting medicinal plants, preparing drugs, and performing procedures on dead animals or fruits, melons, leather bottles, and bladders. When the teacher found his pupil sufficiently trained, he submitted him for certification by the ruler, whose approval was necessary before the graduate could be considered a full-fledged physician. In many ways, the student's final commitment resembled closely the Hippocratic Oath of Greece.

Dedicate yourself entirely to helping the sick, even though this be at the cost of your own life. Never harm the sick, not even in thought. Endeavor always to perfect your knowledge. Treat no women except in the presence of their husbands. The physician should observe all the rules of good dress and good conduct. As soon as he is with a patient, he should concern himself in word and thought with nothing but the sufferer's case. He must not speak outside the house of anything that takes place in the patient's house. He must not speak to a patient of his possible death if by so doing he hurts the patient or anyone else. In the sight of the gods you are to pledge yourself to this. May the gods help you if you follow this rule. Otherwise, may the gods be against you.

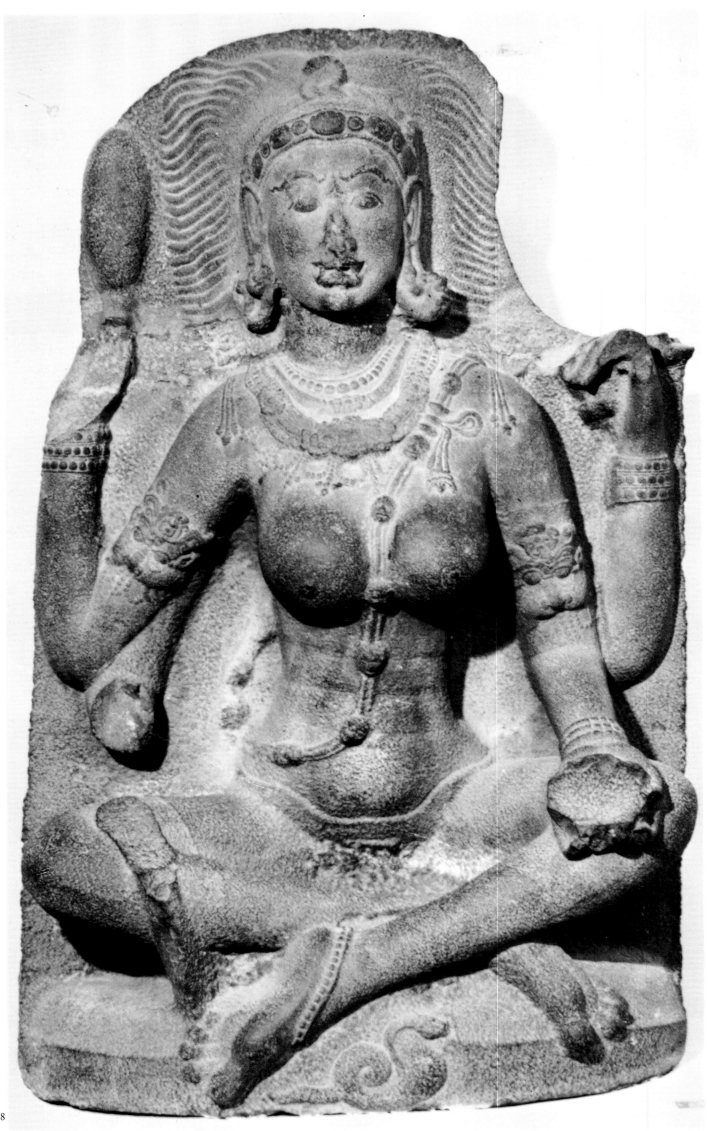

188

Health and hygienic measures were different in various periods of Indian history. For instance the public baths and highly developed water systems during the early Indus valley civilization were not matched by succeeding peoples.

Judging from the written records, epidemics and illnesses must have been frequent throughout India's history; there is evidence for malaria, dysenteries, cholera, smallpox, typhoid fever, plague, leprosy, tuberculosis, as well as a multitude of other catastrophic diseases such as mental illness, blindness, hepatitis, pulmonary affections, neurological disorders, parasitic infestations, and other pathologic conditions of the organ systems.

Traditional medicine recognized the dangers of remaining in an area where a plague or epidemic was raging, and caution was urged in choosing water and food. Smallpox was countered by inoculating people with pus from a smallpox skin boil by puncture or scarification to prevent the full-blown illness.

It is difficult to ascertain when hospitals were first begun. Among inscriptions dating from the third century B.C. by Asoka, the great ruler of the Mauryan dynasty, are statements that hospitals had been established, some for humans and others for animals. According to the scribe of the Asoka *Samhita*, there were elaborate dispensaries with their own compounds, set apart from the buildings of state. One building was usually a maternity facility where patients could stay throughout delivery and postpartum care. A second structure contained separate areas for apprentices to examine patients before reporting to the court physician, a pharmacy for the preparation and dispensing of medications, and an operating room set apart from areas sick patients frequented.

A century later, King Duttha Gamani is said to have listed among his good deeds the founding of eighteen hospitals for the poor. Whether these were true hospitals and not just facilities for custodial and outpatient care of the indigent is not clear. Certainly the account of Megasthenes, ambassador from the eastern Greek Seleucid king (inheritor of a segment of Alexander the Great's empire) suggests that there were hospitals for the rich and royal in the great city of Pataliputra.

Charaka summarized all the attributes of a good hospital, including location in a breezy spot free of smoke and protected from the sun, smells, and objectionable noises. Details of equipment needed were described even to the extent of proper brushes and brooms. He also discussed an appropriate food supply and the availability of drugs, privies, and cooking areas. The personnel should be clean, well-behaved, and able to wash and care for the patients. The well-being of the ailing was also considered, with provision for attendants who could distract the patient by recitation, conversation, and entertainment. The hospital that he pictured was easily a model for all to emulate in any time, but we do not know whether Charaka's principles represent an actual situation or simply an ideal to be hoped for.

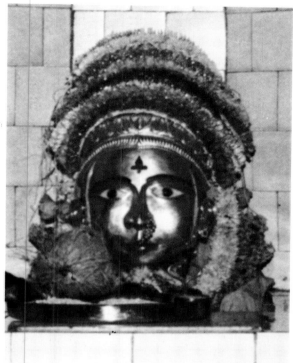

189

188 *Stone relief (c. 10th–11th century) showing one of the Seven Mothers, who were both ogresses and protectresses of children. Although women acted as midwives and were accepted as knowledgeable in drug lore, they were not considered fit for higher learning in ancient times. Musée Guimet, Paris*

189 *Head of Shri Sitala Devi, the smallpox goddess. Variolation to produce mild case of smallpox as protection against more severe attack may have originated in India.*

Ancient China

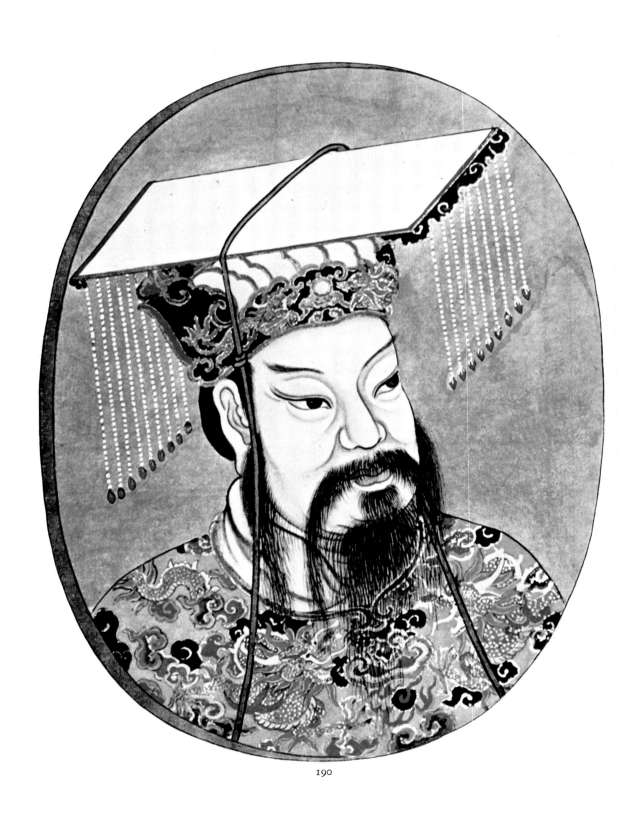

In ancient Chinese cosmology, the universe was created not by divinities but self-generated from the interplay of nature's basic duality: the active, light, dry, warm, positive, masculine *yang* and the passive, dark, cold, moist, negative *yin*. All things, animate and inanimate, and all circumstances were a combination of these fundamentals. The ultimate principle of the universe was the *tao*, "the way," and it determined the proper proportions of *yin* and *yang* in everything. Anything that altered the natural relation of *yin* to *yang* was considered bad, and right living consisted of carefully following the *tao*. If one observed the *tao* by moderation, equanimity, and morality, as taught in the *Tao-te Ching*, by Lao-tzu (sixth century B.C.), one would be impervious to disease and resistant to the ravages of aging; disregard of the *tao* led to illness, which was not so much a punishment for sin as the inevitable result of acting contrary to natural laws. However, illness also could be caused by forces beyond one's control: "Wind is the cause of a hundred diseases," and atmospheric conditions could upset the harmonious inner balance of the *yang* and *yin*. One had to be alert to this possibility and combat its effects as well as modify internal imbalances of the vital forces. Longevity and health were the rewards.

Chinese medicine, in league with Taoism, was focused on the prevention of illness; for, as the legendary Huang Ti, father of Chinese medicine, observed, "the superior physician helps before the early budding of disease." Although Taoist hygiene called for temperance and simplicity in most things, sexual mores were governed by the *yin-yang* aspect of Chinese philosophy. Ejaculation in intercourse led to diminution of a man's *yang*, which, of course, upset the inner balance of his nature. On the other hand, one was strengthened by absorption of the *yin* released by the orgasm of one's female partner—unless she was over thirty, the point where female essence lost its efficacy.

The *tao* was important in Confucianism also, as the path of virtuous conduct, and for centuries the precepts of Confucius (K'ung Fu-tzu, 550–479 B.C.) set the most prevalent standards of behavior. In early Chinese philosophy, there was a tendency to accept and combine aspects of all religions and to make way for new ideas. Nevertheless, the ancient Chinese were profoundly conservative once an institution, custom, philosophy, mode of dress, or even a furniture style was firmly established, and it remained relatively unchanged over centuries. As Confucius said: "Gather in the same places where our fathers before us have gathered; perform the same ceremonies which they before us have performed; play the same music which they before us have played; pay respect to those whom they honored; love those who were dear to them."

Although ancient China's development was relatively isolated, there was early contact with India and Tibet. Buddhism came to China from India, and medical concepts and practices were an important part of its teachings. The gymnastic and breathing exercises in Chinese medical methodology also came from India and were closely related to the principles of Yoga and to aspects of Ayurvedic medicine. There were also contacts with Southeast Asia, Persia, and the Arabic world. In the second century B.C., the Chinese ambassador Chang Chien spent more than a decade in Mesopotamia, Syria, and Egypt, bringing back information on drugs, viticulture, and other subjects. Over the centuries, knowledge of humoral medicine and of numerous new medicaments filtered into China. The introduction of the wisdom of the Mediterranean world was greatly facilitated in the fifth century by the expulsion and wide dispersion from Constantinople of the heretical Nestorian Christians. The mother of Kublai Khan (1216–94), founder of the Mongol dynasty, was a Nestorian and asked the Pope to send European doctors to China.

EARLY MEDICAL WRITINGS

Classical Chinese medicine was based primarily on works ascribed to three legendary emperors. The most ancient was Fu Hsi (c. 2900 B.C.), who was said to

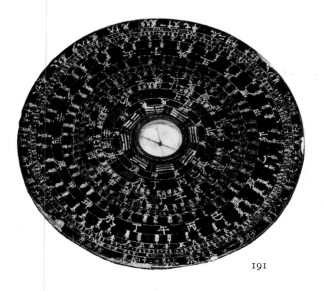

191

190 *Portrait of Huang Ti, the Yellow Emperor (c. 2600 B.C.), legendary author of the* Nei Ching, *a medical compendium that was the standard work for thousands of years.*

191 *Innovators in many fields, including physics, the Chinese used practical instruments such as the magnetic compass along with astrological and geomantic calculations to determine building sites favorable to the gods. Wellcome Institute for the History of Medicine, London*

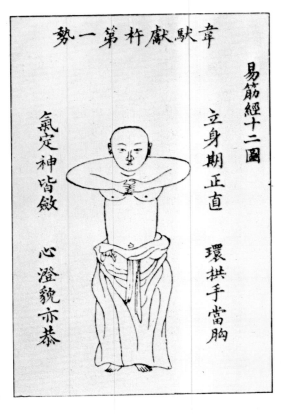

易筋經十二圖

韋馱獻杵第一勢

立身期正直　環拱手當胸

氣定神皆斂　心澄貌亦恭

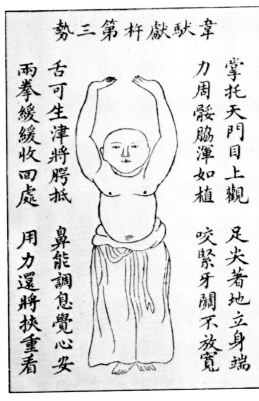

韋馱獻杵第三勢

掌托天門目上觀　足尖著地立身端

力周骽脅渾如植　咬緊牙關不放寬

舌可生津將腭抵　鼻能調息覺心安

兩拳緩緩收回處　用力還將挾重看

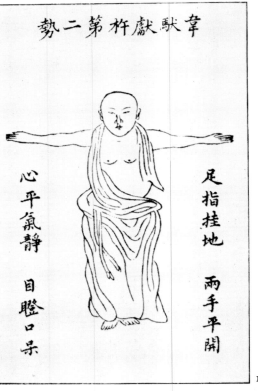

韋馱獻杵第二勢

足指挂地　兩手平開

心平氣靜　目瞪口呆

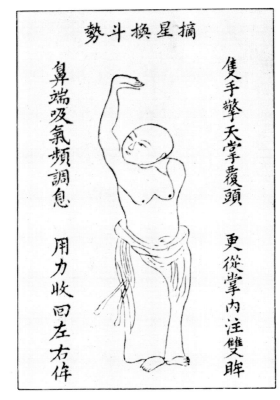

摘星換斗勢

隻手擎天掌覆頭　更從掌內注雙眸

鼻端吸氣頻調息　用力收回左右侔

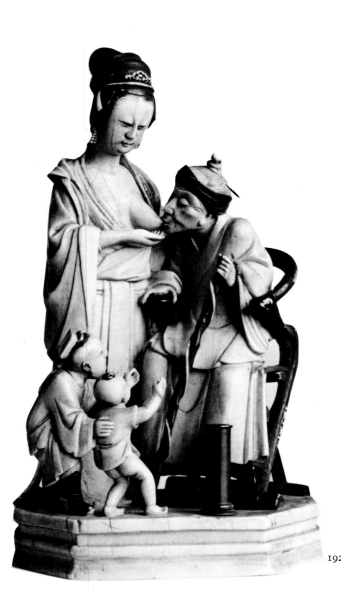

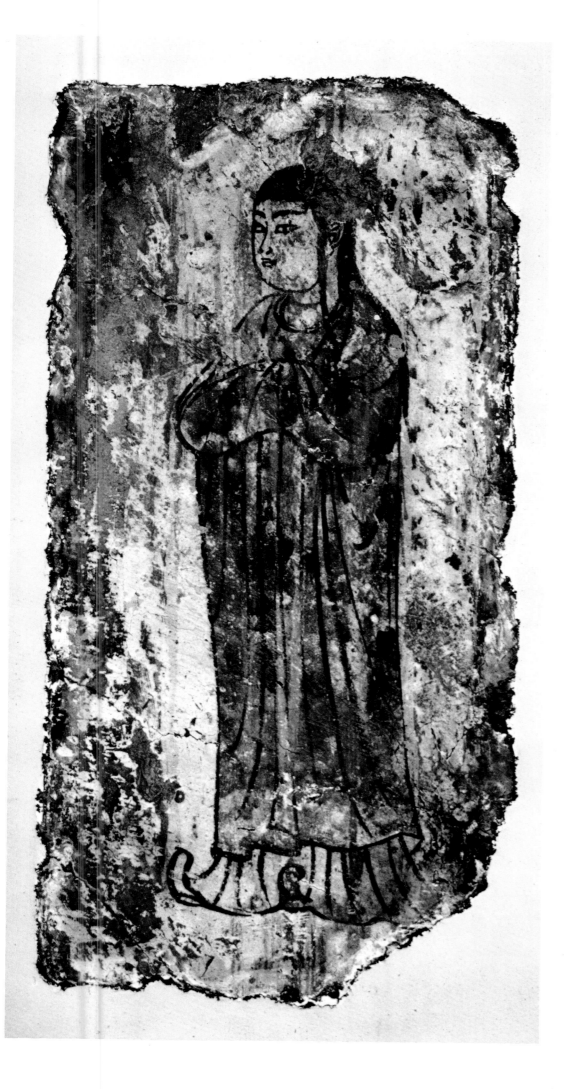

192 *Carved ivory group illustrating the Confucian principle of filial piety. Woman breast-feeds aged grandfather before her own hungry children, who were weaned quite late in China. Courtesy of the Wellcome Trustees, London*

193 *Book pages of breathing exercises based on Kung-fu (medical gymnastics) that may have developed from early contacts with India and the principles of Yoga.*

194 *Worshiper from the Nestorian Christian temple at Qarakhocho (Turfan), Sinkiang, of the late 9th century. The Chinese accepted the simultaneous presence of different religions: Taoism, Christianity, Islam, and others. Museum für Indische Kunst, Berlin*

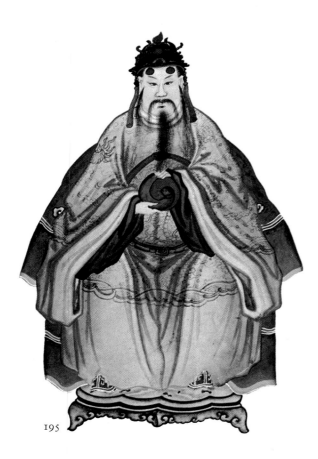

195 *Portrait of Fu Hsi (c. 2900 B.C.), most ancient of the legendary emperors upon whose works classical Chinese medicine was based. The* pa kua *symbol, which he is said to have originated, is supposedly capable of representing all possible* yin-yang *conditions. Courtesy of the Wellcome Trustees, London*

have originated the *pa kua*, a symbol composed of *yang* lines and *yin* lines combined in eight (*pa*) separate trigrams (*kua*) which could represent all *yin-yang* conditions. This system is followed even today in the *I Ching* (*Book of Changes*), though as a game or superstition in the West.

Shen Nung, the Red Emperor (Hung Ti), compiled the first medical herbal, the *Pen-tsao* (c. 2800 B.C.), in which he reported the effects of 365 drugs, all of them personally tested. One legend explains that a magic drug made his abdominal skin transparent, so he could observe the action of the many plants he evaluated. Another story tells that he cut open his abdomen and stitched in a window. Shen Nung is also said to have drawn up the first charts on acupuncture, a medical procedure presumably even older than the legendary emperors.

The fame of Yu Hsiung (c. 2600 B.C.), the Yellow Emperor (Huang Ti), rests on his great medical compendium, the *Nei Ching* (*Canon of Medicine*). Transmitted orally for many centuries, this seminal work was possibly committed to writing by the third century B.C. Its present form dates from the eighth century A.D., when the last extensive revision was done by Wang Ping. The major portion of the *Nei Ching*, the *Sun-Wen* (Simple Questions), records the discourse of the Yellow Emperor with Ch'i Po, his prime minister, on virtually all phases of health and illness, including prevention and treatment. The section called *Ling-Hsu* (Spiritual Nucleus), deals entirely with acupuncture. Yu Hsiung also was said to be responsible for another great compendium, *The Discourses of the Yellow Emperor and the Plain Girl*, which thoroughly covered the subject of sex from the Taoist point of view.

Among other notable sources for ancient medical lore, one might mention the *Shih Ching* (*Book of Odes*), which perhaps predates Homer's epics, and the *Lun-yü*, discourses of Confucius probably written down shortly after his death, which affected patterns of behavior for many generations.

During the long Chou dynasty (c. 1050–255 B.C.), a lengthy compilation of medical works, *Institutions of Chou*, was completed and became the criterion for subsequent dynasties on the duties and organization of physicians. In the Han dynasty (206 B.C.–A.D. 220), there was a noted clinical author named Tsang Kung, who pioneered in the description of many diseases, including cancer of the stomach, aneurysm, and rheumatism. Chang Chung-ching, the Chinese Hippocrates, in the third century A.D., wrote the classic treatise *Typhoid and Other Fevers*.

Ko Hung, a famed alchemist and a careful observer, wrote treatises describing beriberi (a vitamin B deficiency), hepatitis, and plague, and gave one of the earliest reports on smallpox: "As the New Year approached there was a seasonal affection in which pustules appeared on the face and spread rapidly all over the body. They looked like burns covered with white starch and reformed as soon as they were broken. The majority died if not treated. After recovery purplish black scars remained."

Sun Szu-miao (A.D. 581–682) wrote *Ch'ien Chin Yao Fang* (*A Thousand Golden Remedies*), which summarized in thirty volumes much of the known medical learning, and he headed a committee which produced a fifty-volume collection on pathology. An extensive codification of forensic medicine, *Hsi Yuan Lu*, was done in the Sung dynasty and became the prime source for knowledge of medical jurisprudence.

ANATOMY AND PHYSIOLOGY

Ideas of anatomy in ancient China were reached by reasoning and by assumption rather than dissection or direct observation. Since the doctrines of Confucius forbade violation of the body, it was not until the eighteenth century, long after Vesalius, that the Chinese began systematic, direct anatomical studies. Even as late as the nineteenth century, in the Viceroy's Hospital Medical School, anatomy was taught by diagrams and artificial models rather than dissection.

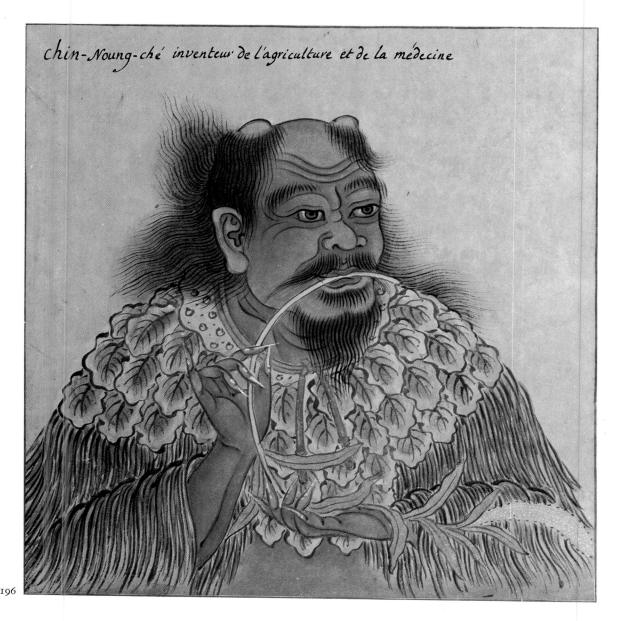

chin-Noung-ché inventeur de l'agriculture et de la médecine

196

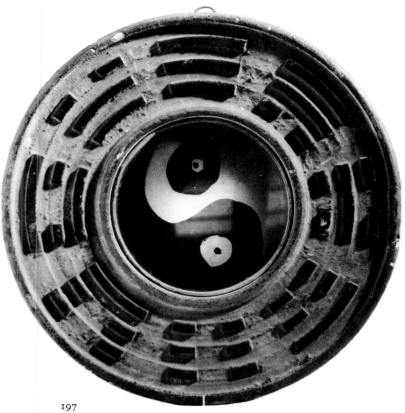

197

196 *Portrait of Shen Nung (c. 2800 B.C.), called the Red Emperor after his talisman fire, compiled the* Pen-tsao, *the first medical herbal, containing 365 drugs he had tested on himself. Courtesy of the Wellcome Trustees, London*

197 *The pa kua symbol, which represents the basic* yin-yang *(female–male) dichotomy in the universe and includes the eight trigrams of all possible combinations of the two. Musée de l'Homme, Paris*

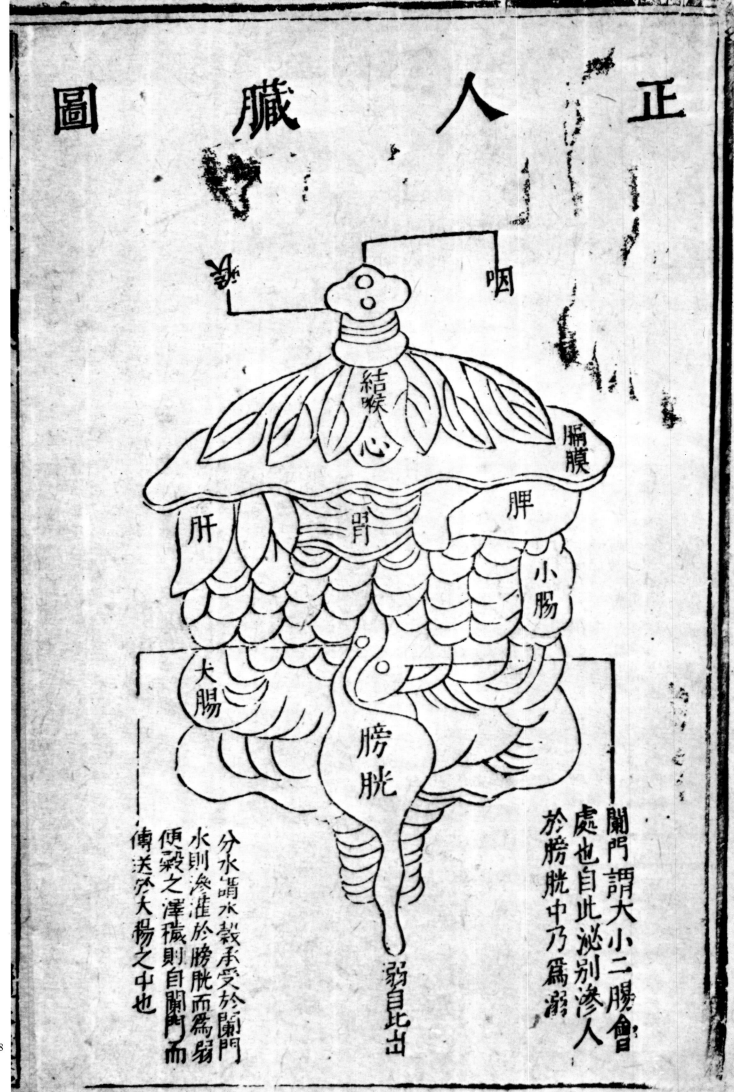

正人臟圖

咽

結喉

心

膈膜

脾

肝

胃

小腸

大腸

膀胱

溺自此出

闌門謂大小二腸會
處也自此泌別滲入
於膀胱中乃爲溺

分水消水穀承受於闌門
水則滲渗於膀胱而爲溺
便穀之澤積則自闌門而
傳送於大腸之中也

Physiological functions were constructed into a humoral system much like Greek concepts of the sixth century B.C. and Galenic views of the second century A.D., except that there were five instead of four essential humors. (The number five had mystical value for the Chinese and was used for most classifications: five elements, five tastes, five qualities, five kinds of drugs, five treatments, five solid organs, five seasons, five emotions, five colors, etc.) The medical compendium *Nei Ching* stated that each emotion had its seat in a particular organ. Happiness dwelt in the heart, thought in the spleen, sorrow in the lungs, and the liver housed anger as well as the soul.

Ideas in the *Nei Ching* concerning movement of the blood ("All the blood is under control of the heart." "The blood current flows continuously in a circle and never stops.") have been thought to approach an understanding of its circulation antedating Harvey by thousands of years; however, some body vessels were believed to convey air, and there is little evidence that commentators perceived the blood-carrying vessels as a contained system.

DIAGNOSIS

The Chinese methods of diagnosis included questioning, feeling the pulse, observing the voice and body, and in some circumstances touching the affected parts. In almost all times and cultures physicians have used a similar approach, for all healers have sought to know as much as possible about a patient in order to understand his or her illness and advise treatment. However, in some respects ancient physicians saw each patient more completely as a reflection of his surroundings (indeed, the entire universe) than does the doctor of today. The Chinese doctor wanted to learn how the patient had violated the *tao*, and to do this he took into account the patient's rank; changes in his or her social status, household, economic position, sense of well-being, or appetite; the weather; and the dreams of the patient and his or her family.

Perhaps the most important diagnostic technique of the ancient Chinese was examination of the pulse. The physician felt the right wrist and then the left. He compared the beats with his own, noting precise time as well as day and season since each hour affected the nature of the pulsations. Each pulse had three distinct divisions, each associated with a specific organ, and each division had a separate quality, of which there were dozens of varieties. Moreover, each division or zone of the pulse had a superficial and deep projection. Thus literally hundreds of possible characteristics were obtainable. In one treatise, *Muo-Ching*, ten volumes were necessary to cover all the intricacies of the pulse.

A patient had only to extend his or her arm through drawn bed curtains for the physician to determine the symptoms, diagnosis, prognosis, and proper treatment by intensive palpation of the pulse. Whenever possible the examiner also felt the skin of the ill person. However, it was considered bad form for a man to intimately examine a woman, so special ceramic, ivory, and wooden dolls were pointed to by the invalid to indicate where discomfort was felt.

TREATMENT

According to the *Nei Ching*, there were five methods of treatment: cure the spirit, nourish the body, give medications, treat the whole body, and use acupuncture and moxibustion. The physician had to put the patient back on the right path, the *tao*. Assuming that specific mental states caused changes in specific organs, the healer linked certain objectionable behavioral and constitutional factors with illness and attempted to have the patient rectify these. For instance, dissolute and licentious ideas led to diseases of the lungs, but acting out such thoughts brought on heart trouble. A doctor had to determine the cause of disharmony in the body and act accordingly.

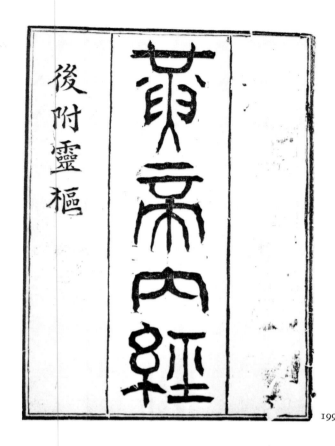

199

198 *Anatomical drawing of the intestines from* Trong Jim Tchou King *by Dr. Oang Oé-Té. Ms. Chinese 5341, Bibliothèque Nationale, Paris*

199 *Title page of late edition of the* Nei Ching *by Huang Ti (c. 2600 B.C.), which summarized all the medical knowledge of the period in dialogues between the Yellow Emperor and his prime minister. Courtesy of the Wellcome Trustees, London*

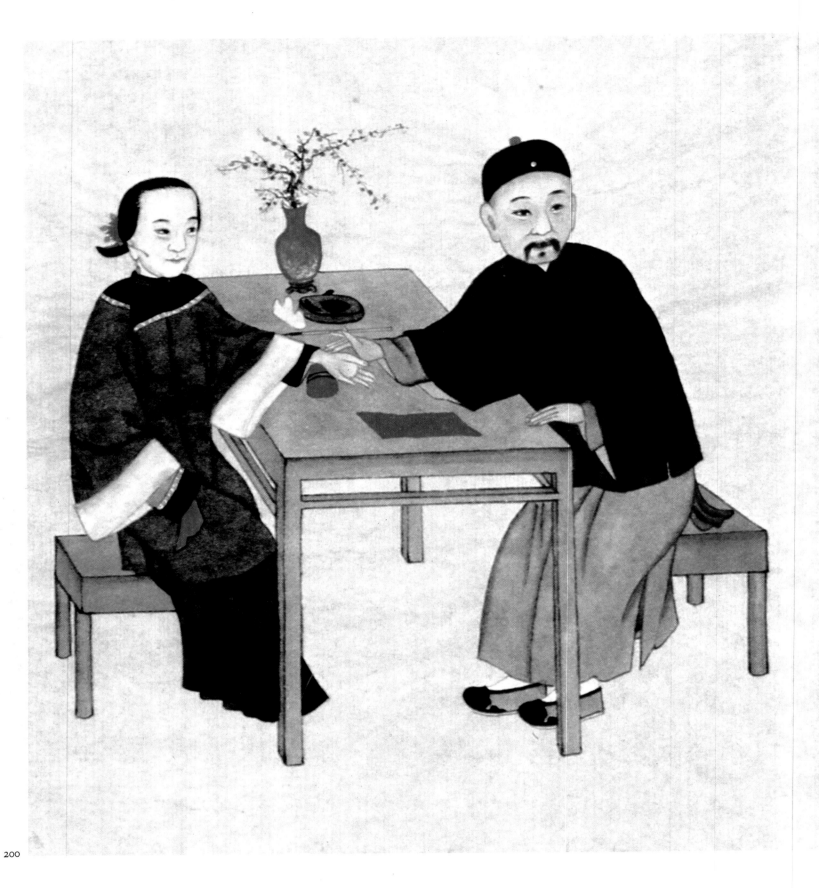

200

200 *Doctor shown examining patient by feeling the pulse, perhaps the most important feature of ancient Chinese medical diagnosis. Courtesy of the Wellcome Trustees, London*

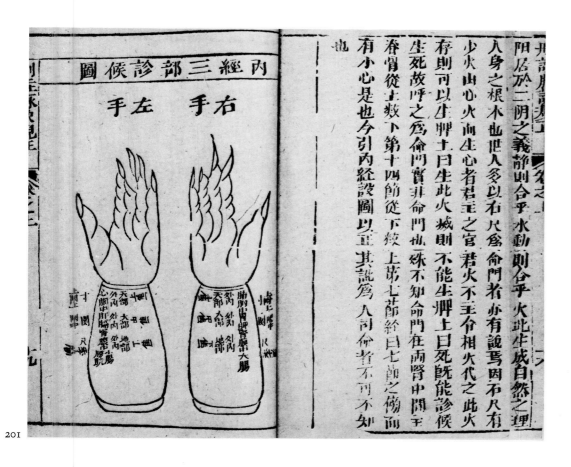

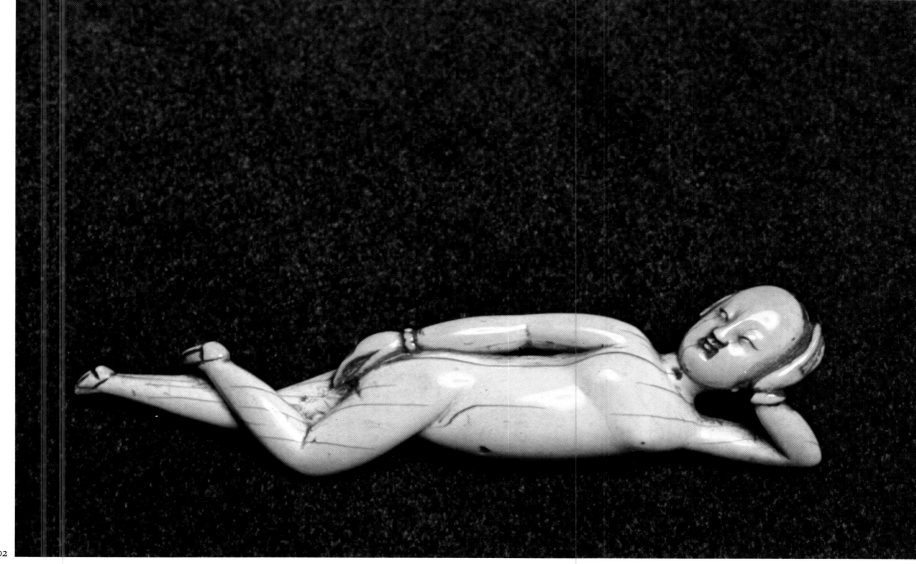

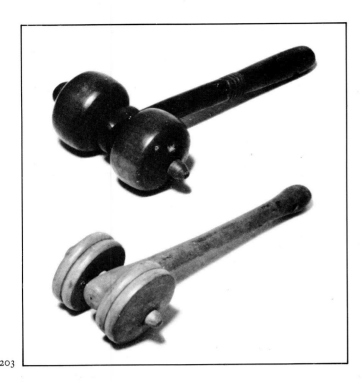

203

203 *Wooden rollers for massaging the abdomen, the Chinese technique for handling the age-old problem of constipation. Courtesy of the Wellcome Trustees, London*

204 *Plant and animal illustrations from an 1883 edition of* Pen T'sao Kang Mu, *compiled by Li Shih-Chen in 1596, considered the finest encyclopedic record of Chinese fauna, flora, and minerals and a valuable reference for the pharmacist. Courtesy of the Wellcome Trustees, London*

205 *Patient shown receiving manipulation of the joints, an important feature of Chinese medical treatment. Courtesy of the Wellcome Trustees, London*

Exercises were developed to keep the body fit and to restore well-being. Hua T'o, the great surgeon, worked out an ingenious system of physical therapy by advising mimicry of the natural movements of animals. Massage—kneading, tapping, pinching, and chafing—was also a regular method of treatment, as were the application of plasters and evacuation of the intestinal tract by cathartics.

In nourishing a patient's body, the physician resorted to complex combinations of foods according to their potential amounts of *yang* and *yin*. Foods also had to fit the seasons, and each of the five tastes had benefits for a particular element of the body: sour for the bones, pungent for the tendons, salty for the blood, bitter for respiration, and sweet for muscle.

MEDICATIONS

The Chinese pharmacopoeia was always rich, from the time of the *Pen-tsao*, the first medical herbal, to the later dynasties when two thousand items and sixteen thousand prescriptions made up the armamentarium. Drugs were considered more likely to be good if they tasted bad. As one would expect, they were classified into five categories: herbs, trees, insects, stones, and grains. The therapeutic minerals and metals included compounds of mercury (calomel was employed for venereal diseases), arsenic, and magnetic stones. Animal-derived remedies, in addition to "dragon teeth" (powdered fossilized bones), included virtually anything obtainable from living creatures: whole parts, segments of organs, urine, dung.

Two plant substances especially associated with China may be singled out. One is ephedra (*ma huang*), the "horsetail" plant described by the Red Emperor, which was used for thousands of years as a stimulant, as a remedy for respiratory diseases, to induce fevers and perspiration, and to depress coughs. Ephedra entered the Greek pharmacopoeia and eventually was disseminated throughout most of the world. It only became a factor in Western medicine in the late nineteenth century after Japanese investigators isolated and purified the active principle, ephedrine, and established its pharmacologic action.

A second medicinal herb, always highly popular among the Chinese, is ginseng ("man-shaped root"). To the Chinese, preparations containing ginseng were almost miraculous in delaying old age, restoring sexual powers, stimulating the debilitated, and sedating the overwrought. In addition it improved diabetes and stabilized blood pressure. In recent years this root has been under scrutiny by Western pharmacologists attempting to evaluate its true benefits. Multitudes in Asia, and even some Westerners, are so convinced of its effectiveness that high-grade wild roots have brought fabulous prices (even reaching thousands of dollars apiece).

Although many items in the Chinese materia medica have either faded into obscurity or been labeled fanciful, others subsequently have been found to possess sound pharmacologic bases: seaweed, which contains iodine, was used in treating enlargement of the thyroid; the willow plant, containing salicylic acid, was a remedy for rheumatism; the Siberian wort has antispasmodics for menstrual discomfort; and mulberry flowers contain rutin, a treatment for elevated blood pressure. Whether opium was used as a drug before quite late in Chinese history is still in dispute.

ACUPUNCTURE AND MOXIBUSTION

These modalities have been an integral part of Chinese medical therapy for thousands of years. The Yellow Emperor is said to have invented them, but they may well have existed long before his time. The aim of these treatments was to drain off excess *yang* or *yin* and thus establish a proper balance, but external energy also could be introduced into the body. In acupuncture the skin is pierced by long needles to varying prescribed depths. Needles are inserted into any of 365 points along the twelve meridians that traverse the body and transmit an active life force

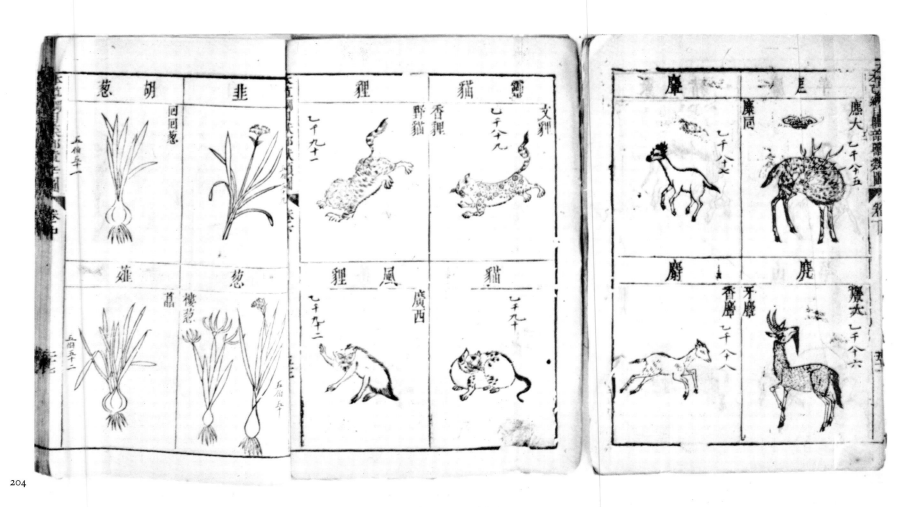

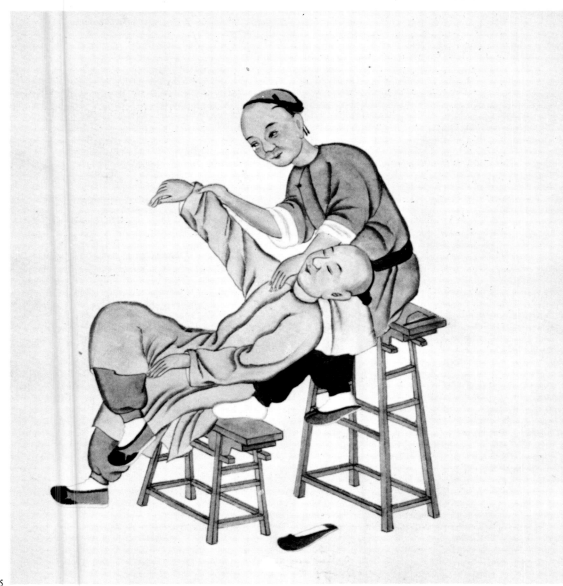

此中國剃頭棚放睡之圖也每日將頭剃完
筋骨疼痛者剃頭者坐于高橙之上其人躺
在剃頭櫈上令其捶拿其快活無比

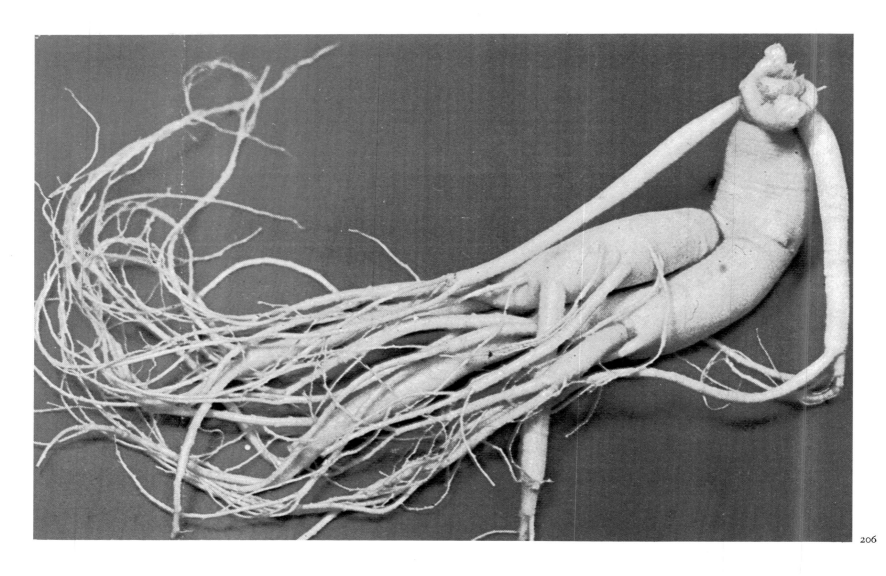

206

206 *Ginseng root, an important ingredient in the rich Chinese pharmacopoeia, ranked with jewels in price and was believed to cure a wide range of diseases, from impotence to tuberculosis.*

207 *Cup fashioned from rhinoceros horn, in powder form a widely accepted aphrodisiac—which may account for pieces removed from lip. Courtesy of the Wellcome Trustees, London*

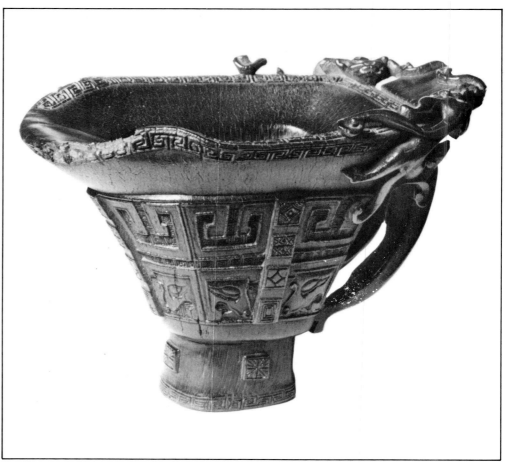

207

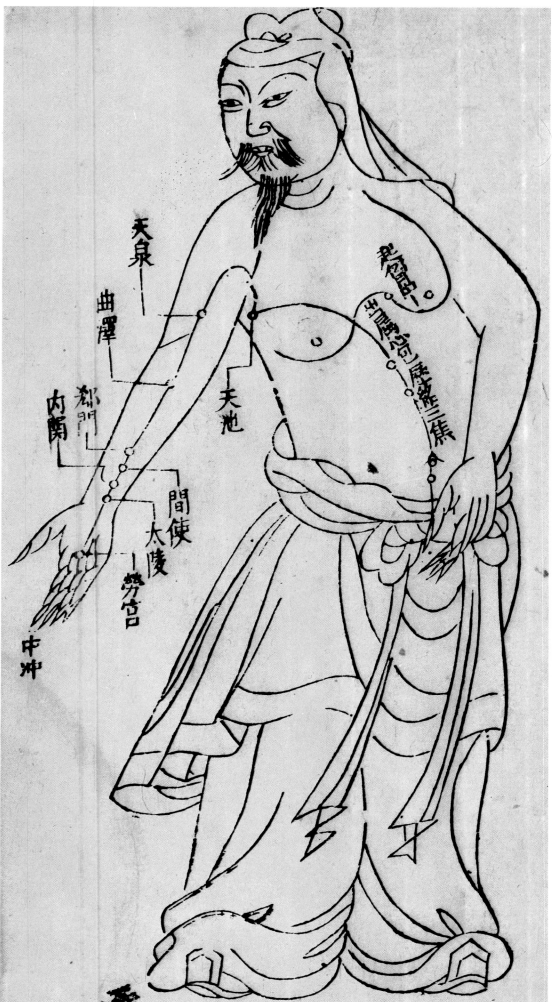

天泉

曲澤

郄門
内關

天池

間使
太陵

勞宮

中衝

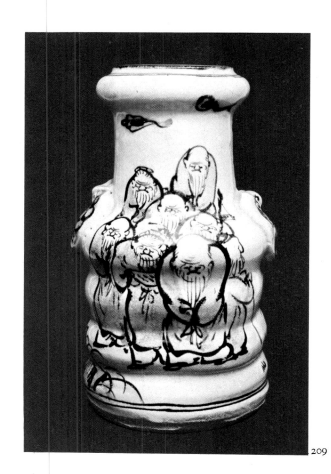

208 *Ming dynasty acupuncture chart showing puncture points along meridians of body which apply to
treatment for various organs, often quite distant from
the point. This important Chinese medical technique
has been in continual use for thousands of years.
Ms. Chinese 5341, Bibliothèque Nationale, Paris*

209 *Ching dynasty apothecary jar used to store
ingredients for herbal medicine heavily relied on by
Chinese doctors. Courtesy of the Wellcome Trustees,
London*

208

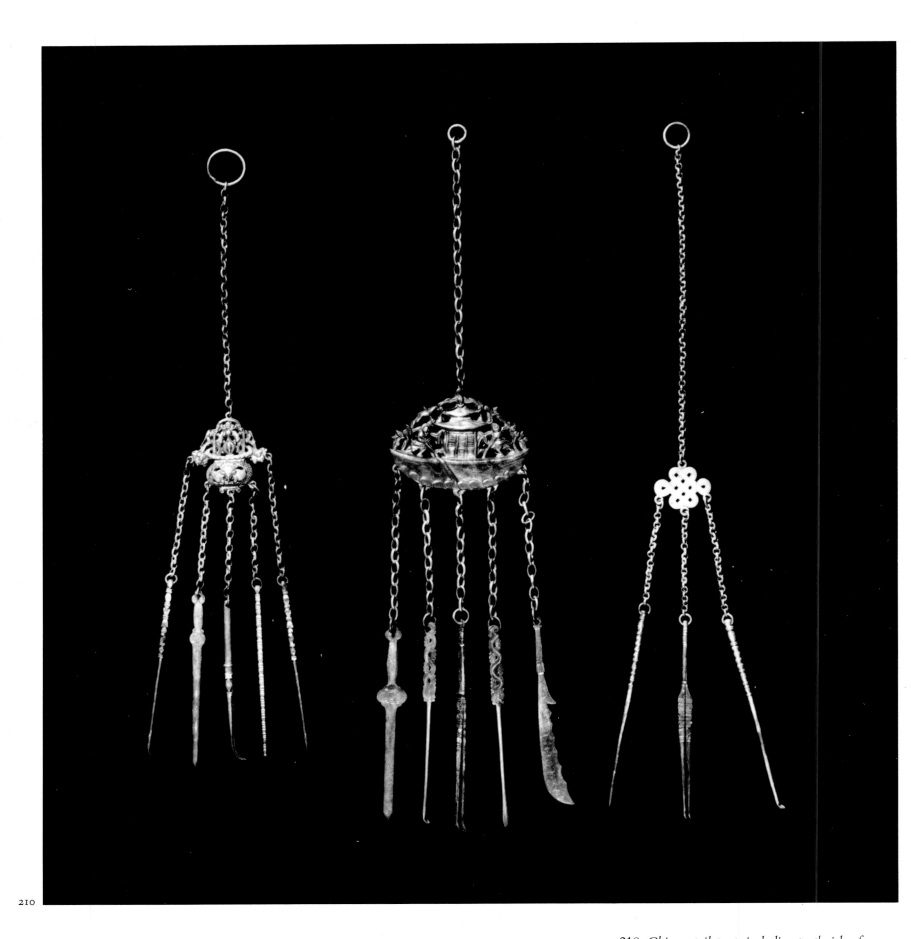

210 *Chinese toilet sets including toothpicks, frequently used by the upper classes for dental care, which also featured cosmetic tooth whiteners. American Museum of Natural History, New York*

called *ch'i*. Each of these points is related to a particular organ. For instance, puncture of a certain spot on the ear lobe might be the proper way to treat an abdominal ailment. Virtually every illness, weakness, and symptom is thought to be amenable to correction by acupuncture.

Acupuncture spread to Korea and Japan by the end of the tenth century A.D., to Europe about the seventeenth century, and recent years have seen a wider interest in this Chinese medical practice in the West. Individual paramedical healers and even some medical practitioners have been swamped with requests for acupuncture, especially for problems apparently little benefited by conventional practices. The eventual acceptability of this practice in standard Western medicine remains to be seen.

Moxibustion is as old as acupuncture, and the same meridians and points govern placement of the moxa. However, in this treatment a powdered plant substance, usually mugwort, is fashioned into a small mound on the patient's skin and burned, usually raising a blister.

Dentistry

The treatment of tooth disorders was confined mainly to applying or ingesting drugs—pomegranate, aconite, ginseng, garlic, rhubarb, and arsenic, as well as animal products such as dung and urine. The *Nei Ching* classified nine types of toothaches, which included some obviously due to infections and tooth decay. Like the Mesopotamians and Egyptians, the ancient Chinese believed that worms were often responsible for dental problems. Toothpicks and tooth whiteners were used, and loose teeth were stabilized with bamboo splints. Gold was sometimes used to cover teeth, but the purpose was decorative rather than protective.

Surgery

Although surgery was not one of the five methods of treatment listed in the *Nei Ching*, the knife was known and used. Hua T'o, one of the few names mentioned in connection with surgery, treated an arm wound of the famous general Kuan Yü by cutting his flesh and scraping the bone. Physicians knew how to deal with wounds, and at least two classics were devoted entirely to their treatment.

The proper attitude toward pain was to bear it without a sign of emotion, and much was made of the insouciance of the general treated by Hua T'o; he played chess while the surgeon operated. Nevertheless, apparently some kind of anesthesia was often used. Wine and drugs like hyoscyamus were probably mainstays, but the use of opium and Indian hemp is still in question.

Eunuchs and Footbinding

Another surgical procedure, though hardly therapeutic, was the frequent castration of certain males seeking advancement at court. Though originally a severe punishment, the total removal of penis and testicles came to be a pledge of absolute allegiance to the monarch, since it released the eunuch from conflict with Confucian admonitions of first loyalty to family and the obligation of siring a son for posterity.

Footbinding is also of medical interest, for it caused the development of artificially clubbed feet. Over a period of one thousand years, every young girl of proper family willingly permitted herself to be crippled by her mother and aunts to achieve the tiny foot of ideal feminine beauty. Her toes were gradually folded under the sole, and by increasingly tight bandaging her heelbone and forefoot were brought closer together. Without Golden Lotuses, as the best-shaped bound feet were called, a girl was unmarriageable, nor was the life of a courtesan open to her, for tiny feet were a woman's most desirable feature.

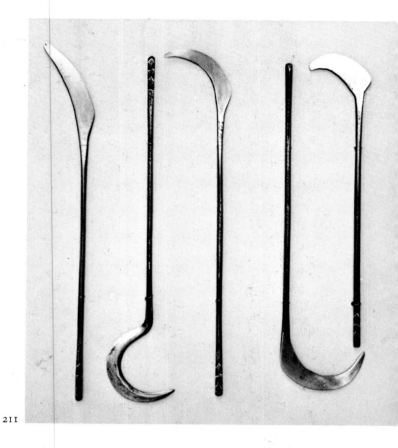

211

211 *Steel surgical knives used for operating on hemorrhoids and varicose veins. Courtesy of the Wellcome Trustees, London*

212 *(Overleaf) Two sections of an 1884 triptych showing the tortured last hours, after eight days of fever, of the great Japanese clan leader Taira Kiyomori (1118–81), who is tormented by Ema, King of Hell, and fierce demons. Collection Walton Rawls, New York*

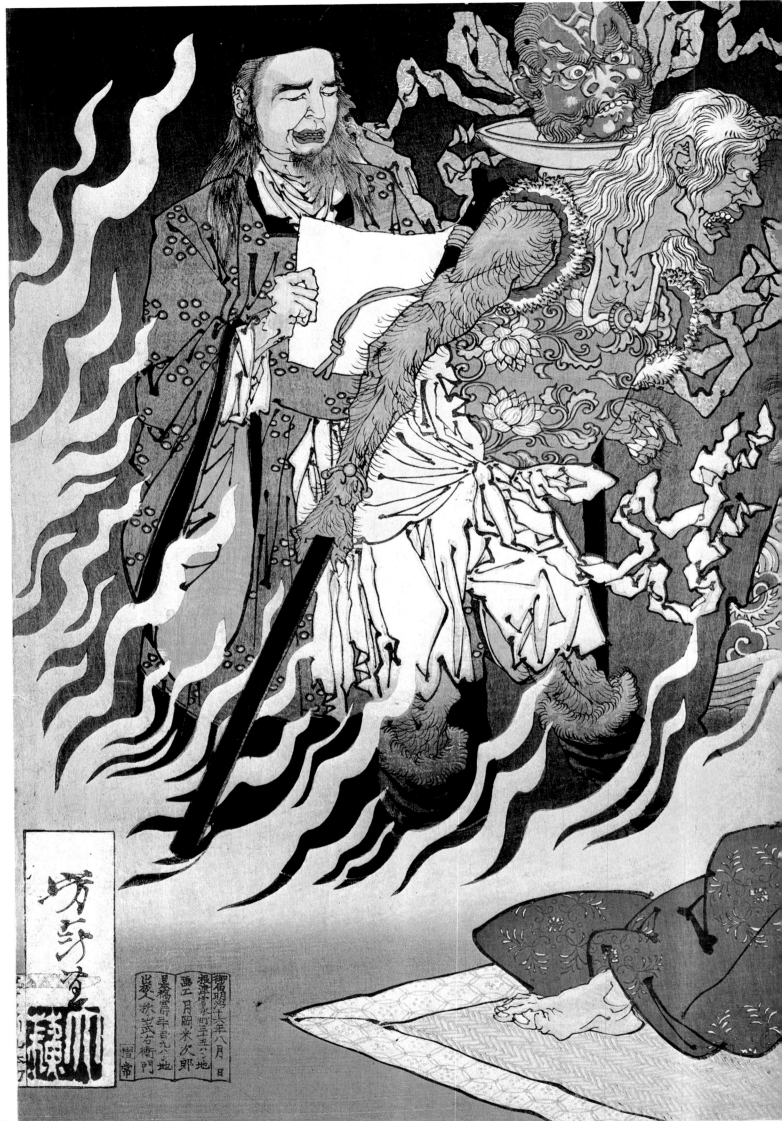

212

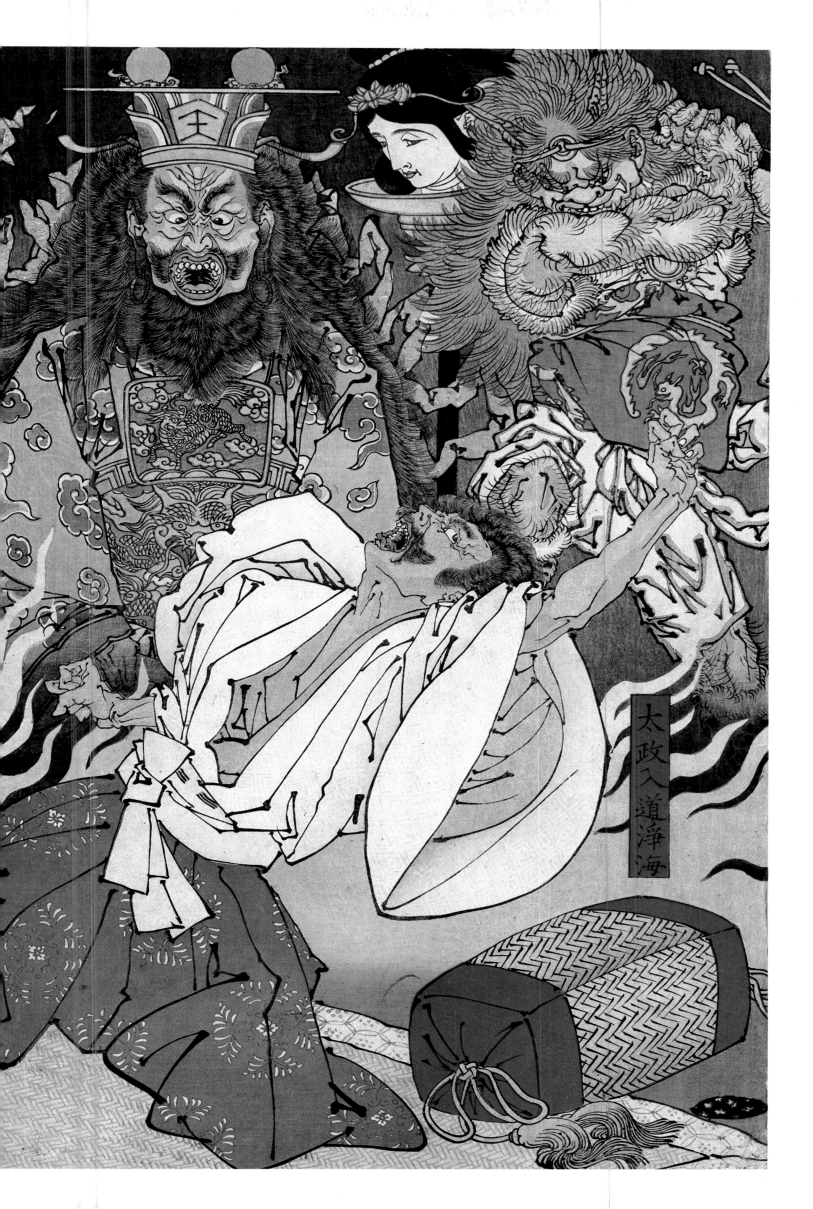

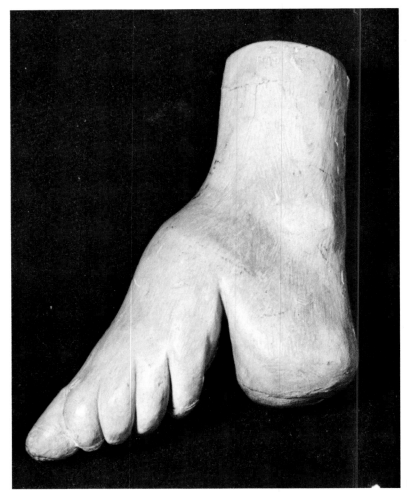

213 *Cast of Chinese woman's bound foot, showing compression of arch and folding under of toes to form the "Golden Lotus" of ideal female beauty. Courtesy of the Wellcome Trustees, London*

214 *Female diagnostic figure in ivory, showing bound feet and fatty development of legs and thighs thought to be voluptuous by the Chinese. Courtesy of the Wellcome Trustees, London*

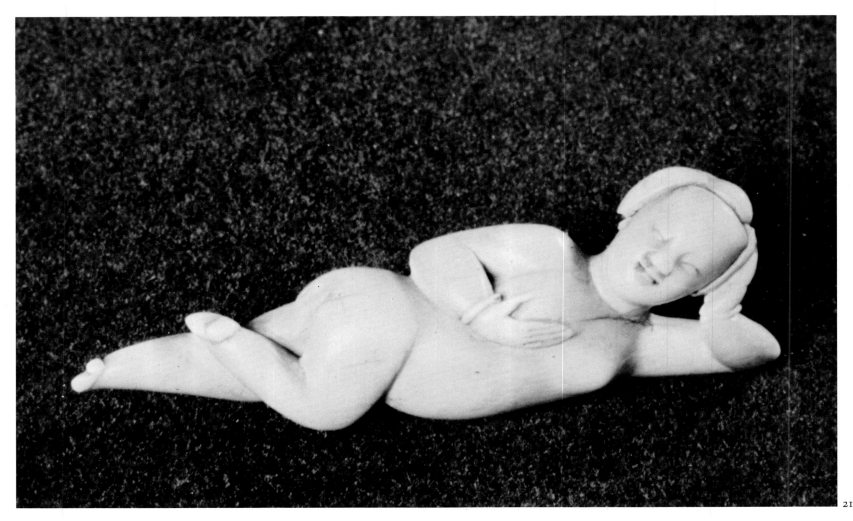

For a man, a bound-foot wife had profound sexual significance, but she was also a status symbol inasmuch as her helplessness indicated that he was wealthy enough to support a woman, or women, in idleness. There was also an advantage to him in her restricted mobility, for it kept her home and made illicit amorous adventures difficult. Although China's Manchu conquerors forbade the practice in the nineteenth century, it was not until the early twentieth that footbinding was completely abandoned.

DISEASES

Some epidemic diseases were understood well enough to allow the development of protective measures. In the eleventh century, inoculation against smallpox was effected by putting scabs from smallpox pustules into the nostrils, a method which may have come from India. Wearing the clothing of someone who had the disease was another means of prevention. The relationship of cowpox (as a protective) to smallpox may have been perceived, since ingesting powdered fleas from infected cows was also recommended to stave off smallpox. But other devastating pestilences were neither understood nor held in check. During the Han dynasty an epidemic of what appears to have been typhoid fever killed two-thirds of the population of one region.

Precise descriptions of leprosy in the *Nei Ching* and later works attest to the diagnostic accuracy of the early Chinese healers, but their explanation of the disease's causes and their treatment follow preconceived notions of the time. "The wind and chills lodge in the blood vessels and cannot be got rid of. This is called *li-feng*. For the treatment prick the swollen parts with a sharp needle to let the foul air out." Fourteenth-century writings referred to chaulmoogra oil, a pressing from seeds of an East Indian tree, as a specific for leprosy, and this oil remained the principal antileprous drug even in the West until recent decades.

An illness that may have been tuberculosis was recognized as contagious: "Generally the disease gives rise to high fever, sweating, asthenia, unlocalized pains making all positions difficult and slowly bringing about consumption and death, after which the disease is transmitted to the relations until the whole family has been wiped out."

Venereal diseases, although not well differentiated, received a variety of therapies, including the use of metallic substances for internal medication. In the *Secret Therapy for the Treatment of Venereal Disease*, the seventeenth-century physician Chun Szi-sung reported using arsenic, which, until the development of penicillin, was the modern medication for venereal disease, in the form of Salvarsan and derivatives synthesized by Paul Ehrlich.

There seem always to have been places in China where the sick poor could go for medical care. With the advance of Buddhism in the Han and T'ang dynasties, in-patient hospitals staffed by physician-priests became common. However, in the ninth century, when anti-Buddhists were in control, hospitals as well as 4,600 temples were destroyed or emptied. Nevertheless, by the twelfth century hospitals had again become so numerous that virtually every district had at least one tax-supported institution. The upper classes preferred to be treated and cared for in their homes, thus leaving public hospitals to the poor and lower classes.

THE PRACTITIONERS

In the *Institutions of Chou*, compiled hundreds of years before Christ, the hierarchy of physicians in the kingdom was delineated. The five categories were: chief physician (who collected drugs, examined other physicians, and assigned them); food physicians (who prescribed six kinds of food and drink); physicians for simple diseases (such as headaches, colds, minor wounds); ulcer physicians (who may have been the surgeons); and physicians for animals (evidently veterinarians).

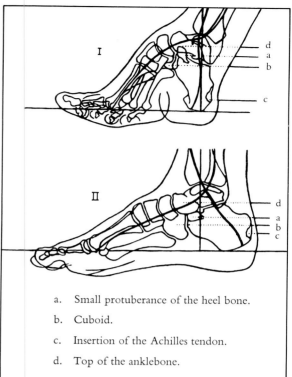

a. Small protuberance of the heel bone.

b. Cuboid.

c. Insertion of the Achilles tendon.

d. Top of the anklebone.

215

215 *X-ray comparison of bound and normal foot, showing displacement of bones resulting from this unusual thousand-year-old custom.*

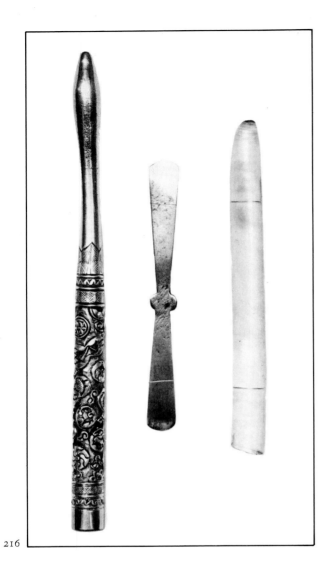

216

一子九歲

毒湧掀腫痘形十六

217

Physicians were also rated according to their results, and as early as the Chou and T'ang dynasties each doctor had to report both successes and failures—to control his movement up or down in the ranks. In the seventh century A.D. examinations were required for one to qualify as a physician, some four centuries earlier than the first licensing system in the West.

Medical knowledge was thought of as a secret power that belonged to each practitioner. Whereas in other societies, both advanced and primitive, closely knit guilds might control the spread of medical lore, the Chinese physician kept his secrets to himself—passing them on only to sons or, sometimes, specially selected qualifiers. In early times, a physician gave his services out of philanthropy, for since the original healers were rulers, sages, nobles, and, perhaps, priests, economic and social incentives were absent. Later, direct fees or salaries were instituted, and the court and certain prosperous households kept physicians on retainer.

Formal schools may have existed as early as the tenth century, and in the eleventh century an organization for medical education was set up under imperial auspices. Under the Ming dynasty in the fourteenth century, the school system became fixed. It changed little over the next centuries, except for a gradual decline, and by 1800 there was only one medical school left in Peking.

Teachers were held strictly accountable for the performance of their students, and fines were imposed if the professor failed to enforce attendance or if his pupils did poorly on exams. The examination system was complex: a pyramidal structure provided a process of elimination which continued until those with the highest scores emerged. The top students could be heart doctors, the next level were assistant examiners, and lower scores could mean limited assignment in teaching.

Specialization may have occurred early. While physicians and apothecaries were separate for a long time, they were both regarded as healers. In the Chou dynasty there were nine specialties, and they grew to thirteen by the Mongol period, early in the fourteenth century. The subdivisions became even more complex, with doctors for the great blood vessels, small vessels, fevers, smallpox, eyes, skin, bones, larynx, and mouth and teeth. There were also gynecologists, pediatricians, and pulsologists for internal diseases, external medicine, the nose and throat, and for children's illnesses. Some healers specialized in moxibustion, acupuncture, or massage. Even the experts in incantation and dietetics were considered medical specialists and were often held in higher regard than other doctors; surgeons were generally of low rank. Furthermore, each of the practitioners in each category had assistants and students—all of whom had to qualify by examination.

Obstetrics was in the hands of midwives for many centuries; it is not known when the first women doctors were in practice. One female physician is mentioned by name in documents from the Han dynasty (206 B.C.–A.D. 220), but women may have been doctors at an earlier date. By the fourteenth century women were officially recognized as physicians.

Throughout the Ming dynasty (1368–1644), the practicing medical theorists could be divided into six main philosophic schools. The *Yin-yang* group focused on insufficiencies of one of these forces. The *Wen-pou* doctors attributed illnesses to a preponderance of *yang* and frequently prescribed ginseng and aconite. The Radical group used drastic medication. The Conservatives relied entirely on the authorities of the past, reedited the classic works, and made no deviations from strict authoritarianism. The Eclectic physicians, as their name implies, used a variety of principles from the other sects. The sixth school based all therapy on bringing the five elements and six vapors into harmony.

SPREAD OF CHINESE MEDICINE TO KOREA, JAPAN, AND TIBET

Ancient Chinese medicine was well-developed long before the beginning of the Christian era, and its influence appears to have spread into adjacent Korea by the

216 *Set of instruments used for immunization against smallpox. Dried smallpox scabs were ground to powder and blown into nostrils through silver tube such as one shown. Courtesy of the Wellcome Trustees, London*

217 *Girl with smallpox, accurately delineated by artist at a time when disease was known to be contagious and thoroughly described in medical literature. Bibliothèque Nationale, Paris*

218 *Figure of Pien Ch'iao, author of* Secrets of the Pulse *(6th–5th century* B.C.*), the first noteworthy medical man mentioned in Chinese history and one of the Eight Immortals. University of Kansas Medical Center, Lawrence*

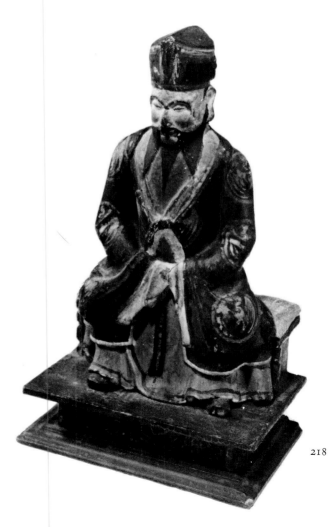

218

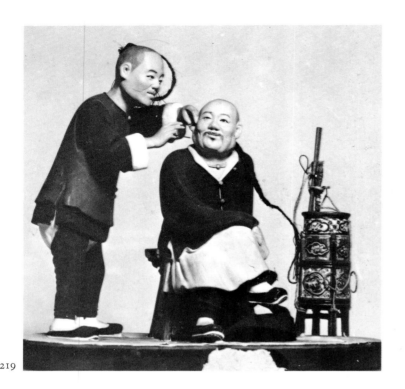

219

219 *Model figures showing Chinese street barber cleaning out ears of client. Like his Western counterpart, he performed numerous services other than cutting hair. Courtesy of the Wellcome Trustees, London*

220 *Carved wooden sign inscribed "Doctor for treating miscellaneous diseases," but strings of extracted teeth seem to indicate that numerous patients came for dental problems. Courtesy of the Wellcome Trustees, London*

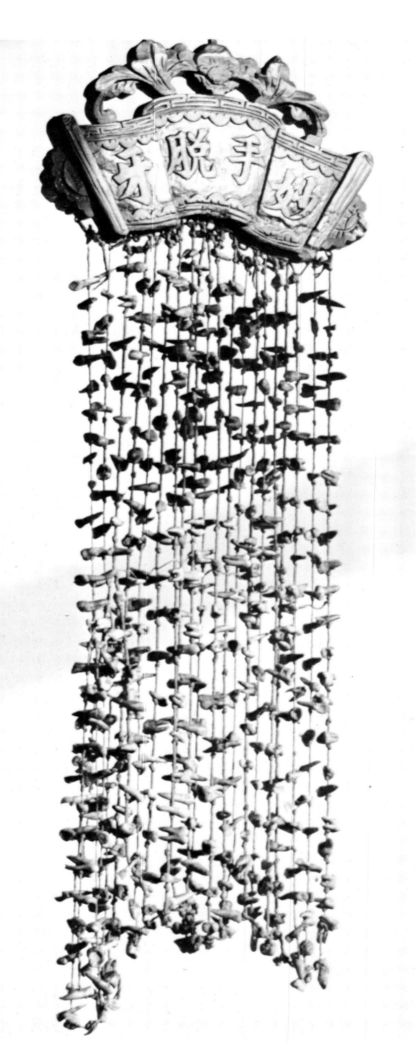

220

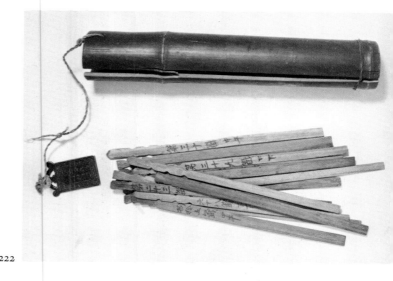

222

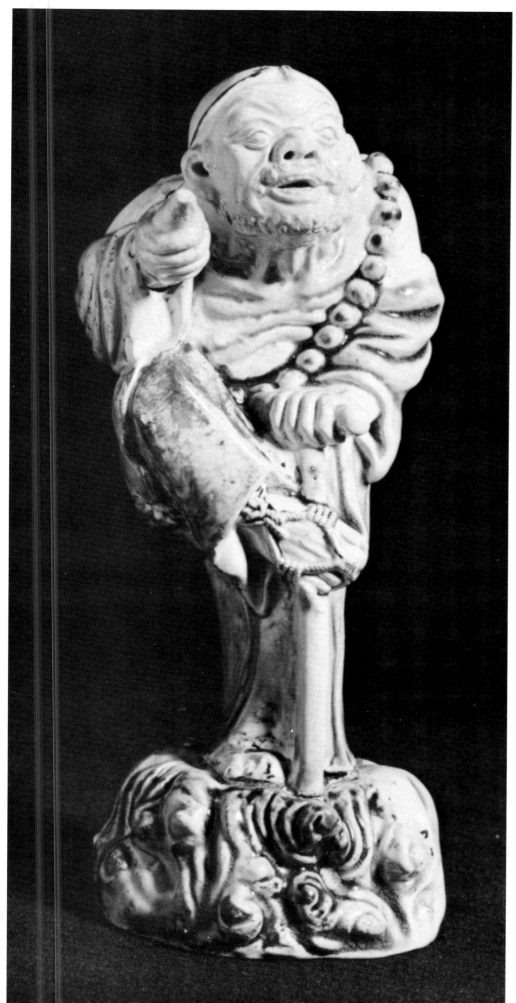

221

221 *Pottery figure of Li T'ieh Kuai, one of the Eight Immortals, here depicted as a beggar leaning on a crutch and carrying a gourd of "magic medicines" on his back. Courtesy of the Wellcome Trustees, London*

222 *Bamboo container with numbered sticks, employed at Medicine Temple to shake out number of prescription to be used in treating ailment of the suppliant. Courtesy of the Wellcome Trustees, London*

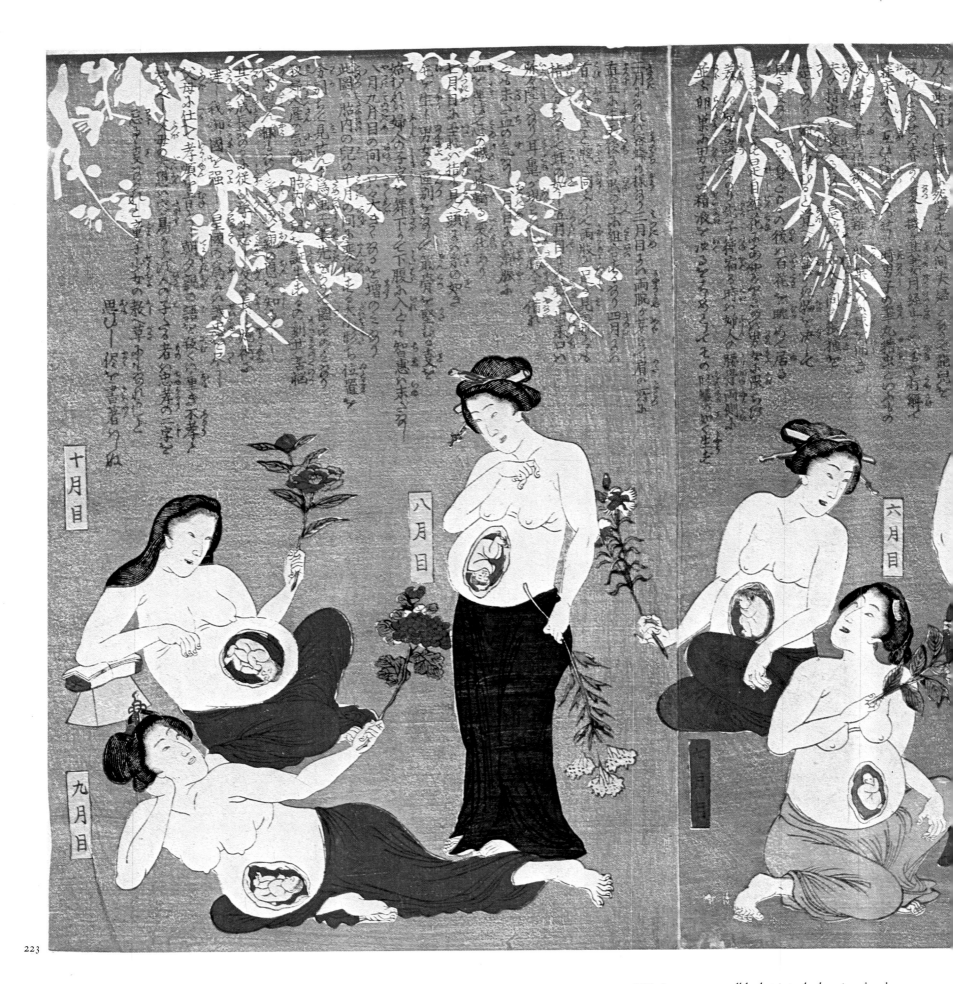

223

223 *Japanese woodblock triptych showing development of fetus, right to left, set in scheme of changing seasons. National Library of Medicine, Bethesda*

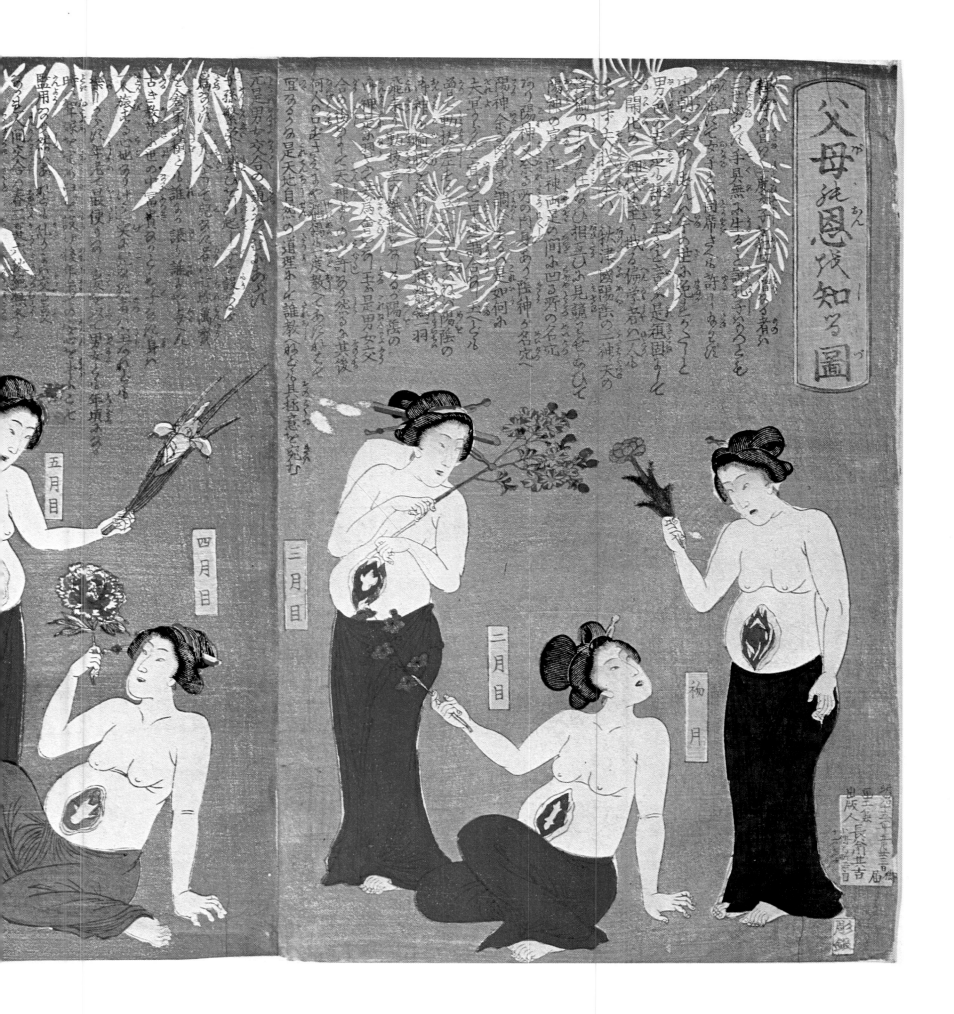

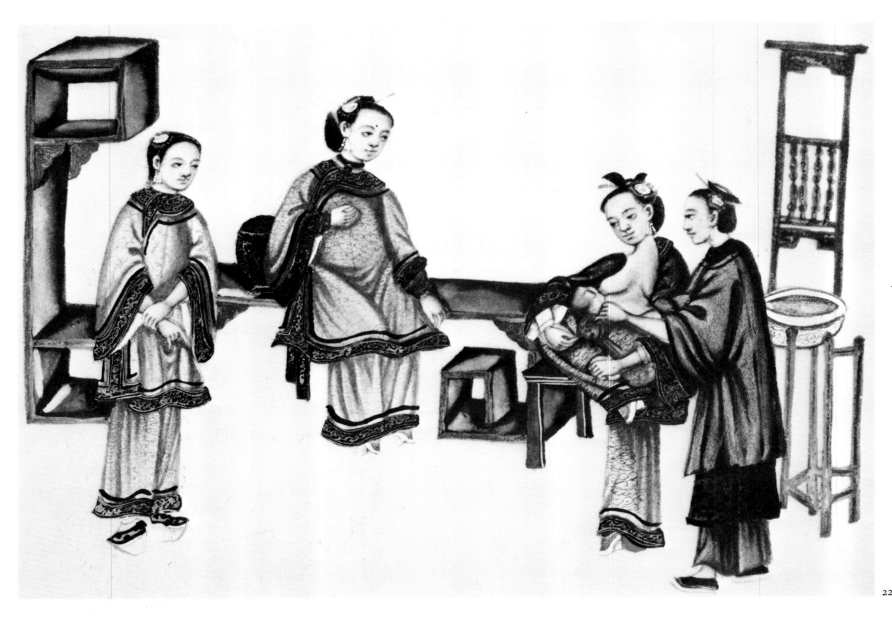

224

224 *Watercolor of Chinese mother nursing newborn child, supported by servant as she cradles baby in crook of upraised leg. Courtesy of the Wellcome Trustees, London*

225 *Watercolor of birth scene, showing mother receiving support and restorative drink from servants —clearly identified by size of feet. Courtesy of the Wellcome Trustees, London*

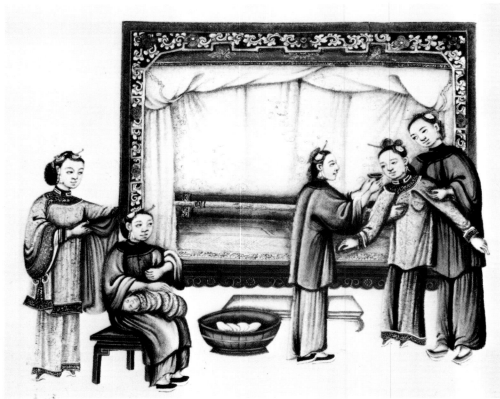

225

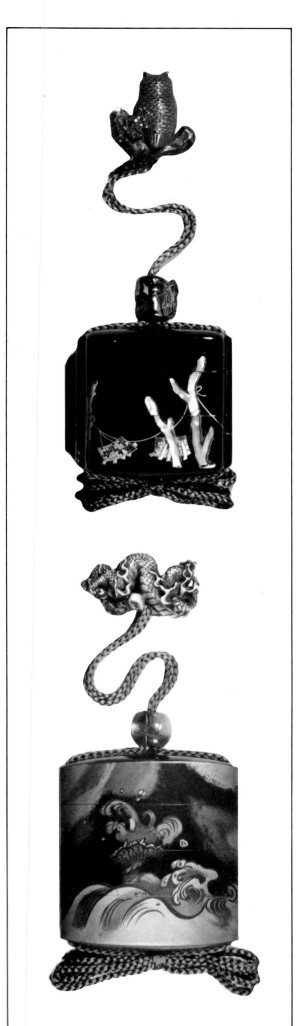

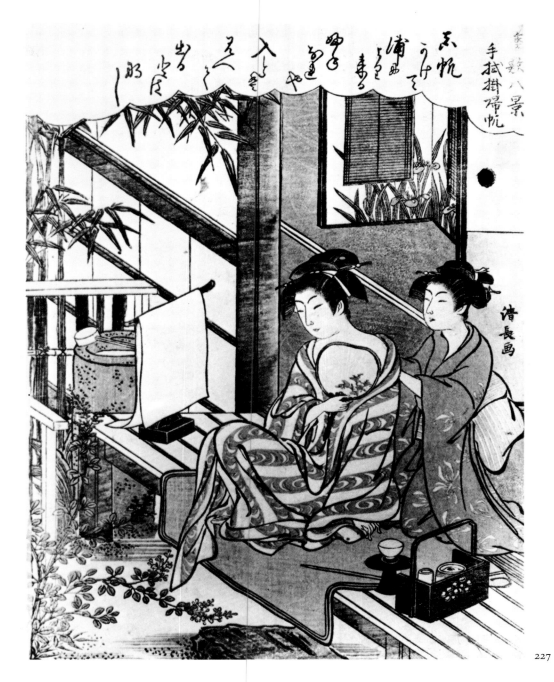

226 *Japanese lacquered* inro *medicine box with* netsuke *toggle (18th–19th centuries), designed with several compartments to provide a selection of medicaments when traveling. Semelweis Orvostörténeti Muzeum, Budapest*

227 *Japanese woodblock print by Kiyonaga (16th century) showing woman receiving massage, probably a heritage of Japanese espousal of Chinese medical systems. Collection Camondo, The Louvre, Paris*

228 *Japanese papier-mâché doll (c. 1880) used to demonstrate 660 treatment points in adaptation of Chinese acupuncture methodology. The Japanese also used these points in moxibustion, treatment by burning powdered mugwort on skin. Peabody Museum, Salem*

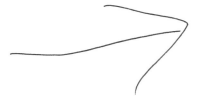

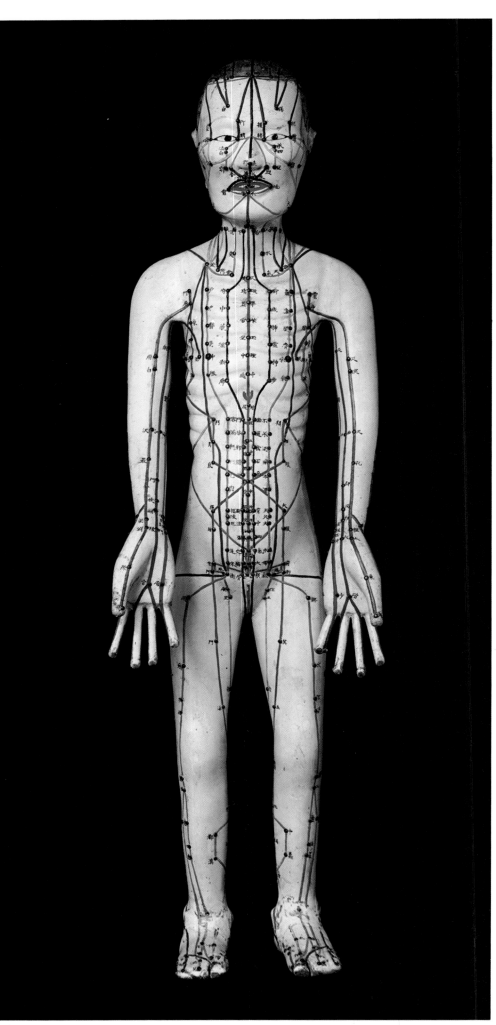

228

sixth century A.D. At that time, after a severe epidemic had ravaged Japan, Korean doctors who were invited to counsel Japanese physicians introduced them to Chinese medical classics and commentaries. By the seventh century, Japanese scholars and doctors were going directly to China for their information and experience. In the eighth century, a Chinese Buddhist monk named Chien Chen came to Japan and achieved a prominent position in the imperial court at Nara, where, given the Japanese name Kanjin, he taught, practiced medicine, and translated Chinese materia medica. Late in that century, Chinese medicine was well-established in Japan, and a medical school based on its methodology was founded by the Japanese physician Wake Hiroya. Early in the next century (806–10), the Emperor Heijo vainly attempted to combat foreign influence and restore traditional Japanese medical practice, but the methods of Chinese healing were too firmly entrenched. In the tenth century, acupuncture reached Japan, followed by moxibustion (the word moxa is Japanese), and the full complement of Chinese medicine was accepted in Japan.

With medical training closely based on Chinese systems, the Japanese exacted exceptionally intensive and prolonged study before permitting entrance into the profession by governmental examination. As in ancient China, high social standing was a requirement for admission to medical school, but separate instruction by assigned teachers was apparently also arranged to accommodate the more lowly.

The authority of Chinese medicine, not to mention Chinese culture and philosophy, moved east as well as west by the seventh and eighth centuries. However, Arabic and Indian missionaries of Islam and Buddhism made influence a two-way exchange as they traveled to China seeking converts. Since their missions necessitated the translation of Sanskrit and Arabic writings into Chinese and vice versa, medical knowledge inevitably was passed back and forth. Consequently, the crossroads areas of Southeast Asia and Tibet developed a medical system combining aspects of Chinese, Indian, and Arabic practice. Arabic influence, which stemmed in part from Greek teachings, was evident in the doctrine of four humors (phlegm, blood, bile, and wind), whereas Indian ideas were seen in the Yogic placement of the soul in the core of the spinal column and reliance on breathing exercises.

Traveling Buddhist priests, who were quite successful in spreading their faith, for a long time also practiced medicine. During this early period, the two wives (one Chinese) of a Tibetan king converted him to Buddhism, and thereafter scholars were invited to bring Chinese writings into Tibet, which resulted in collections in Tibetan called *Kanjur* and *Tanjur*, the latter containing medical information. In the thirteenth century, the Mongol conqueror Kublai Khan wanted this body of knowledge available again in Chinese but was unable to carry through the translation. Nevertheless, his grandson in the next century arranged for scholars from Tibet, Mongolia, and Central Asia to accomplish the task. Ironically, while the Mongols were in control they allied themselves with non-Chinese such as Uighars, Jews, Christians, and Moslems, and they preferred Arabic medicine to Chinese.

GREECE
AND ROME

Cretan and
Mycenaean Medicine

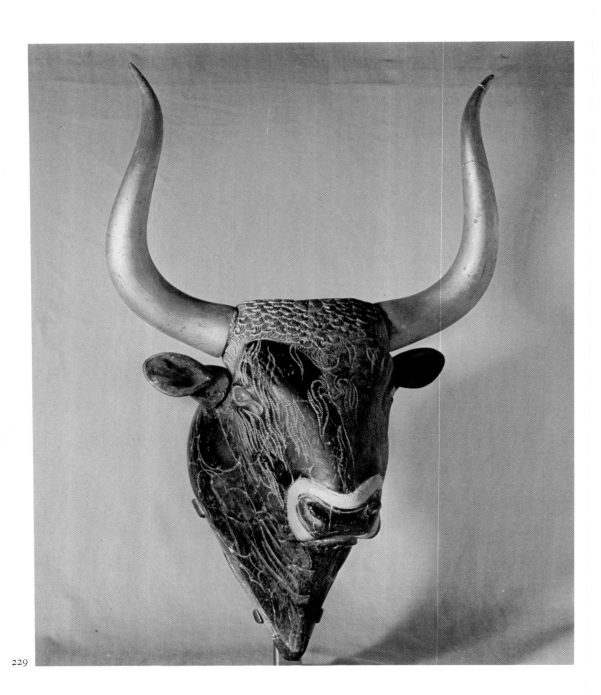

229

W HEN Greek medicine is mentioned, the name of Hippocrates is usually called to mind as the personification of a rational, nonreligious approach to medical practice. But Hippocrates did not in the fifth century B.C. spring fully formed from the forehead of Zeus like the mythological Athena. For hundreds of years the Greeks had had contact with and cross-fertilization from numerous other ancient peoples—for example, the Egyptians—and in the centuries before Hippocrates there were many developments in medical experience, knowledge, and understanding, both on the mainland of Greece and the islands of the Aegean Sea, which were important to the evolution of Hippocratic medicine. Furthermore, after Hippocrates, great men, influential doctrines, and extraordinary advances in knowledge continued to enhance Greek civilization.

For clarity, we will divide the periods of Greek medicine into Cretan-Mycenaean, Mythologic, Pre-Hippocratic (The Philosopher-Scientists), Hippocratic, and Post-Hippocratic (Alexandria and the Medical Sects), treating each division separately.

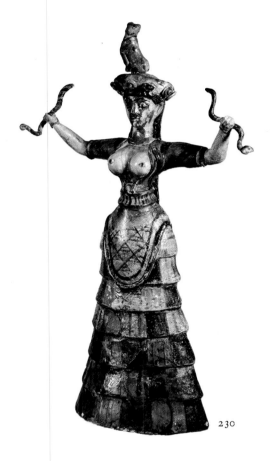

230

A little more than a century ago, virtually everything we knew of the most ancient Greeks came from their traditions, legends, and epic poems such as the *Iliad* and *Odyssey* of Homer and the *Theogony* of Hesiod. How much was based on historical fact was unknown until 1870, when Heinrich Schliemann discovered and began excavating the site of Troy—located almost solely from clues in Homer's epics. Encouraged by Schliemann's astounding discoveries at Troy and elsewhere, Sir Arthur Evans began to dig in Crete at Cnossus in 1900. His excavations proved equally spectacular, for they showed evidence that the site had been occupied by a well-developed culture before 3000 B.C., that Cnossus had been destroyed (possibly by earthquake) about 1500 B.C., and that after being magnificently rebuilt the palace had been laid waste again around 1400 B.C., this time probably by a maritime invasion from the Greek mainland across the Mediterranean Sea.

Based on the fabulous artifacts recovered from the ancient sites, archaeology had made it clear that the hoary legends and epics had been created within a framework of historical truth. The ruins of the palace at Cnossus provided evidence of an advanced culture that had flourished some two thousand years before Christ, the first high civilization of the Aegean—and the West. Named Minoan after the legendary King Minos, this civilization is reputed to have developed a maritime power which reached across the Mediterranean and a pictographic script now known as Linear A, a language still not understood. The Minoans seemed to have reached the height of their prosperity and civilization about 1600 B.C., by which time their maritime rivals the Mycenaeans on the Greek mainland had overtaken them and made their fortified city-state Mycenae the mercantile center of the ancient world. Roughly contemporary to the Minoan, Mycenaean civilization through trade contact had been greatly influenced by Cretan culture. Late evidence in Cnossus of a new script, Linear B, which probably came from the mainland, suggests the presence of Mycenaeans and points to their responsibility for the final destruction of Cnossus about 1400 B.C.

The Mycenaean fortress-citadels of about the twelfth century B.C. were the settings for Homer's epics the *Iliad* and the *Odyssey*. Historical details of that time had been passed down to Homer in the mid-ninth century B.C. through oral tradition. Although medical information is incidental, so much of the daily life of these ancient Greeks is included that many studies have attempted to piece together an accurate picture of the period. However, details of Homer's own times are probably mingled with the poems' legends about the Mycenaean era. Nevertheless, despite challenges to the accuracy of Homer's picture of ancient life, there is enough archaeological and other confirmation that a reasonably faithful view of Aegean medicine can be presumed to exist in the epics. It is, therefore, called Homeric Medicine.

229 *Bull's head rhyton in black steatite with inlaid shell and rock crystal (c. 1550 B.C.), found in Little Palace at Cnossus. A recurring image and cult symbol, the bull was highly significant in Cretan civilization. The island's most famous legend is of the Minotaur, a monster with the head of a bull and the body of a man. Archaeological Museum, Heraklion, Crete*

230 *The Snake Goddess, in faience, from the Palace at Cnossus (c. 1600 B.C.). One of several similar figures, this may instead represent a priestess of the important mother-goddess cult of ancient Crete. Archaeological Museum, Heraklion, Crete*

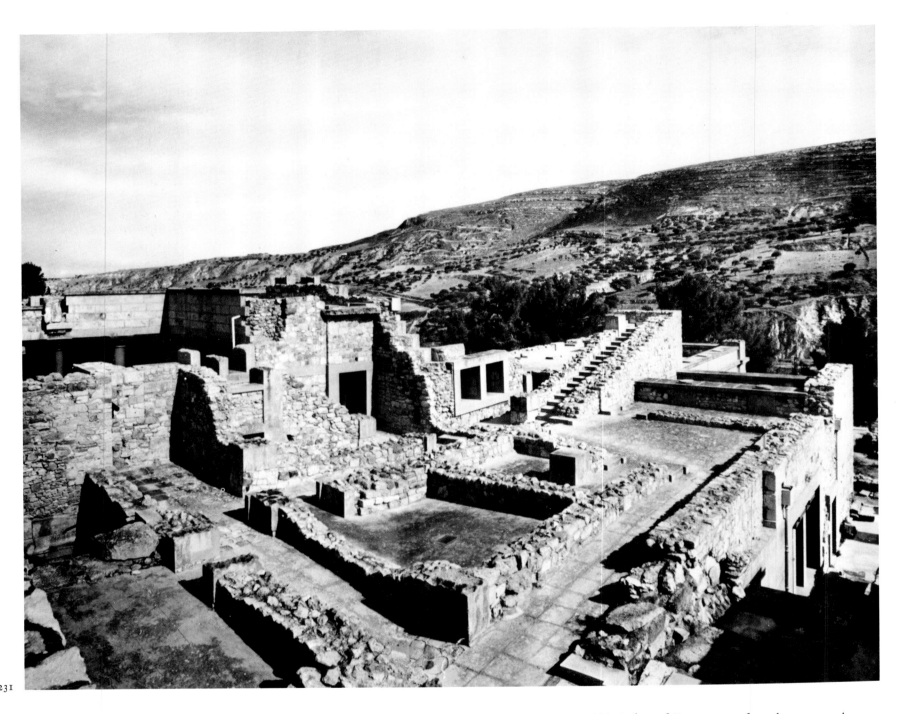

231

231 *Palace of Cnossus seen from the west-southwest. Excavated by Sir Arthur Evans in 1900, the palace had many rooms, running water, and well-engineered drainage systems.*

232 *Clay figure, possibly a mother-goddess (c. 1100– 1000 B.C.), wearing "horns of consecration" on head and with movable legs, found at sanctuary on Mt. Dikte, Crete.*

233 *Cretan-Mycenaean-period figure in terra-cotta from Boeotia, said to represent a goddess of animals. The Louvre, Paris*

234 *Marble figure from Amorgos (c. 2500–1100 B.C.) of a type found in tombs of the Cyclades islands of the south Aegean and thought to symbolize a nature goddess. National Archaeological Museum, Athens*

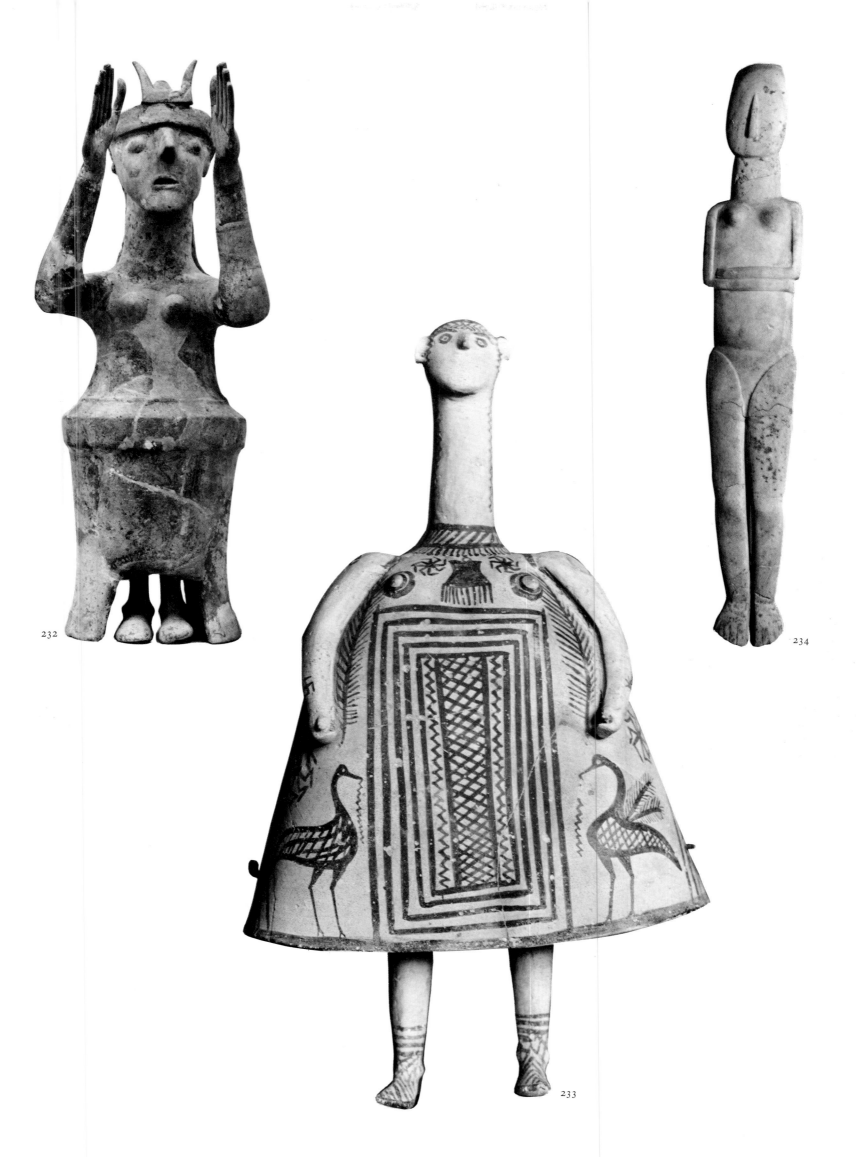

232

233

234

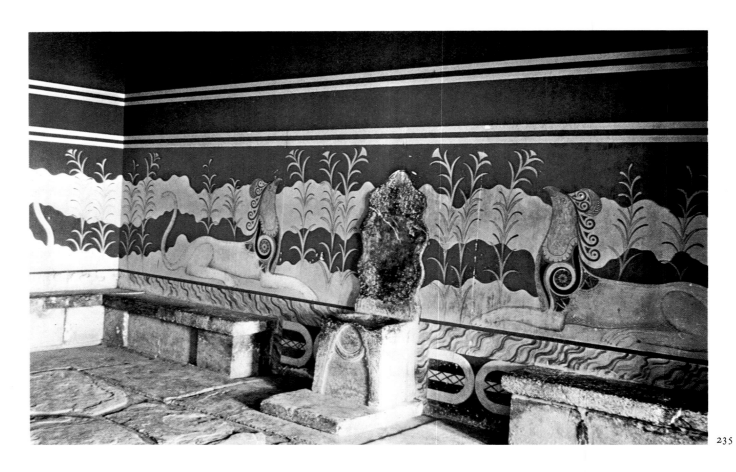

235

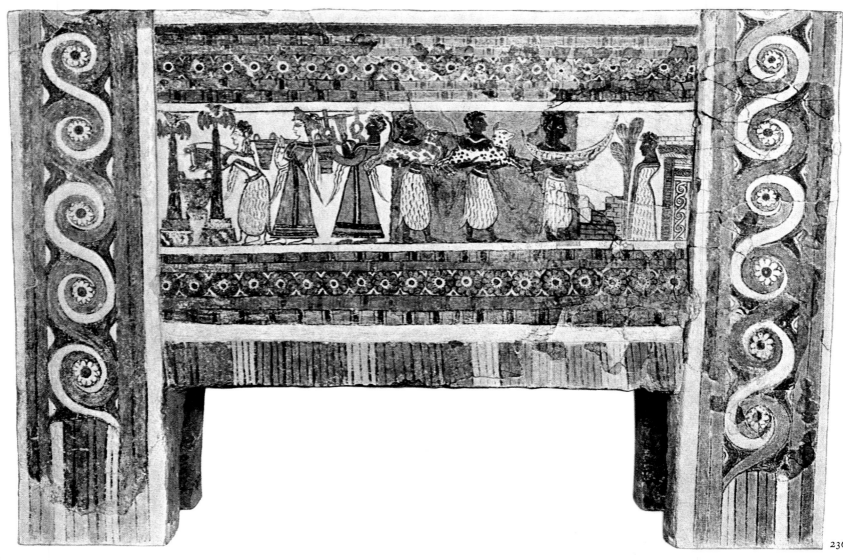

236

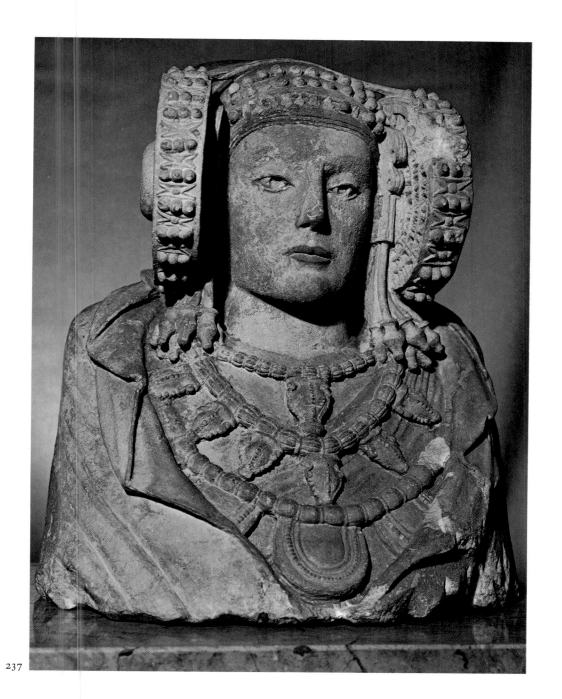

237

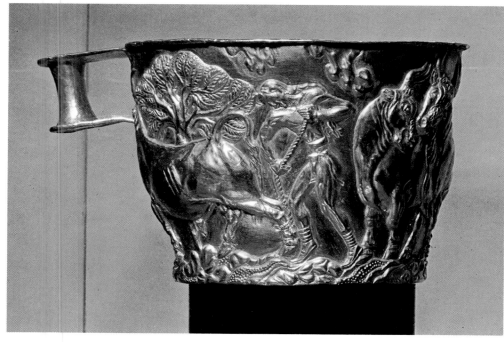

238

235 *Throne room of the Palace of Cnossus (c. 1500 B.C.), restored, which gives a good impression of the level of civilization that once thrived there.*

236 *Painted limestone sarcophagus (c. 1400 B.C.) from Hagia Triada, Crete, with one side showing women pouring libation (at left), and men bringing offerings of calves and boat model to figure before altar, or tomb (at right). Archaeological Museum, Heraklion, Crete*

237 *Cretan–Mycenaean ornamental style seen on regal Iberian figure (4th century B.C.), from Elche, Spain, which demonstrates wide-ranging influence of the maritime cultures of the eastern Mediterranean. The Louvre, Paris*

238 *Gold cup in Minoan style (c. 1500 B.C.), from a tomb at Vaphio, near Sparta, with repoussé figures of tame bulls and wild bulls being captured in nets and tethered. National Archaeological Museum, Athens*

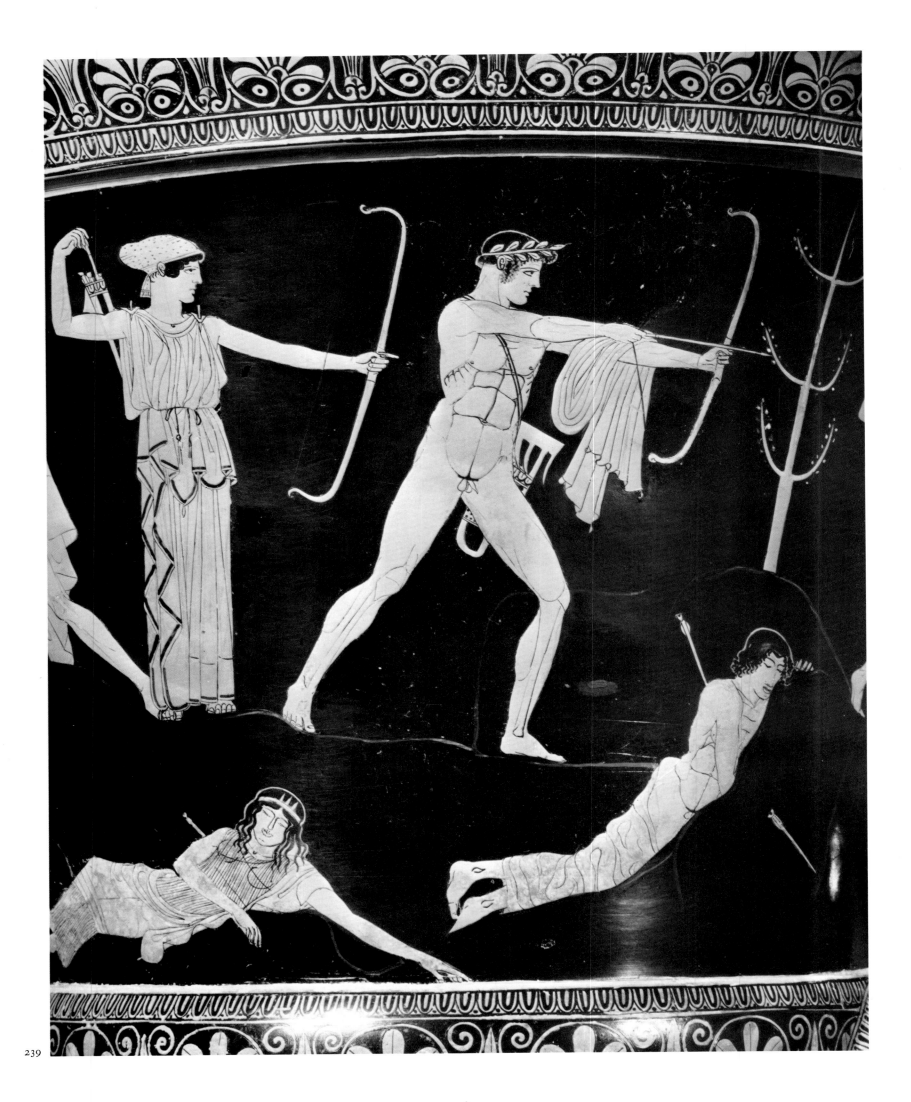

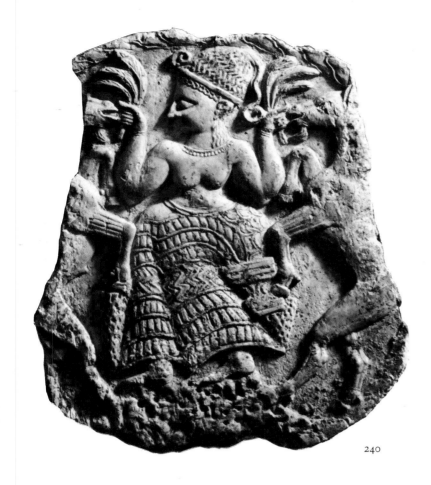

UNDERSTANDING OF HEALTH AND DISEASE

Virtually any of the Greek gods could cause disease. Apollo and his sister Artemis (both children of Zeus) could shoot certain "arrows" which would bring on illness or widespread pestilence and others which would produce the deterioration and death of old age. The *Iliad* opens with an epidemic sent by Apollo, and the accepted means to end it calls for discovering what has offended which god (often determined through the services of a soothsayer), and then by prayer, sacrifice, and purification to try to appease the alienated deity.

Nonetheless, natural causes of disease were recognized and rational methods of healing were most important. Furthermore, what was known of human anatomy and physiology was more rational than superstitious or religious. Even at that, anatomical knowledge was limited (derived chiefly from butchering, sacrifices, and battle injuries), for apparently dissection was not practiced. Yet many rudimentary and fundamental facts were probably well known: for instance, that breathed air went through the windpipe; the heart was a beating organ; the throat carried down food and drink by swallowing; the rectum, bladder, buttocks, and pelvic bones had precise topographical relationships to each other.

The life force, *thymos*, was in all parts of the living organism. Maintained by factors that came from outside (such as food, drink, and air) as well as actions of internal body environment (such as movements of body fluids, including blood), *thymos* could also escape from wounds and by exhalation, leaving the body at death.

The *psyche*, the soul or individual personality, was the spirit which went to the underworld after death. Whether the Homeric Greek considered consciousness to reside in the chest and diaphragm, as has been suggested, or actually in the head is a matter of interpretation. Nevertheless, the heart was the site of consciousness in ancient Egypt and in Greece by the time of Aristotle, in the fourth century B.C.

METHODS OF HEALING

For the most part, medical treatment was restricted to external injuries and wounds. On the battlefield, weapons that pierced the body were extracted,

239 *Calyx-crater (c. 455–450 B.C.) by the Niobid Painter, found at Orvieto, possibly shows the deities Apollo and Artemis shooting arrows that brought disease to mankind, a manifestation of the widespread ancient idea that sickness was punishment by the gods. The Louvre, Paris*

240 *Mainland Mycenaean ivory bas-relief fragment (c. 1500–1400 B.C.) perhaps of a fertility goddess, in the dress and posture often seen in the Minoan mother-goddess cult figures of island Crete. The Louvre, Paris*

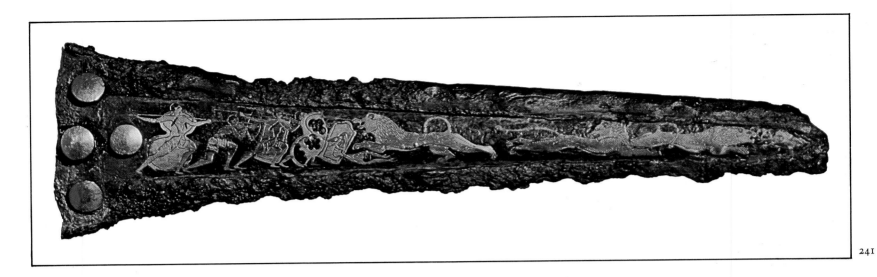

241 *Bronze dagger (c. 1570–1550 B.C.), inlaid with gold and silver, excavated by Schliemann at Mycenae. Since the hunters wear belted shorts in Cretan style, some infer that Mycenaean culture was influenced by Crete, but no similar blades have been found in Crete. National Archaeological Museum, Athens*

242 *Terra-cotta figure of Middle Minoan man with dagger stuck in belt (c. 2000–1850 B.C.), found in sanctuary of Mt. Petsofa, Crete. Archaeological Museum, Heraklion, Crete.*

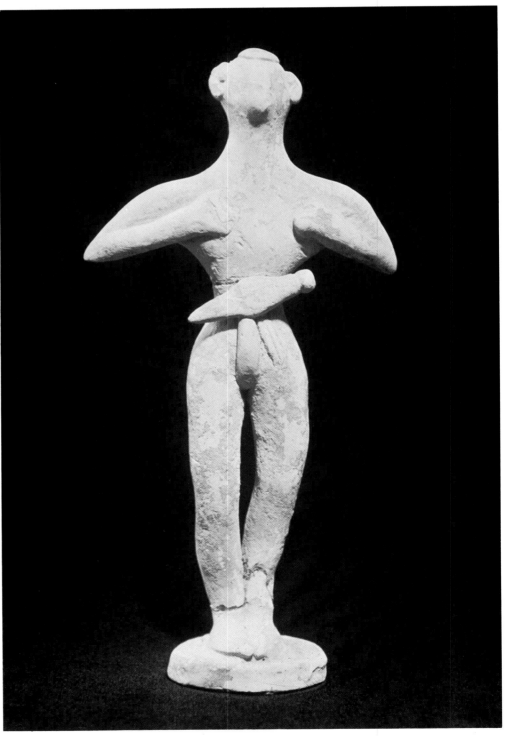

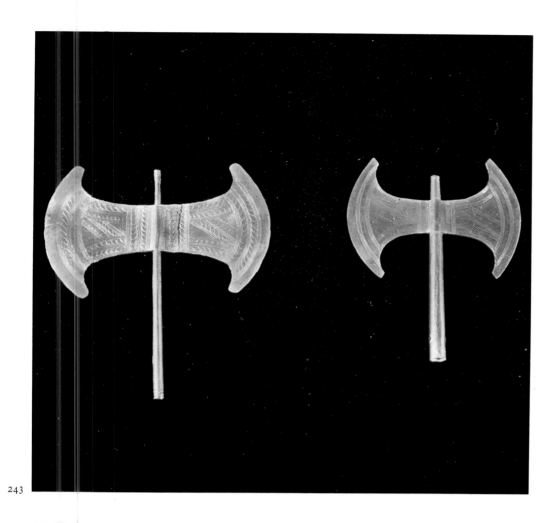

243 *Gold double ax symbols (c. 1500 B.C.) found in cave at Arkalochori in eastern Crete. The double ax is among the most pervasive of Cretan emblems, possibly signifying authority.*

244 *Painted clay bathtub–sarcophagus (c. 1350 B.C.) from Pachyammos in northern Crete. Early Cretans were often buried in household furnishings such as bathtubs and chests.*

243

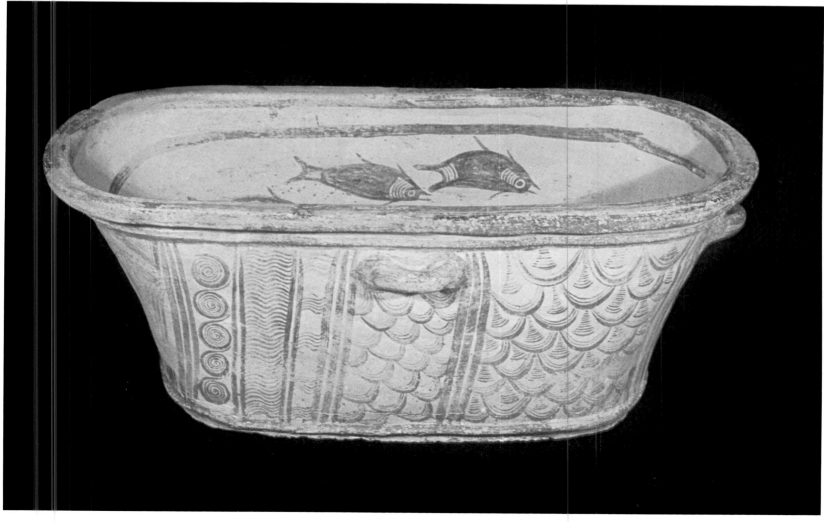

244

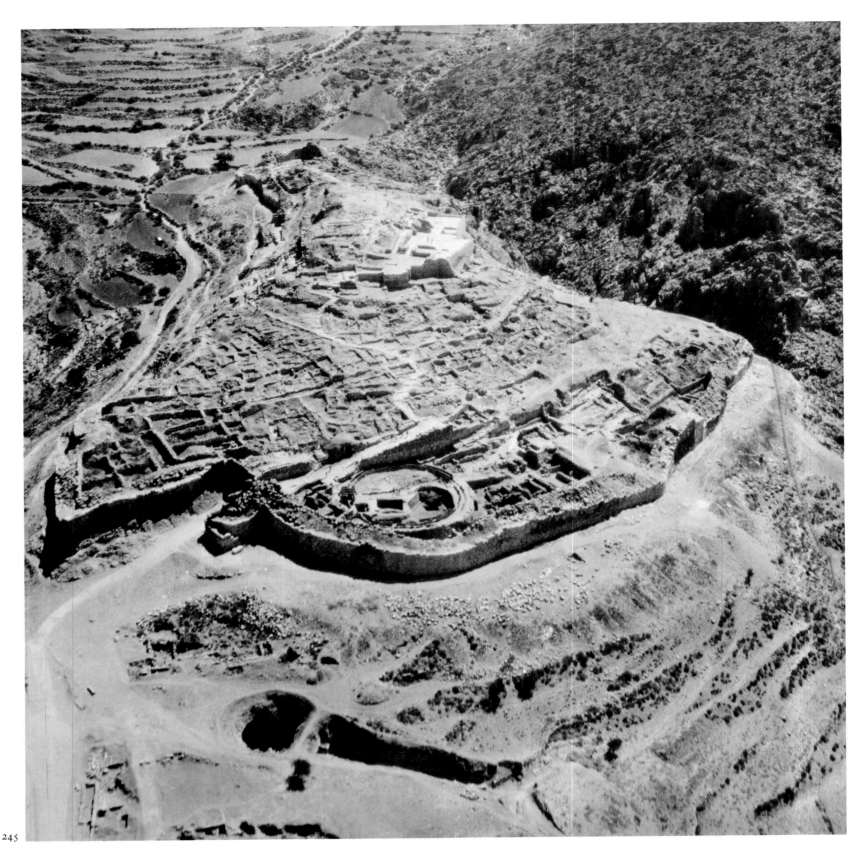

245

245 *Aerial view of the Citadel of Mycenae*

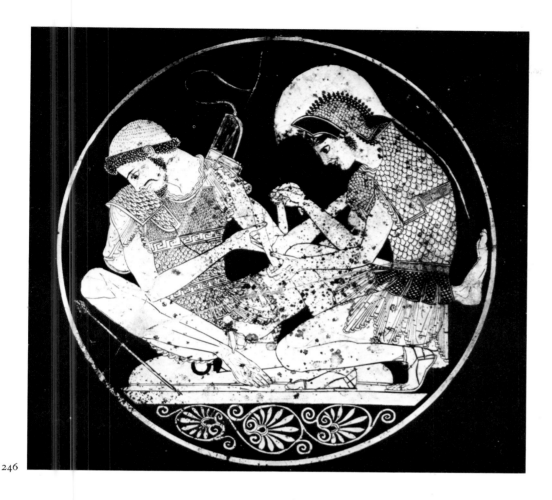

246 *Detail from bowl of Sosias (c. 50 B.C.) showing Achilles bandaging the wounds of Patroclus, a typical battlefield scene of warriors caring for the injuries of others. Staatliche Museen, Berlin*

hemorrhage was stopped by bandaging, and wounds were washed and picked clean of debris. Medicaments were used chiefly, though not exclusively, for local application and were usually sprinkled in powdered form. *Pharmaka*, the name broadly applied to drugs, covered substances used for magic, for poison, or for curing, but the locally applied medications were intended to soothe, relieve pain, dry the secretions, and hasten healing.

THE HEALERS

Just as in mythology gods treated one another, in the *Iliad* and *Odyssey* warriors helped each other survive their wounds and sicknesses. Among the warrior-lords mentioned were some who had special knowledge, as for example Machaon and Podalirios, sons of the chieftain Asclepios. Both of them treated wounds, but Machaon's name was continued through subsequent centuries as the father of surgery. Podalirios was later enshrined as the father of internal medicine, but this was not based primarily on his activities in the *Iliad*, for he cleansed and sprinkled medicaments on wounds just as his brother Machaon did. However, a need among later practitioners of medicine for an ancient patron from whom to take a semidivine image led to a fictionalization of the skills of Podalirios in treating internal diseases—creating a place for him alongside Machaon, the ancestor of surgeons.

There were others besides the warrior-nobles who were skilled physicians. Apparently these healers, although of the class of craftsmen, were singled out together with others of special skills for recognition and esteem. Emmaeus is quoted as saying: "Who would take it on himself to extend hospitality to a wandering stranger, unless he were one of the itinerant workers for the people, a diviner, a physician, a carpenter, or a minstrel?"

The gods and the practitioners throughout early Greek history were together engaged in treating the sick, and the healing gods gradually became enshrined in special temples, of which the most famous were those dedicated to Asclepios.

Greek Mythology and the Temples of Asclepios

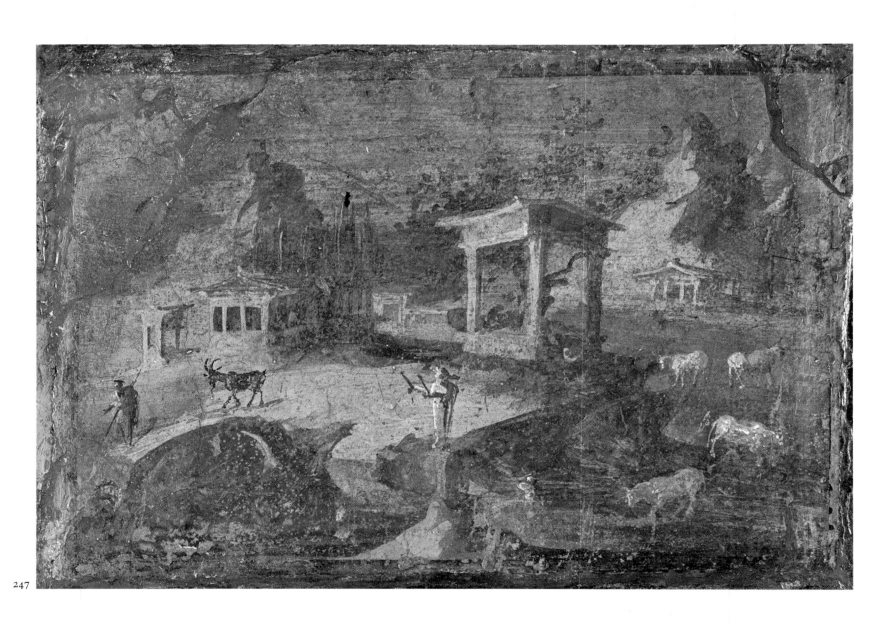

As in Mycenaean times, both religious and secular medical practice continued to operate side by side. Physicians frequently contributed to the Asclepieian temples, and columns of the temples were sometimes inscribed with the names of honored physicians.

Although the temples and cult of Asclepios eventually became the principal focus of religious medicine, a long and mythological heritage had preceded. The ancient gods of the earth and underworld, with animal agents such as snakes and moles, were often healing forces, and Asclepios may have been the later personification of some of these older gods.

The legendary Melampos (c. 1500 B.C.) gained fame as a healer when he cured the mad women of Argos, among whom were daughters of the king of Tiryns, a citadel like Mycenae. His method of first stimulating the women to even further wild behavior is said to have foreshadowed the Dionysian mysteries involving orgiastic rites. He then employed the drug black hellebore, which has a number of actions depending on how much is given—narcotic, diuretic, cathartic.

Amphiaraos was one of the most famous descendant divinities of Melampos. He may have originated as a local subterranean demon known in Thebes, Athens, and especially in Oropos where he apparently became a sort of competitor to Asclepios. Tromphonios was another supernatural physician from the underworld, whose ministrations were sought in caves and whose healing powers were conveyed through snakes, which go back to early times as symbols of regeneration and therefore of cure.

More in the orbit of Olympian gods was Orpheos, whose music and poetry had power over the soul, and who once may have lived as a mortal in Thrace about 1300 B.C. A religious sect developed around him involving a belief in reincarnation and asceticism (celibacy, vegetarianism, exercises). The philosophic medical center of Pythagoras (fl. c. 530 B.C.) was intimately connected with Orphic mysticism.

Of course, almost every god in the Greek pantheon, as well as many demigods and heroes, seems to have had some association with illness and health. Hera, Zeus's wife and goddess of the home, was a protector of women in childbirth. Athena, the goddess of wisdom, also had temples dedicated to her as a healer and was sometimes referred to as a patroness of the eyes.

Chiron was a half brother of Zeus, sharing the same father, the Titan Cronos, from whom the Olympian Zeus wrested power over the universe. Half human, half horse, he had a special place as a patron of healing. There were legends as late as the Middle Ages of his having imparted secrets of medicinal plants to Apuleius, the compiler of a famous herbal. His knowledge of the healing properties of herbs was said to have been conveyed to him by Artemis. Pindar's poetic stories indicate that Chiron, in addition to performing magic cures by incantations, also administered drugs, soothing applications, and surgery, from which we may infer their use in the author's own time (518–438 B.C.). Chiron was indeed the godhead of medical teachers, for his pupils were said to include Melampos, Achilles, and Asclepios. However, it was Apollo who became identified as the principal divinity controlling illness. The legend that Asclepios was Apollo's son may have helped him to eventual predominance as god of healing.

The *Iliad* speaks of Asclepios as a warrior-king contributing ships and men to the Trojan war. It was his two sons Machaon and Podalirios who were knowledgeable in the healing arts. Nevertheless, by the time of Hesiod (700 B.C.?), about two centuries after Homer, Asclepios was considered the principal god of healing. Hesiod's version of Asclepios's birth and elevation has remained the best known, although it is not clear whether he created or simply reported it.

The story is that Coronis, a mortal woman, either voluntarily or unwillingly, succumbed to the sun-god Apollo, but while pregnant with the god's child she married Ischys, to whom in some versions she had been betrothed. Apollo killed Ischys while his sister Artemis slew Coronis, but before her body was burned on the funeral pyre Apollo snatched the babe Asclepios, bringing him to the mountain

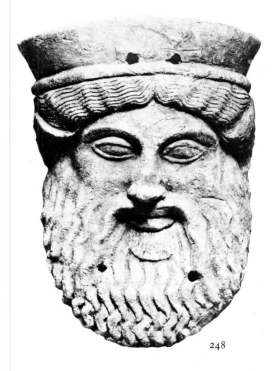

248

247 The Sacred Landscape, *a wall painting from Pompeii (c. A.D. 63–79). Although not Greek, this imaginary scene reflects the Romans' respect for and adaptation of ancient Greek mythology and ideas. Museo Archeologico Nazionale, Naples*

248 *Terra-cotta mask (c. 450 B.C.), from Boeotia, of a type associated with the earliest Dionysian fertility rites, ceremonies that ultimately evolved into Greek drama. Collection Norbert Schimmel, New York*

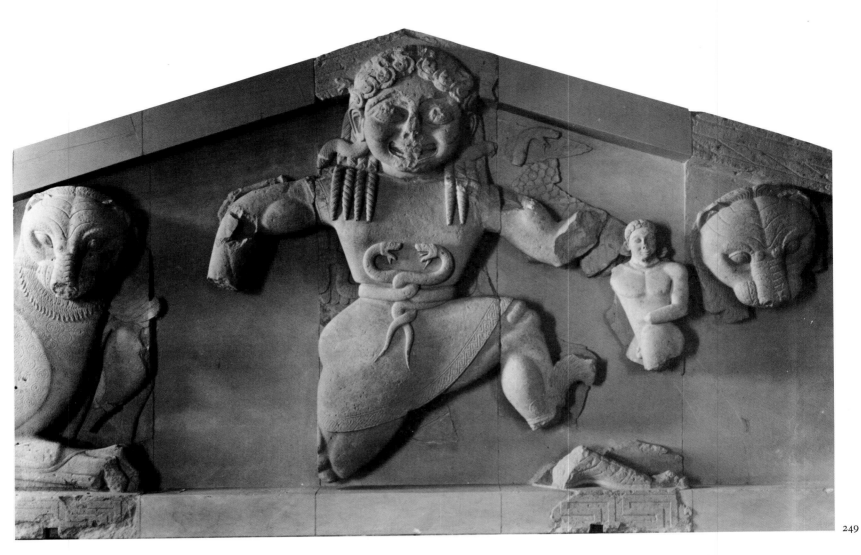

249

249 *The Gorgon Medusa, from the pediment of the
Temple of Artemis at Corfu (c. 600–580 B.C.),
probably there to scare off evil spirits, since a Gorgon's
glance was capable of turning someone to stone.
Archaeological Museum, Corfu*

250 *Bronze helmet (c. 9th–7th century B.C.) decorated with ancient medical symbol of twined snakes,
which may have offered symbolic protection to the
wearer. Collection Norbert Schimmel, New York*

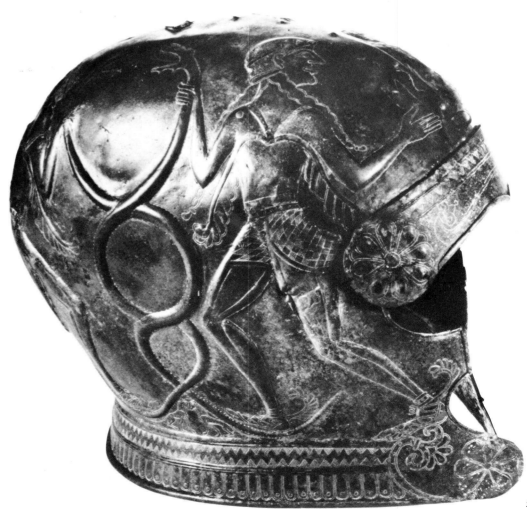

250

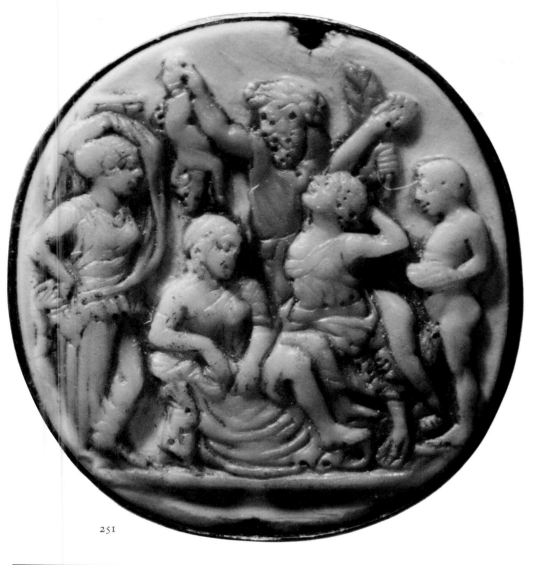

251

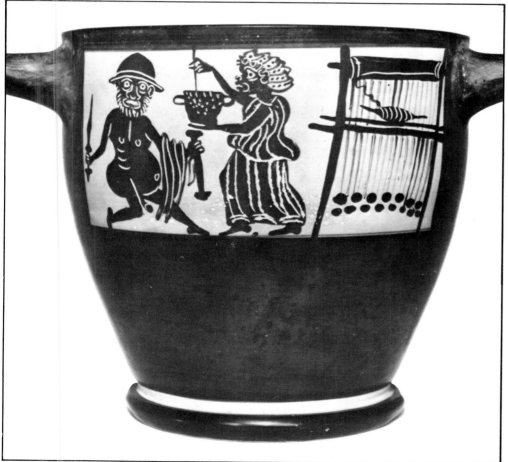

252

251 *Archaic cameo (c. 7th–6th century* B.C.*) showing famous healer Melampos treating mad daughters of King Proetos by spilling pig's blood on their foreheads. The Louvre, Paris*

252 *Detail from Greek drinking vessel showing Circe offering Odysseus the same potion she had used in turning his men to swine. However, Odysseus had been given a protective herb medicine by Hermes and was able to outwit her. Ashmolean Museum, Oxford*

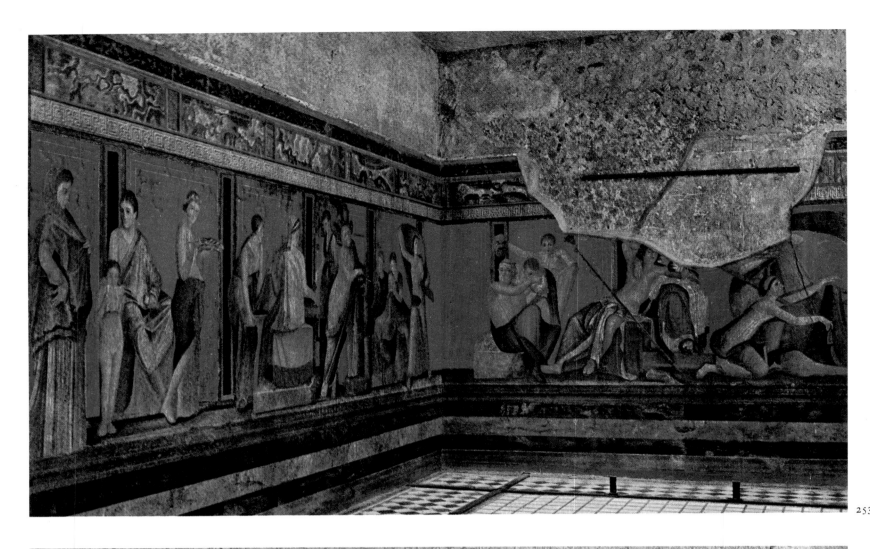

253

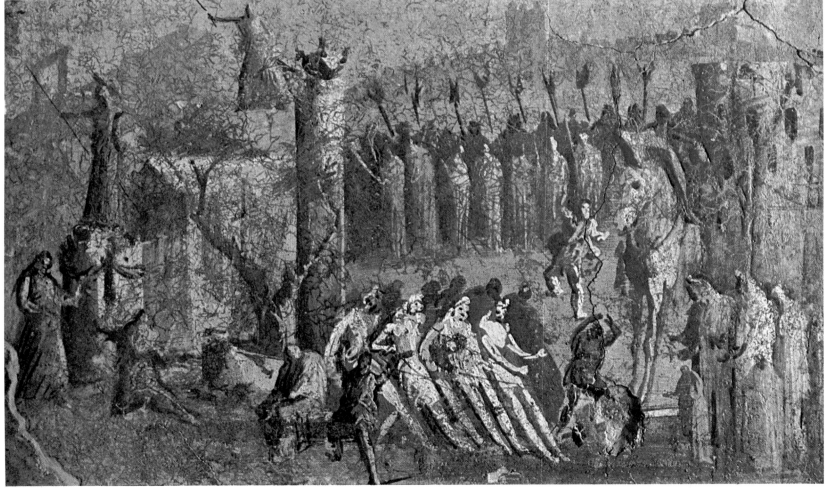

254

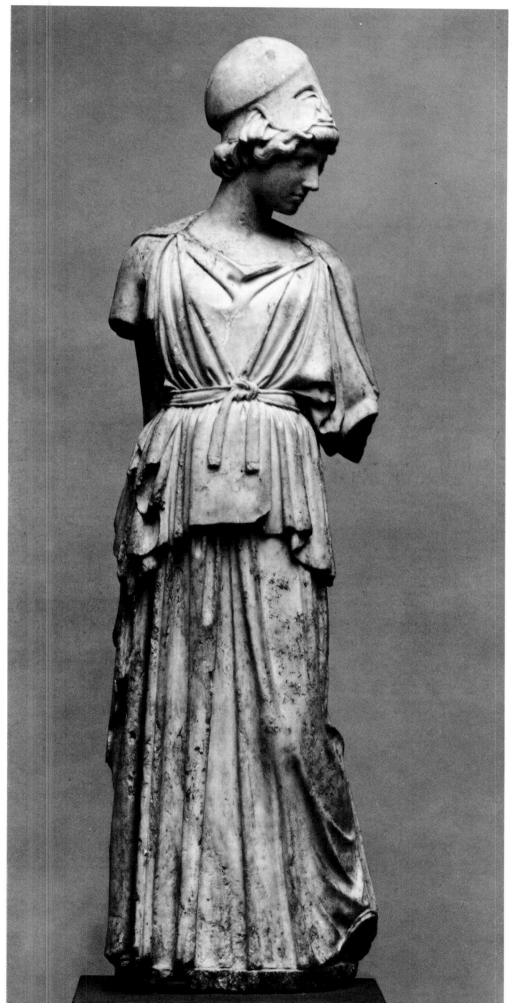

255

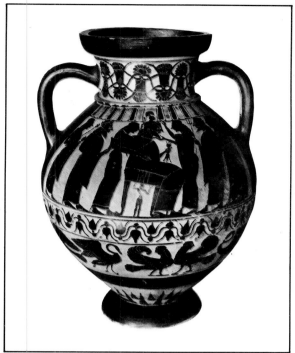

256

253 *Dionysian mystery cult depicted in Pompeian Villa of the Mysteries (c. 50 B.C.). Although not fully understood today, this Roman cult was based on ancient Greek worship of Dionysos, god of wine and fertility.*

254 *Wall painting (c. A.D. 63–79) from Pompeii illustrating Trojan Horse story from* Iliad, *which also tells that medical god Asclepios had been a warrior-king in Trojan War. Museo Archeologico Nazionale, Naples*

255 *Marble statue of Athena (c. 6th–5th century B.C.), daughter of Zeus and patron goddess of Athens and of the eyes. Städtische Galerie Liebighaus, Museum Alter Plastik, Frankfurt*

256 *Attic-style Greek vase (c. 7th century B.C.) depicting Athena's birth from forehead of Zeus, whose wife Hera was the protectress of mothers in childbirth. The Louvre, Paris*

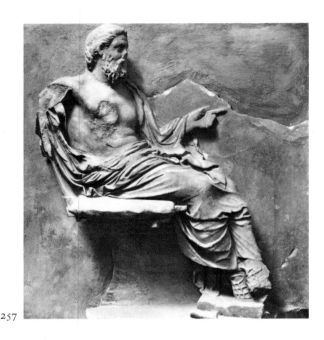

257

257 *Asclepios, god of healing, shown on a metope from the Temple of Asclepios at Epidauros (c. 4th century B.C.), one of the most famous of the healing temples. National Archaeological Museum, Athens*

258 *Three principal healing deities—Apollo, the centaur Chiron, and Asclepios—shown in Pompeian wall painting (c. 1st century A.D.). Apollo, the father of Asclepios, had entrusted the boy to Chiron for educating. Museo Archeologico Nazionale, Naples*

259 *Asclepios and his family depicted on votive tablet (c. 370–270 B.C.) found at Thyrea in Argolis. His sons Machaon and Podalirios became patron gods of surgeons and physicians. His daughters Hygeia and Panacea became goddesses of health and remedies. National Archaeological Museum, Athens*

260 *Detail of the marble Apollo from the west pediment of the Temple of Zeus at Olympia (c. 460 B.C.). Apollo, patron deity of medicine, was the father of Asclepios, who eventually replaced his sire as god of healing. Archaeological Museum, Olympia*

retreat of Chiron, the centaur, who raised the child and taught him all there was to know about the healing arts, especially in regard to plants and medicines. When the boy grew to manhood he had become so skillful that he even brought a dead man back to life. Zeus, the chief Olympian god, fearing that the afterworld would be depopulated if Asclepios continued to resurrect people, struck down the healer with a thunderbolt. Asclepios was then brought into the heavens as a deity.

By the time of Pindar, the unfairness of the gods in the plot had become unacceptable, and so alterations were made in the legend to fit the changed notions of morality. Coronis was turned into an adulteress who deceived both Apollo and her husband, thus deserving her treatment. Asclepios's punishment was made acceptable by having him perform the resuscitation for a fee rather than a noble purpose. This revision also showed that every physician, even Asclepios, should be punished for *hubris*, the sin of aspiring to what belongs to the gods; that nature must not be thwarted; that physicians are mercenaries—perhaps an indication of common attitudes of the time.

Asclepios had a large family, most of whom had health and medical functions. His wife Epione soothed pain, and his daughter Hygeia was the deity of health who came to represent prevention of disease. Panacea, another daughter, represented treatment. The boy Telesphoros who normally accompanied him stood for convalescence.

The healing temples of Asclepios originated about the sixth century B.C., apparently in Thessaly—either in Tricca (according to both the *Iliad* and Hesiod) or in Epidauros (on the basis of archaeological evidence). By the fourth century B.C. temples were in many places on the mainland, including the Argolid, Mantinea, Gortys, Cyllene, Corinth, Aegina (just off the coast), Athens (following a plague in 410 B.C.), and Piraeus. Asclepios was not recognized on the island of Cos, the birthplace of Hippocrates, until the fourth century B.C.—first as a sort of healing partner with Apollo. This was after Hippocrates had died, so there could have been no connection with local medical practice on Cos during his lifetime. After the temple to Asclepios was established, it flourished for centuries, indeed outlasting the Hippocratic teaching group on the island.

Two of the most famous temples to Asclepios (established in the fourth century B.C.), second only to that of Epidauros, were in Pergamon on the coast of Asia Minor and on the nearby island of Rhodes. Delos and Lebera also established temples soon after. There was a rapid spread of the cult throughout the Greek world—east to Ephesos and beyond, south to Crete and Africa, west to Taras (Tarentum) and Syracuse. In Egypt, the divinity of Asclepios became mingled with that of the deified Imhotep, as Asclepios-Imhoutes. After the death of Alexander in 323 B.C., the strong support by the ruling Ptolemies for the god Serapis as the healing divinity seems to have been followed by another merger with Asclepios. Apparently the legend was so persuasive, and Asclepios so satisfied the need for a personal, compassionate divinity, that he inherited, replaced, or merged with the power and influence of each local healing god, wherever the Asclepieian rites were introduced.

The first temple to Asclepios in Rome was erected in 295 B.C. According to the story, a request was brought to the temple in Epidauros for help in stopping the plague then raging in Rome. The Epidaurian snake came out of the temple precincts, boarded the waiting ship, sailed to the island in the Tiber, and there disembarked. A temple was built on the spot, and the epidemic ended.

Each Asclepieian temple was a conglomeration of buildings and areas, depending in size and opulence on its wealth and influence. The dominant structure was usually the main temple, in which a statue of the god was given a prominent place. The Epidaurian statue is said to have been huge and awe-inspiring with its gold and ivory decorations. Statues of various members of the family of Asclepios were often to be seen either in the temple or within its compounds. Somewhere in the precincts, on the entrance gates or before the portals, were

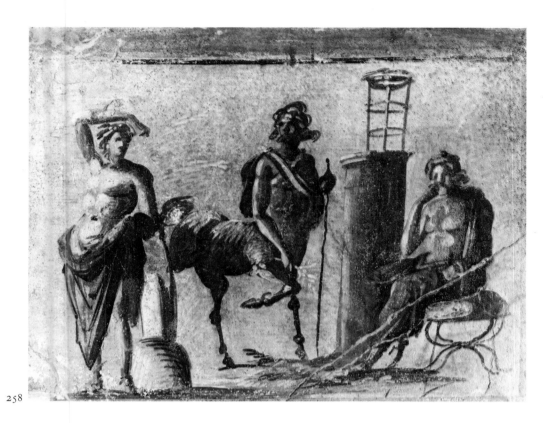

258

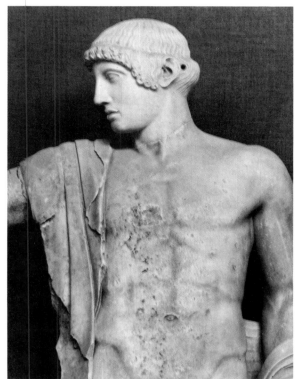

260

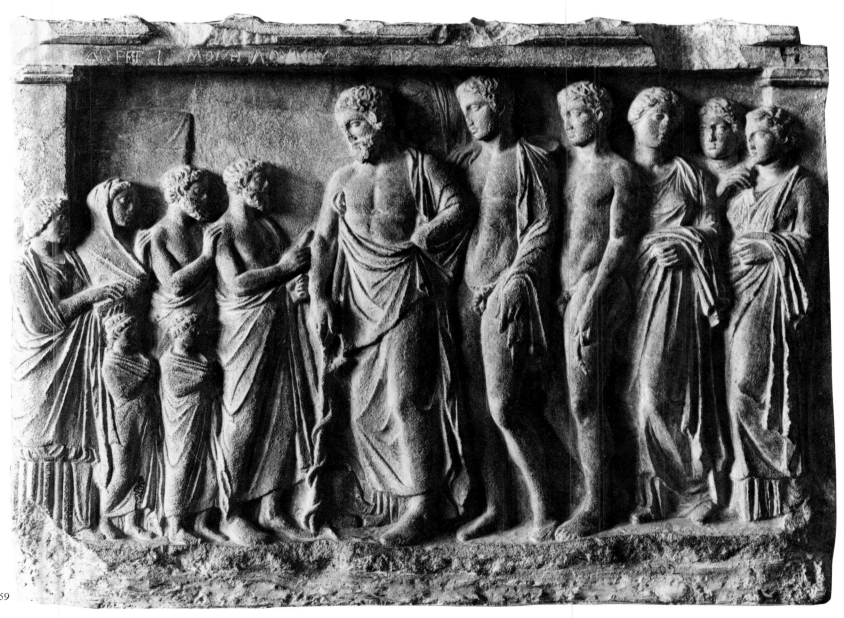

259

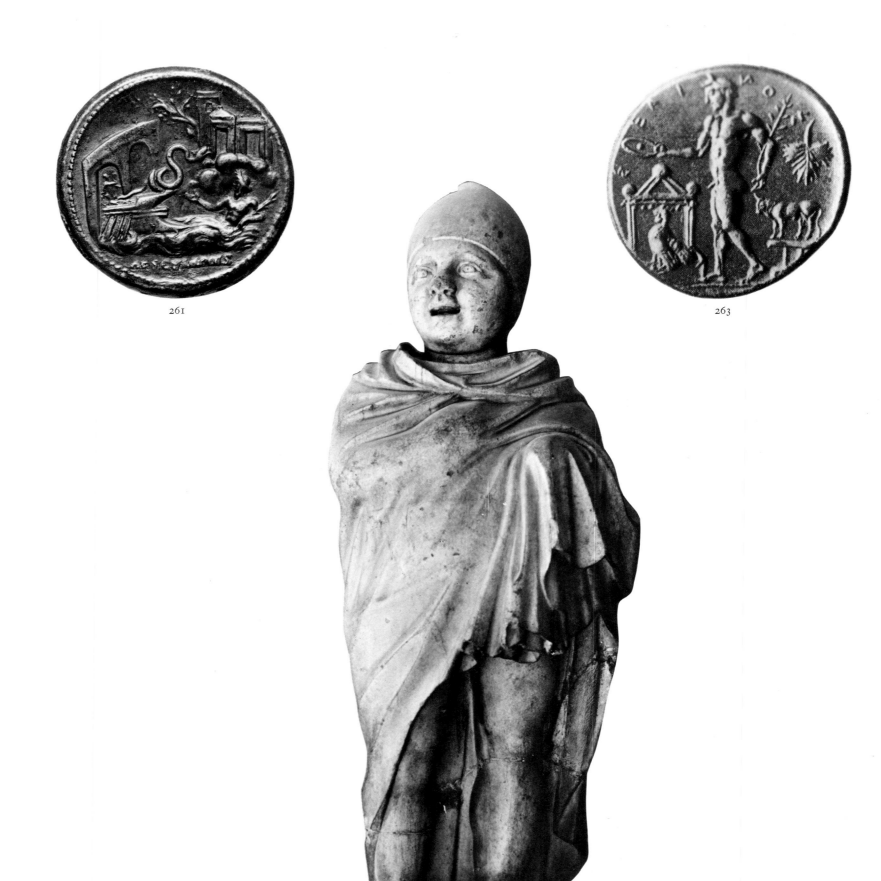

261

263

262

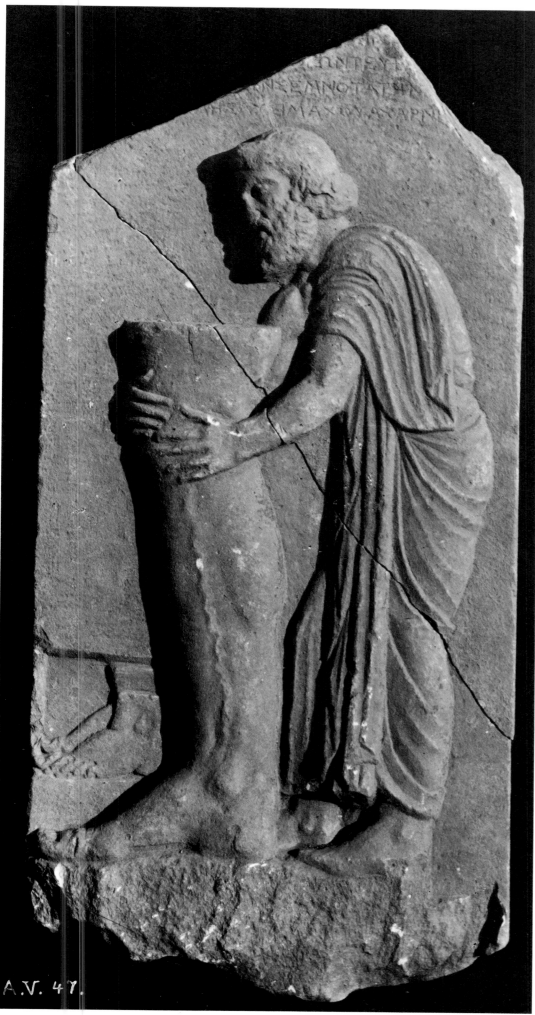

261 *Roman coin (c. 291 B.C.) depicting arrival of Epidaurian serpent on island in the Tiber to end raging plague and to found first temple to Asclepios in Rome. The Louvre, Paris*

262 *Statue of Telesphoros, the boy often depicted in the company of Asclepios, thought to represent convalescence. The Louvre, Paris*

263 *Greek coin showing river-god Silenus sacrificing at altar of Asclepios (represented by cock) in celebration of ending of malaria epidemic by Empedocles, who diverted one river to clear another which was stagnant. British Museum, London*

264 *Votive tablet dedicated to Asclepios, probably in gratitude for relief from varicosities shown on leg. National Archaeological Museum, Athens*

264

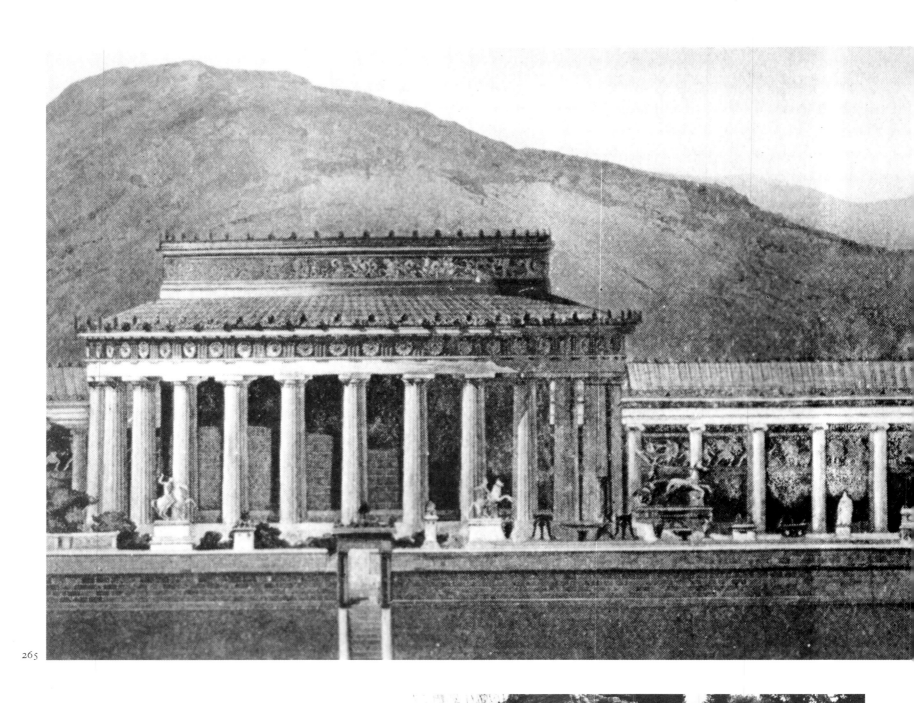

265

266

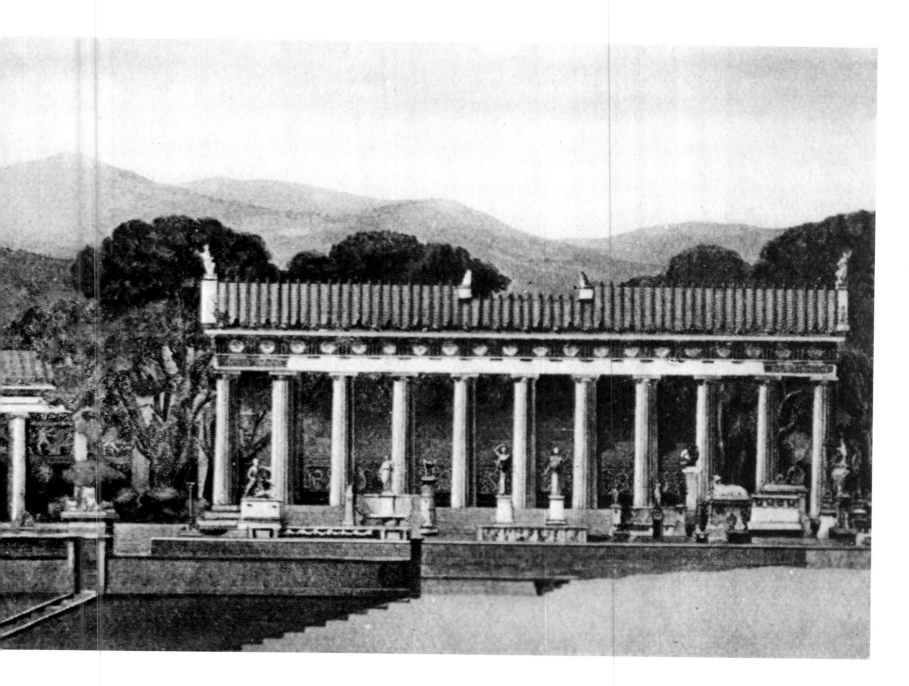

265 *Artist's reconstruction of Temple of Asclepios at Epidauros; this and the Asclepieian at Pergamon were the most opulent of the healing temples. Between Tholos, on* left, *and temple, on* right, *was* Abaton, *where patients slept and dreamed during cure.*

266 *Ruins of the Temple of Asclepios (c. 4th century* B.C.) *on the Acropolis, Athens. One of about 200 such sanctuaries throughout the Greek world now known to us.*

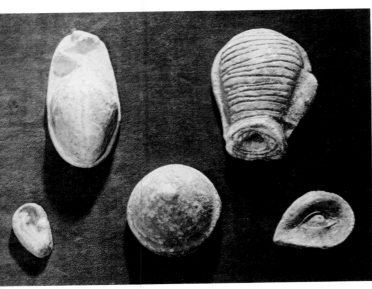

267

267 *Terra-cotta votives from an Etruscan temple at Veii (c. 6th century B.C.), a common type of offering to gods for relief from localized ills, in these instances of the vagina, uterus, breast, ear, and eye. University of Kansas Medical Center, Kansas City*

tablets describing earlier miraculous cures and votive offerings which expressed gratitude for successful results. A round building, the *tholos*, contained water for purification, sometimes in a pool or bubbling from a sacred spring. Here, too, paintings and decorations were frequent.

The most important structure to the ailing suppliant was the incubation site, the *abaton*, where the actual cure took place in the worshiper's dreams. All the preparations and anticipations were prelude to what happened within the *abaton*, where the patient went to sleep until he was visited by the god.

The large temple compounds like that at Epidauros might have included a theater, stadium, and gymnasium, serving to entertain, soothe, and otherwise affect people's spirits. Often inns and temporary housing were also necessary, though usually situated outside the boundaries of the complex. The Asclepieian temples were extremely popular among both rich and poor. Rather than forerunners of hospitals, they seem to have been in modern terms a mixture of religious shrine and health spa.

The ceremony itself, begun after sundown, was surrounded by well-developed rituals which, together with the impressiveness of the buildings, the diversions outside, and the influence of many successful case histories, put the visitor into a mental state receptive to the healing ministrations of the priests and staff.

Prior abstinence from specific foods and wine or even fasting could be required, and a clean white robe was to be worn after ritual bathing. A gift or sacrifice to the god Asclepios followed, which might be food, an animal, or some other evidence of obeisance. In later times, a rooster came to be particularly common as a donation to Asclepios; its special significance may have derived from Zoroastrianism, where the crowing of a cock was believed to drive off evil spirits and prevent illness.

The suppliant was now ready for the vital part of the ceremony: incubation. He or she would lie on a pallet, usually of skins, and await a visit by the god. There appears to be little evidence that drugs induced the somnolence or half-awake state in which worshipers found themselves. During the night, the priest, dressed as Asclepios, accompanied by his daughters, servants, assistants, and snake or dog, would make his "rounds" (in the semidark), moving from sleeper to sleeper, administering the cure or giving advice. Usually the impressive retinue carried medicines, bandages, and other accoutrements of physicians in the world outside the temple. The patient was treated by the god, by his assistants, or by an accompanying snake or dog which might lick the affected part. To treat a woman's sterility, a snake was placed on her abdomen, and in one situation, a woman dreamed that a large snake had intercourse with her. Other animals also participated in the curing process, including a sacred goose which would bite a boil. The divinity used a variety of treatments: laying on of hands, applying a medication, performing a surgical operation, or giving instructions or advice.

By morning the visitor expected to be cured. Sometimes it took longer, and the person might have to remain in the precincts or nearby for days. In any case, before departing from the temple, the cured person was expected to leave a sign of his gratitude—a modest token if poor, a sumptuous gift if rich.

A great many different techniques were used by the god, but most often they were clearly based on the usual practices of the secular doctors and the folklore of the day. Sometimes the precise actions in regular surgical operations were employed, with blood dripping on the floor and assistants holding the patient while the god-physician operated. Even conservative, nonoperative surgery was practiced, in one instance countering the advice of a person's physician for surgical drainage of an abscess on the chest. He was told the pus would later break out by itself, thus draining the chest.

Not all methods used were copies of the rational procedures of physicians. Some were magical and fantastic. Also a vicarious kind of treatment was occasionally reported, whereby one person could sometimes stand in for another,

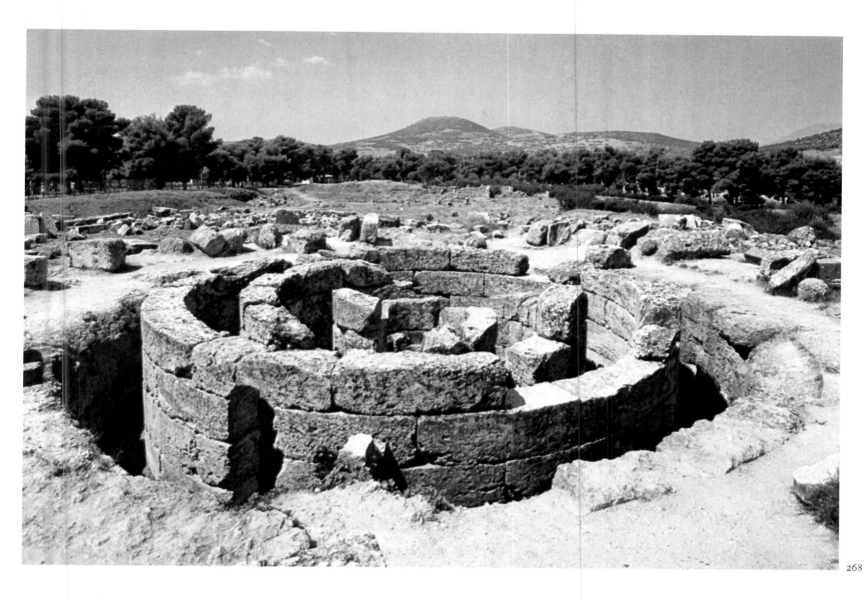

268 *Restored* Tholos *of Temple of Asclepios at*
Epidauros (c. 360 B.C.*). Designed by Polycleitos the*
Younger and used as a place for sacrifices to the god–
physician.

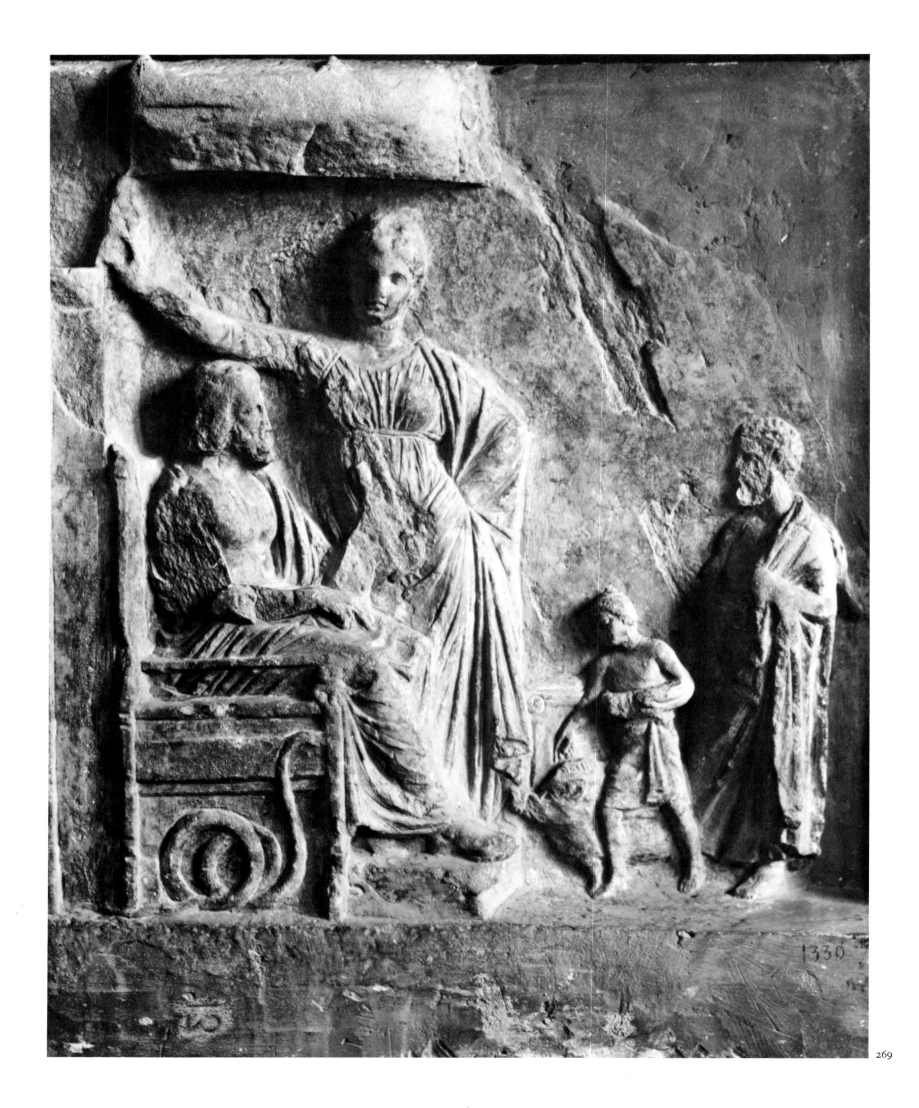

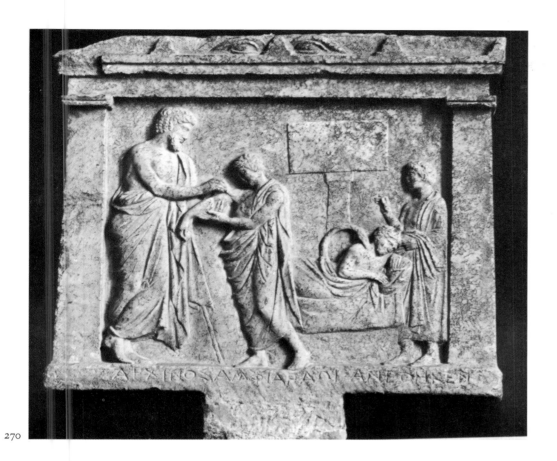

270

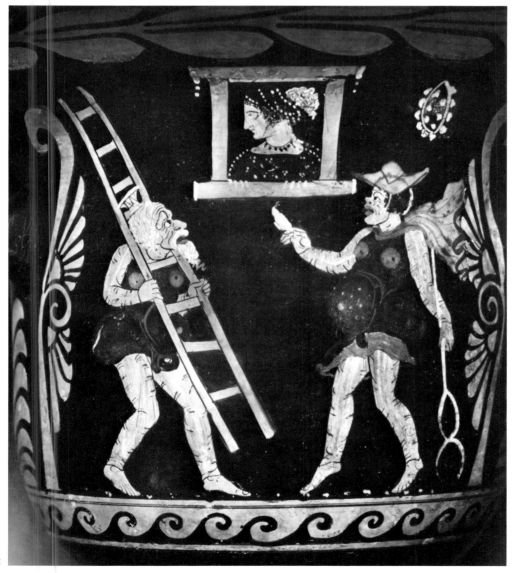

271

269 *Bas-relief (c. 4th century* B.C.) *showing the god of healing Asclepios and his daughter Hygeia, goddess of health, who was also worshiped at Epidauros and Pergamon, the two major sites of Asclepieian influence. National Archaeological Museum, Athens*

270 *Bas-relief (c. 400–350* B.C.) *thought to show scene in Asclepieian temple where physician-god, daughter Hygeia, and symbolic snake cured patients during sleep of* incubatio. *National Archaeological Museum, Athens*

271 *Scene from Phylax play depicted on Greek vessel of late 4th century* B.C., *typical of diverting entertainment available at temples of Asclepios throughout Greek world. Vatican Museums, Rome*

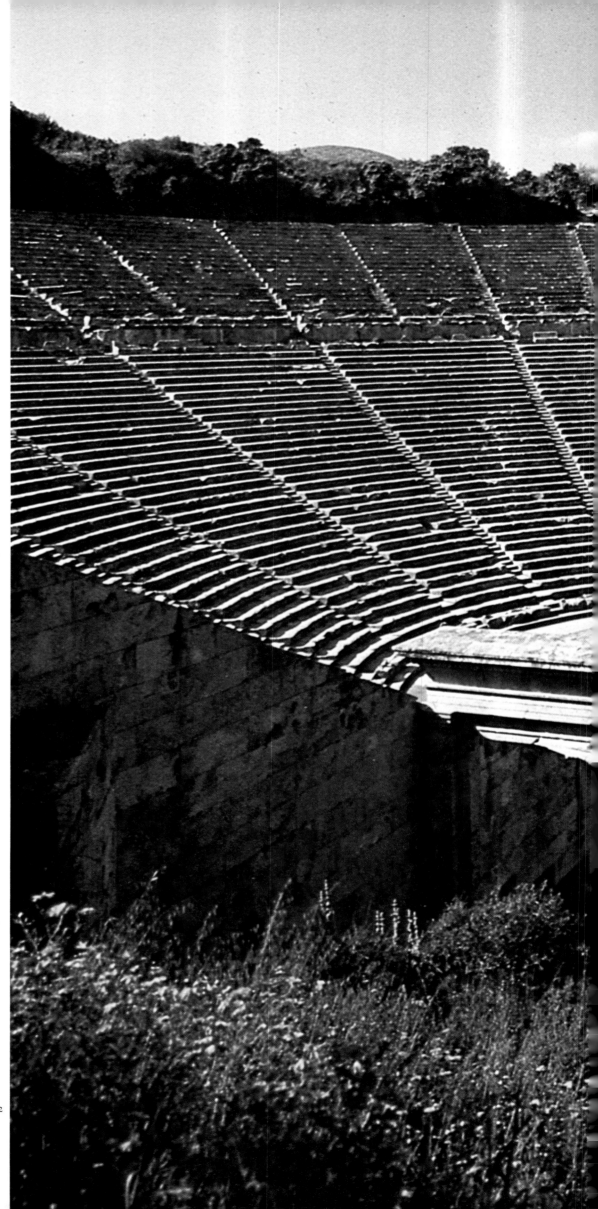

272 *Theater of the Temple of Asclepios (c. 360 B.C.) at Epidauros. Theaters were common at Asclepieian sanctuaries, where their purpose may have been to distract and soothe the ill and worried suppliants.*

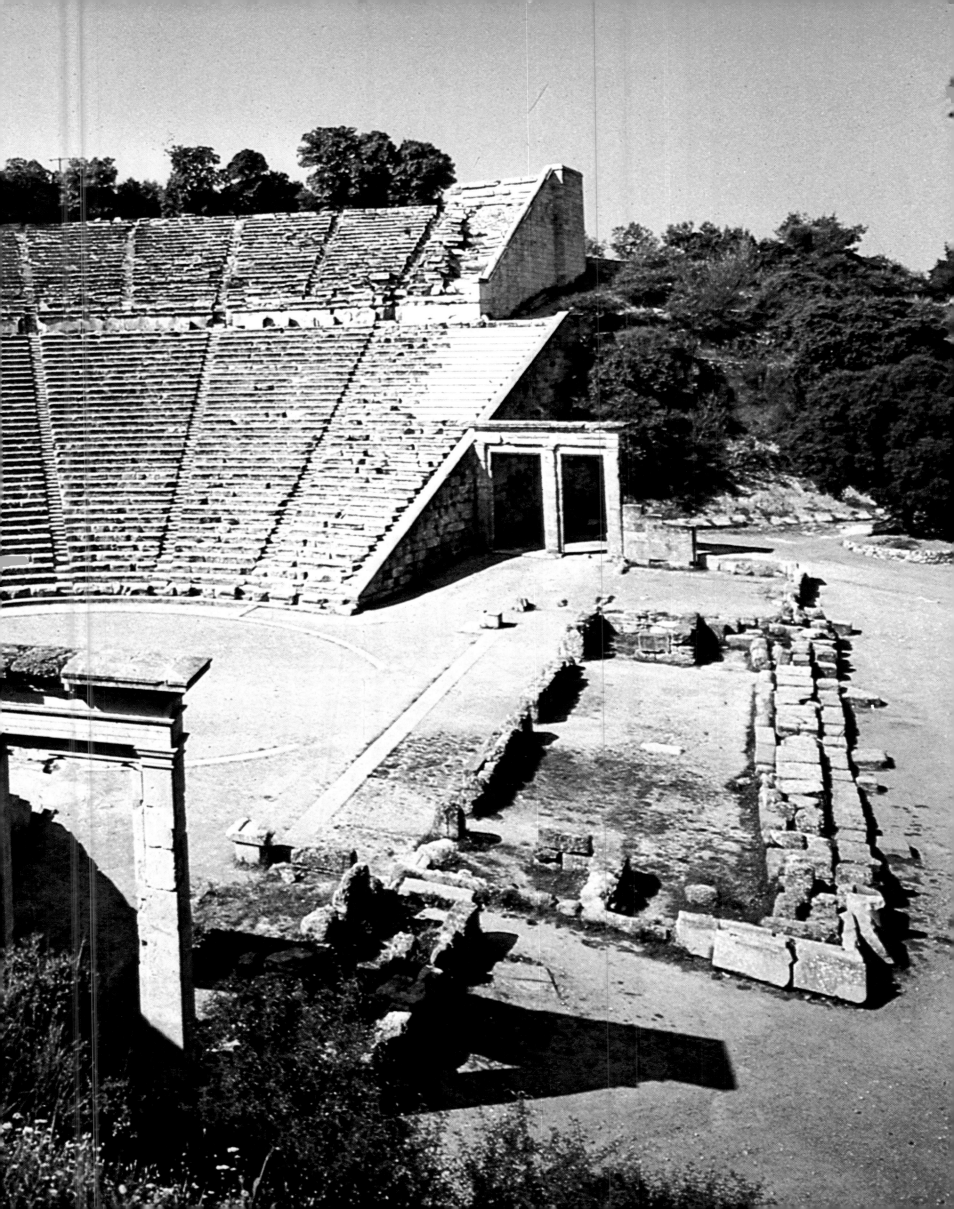

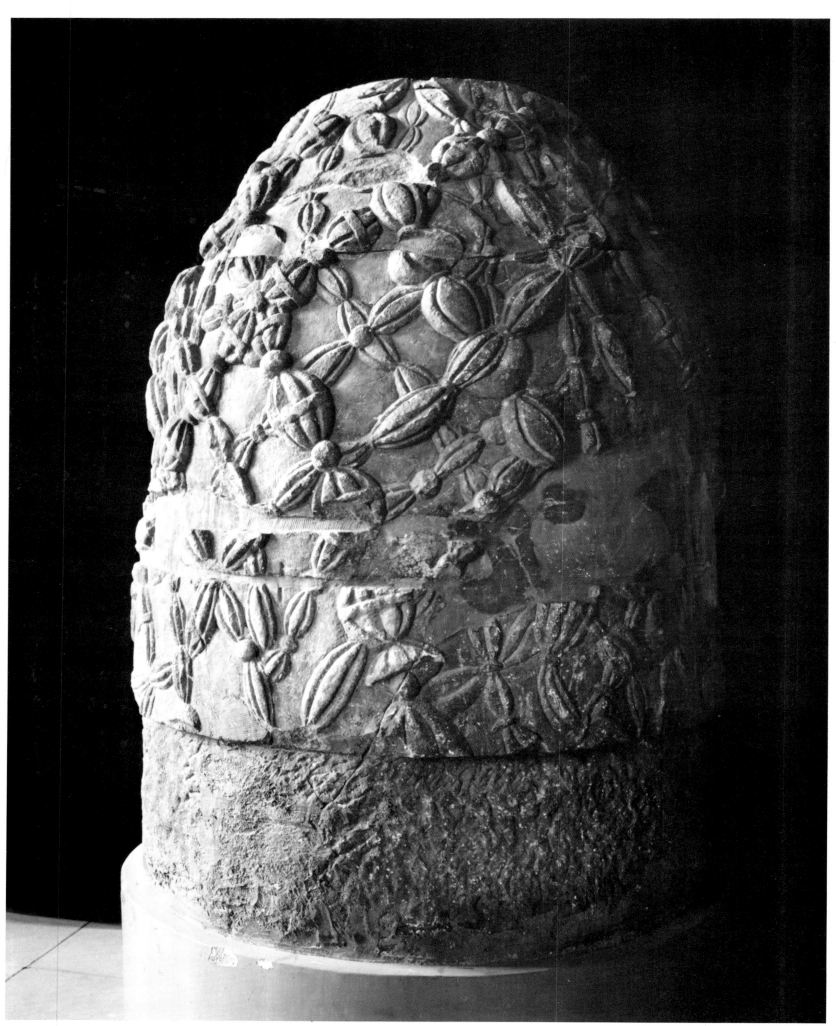

273

going through the incubation so that the other might be cured. Even cure at a distance was supposed to have occurred.

Many types of illness were treated, but the vast majority were of a kind that might be psychically based. Blindness, muteness, and lameness were sometimes cured by what may be characterized as miracle methods, such as bathing in a sacred spring, or by surprise techniques, such as snatching away a boy's crutches in hopes he would instantly chase the thief before remembering he was lame. A particularly ironic cure of blindness was effected on Phalysios by sending him a special tablet at which he was to look. When he looked his sight was restored, but he was shocked to read an order for him to give an exorbitant gift to the temple. Barrenness, impotence, headache, and skin diseases also made up a large part of the list of symptoms reputed to have been cured.

Clearly the most important ingredient in the effectiveness of the temple cure was faith. The suppliant's belief in the efficacy of the god was aided by accounts of cures on tablets and probably by oral descriptions given by temple assistants. Also a feeling of relaxation was engendered by music and comfortable surroundings. The religious and spiritual atmosphere was inspiring, and the appearance and ministrations of the priest acting as Asclepios, with his accompanying retinue, were doubtless impressive.

It is not astonishing that the healing cult of Asclepios was so popular and lasted for so many centuries when one considers that secular physicians had few specific or effective remedies for the organic diseases of the time. Furthermore, since it was considered prudent and moral to refuse to treat the hopeless (to do otherwise was criticized as fraud), the patients had no other pathways open except to charlatans or the temples. Since there must have been instances in which illnesses deemed incurable by physicians were actually psychically based, word of a dramatic success in the temple would surely be spread widely and give hope to numerous sufferers.

It is difficult to know how much of the temple healing was believed by the priests themselves, how much was deliberate deception. In any case, the temples continued to be a haven of hope to the sick even as some physicians were elsewhere using the rational, nonreligious means that were available to them.

273 *Marble* omphalos *from Temple of Apollo at Delphi, which marked center (navel) of earth, where Pythian oracle uttered prophecies and suppliants worshiped patron deity of medicine. Archaeological Museum, Delphi*

Pre-Hippocratic Medicine
The Philosopher–Scientists

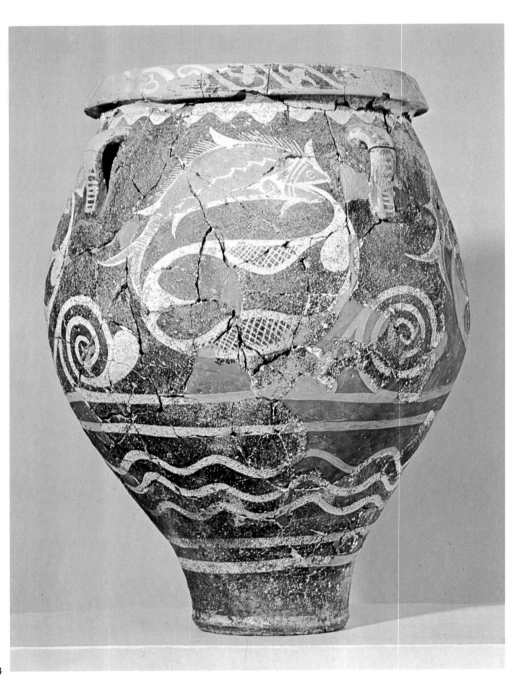

274

GREEK secular, rational medicine, which reached its summit in the time of Hippocrates, was undoubtedly preceded by a long tradition. But we do not know precisely the nature of medicine, or even science, in the centuries between the Homeric period of the ninth or eighth century B.C. and the advent of the philosopher-scientists in the sixth century. Interchanges among Crete, Mycenae, Egypt, and Asia had always contained interlacings of religious and empiric healing methods, so it is likely that this cross-fertilization continued. A few bits of information from Hesiod's *Works and Days* of the eighth century suggest the prevalence of a kind of folk medicine which combined basic hygienic rules with pragmatic use of foods and plants, but it also included religious and magical associations. Therefore, when one comes upon the sixth century—about which we have direct and indirect information on the philosopher-scientists—one is impressed by what appears to be a sudden new approach: an attempt to give all phenomena natural rather than supernatural explanations.

By the time of Thales (640?–546 B.C.), the first true scientist-philosopher of the Greeks, his birthplace Miletos on the Aegean west coast of Asia Minor had become a great port of trade, with an international population and exceptional thinkers and teachers. It was on the periphery of the Greek world, and in that sense typical of the areas in which the new philosophies seem to have developed: the Aegean islands, the Asiatic coast, and Italy and Sicily, in centers which must have been growing over centuries.

Meanwhile, the practice of medicine was probably carried on by itinerant craftsmen, as in Homer's time. Information was transmitted orally from generation to generation, and by the time of Hippocrates (mid-fifth century B.C.) practitioners were engaged in a variety of methods of differing effectiveness. At the same time, medical teaching groups, or "schools," were developing throughout the Greek world and were heirs of both the empiric tradition and the philosophic inquiries of the philosopher-scientists.

Our information about Thales is based on what others wrote about him and quoted from his teachings. ("What is difficult? To know thyself. What is easy? To advise another.") The man who emerges from these accounts had an extraordinarily wide range of interests and a profound effect on his contemporaries and followers. It is no wonder that he was considered among the seven greatest sages.

Thales believed that the basic element in all animal and plant life was water, from which came earth and air. He made many contributions to mathematics, astronomy, navigation, and geometry, and is said to have developed several of the geometric theorems later used by Euclid. The most significant attribute of his work, for which he has been called the "Father of Science," is that his explanations of phenomena did not fall back on supernatural agency. Although he accepted the idea of a God, he did not use religious means to seek or establish the natural processes of the universe or of humans.

At Miletos, two especially influential thinkers followed Thales: Anaximander (fl. c. 560 B.C.) and Anaximenes (fl. c. 546 B.C.). Anaximander (extending the rational views of Thales) taught that all living creatures had their beginnings in water. Even man originally came from a water organism. Anaximander also espoused the doctrine that the universe was constituted of opposite forces in balance and that it was governed by universal laws. His pupil Anaximenes considered air rather than water the primary element and therefore the essential requirement for life.

Heraclitos (fl. c. 500 B.C.), the outstanding philosopher of Ephesos, to the north of Miletos, considered fire rather than water or air as the principal element, but he underlined Anaximander's concept of opposites by suggesting that tensions between opposing forces were essential to the universe and to life. Change was the only constant.

By the sixth century B.C., four basic elements had become generally accepted as the components of all substances: water, earth, fire, and air, each of which had

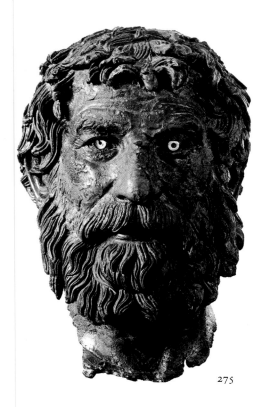

275

274 *Ancient Cretan jar (early 2d millennium B.C.), typical of many Aegean vessels found decorated with images of the sea. From earliest times, the Greeks gained their living from the sea; no wonder early philosophers concluded that all creatures had their beginnings in water. Archaeological Museum, Heraklion, Crete*

275 *Bronze head of a philosopher (early 3d century B.C.), found in the sea off Anticithera, epitomizes ancient philosopher-scientists who were the sources of medical knowledge in the days before Hippocrates. National Archaeological Museum, Athens*

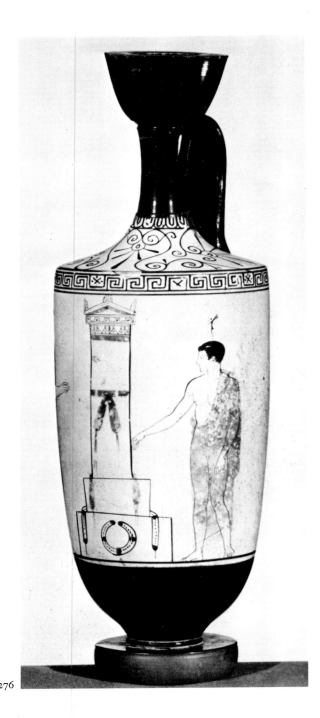

276 *Lecythus by the Achilles Painter (c. 440 B.C.) showing deceased youth before funeral altar with soul hovering above his head. Pythagoreans believed that souls were continually reborn. Collection Norbert Schimmel, New York*

its corresponding characteristic—wet, dry, hot, cold. This doctrine of the four elements and their qualities (later projected into the four humors) continued to affect medical theory for many centuries, even into recent times.

There were many other leaders of what was referred to as the Ionian school because it sprang from the islands and territories to which the ancient mainland Ionians had migrated. Each inquired rationally into the makeup of humans as well as the cosmic environment.

At the western borders of the Greek world in the sixth century, an Italic "school" of philosophers was centered in Sicily and southern Italy. The most famous group was at Crotona, where Pythagoras came to teach. A center of philosophy may have been there before he arrived, but the influence of Pythagoras and the teachings of his followers were to have a profound effect on medicine.

Pythagoras (fl. c. 530 B.C.) was born on the island of Samos just off the coast of Asia Minor, but he emigrated west to Crotona in southern Italy because of his opposition to the tyrant Polycrates. He and his followers formed not only a school of philosophy but also a religious cult that allied itself with the ancient mystical teachings of Orpheos.

The Pythagoreans in the west focused principally on the soul and the spiritual universe, whereas Thales in the east was concerned with matter. Humans were fallen gods eventually capable of returning to divinity, for although the body decayed the soul was continually reborn—even in animals. All life was therefore sacred, and surgical procedures were forbidden since they might interfere with the soul. Their belief in reincarnation resembles some religious ideas developing in India (where the Buddha also lived in the sixth century B.C.).

The basic principle of the Pythagorean universe was not any of the elemental substances but rather the science of numbers, which determined what happened in living creatures as well as in the cosmos. Each number had a special significance beyond its own function in mathematical process. For instance, 1 represented God, 2 stood for matter. Therefore 12 was the universe, divisible by 4 three times. The Pythagoreans also established scientific theories of sound and of musical octaves. Furthermore, as proponents of the mythical teachings of Orpheos, they felt that music should play an important role in their discipline.

Balance in all things was the goal of correct behavior. Opposite pairs of substances and qualities achieved the balance; therefore the number 4 was important to health, and the concept of four elements with four qualities received further impetus, particularly when supported by so influential a school.

As a logical concomitant of Pythagorean beliefs, diet was vegetarian and frugal, but there were a few curious prohibitions against some foods, such as beans. The explanation given by Diogenes Laertius (third century A.D.) was that in mythical times the bean had been a symbol of the head and therefore of the mind, which might have made it taboo to this sect. Cabbage, anise, and squill were recommended to maintain health and treat illness, and external applications of plant substances were also permissible, but the chief Pythagorean therapy consisted of diet, exercise, music, and meditation.

Other "schools" of medicine (that is, associations of philosophers, medical teachers, practitioners, and students) had been developing nearby in Sicily, in Cyrene on the African coast, and in Rhodes, Cnidos, and Cos at the eastern periphery of the Greek world. But Crotona was the most famous of philosophic centers according to Herodotos. Democedes, one of the best-known practitioners among the Greeks, was educated at Crotona, and his reputation increased after he went to Aegina and to Athens. He was persuaded to come to Samos by its ruler Polycrates, but when Samos was taken by the Persians Democedes was brought along to the court of Darius. There chance brought him to the attention of the king, whose ankle injury he was able to treat successfully, as well as his daughter's abscessed breast. We do not know his method of treatment, but Egyptian physicians had previously been unsuccessful in relieving the king's difficulties.

186

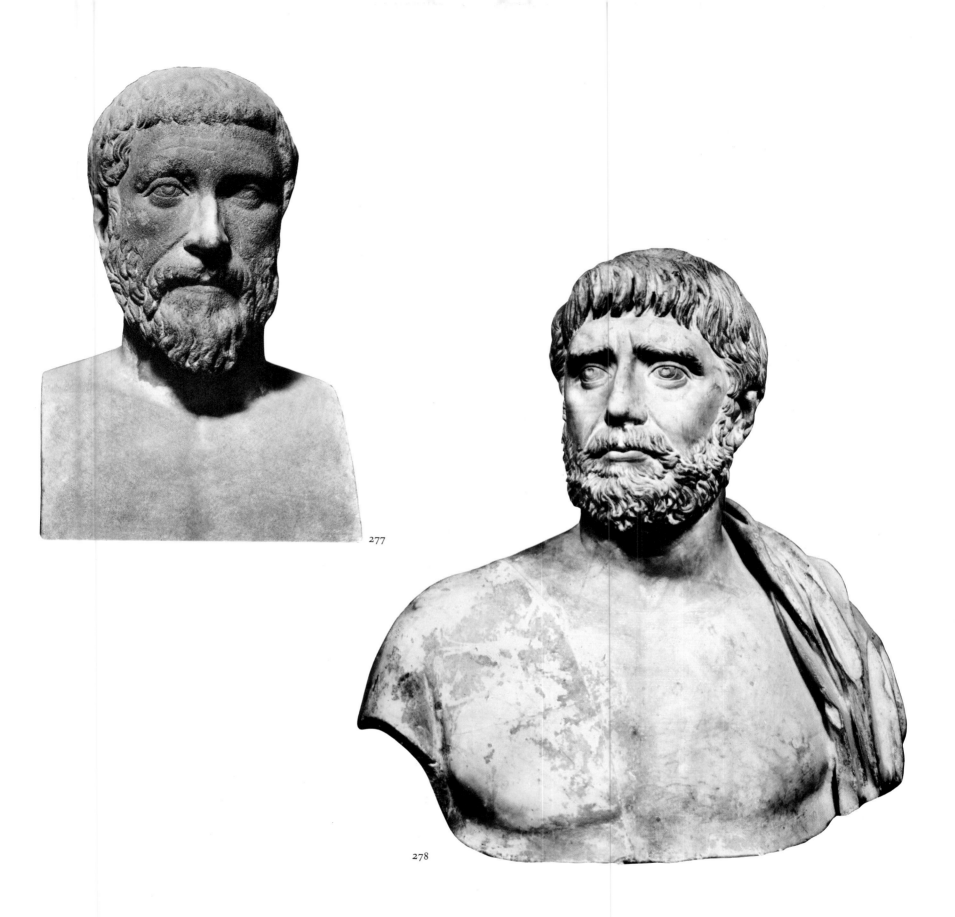

277

278

A younger member of the Crotona school (possibly of the fifth century B.C.) was Alcmaeon, whose principal focus was on man, not the cosmos. His book *Concerning Nature* may be the beginning of Greek medical literature, but only a few fragments survive. Works by a number of later writers—especially Aristotle—are the principal sources for what was contained in Alcmaeon's teachings. He held a general philosophic attitude: health is harmony; disease is a disturbance of the harmony. But he also believed that investigation (including dissection), not just philosophy, was needed in order to understand the body. His combination of direct observation and experimental testing stands out as unique in his time.

Although many remarkable facts emerged from his dissections (probably on

277 *The philosopher-scientist Pythagoras, founder of a "school" with profound influence on early medicine, as seen in a Roman copy of a Greek bust. Museo Capitolino, Rome*

278 *Thales of Miletos, the first true scientist-philosopher of the Greeks, who taught that water was the basic element in life. Roman copy of a Greek bust. Museo Capitolino, Rome*

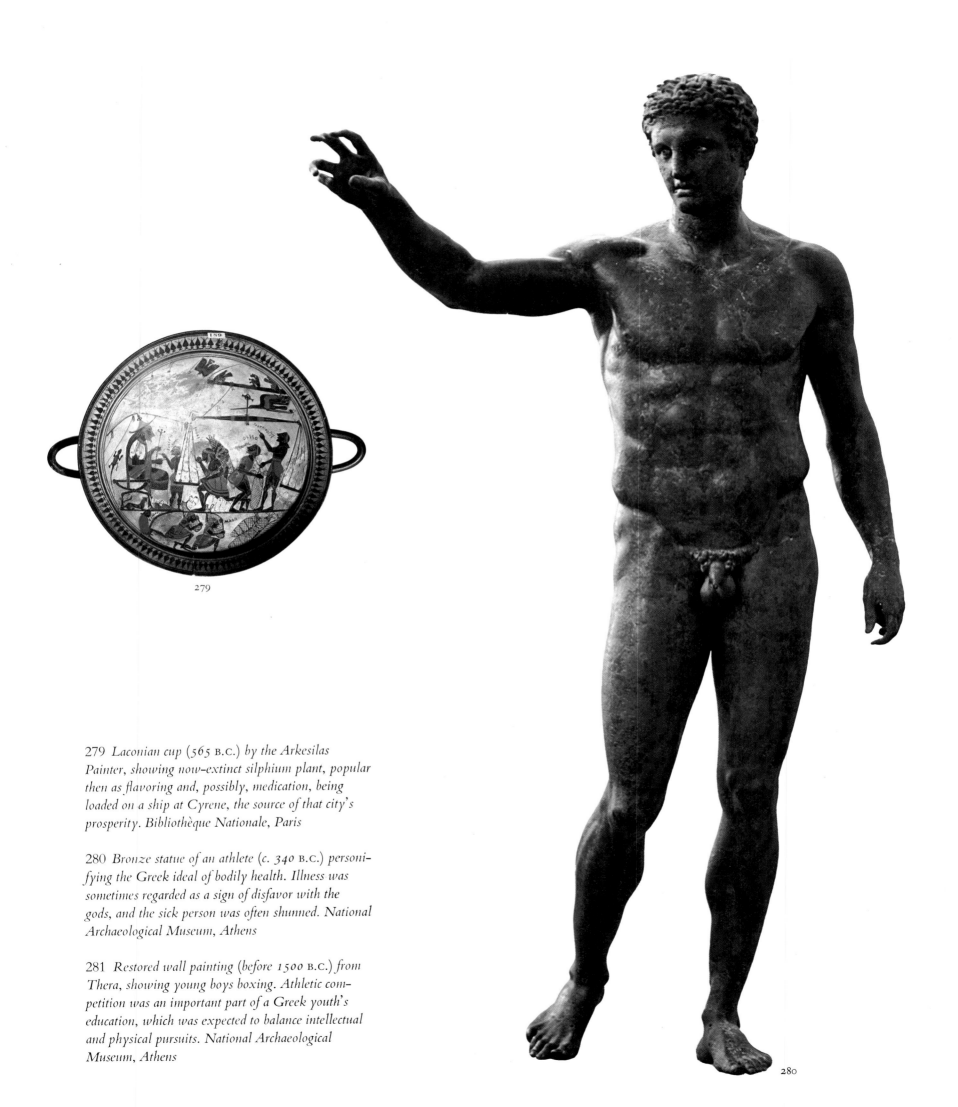

279 *Laconian cup (565 B.C.) by the Arkesilas Painter, showing now-extinct silphium plant, popular then as flavoring and, possibly, medication, being loaded on a ship at Cyrene, the source of that city's prosperity. Bibliothèque Nationale, Paris*

280 *Bronze statue of an athlete (c. 340 B.C.) personifying the Greek ideal of bodily health. Illness was sometimes regarded as a sign of disfavor with the gods, and the sick person was often shunned. National Archaeological Museum, Athens*

281 *Restored wall painting (before 1500 B.C.) from Thera, showing young boys boxing. Athletic competition was an important part of a Greek youth's education, which was expected to balance intellectual and physical pursuits. National Archaeological Museum, Athens*

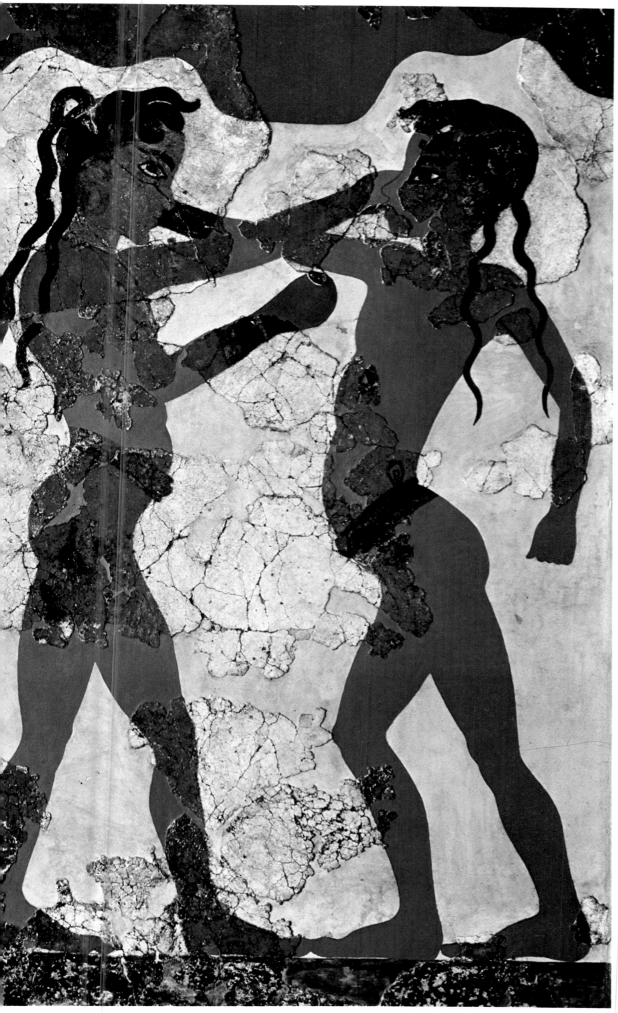

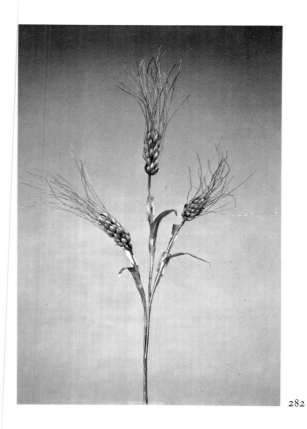

282 *Wheat reproduced in gold (4th–3d century* B.C.), *found near Syracuse, Sicily, one of the great preHippocratic centers of medical learning. Collection Norbert Schimmel, New York*

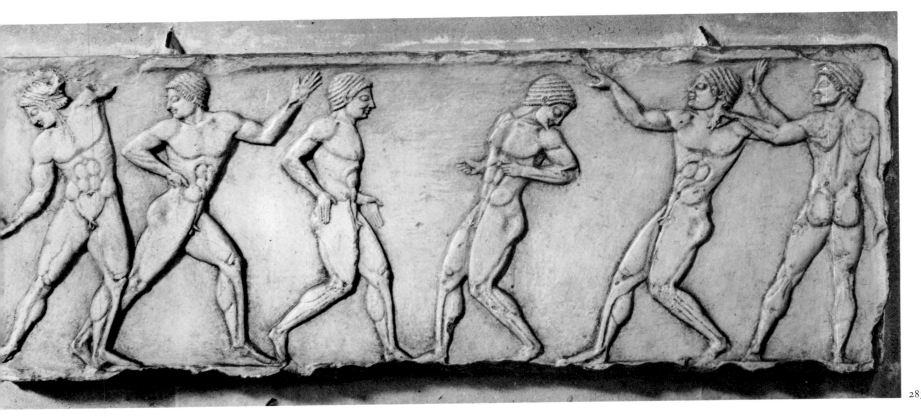

283

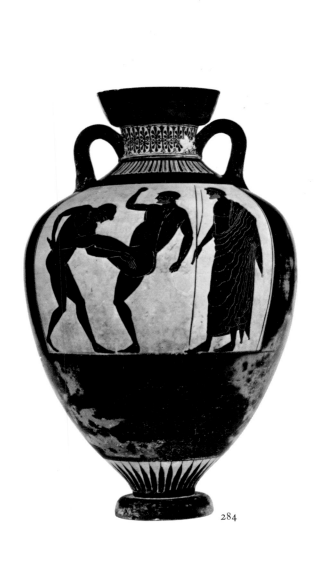

284

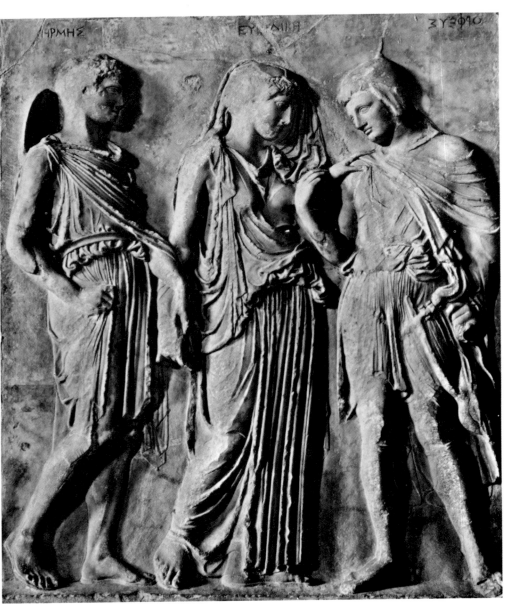

285

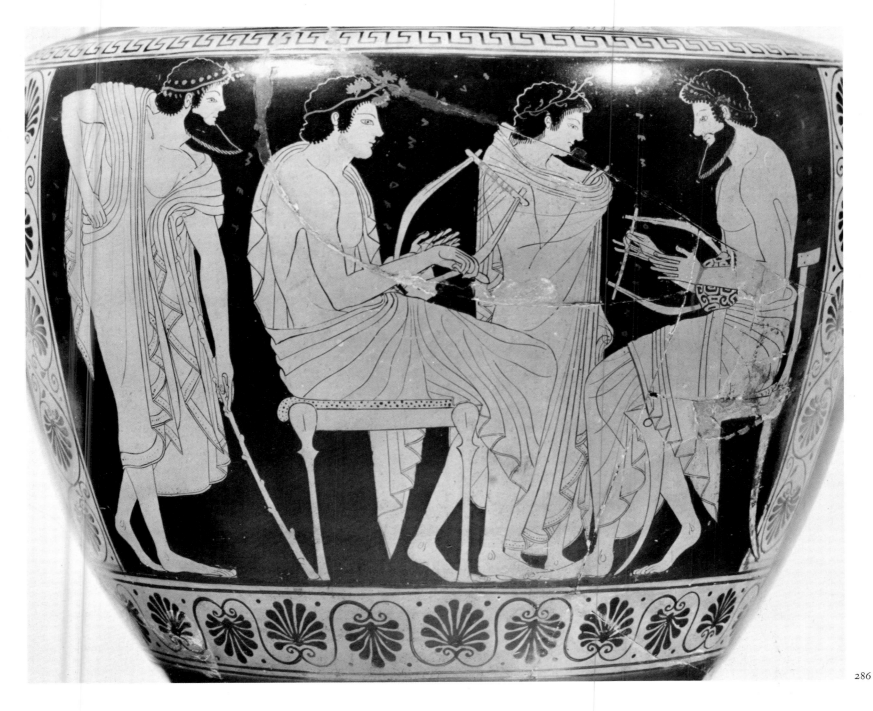

286

283 *One of three reliefs, showing Greek youth at athletics, on a statue base (late 6th century B.C.) found in a wall built in Athens by Themistocles in 479–478 B.C. Athletics was more than just entertainment. National Archaeological Museum, Athens*

284 *Two youths practice wrestling, while their teacher, possibly a gymnast, observes, on black-figured Panathenaic amphora (500–490 B.C.) attributed to the Kleophrades Painter, from Vulci. Rogers Fund, Metropolitan Museum of Art, New York*

285 *Votive relief (5th century B.C.) showing Orpheus and Euridyce with Hermes. The disciples of Pythagoras were also followers of the mythological Orpheus, emphasizing music and mathematics in their doctrines. Museo Archeologico Nazionale, Naples*

286 *Music lesson shown on red-figured vase by Phintias (6th century B.C.). Music was an element in Pythagorean medical therapy, and youth on crutch may have been there for health benefits. Staatliche Antikensammlungen, Munich*

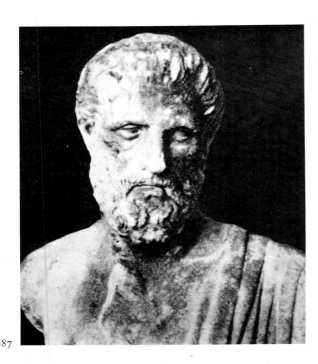

287

287 *Statue, once thought to represent Hippocrates, found on Isle of Cos, where one of the great medical centers of antiquity gained fame late in the 5th century* B.C. *Cos Museum, Cos*

288 *Roman copy of a Greek sculpture of Democritos, who taught that all matter was composed of "atoms." He was called the laughing philosopher because he advised good cheer. Museo Capitolino, Rome*

289 *This bust, also once thought to be a portrait of Hippocrates, is now considered to be of Chrysippos, one of the outstanding leaders of the Cnidian "school." Museo Capitolino, Rome*

animals), his most striking contribution was to establish the connection between the sense organs and the brain. Even the optic nerves and their chiasm (crossing) were clearly delineated. Going further he concluded that the brain was the organ of the mind, not only perceiving sensations but also responsible for thought and memory. About a century later, Aristotle, one of the greatest philosopher-scientists in history, disagreed entirely with Alcmaeon, believing instead that the heart was the center of sensation.

Alcmaeon was also a hostage of his age. For instance, he speculated that sleep occurred when the blood vessels in the brain were filled; withdrawal of blood from the brain caused waking. Along with his careful dissections of the eye and demonstrations of the pathways connecting the brain and the eye, he reported that the eye contains both water and fire. However, he condemned the commonly accepted belief of the time that semen originated in the brain. His doctrine of the balancing of opposite qualities and its effect on health were in agreement with Pythagorean teachings. But the breadth of his detailed examinations and rational concepts opened a new view on the acquisition of medical knowledge. He can be called virtually the first medical scientist.

Further south in Sicily another Greek Italic center of medicine flourished. The best-known member of this group was Empedocles (c. 493–c. 433 B.C.). Many fragments of his writings survive, and much other information about him is contained in later commentaries. From these sources historians have obtained a picture of an aristocratic leader of enormous egotism but also of exceptional knowledge and ability. He went about dressed in purple finery and decorated with flowers, boasting in verse of his own godlike nature and power of accomplishment. Yet, he did work prodigious feats for his city and its citizens. During a time when it was still possible for one person to encompass many fields he seemed to outdistance anyone else in being many-sided. Poet, statesman, priest, philosopher, scientist, physician—he excelled in all.

His treatises were written in verse, a common practice, and he preached the Pythagorean doctrines concerning purity of mind, body, and behavior, as well as the virtues of regulated, temperate diet and exercise. His teaching that gained the widest influence was the concept that all things inanimate and animate were comprised of four basic elements: water, air, fire, and earth. Although this belief was accepted before Empedocles, he is often credited with its origination.

The elements according to Empedocles are joined together during life and separate after death. Substances are formed by attraction and repulsion of the elements in different proportions. He saw that the element air had substance and could exert pressure. The flow of blood through the body was connected in some way with propulsion by air. Respiration occurred not only through the nose and mouth but also through respiratory pores in the skin; after Hippocrates, a system of medicine called Methodist was developed from this idea. Even today some speak of the opening of the pores in hot weather and their closing in the cold.

The theories espoused by the followers of Empedocles led to further elaboration and were a step toward the concept that matter is composed of atoms. For instance, Anaxagoras (c. 500–c. 428 B.C.) held that each element was composed of many small invisible particles or seeds which were released from a food by digestion and then reconstituted into components of the body—such as bone and muscle. However, it was Democritos and Leucippos later in the fifth century B.C. who advanced the fully developed theory that all matter is made up of atoms of different size, weight, shape, and position. All animate and inanimate objects were originally created by the collisions and combinations of atoms. Democritos also dealt with diet, health and illness, and his speculative writings had a great influence on medical as well as scientific thought.

Of the other philosopher-scientist groups flourishing in the sixth and fifth centuries, two of the most important in influence were at Cnidos on the Asia Minor shore, and at Cos on an island off the coast. However, their fame may have come late in the fifth century B.C. because the historian Herodotos, who wrote in the mid-fifth century, spoke of the "schools" at Cyrene in Africa and Crotona in Italy but made no mention of either Cnidos or Cos.

It was on Cos that Hippocrates lived and taught. The writings of the Coan teachers, presumably by Hippocrates or by others of his time, are called the *Corpus Hippocraticum* and will be considered in a later section.

Neighboring Cnidos on the mainland was the location of a group of teachers and students that was probably as important as Cos and slightly older. The "Cnidian Sentences" was a collection of medical treatises which has not survived and is only known to us by mention in the *Corpus Hippocraticum* and through later commentators on Hippocrates, especially Galen in the second century A.D. Scholars consider it probable that some writings attributed to Hippocrates actually came from Cnidos.

For a long time historians have assumed that Cos and Cnidos were rival centers, but more recent analysis suggests that the two groups may not have been much different or even competitive. Nevertheless, a summary of the attitudes which scholars heretofore have believed were prevalent at the two locations may help clarify medical principles in the Greek world.

In Cnidos diseases were supposed to have been elaborately categorized according to the organ affected, a system with some resemblance to the practice in the Mesopotamian lands east of Cnidos. Treatments which were linked with and listed with each disease were simple and sparse.

In contrast, the Hippocratists, it was assumed, made virtually no classifications and used empiric rather than theoretical bases for the management of patients. With respect to treatment, however, Hippocratic methods were not much different from the Cnidian.

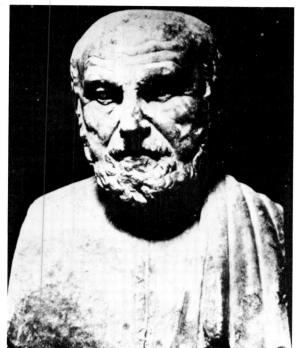

In addition, according to Galen, the system at Cnidos emphasized elaborate diagnosis based on symptoms, so that virtually every symptom was a disease. For instance, there were seven diseases of the bile, twelve of the bladder, and four types of consumption (which usually meant the spitting of blood). Although descriptions of the patient's history were complete and clear, the accent was on the disease rather than the patient (Hippocratic methods emphasized the patient rather than the disease, with great attention paid to observing and evaluating the physical findings). Wherever these Cnidian characteristics are found in the body of the Hippocratic works, they have been attributed by some scholars to Cnidian origin. Two treatises, *On Diet and Acute Diseases* and *On Diseases*, have been particularly singled out as probable contributions from Cnidos.

Some of the outstanding leaders of that school were Euryphon, Ctesias, Chrysippos, Polycrates, Endoxos, and Nichomachos, the father of Aristotle. According to Galen, Euryphon, a great anatomist, was one of the most famous physicians of his time and made many contributions to the "Cnidian Sentences." Ctesias, a younger contemporary of Hippocrates, attained fame as a physician in the Persian court of Artaxerxes Mnemon, and he wrote a commentary on Hippocrates which contained a number of disagreements with the methods and conclusions.

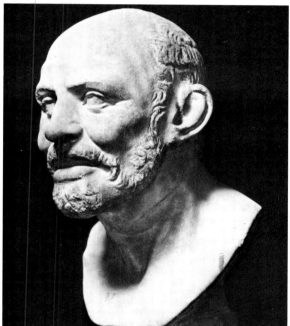

However, the most famous name that has come down to us is Hippocrates of Cos. Whether the teachings with which he has been associated are the work of one man or of many is not known. When the Hippocratic writings were collected in the great library of Alexandria in the fourth century B.C., the works of others were presumably also attributed to Hippocrates. So when we speak of Hippocrates we are probably referring to more than one man. Nevertheless, there is some evidence that he did exist and that he may indeed have been the extraordinary person later generations considered him. In any case, he typifies in his teachings, his life, and his behavior the ideal to which all healers strive and which all patients seek in their doctors.

Before considering the principles and methods of Hippocrates, it is appropriate to describe the common medical practices of his time.

Medicine in
Hippocratic Times

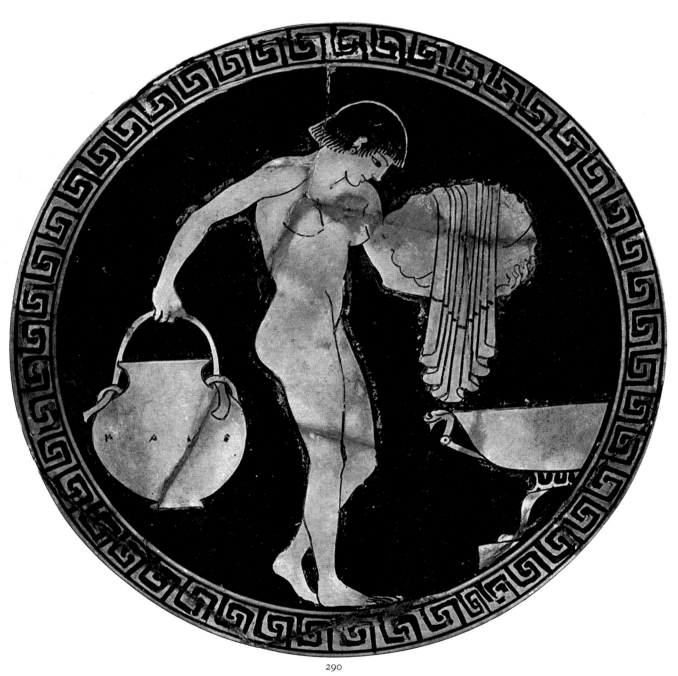

IN the several centuries between the flourishing of Cretan-Mycenaean civilization and the time of the philosopher-scientists, a distinct change had come about in Greek attitudes toward the causes of disease: the teachers and medical practitioners of the time of Hippocrates no longer looked at illness as a punishment by the gods. Nevertheless, a sick person was thereby only a little better off. If the ill patient could be restored to a healthy state, all possible means were employed. But if he could not be cured or at least improved, he was virtually abandoned by the physician as well as his neighbors. Illness was indeed still a curse—of man if not of the gods.

The Stoics (in the fourth and third centuries B.C.), who preached virtue rather than health as the highest good, also considered illness an evil to be avoided at all costs. As a matter of fact, suicide was justified for illness under their code. Nevertheless, the position of the sick person was now better in that—unless his condition was considered hopeless—he was the focus of healers who looked upon him as a victim of natural causes within and outside his body, deserving, therefore, of rational methods of management.

EDUCATION

In his early years, a Greek youth was urged to be athletic, but at about the age of eighteen he was directed more to intellectual pursuits: philosophy, rhetoric, science, and—significantly—medicine. The educated man was expected to be acquainted with all fields of knowledge, and it was only natural for physicians to pursue all branches of medicine, both medical and surgical. Specialization had not yet appeared, although Herodotos had mentioned that a well-advanced system had already developed in Egypt.

By the time of Hippocrates the Greeks had developed a hypothetical system which explained the mechanism of illness in terms of four basic humors of the body. One can detect a clear progression of ideas in Greek metaphysics that led to this system: the teaching that four basic elements (water, air, fire, and earth), each with its specific quality (moist, dry, hot, and cold), comprise the entire universe; the concept that pairs of opposites (with concomitant emphasis on the number 4) were to be kept in equilibrium to achieve harmony in the cosmos and health in the microcosm of man; the special effects on the body and mind of the seasons, which were at first three and then four; the visible secretions of the body, also at first three (blood, phlegm, and bile) and then four by separating bile into yellow and black. Ultimately, some kind of hypothesis was required to organize these concepts, for as Peter Medawar, a Nobel Laureate of the twentieth century, has said, "Science without the underpinning of hypothesis is just kitchen arts."

The key principle was that all body fluids were composed of varying proportions of blood (warm and moist), phlegm (cold and moist), yellow bile (warm and dry), and black bile (cold and dry). When these "humors" were in balance the body was in health; excess or deficiency of one or more caused illness. There were three stages of disease: a change in humoral proportions caused by external or internal factors; the reaction of the body to this by fever or "boiling"; the resultant crisis when the disorder ended through discharge of the excess humor—or by death. The emanations or humors of the body were often seen during illness (blood, phlegm from the nose, vomit, fecal matter, urine, sweat), and frequently an illness did suddenly disappear after reaching a crisis—the discharge of one of the humors.

In attitudes toward mental disease, the Greeks like other peoples showed a gradual development from belief in supernatural or demoniac causes to more rational explanations. By the fifth century B.C. the mind and its derangements were clearly located in the brain. Yet even Plato, a contemporary of Hippocrates, classified madness mythologically into four main types: prophetic (mediated by Apollo); ritualistic (as in the Dionysian ceremonies); poetic (inspired by the Muses); erotic (under the influence of Aphrodite and Eros).

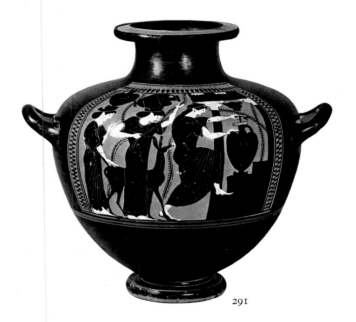

291

290 *Painted medallion from Athenian cup (early 5th century B.C.), attributed to Onesimos, school of the Panaitos Painter, found at Chiusi in Etruria. Girl preparing to do laundry illustrates importance of personal cleanliness in ancient Greece. Musées Royaux d'Art et d'Histoire, Brussels*

291 *Greek hydria, or water pot (c. 520 B.C.), in the style of the Nikosthenes Painter, shows women filling jugs with precious water, often in short supply, for use at home. Museo Nazionale di Villa Giulia, Rome*

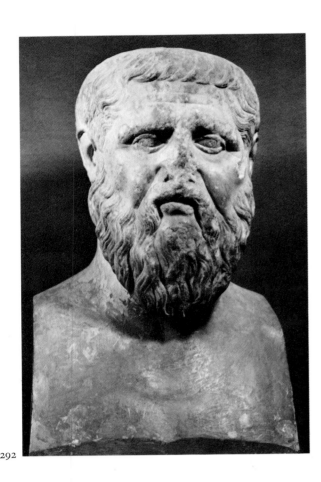

292 *The philosopher Plato, apparently a contemporary of Hippocrates, in 3d-century A.D. copy of 4th-century B.C. statue. His teachings on immortality, universal ideals, and balancing body and mind descended from Pythagorean doctrines, which were in consonance with those of the Dionysian-Orphic sects. The Louvre, Paris*

THE PRACTITIONERS

As in Mycenaean days described in the Homeric epics, the physician of the sixth and fifth centuries B.C. was still of the class of craftsmen, although his status was enhanced because of the exceptional emphasis placed on health by the Greeks. An upper-class freeborn physician usually treated his own kind, for which he received fees. His assistants and slaves might attend to *metics* (resident aliens) and slaves, but there were no rules in this respect. Those who could afford to pay for treatment probably had access to experienced practitioners, but the poor had little open to them. This may account in part for the rise and extension of the Asclepieian temple as a doorway of medical treatment for all. Of course, magical medicine, which was respected by even the philosophers Plato and Theophrastos, was available to all—rich and poor, slave and free. In general, physicians cast a clinical rather than a political or economic eye on the patient, and treatment was the same for poor and rich. The physicians themselves came principally from the class of aristocratic citizens or from the *metics,* who also supplied the freedmen, traders, artisans, and farmers.

The training system was by apprenticeship, and apparently for a fee the neophyte received instruction, participated in the care of patients, assisted and nursed as needed, and performed menial tasks in maintaining the equipment as required by the teacher. This may not have been much different from the practice in our recent past of a young physician's assisting an established practitioner in his office, staying in his place at the bedside of desperately ill patients as well as performing other tasks.

The office (*iatreion*) of a Greek physician was often in the vicinity of a temple of Asclepios in regions where they existed. Most often the office was a temporary location for medical activities because the majority of physicians were itinerant, traveling from city to city, carrying drugs and instruments, setting up in a suitable house near the market place where patients could even stay a day or longer for a procedure that required special attention. Most often, however, the physician went to the home of the patient, especially if he was rich. Even operations were often performed there—as was still customary in the nineteenth and early twentieth centuries in the West, when tonsillectomies were frequently performed in the home.

Payment was expected, but not necessarily for every service. Fees were often set and given in a lump sum in advance, a procedure advised in the Hippocratic writings but coupled with a precaution to avoid discussion of fees if the patient was acutely ill or worried about finances. "I advise making no excessive demands, but to take into account the means and income of the patient. In certain circumstances, the physician should give treatment for nothing. It is better to reproach those who escape than to bellow at those who are in danger."

By the time of Hippocrates in the mid-fifth century B.C., a multiplicity of practicing healers had come upon the scene. The question of who were charlatans and who were bona fide contributors is difficult to answer. There was no system of licensure or certification before 300 B.C., and anyone except a woman could take the title of physician.

That women did not qualify as medical practitioners would be expected in a culture which relegated them to secondary status. In Athens, wives rarely appeared in public, almost never showed themselves at feasts or social events, and were confined principally to household duties for all of their lives. In Sparta, presumably, they had a measure of greater freedom, but in that society in which everyone's function was to serve the state women were mainly breeders. One group of women in Greek society who did succeed in becoming relatively free spirits were the hetaeras who entertained men. Not exactly prostitutes, although their favors were for sale, they were like the "adventuresses" of more recent times who lived by their wits.

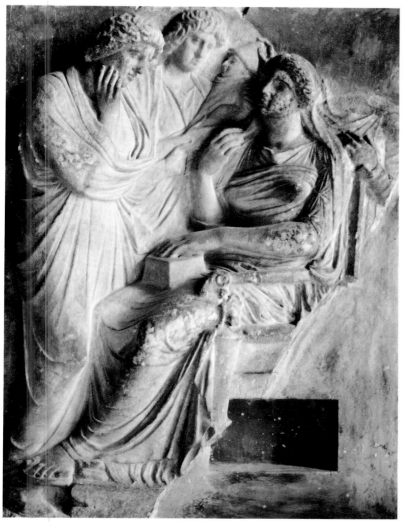

293

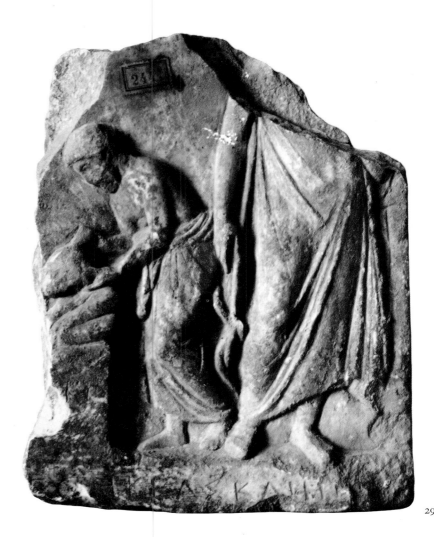

295

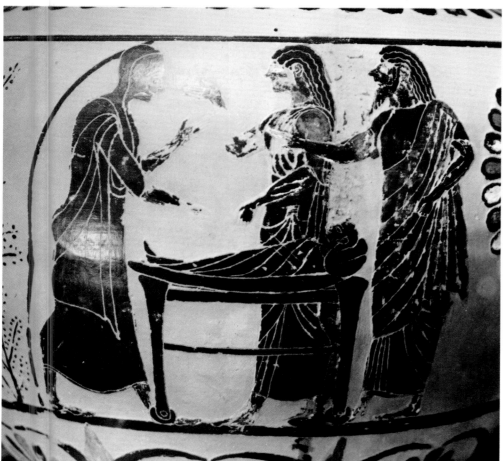

294

293 *Funerary stele (c. 4th century B.C.) of a young mother and child who both died in childbirth, evidently the loved ones of a wealthy family. National Archaeological Museum, Athens*

294 *Hydria with a painted scene of the god Hermes as an infant asleep in swaddling clothes, a custom of ancient origins still practiced in some parts of the world. The Louvre, Paris*

295 *Bas-relief fragment showing doctor performing operation on patient's head while Asclepios, the patron god of medicine, looks on. National Archaeological Museum, Athens*

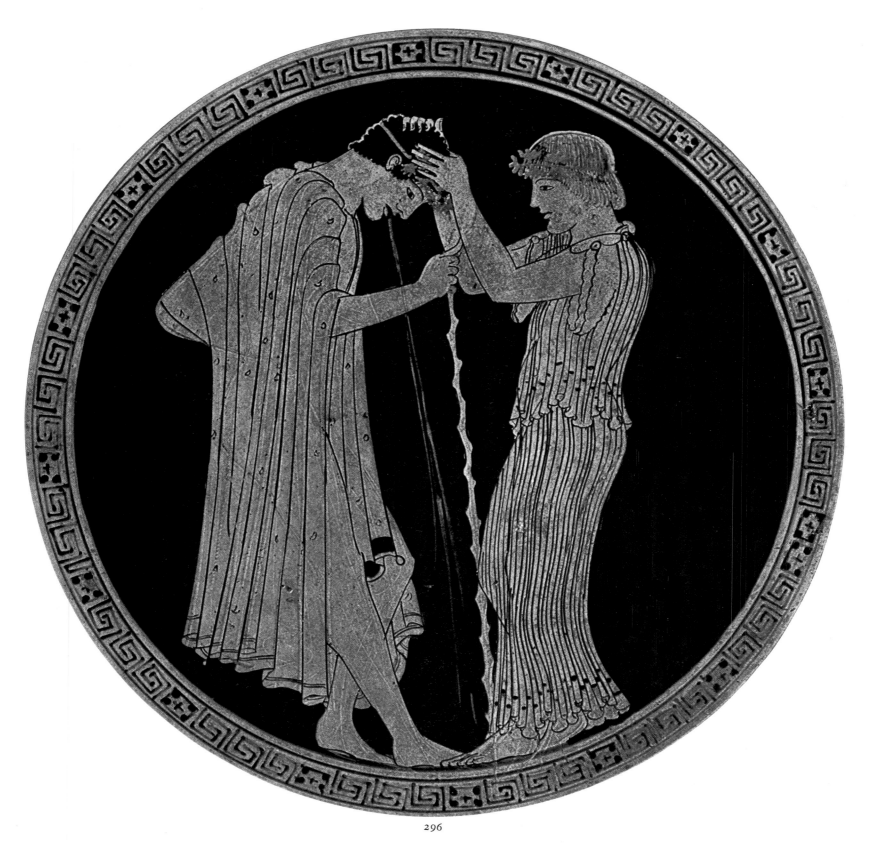

296

296 *Interior medallion of a cup done by the Brygos Painter (c. 490–480 B.C.), showing man vomiting— one way to rid the body of excess humors. Martin von Wagner Museum, Würzburg University*

The methods of treatment were general and local. Regimens consisted of diet, daily exercise, and temperate behavior in eating, drinking, sleeping, and sexual indulgence. This therapy was probably only suitable for the upper class, for the common workingman had neither the time nor financial security to embark on daily activities just to keep fit. During illness a sparse diet was the usual prescription. This restricted intake (sometimes consisting of only gruel, water, vinegar, and honey) has been evaluated in recent times as highly deficient and therefore probably harmful to the patients. Even the regular diet of the healthy Greek in those days may have been rather frugal.

Numbers in relation to the day of illness were important considerations. In the Pythagorean teachings of the sixth century B.C., the three- or four-day intervals between chills were significant. As in Mesopotamian cultures, the number 7 was also of medical interest: the menses occurred at four times seven intervals. Pregnancy lasted forty times seven days.

What we consider today branches of medicine (such as surgery, internal medicine, and obstetrics) were all combined as one in the healing art. Thus dental illnesses were also treated by the physician, who probably included among his methods the fixation of loose teeth with gold wire, an Etruscan practice.

Wounds and sores were cleansed and sprinkled with many kinds of mineral substances and mixtures of plant extracts, most of which included wine. The purposes were to soothe and presumably to hasten healing, but cloth stuffings placed within and around the open wound may have caused infection and pus. Since the sudden discharge of pus often is followed by the healing of a vexatious boil, sore, or wound, the encouragement of draining pus in a wound came to seem desirable. This belief, later memorialized in the Middle Ages as "laudable pus," represented a common attitude for centuries before and after the Greeks.

Although medicaments were used most often for external application, some drugs were taken internally to produce purging or vomiting, to rid the body of the excess humors. Enemas were also used. These practices had been common in other regions of the world for centuries. Herodotos reported, for example, the Egyptian custom of regularly cleansing the intestinal tract to maintain health, not just when ill.

Injuries to the bones and joints must have made up a substantial part of medical practice. The manipulations to reduce dislocations and fractures achieved a high degree of sophistication, sometimes with the employment of mechanical devices. Effective and complex techniques of bandaging all parts of the body are also to be found in the works of Hippocrates and in the numerous later commentaries. The cautery evidently was effectively used by the Greeks to treat infections, wounds, and tumors. In addition, their careful and extensive use of operative surgery with the knife is most impressive. The juice of the opium poppy and of mandragora (hyoscyamus) for anesthesia and pain relief were probably also commonly available among the Greeks.

Human and veterinary medicine were separate, especially since man was the only creature with a soul, but the anatomic and physiologic information obtained from animals in the kitchen, the butcher shop, and the hunt were applied to the human body. Furthermore, it seems that regular physicians cared for animals too, especially horses.

It was apparently on Cos that physical examination was brought to a high art. No detail of a patient's appearance and function was to be omitted. Moreover, his way of life, his emotional state, surroundings, and behavior were carefully examined. The climate and customs of his city and country were also part of the medical examination.

When all the information had been obtained and the responses of the sick person evaluated, the Coan physician apparently made a judgment on whether the

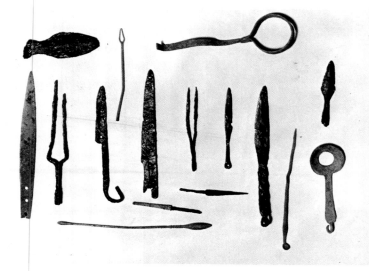

297

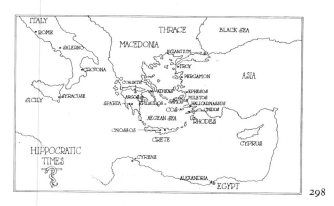

298

297 *Medical instruments—forceps, knives, and probes—of ancient Greece, with which the physicians of Hippocratic times did careful and extensive surgery on external parts, using opium and mandragora as anesthetics. Archaeological Museum, Epidauros*

298 *Map of the eastern Mediterranean in the time of Hippocrates*

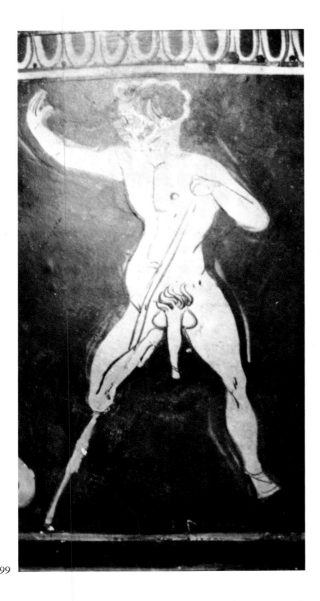

299

299 *Greek-influenced Etruscan vase (2d century* B.C.) *with crippled satyr depicted using crutch, probably representing a typical way that ancient Greeks dealt with this problem. The Louvre, Paris*

300 *Charioteer (c. 470* B.C.), *from a votive group attributed to Sothadas, offered by Polyzalos of Gela to the god Apollo, early patron of healing. Found in the Sanctuary of Apollo at Delphi. Archaeological Museum, Delphi*

301 *Tombstone of the Athenian physician Jason (2d century* B.C.), *shown examining a patient by palpating his abdomen. A giant cupping-glass is seen on the right. British Museum, London*

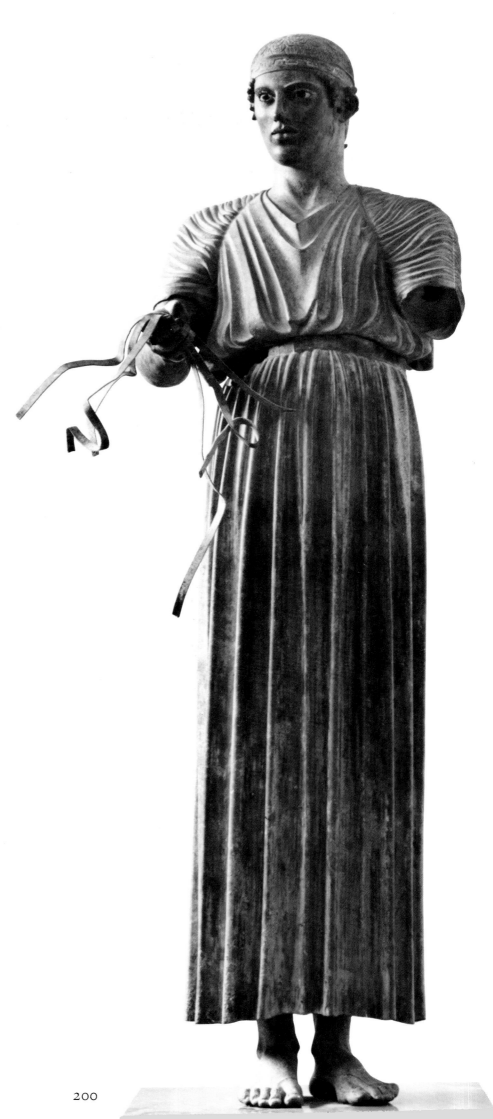

300

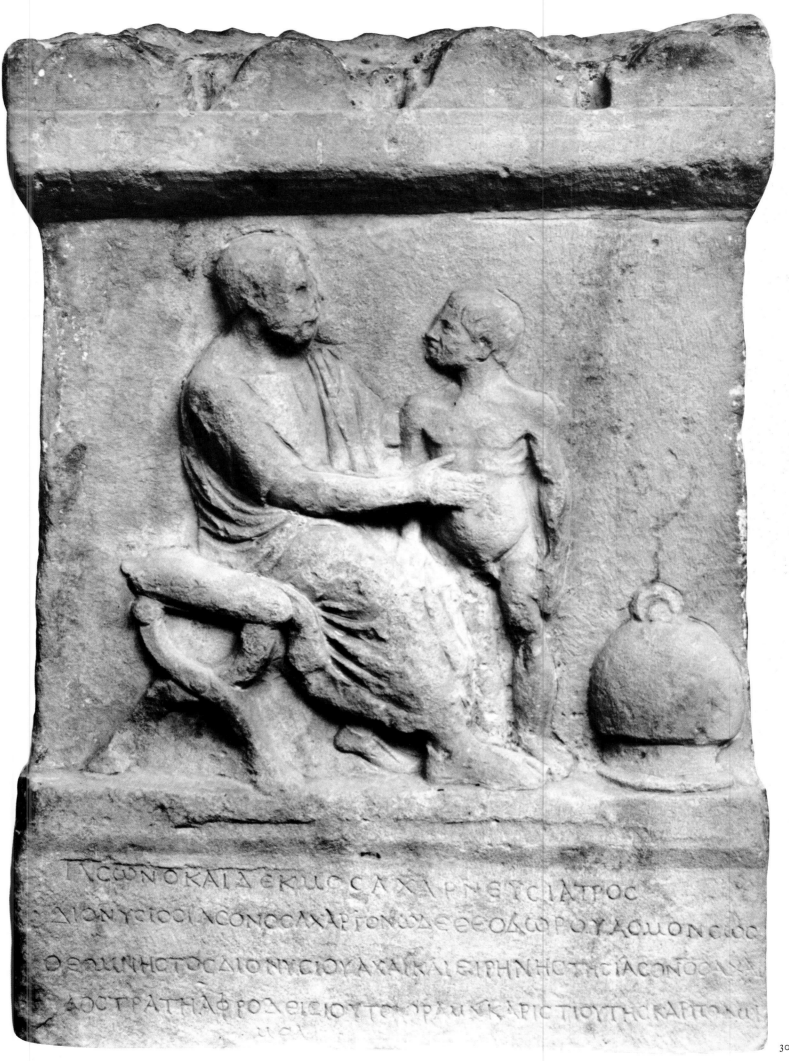

301

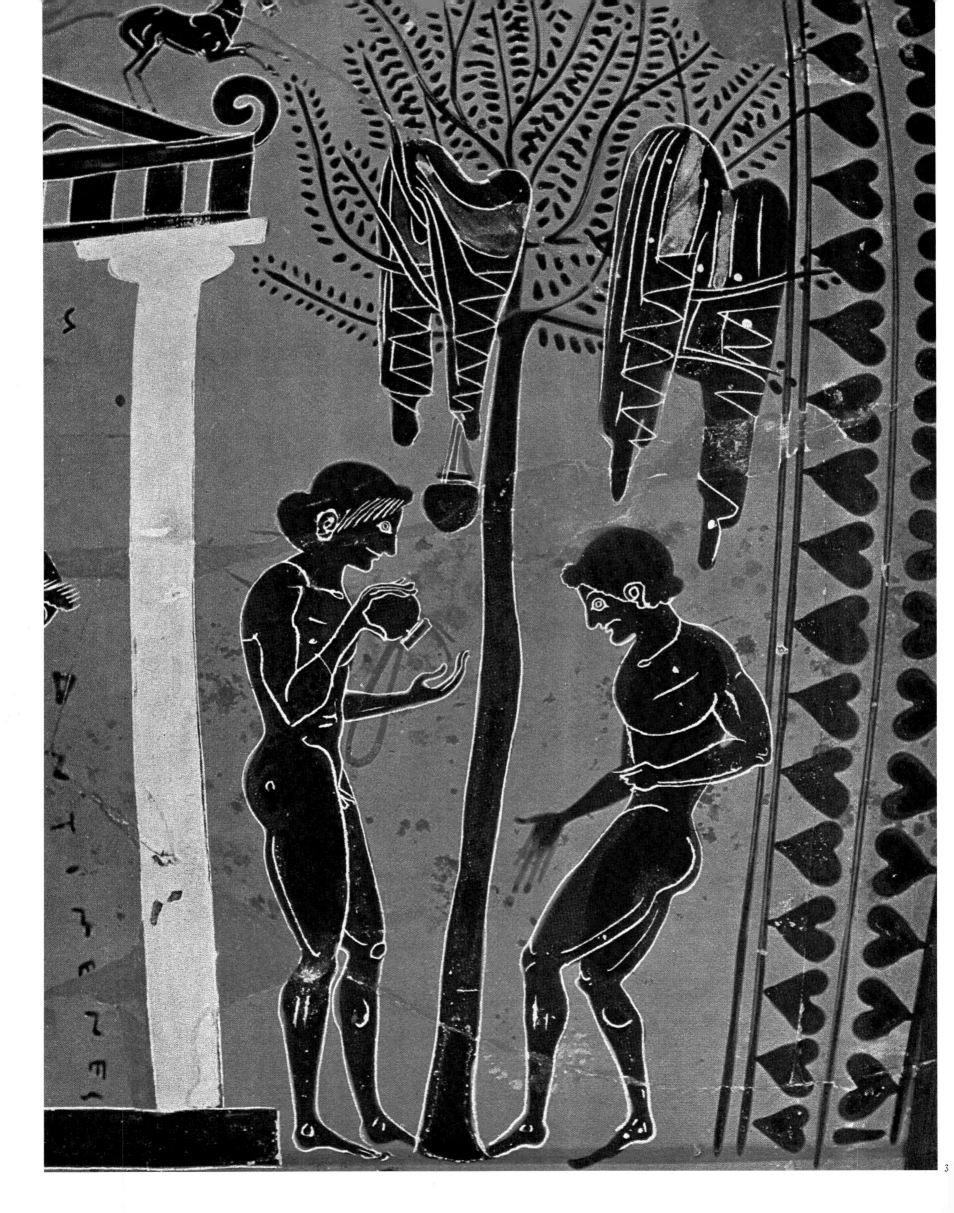

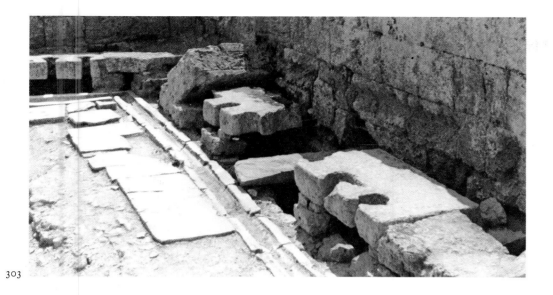

303

patient would get well (prognosis) and then on what should be done. The explanation for a sickness or the type of disease it represented was subordinate to the outlook. For in a society where the physician traveled from place to place, his reputation was doubtless based more on how he predicted the outcome of an illness than on diagnosing what was wrong. Furthermore, at a time when therapy was limited, the prognosis might be the only contribution a physician could make.

PUBLIC HEALTH AND HYGIENE

The Hippocratic writings used the word "endemic" to cover those diseases which were always present in an area because of climate, water, agriculture, nutrition, and customs. Among them were what we would today call "colds," pneumonia, gout, cirrhosis, mumps, tuberculosis, malaria, and diarrheal diseases. From the reports available it is difficult to identify with certainty the acute diseases with skin rashes (exanthemata) such as smallpox, measles, chicken pox, and scarlet fever. Some other descriptions may be interpreted as representing diphtheria, although they may have referred merely to severe infections of the mouth and neck.

For the bulk of the population, the houses were cramped, closely packed, poorly ventilated, and little better than hovels. The homes of the rich, however, were built with consideration for health in the choice, if possible, of a location far from swamps, where the sun was warm and the breezes mild. But the cities for the most part were laid out in squares, with row on row of small, poor dwellings. The streets were narrow and mired in filth. Since most people walked about outside in sandals, it is not surprising to learn that each man, whenever possible, washed his feet on entering his home. Bathing was frequent in the public baths as well as at home, usually in tubs (somewhat resembling large washbasins) and in showers that were created by running water through holes or spigots in an elevated wooden tub.

Water was always precious in Greece, never reaching the abundance achieved in Rome, a fact that may account for the reputation of the Greeks as connoisseurs of water, which they drank as often as feasible and with gusto. They also drank wine (considered of high quality in antiquity) but it was most often diluted with water. Resins used to prevent stored wine from turning to vinegar added a unique taste that came to be appreciated and later preferred by some—even to this day. Drunkenness was apparently not a major health problem in a culture which accented moderation. Yet at feasts of aristocratic citizens great quantities of wine were apparently consumed.

Thus there was a marked contrast between personal hygiene and public sanitation; between lofty philosophic moralizing and oppressive social organization; but also between the limited knowledge of the time and the brilliant, rational application of sensible principles to healing the sick.

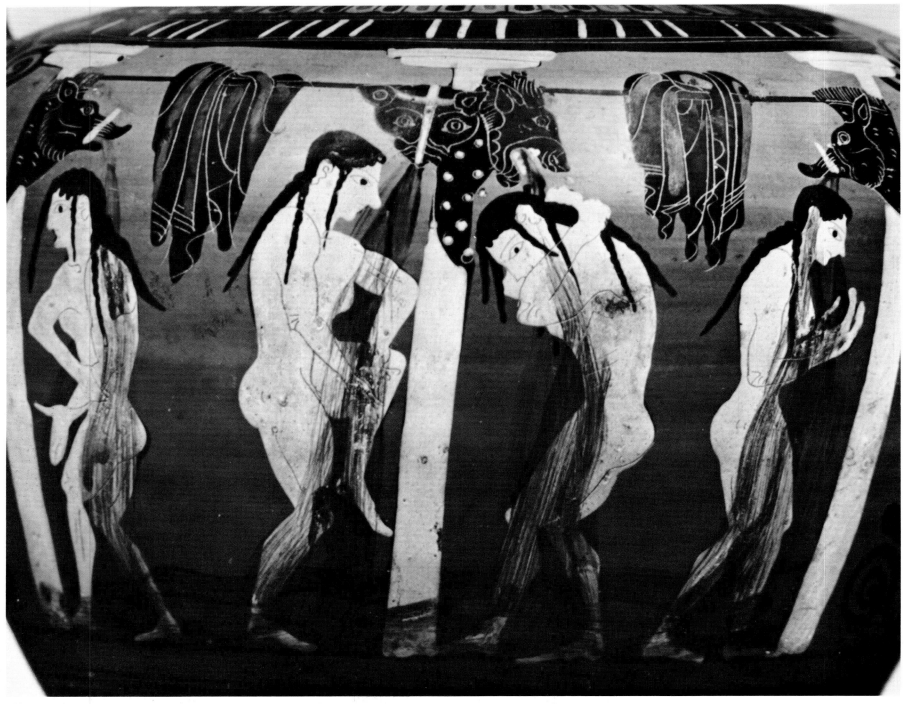

304

304 *Attic vase (c. 6th century B.C.) showing young women enjoying the luxury of a shower under streams of water issuing from decorative shower heads. Staatliche Museen, Berlin*

305, 306 *Exterior decorations by the Antiphon Painter on a cup (c. 490–480 B.C.) found at Vulci, showing scenes of drinking and drunkenness—not a major health problem among the ancient Greeks. Collection Norbert Schimmel, New York*

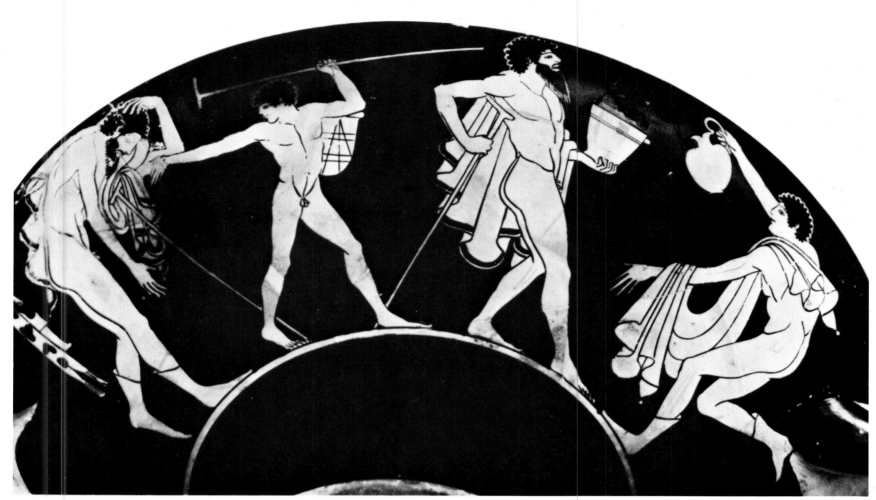

305

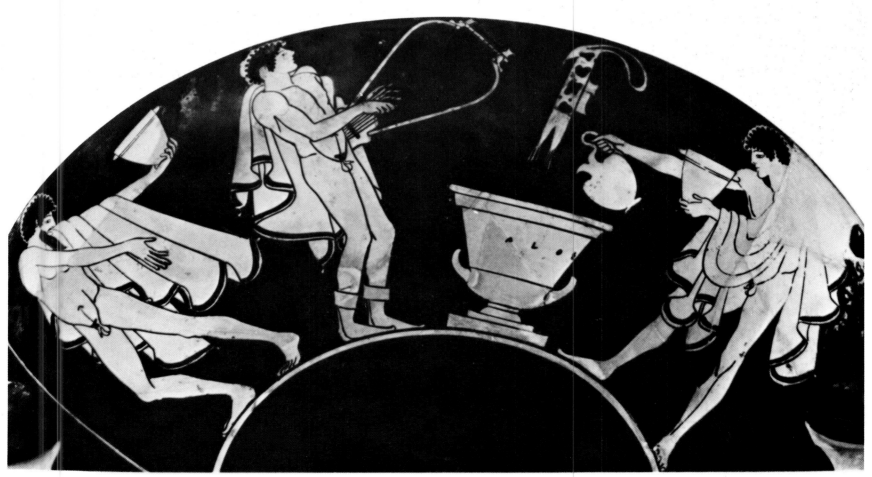

306

Hippocrates

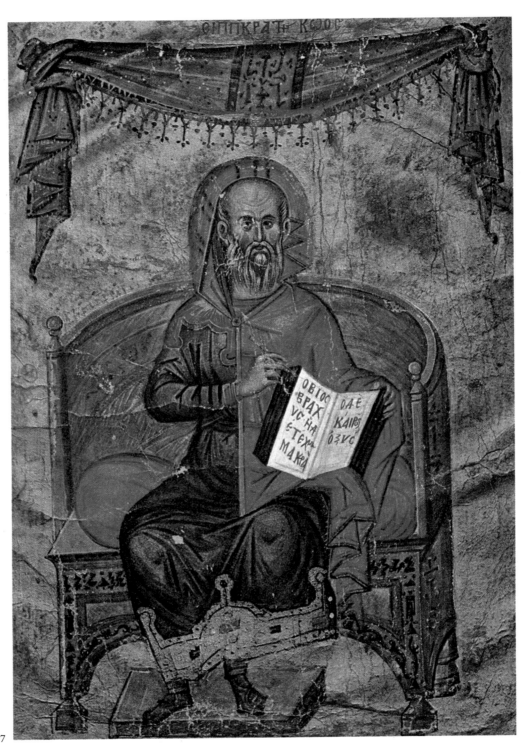

307

O VER many centuries, the warrior heroes, the medical craftsmen, and the gymnasts of ancient Greece had accumulated a store of pragmatic information on maintaining health; the philosopher-scientists had championed secular causation in the cosmos and had developed rational theories and methods of treatment. In the fifth century B.C. this lengthy development of Greek medicine was capped by and epitomized in Hippocrates. From then on into modern times, medicine in the Western world and in parts of the East would be continually under the influence of the teachings of the man (or men) referred to as Hippocrates.

WHO WAS HIPPOCRATES?

Some facts have been generally accepted. Hippocrates did exist (although some scholars dispute even this) and was well known in the Greek world. Apparently born about 460 B.C. on the island of Cos, he died about 370 in Thessaly. He was a teacher on Cos, an itinerant practitioner of medicine, and the presumed author of a number of treatises. Precisely which parts of the Hippocratic Collection were actually written by him is not altogether established, but some reasonable attributions have been made on the basis of style, content, and what is known of attitudes and practices of rival teachers.

There were other prominent physicians of the time who were probably as well known. Chrysippos (whose statue was long thought to represent Hippocrates) was a later philosopher-physician of great reputation. Euryphon of Cnidos, a contemporary, seems to have been at least as famous and has often been considered an important contributor to the "Cnidian Sentences." Another famous physician of Cos, but later than Hippocrates, was Praxagoras, whose student Herophilos became an outstanding, influential figure as an anatomist and author in the Alexandrian school of the late fourth century B.C. Hippocrates, Chrysippos, and Praxagoras have sometimes been grouped as proponents and innovators of dietetics as a method of treatment.

But it was Hippocrates whose name shone ever brighter in subsequent years. Facts were embellished, stories told, and legends created. Some may have been true, some may have contained germs of truth, but others were wholly fabricated. A few of these legends may be worth mentioning because they indicate the types of achievement that appealed to the minds of the centuries following Hippocrates.

In Macedonia he cured the king of what had been diagnosed as phthisis (a progressively debilitating condition) but was perceived by Hippocrates as psychological in origin, a situation missed by Euryphon, the leading physician of Cnidos.

In Abdera, Hippocrates was asked to cure Democritos of presumed madness—thus illustrating his prowess but also enhancing his image as a philosopher to have communicated with the great Democritos, who introduced the atom into science. Invited to Asia Minor to stop the plague, he chose to remain home and help his own people. His patriotism was similarly shown by the tale of his rejecting a request from King Artaxerxes because the Persians were enemies of Greece. (The wars with Persia occurred just before the decades in which Hippocrates lived.)

Even fantastic legends arose. For example, on his tomb a beehive produced honey which had exceptional curative powers. Despite proof that there were no Asclepieian temples on Cos at the time, a rumor once started that Hippocrates had set fire to the temple to preserve his own primacy there.

Concerning his appearance, there have been many attempts to present to the world a noble face and impressive body to go with the physician's other attributes. However, very few Greek statues of the period have survived, so our view of Greek sculpture rests principally on Roman copies. Various dignified antique busts have been said to represent Hippocrates at different times, and likenesses painted and drawn from imagination have also perpetuated a belief in his

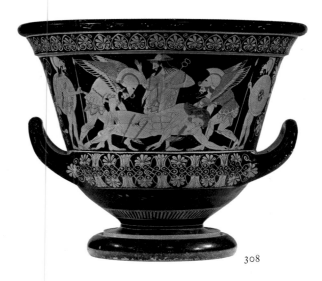

308

307 *Hippocrates, as envisioned by a Byzantine artist in the 14th century, became the most famous name of ancient Greek medicine and was associated with an influential collection of writings called* Corpus Hippocraticum. *From Greek Ms. (c. 1342) 2144, f. 10 v., Bibliothèque Nationale, Paris*

308 *Red-figured calyx-crater (c. 515 B.C.) by Euphronios, showing the dead Sarpedon being carried off the battlefield by Thanatos and Hypnos. For Greek warriors, medicine was often learned in action. Bequest of Joseph H. Durkee. Gift of Darius Ogden Mills and C. Ruxton Love, by exchange, 1972. Metropolitan Museum of Art, New York*

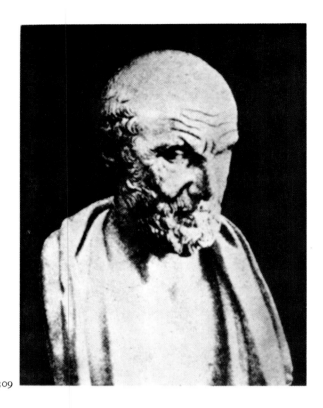

309 Roman copy of a Greek statue of Chrysippos, a famous physician who lived after Hippocrates, formerly thought to be a portrait of Hippocrates. British Museum, London

310 Marble statue found near the Odeion on Cos, another of the many presumed representations of Hippocrates, but it may be of an unknown citizen of late Hellenistic times. Cos Museum, Cos

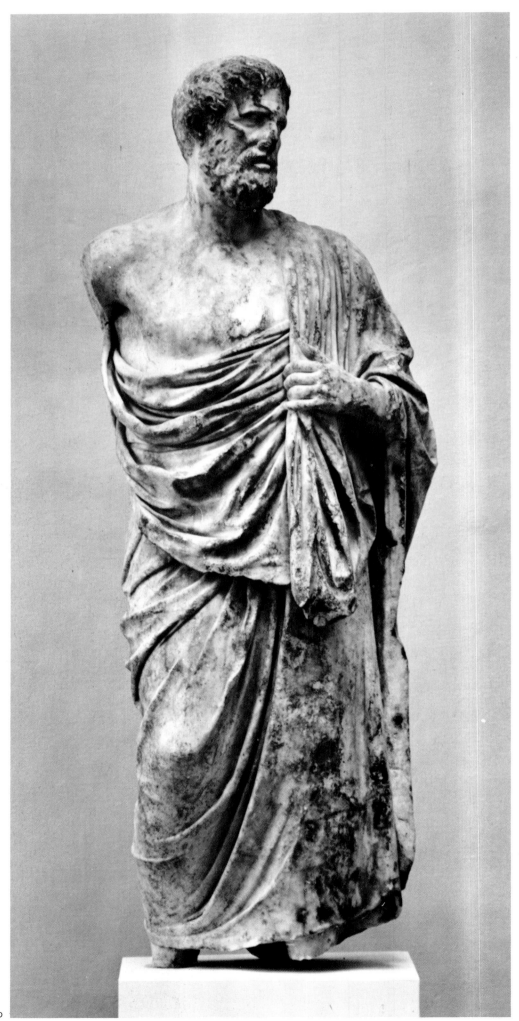

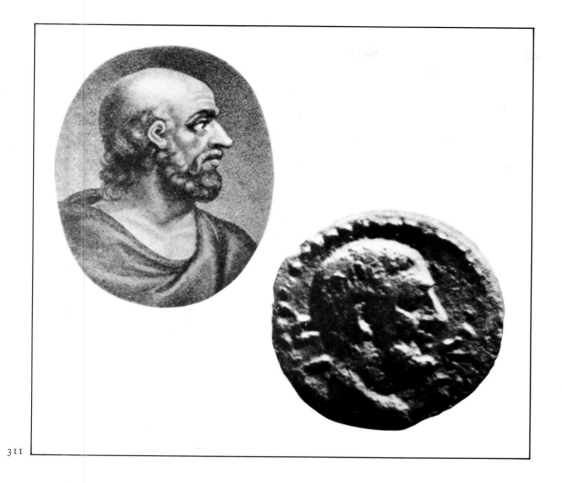

311

311 *Roman coin (1st century* A.D.*) from the island of Cos, now in British Museum, compared to likeness of Hippocrates, published in 1809, taken from ancient gem. National Library of Medicine, Bethesda*

312 *Site of the Plane Tree of Hippocrates on the island of Cos, in the shade of which the great teacher is said to have instructed his many pupils.*

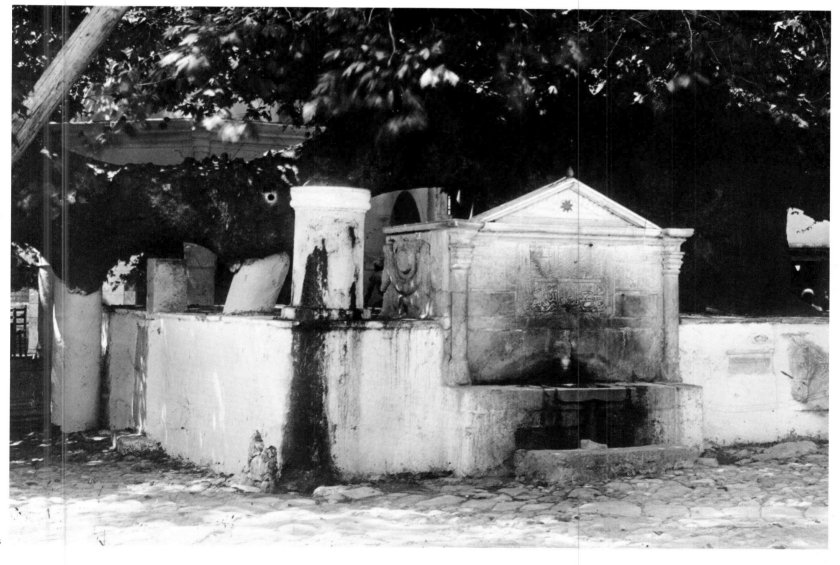

312

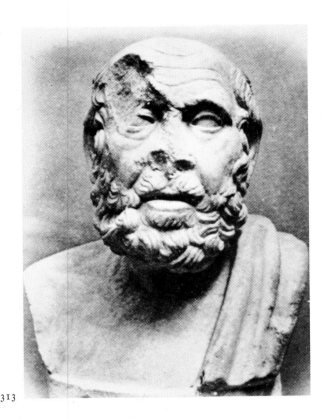

313 *Roman copy of a Greek statue, found near Ostia in 1940, now widely thought to be a true likeness of Hippocrates. This head bears a close resemblance to one on a coin from Cos marked Hippocrates. Museo della Via Ostiense, Rome*

314 *Bath therapy shown in 14th-century miniature by Pietro da Eboli from De Balneis Puteolanis, based on same treatment advocated by Hippocrates and his followers nearly 1,800 years earlier. Ms. 1474, Biblioteca Angelica, Rome*

impressive appearance. Aristotle indicated that Hippocrates was of short stature, so there was all the more reason to seek a handsome, outstanding face to portray the greatest physician of all time. Recent studies have yielded coins from Cos with profiles bearing the name of Hippocrates, which a sculpted head found in a cemetery in Ostia seems to resemble. These are now accepted by almost all as the likely appearance of Hippocrates.

What Did He Write?

The works of Hippocrates compiled under the title "Hippocratic Collection" or *Corpus Hippocraticum* almost certainly include writings by many authors from Cos, Cnidos, Sicily, and perhaps elsewhere. The Collection was assembled in the fourth century B.C. at the great Library in Alexandria, where an extraordinary center of learning had been established by Ptolemy, one of Alexander's generals, who started a ruling Greek dynasty in Egypt that was ended when the Romans under Octavian overthrew Cleopatra VII in 30 B.C. The intention of the Ptolemies was to collect the entire sum of human knowledge in the Library, and the works of Hippocrates were undoubtedly sought out. As his name became increasingly famous it is likely that more and more medical contributions were assigned to his authorship. Since it is virtually impossible to determine which treatises were genuinely by Hippocrates, the custom has arisen to refer to the entire Collection as writings of the Hippocratists or Hippocratics, thus leaving the authorship undetermined. When we use the name Hippocrates we refer not only to the man but to any others who made important contributions to the *Corpus Hippocraticum*.

The total number of works in the Collection has been variously estimated, depending on how one counts the treatises and the books of which each treatise is composed. The books number about seventy-two and the treatises about fifty-nine, but the subject matter is not arranged in any coherent plan. Therefore, each summary of the Collection is forced to reassemble the works according to its perception of relatively similar topics. Although we cannot classify all the information under specific headings we would use today, we can extract and categorize a few general beliefs found in the collection.

Anatomy—Anatomical details are relatively sparse and there is no truly systematized presentation. Information on most of the viscera is scanty, but the heart is somewhat more completely dealt with. The pericardium, the muscular ventricles, the heart valves, the different contracting times of auricles and ventricles, and the great vessels are mentioned. Nerves are considered hollow and are confused with ligaments. Differences between arteries and veins are not understood.

Physiology—The innate heat of the body necessary for life comes from the *pneuma* of the air and is taken in by the lungs. Air along with blood fills the arteries. Sight depends on the lens and the vitreous humor (the gel that occupies the eyeball). The retina is not understood as the organ of sight. The four humors corresponding to the four elements are the physiological bases of body function. Harmony of all parts is necessary to health.

General Pathology—Causes of illness are either immediate due to internal difficulties or remote because of outside influences, especially climate, personal hygiene, diet, activity, and surroundings. Diseases have three stages: degeneration of the humors, coction (a cooking process), and crisis with the evacuation of offending humors. Over forty case histories are summarized in descriptions so superb that we can make good inferences even today on the type of illness presented.

Therapy—The repeated advice is to avoid interfering with the course of the illness except at the proper time indicated by natural signs. One must assist nature in doing the cure. "Timidity indicates incapacity; rashness is evidence of unskillfulness." Relatively few drugs are used, certainly not as many as were

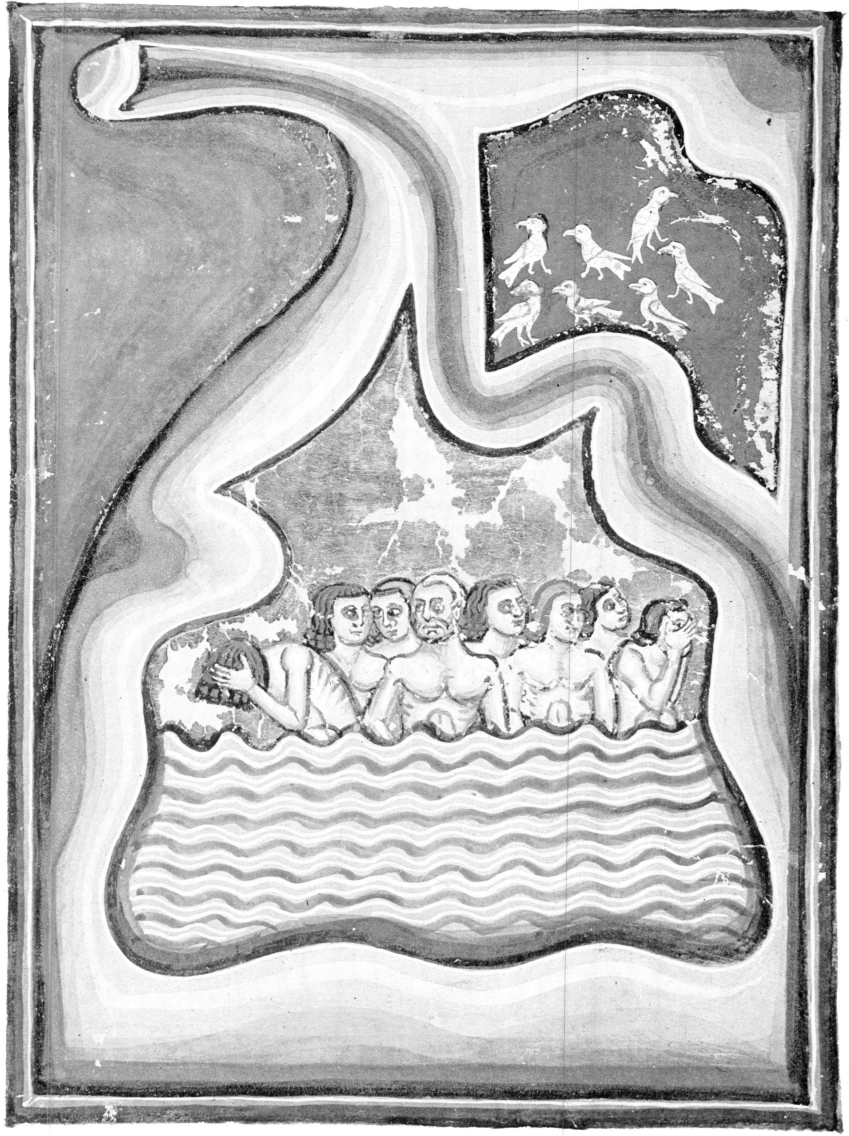

314

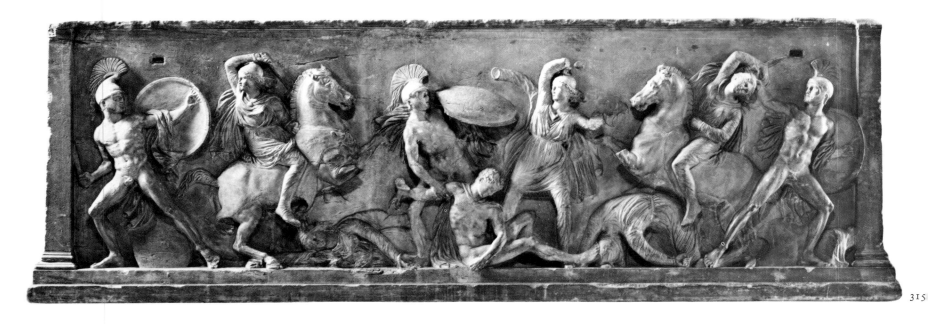

315

315 *As seen on this marble Amazon sarcophagus (c. 310 B.C.), war injuries were common experiences to the ancient Greeks, and they developed a variety of treatments for wounds. Kunsthistorisches Museum, Vienna*

316 *Long-term influence of the teachings of Hippocrates (in this case, reducing a dislocation of the knee), as seen in an 11th-century Byzantine copy of a 9th-century codex,* Commentaries of Apollonios of Chition on the Peri arthron of Hippocrates. *Biblioteca Medicea-Laurenziana, Florence*

317, 318 *Reducing dislocations of the spinal column (above) and the elbow (below), as illustrated in an 11th-century Byzantine copy of a 9th-century Greek codex,* Commentaries of Apollonios of Chition on the Peri arthron of Hippocrates. *Biblioteca Medicea-Laurenziana, Florence*

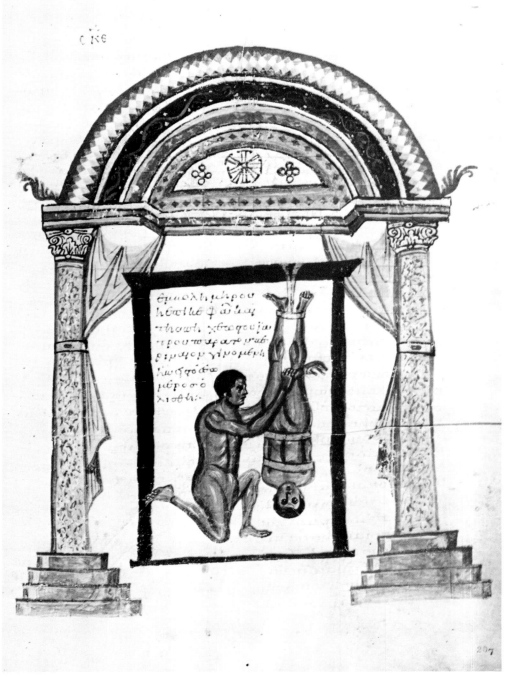

316

supposedly given on Cnidos or in the Western world in subsequent centuries. Laxatives and emetic herbs are the principal agents, as was the custom in Egypt. Narcotics, however, are also advised. Much emphasis is placed on regimens, including baths, inunction, and diet (usually quite simple and limited). Cupping, scarifications, and bleeding are also part of therapy, but they do not seem to be important.

Diagnosis—Very few names of diseases are mentioned and no special syndromes are presented. The condition of the patient is the important thing to the Hippocratists, and inquiry is made into details of his past and present behavior as well as his complaints. The patient's appearance is observed in detail, including his body makeup and excretions. Vaginal examination is practiced, and probes and speculums (instruments to hold open) are used to examine orifices. An ear is held against the chest to hear the breathing sounds, but the heart sounds seem not to have been well described. Palpation discloses the temperature as well as characteristics of parts of the body. The pulse is noted but not made much of, in contrast to the great emphasis on describing the pulse in later times. Even smelling and tasting are advised to give the doctor a complete picture of the patient's condition.

Prognosis—Almost all the information obtained from questioning the patient and examining him is considered. "In order to prognosticate correctly who will recover and who will die, in whom the days will be long, in whom short, one must know all the symptoms, and must weigh their relative value." The traveling physician could gain the patient's confidence and make his reputation by accurately predicting the outcome of an illness.

Surgery—Probably the most thorough treatises in the Collection are on surgery. Many conditions are treated by operative, manipulative, and more conservative means. Fractures and dislocations of all types are given much attention, as are wounds of the skull, which come in for particularly detailed analysis and treatment. Wounds of all kinds are carefully described and treated by a variety of methods, including local drugs, applications, insertions, and bandages. The injuries of war figure prominently: "He who desires to practice surgery must go to war."

Hemorrhage is controlled by positioning the part, compression, and mere watching. Cauterization is mentioned a number of times. "What drugs fail to cure, that the knife cures; what the knife cures not, that the fire cures; but what fire fails to cure, this must be called incurable." This concept is actually more ancient than Hippocrates, appearing even in Indian medicine. Later, in the Middle Ages, it was to become an important principle of Arabic medicine. Ligation of blood vessels is not spoken of at all.

Operative techniques are reported in detail, including preparation of the patient, table, light, instruments, and assistants. Tumors, fistulas, ulcers, and hemorrhoids are among the diseases treated by surgery, but very little is said of hernias. Almost all of the writings on surgery have been attributed to Hippocrates the man because they are clear, consistent, and pragmatic.

Gynecology and Obstetrics—The treatises on gynecology and obstetrics are a diffuse mixture of accurate observations and inaccurate suppositions. The head presentation at birth is understood to be normal, and the breech (feet first) position is known to require turning of the baby before delivery; however, the fetus is thought to initiate its own delivery. Some diseases of the uterus are well described, but it is thought to wander about in the abdomen. Delivery is performed with the patient kneeling or on a stool, and gradual expulsion of the placenta is advised, although its anatomy is poorly understood. Newborns of a seventh-month delivery are more likely to survive than those of the eighth month (possibly another example of emphasis on the number 7). "Semen" that produces a female child comes from the left ovary, whereas male-producing "semen" comes from the right. Some of the

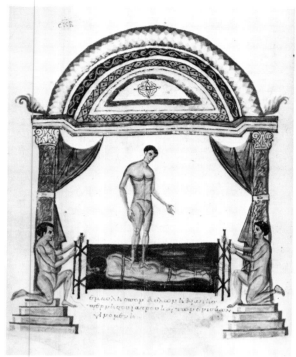

317

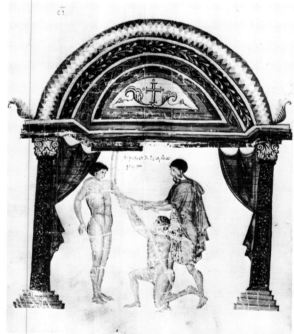

318

213

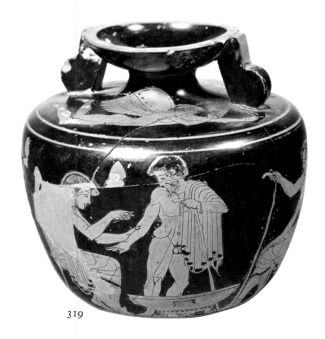

319 *Perfume vessel of the time of Hippocrates, with decorations attributed to the Painter of the Clinic (2d quarter of 5th century B.C.), showing physician treating patient's arm, presumably after having bled him. The Louvre, Paris*

319

information and advice is contradictory to that in other parts of the collection, but it is likely that a difference in authorship is responsible.

Mental Illness—Concerning the emotional state of the patient and mental illness in general, the writings are especially astute and accurate in terms of modern understanding. Assignment of the brain as organ of thought and sensation is an important indication of a high state of understanding. Organic diseases such as epilepsy and delirium tremens and the more subtle derangements such as depression and anxiety are discussed with perspicacity. Even the possible medical origin of dreams is considered.

Ethics—On the subject of behavior the writings are exceptional. They deal with who should enter the profession of medicine, how the physician should look and comport himself, and what one should say and do to comfort the patient. He must also observe the following rules for a temperate inner life: not only reticence, but an absolutely well-ordered life, for in that he has the greatest advantage for his good calling.

The physician must have a worthy appearance; he should look healthy and be well-nourished, appropriate to his physique; for most people are of the opinion that those physicians who are not tidy in their own persons cannot look after others well. Further, he must look to the cleanliness of his person; he must wear decent clothes and use perfumes with harmless smells.

The physician must have a certain degree of sociability, for a morose disposition is inaccessible both to those who are well and those who are sick.

THE OATH

I swear by Apollo Physician and Asclepios and Hygeia and Panacea and all the gods and goddesses, making them my witnesses, that I will fulfill according to my ability and judgment this oath and this covenant:

To hold him who has taught me this art as equal to my parents and to live my life in partnership with him, and if he is in need of money to give him a share of mine, and to regard his offspring as equal to my brothers in male lineage and to teach them this art—if they desire to learn it—without fee and covenant; to give a share of precepts and oral instruction and all the other learning to my sons and to the sons of him who has instructed me and to pupils who have signed the covenant and have taken an oath according to the medical law, but to no one else.

I will apply dietetic measures for the benefit of the sick according to my ability and judgment; I will keep them from harm and injustice.

I will neither give a deadly drug to anybody if asked for it, nor will I make a suggestion to this effect. Similarly I will not give to a woman an abortive remedy. In purity and holiness I will guard my life and my art.

I will not use the knife, not even on sufferers from stone, but will withdraw in favor of such men as are engaged in this work.

Whatever houses I may visit, I will come for the benefit of the sick, remaining free of all intentional injustice, of all mischief, and in particular of sexual relations with both female and male persons, be they free or slaves.

What I may see or hear in the course of the treatment or even outside of the treatment in regard to the life of men, which on no account one must spread abroad, I will keep to myself, holding such things shameful to be spoken about.

If I fulfill this oath and do not violate it, may it be granted to me to enjoy life and art, being honored with fame among all men for all time to come; if I transgress it and swear falsely, may the opposite of all this be my lot.

(Translation by Ludwig Edelstein)

In summary, this famous testament contains both affirmations and prohibitions. It begins with pledges to the gods and to teachers as well as future students. The prohibitions are against harm to the patient, deadly drugs, abortion, surgery, sexual congress with the patient or his household, and revelation of secrets discovered while ministering to the sick. The duties are to act with purity and holiness.

The Oath is the most widely known document associated with the name of Hippocrates. Graduating medical students for centuries have stood to swear to its provisions (either unaltered or with modifications). Yet it is probably not a part of the Hippocratic teachings, was not in all likelihood sworn by physicians on Cos, and is at variance with some of the principles and practices of Hippocrates.

One immediate inconsistency is the Oath's prohibition against abortion and contraceptives; the Hippocratic Collection contains a number of allusions to the methods of abortion and the use of pessaries. The interdiction in the Oath against the knife is especially out of keeping with the several treatises that deal at length and in detail with surgical techniques and operating room procedures.

There are possible explanations. It is likely that the Oath was never part of the teachings on either Cos or Cnidos. One view is that it represents a testament of Pythagorean origin antedating Hippocrates but added to the Hippocratic Collection in later centuries. The Oath's main points concur with the Pythagorean prohibitions against taking life in any form within or outside the body; against surgical procedures of all kinds; indeed, against the shedding of blood, in which the soul was thought to reside.

The omission from surgical treatises in the *Corpus Hippocraticum* of any mention of operations for urinary tract stones may be variously interpreted. For instance, it may be that results were ordinarily so unsuccessful that ethical physicians avoided such procedures, or cutters for the stone might have been lowly regarded, but there may be other explanations. Certainly the extensive involvement in many types of surgical activity by physicians on Cos would make untenable a pledge that forbade surgery.

If the Oath is so clearly a non-Hippocratic document, why has it remained steadfastly the symbol of the physician's pledge to his calling? For one thing, the prohibitions against abortion and contraceptives were in easy consonance with the principles of the Christian Church of later centuries. The earliest reference to the Oath is in the first century A.D., and it may have been taken up later to fit the religious ideals of the time. Substitution of God, Christ, and the saints for the names of Asclepios and his family in the invocation would be a simple matter. Furthermore, the principal parts of the Oath that stick in the memory are those in which the physician swears to act in purity and holiness and to conduct himself in a way that generations of people in many lands and different cultures consider ideal behavior for a physician.

THE HIPPOCRATIC METHOD

The rational attitudes expressed in the collected writings, free of religious or supernatural explanations, represent a great advance in medical thinking, but they were only arrived at after centuries of gradual development. Furthermore, even in those lands where the religious and the rational were closely linked, as in Egypt, wholly secular, empiric systems of medicine were also practiced. Yet the consistency of the rational approach shown by the Hippocratic authors and by the philosopher-scientists before them is exceptional.

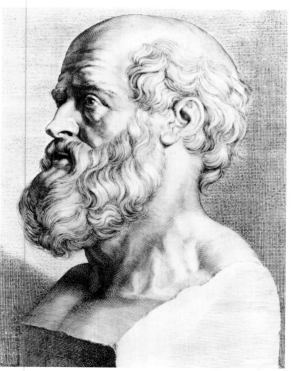

320

320 *Hippocrates, as envisioned in an engraving by Paulus Pontius (1603–58) after a drawing by Peter Paul Rubens from an ancient marble bust. For centuries people have wished Hippocrates to have been of handsome and noble visage. Aristotle, in the 4th century* B.C., *implies that he was short. National Library of Medicine, Bethesda*

The principles of the Hippocratic method may be thus summarized:

1. *Observe all.*

"A great part, I believe, of the Art is to be able to observe." Taking an intensive history was stressed. "Leave nothing to chance, overlook nothing: combine contradictory observations and allow yourself enough time." Hippocrates indicated that a nonmedical person could take a history, but "much of what the physician should know besides, without the patient's telling him, would be omitted."

A particularly well-known description of pulmonary edema (failing circulation in the lung) and fluid in the chest shows close attention to detail, contains the first description of clubbing of the fingers (a sign of chronic disease), and illustrates the use of picturesque, clear phraseology: "Water accumulates; the patient has fever and cough; the respiration is fast; the feet become edematous [swollen]; the nails appear curved and the patient suffers as if he had pus inside, only less severe and more protracted. One can recognize that it is not pus but water. . . . If you put your ear against the chest you can hear it seethe inside like sour wine."

The doctor employed all the senses: sight, hearing, smell, taste, and touch. No finding was too insignificant to be recorded; no emanation from the patient was ignored. Furthermore, the observations were collected without prejudice; that is, before attempting to explain or fit them into the physiological systems of the time. This intellectually unconfined examination lessened the tendency to see what wasn't there or to miss a finding that was not expected—a failing to which observers in all ages are susceptible.

2. *Study the patient rather than the disease.*

The emphasis was on how the patient reacted to his illness, not just on the type of disease. To Hippocrates, the patient's makeup, surroundings, and way of life were all important in evaluating his state of illness and likelihood of recovery. "Observe the nature of each country; diet; customs; the age of the patient; speech; manners; fashion; even his silence; his thoughts; if he sleeps or is suffering from lack of sleep; the content and origin of his dreams . . . one has to study all these signs and to analyze what they portend."

The Hippocratists on Cos opposed the practice of classifying diseases according to the organs affected. Today, with our advanced physiological and anatomical knowledge, we can make such classifications and find them useful—even necessary. On the other hand, we may focus too much on disease and too little on the patient. Francis Adams, himself a nineteenth-century country doctor and a great translator of Hippocrates, expressed it this way: "The great superiority of the ancient savants [the Hippocratists] over the modern was that the former possessed a much greater talent for apprehending the general truth than the latter who confine their attention to particular facts, and neglect too much the observations of general appearances."

3. *Evaluate honestly.*

The courses of over forty patients were described in detail in the Collection. More than half of the patients died, but their case histories were reported faithfully, with accuracy and objectivity. The author did not hesitate to admit the lack of response to treatment, for his expectations (and the patient's) did not exceed the reality that some people get well and others die no matter what is done.

Also, the ancient physician traveling from place to place was interested mainly in prognosis. If he could say with accuracy which of the sick brought to him would survive and which would die, he would be answering what most people wanted to know, even now. "I hold that it is an excellent thing for a physician to practice forecasting. For if he discover and declare unaided by the side of his patients the present, the past, and the future, and fill in the gaps in the accounts given by the sick, he will be the more believed to understand the cases, so that men will confidently entrust themselves to him for treatment."

4. *Assist nature.*

The constant thread throughout the treatises is a reliance on nature. The physician's chief function is to make conditions propitious for the natural forces in the body to reach harmony and therefore health. Even in the surgical treatises the focus is always on restoring. The physician must do what he can do—that is, what has been proved by his past experiences. He must leave alone what he cannot help. "As to diseases, make a habit of two things; to help or at least not to harm."

To be sure, weaknesses may be found in many of the methods of the Hippocratists. For one thing, their anatomical knowledge was scanty and unsystematic. Yet the writings do contain astonishing anatomical detail, as in the sections on wounds, dislocations, fractures, and rectal diseases. Apparently the Hippocratists had sufficient information to deal with what was known of sickness and injury at the time.

A second limitation lay in the lack of specific diagnosis and a sort of nihilism in therapy. The great emphasis on nature taking its course often resulted in a wait-and-see approach. Yet, in addition to dietary and other regimens Hippocrates did use direct methods, as witnessed by the numerous surgical and mechanical techniques in the Collection. However, he recognized his limitations and did only what appeared to be useful.

Another weakness was espousal of the four humors theory. This doctrine, together with many ramifications which had origins long before Hippocrates, was to be a principal basis for medical speculation in subsequent centuries, but Hippocrates used the system chiefly to explain illness in current terms. However, his treatment was not based on that theory alone since extreme remedies were not employed. Furthermore, Hippocrates judged results not on how they fit the theory but only on the outcome. Yet, like Galen much later, Hippocrates had need of a base, a system, a theory, to underlie the knowledge of physiology and illness.

Paracelsus, who will appear in the chapters on the Renaissance, burned the works of Avicenna and Galen to symbolize the need to rely on one's own observations rather than authorities. That principle, however, is part of the Hippocratic method itself. Hippocrates relied on his own observations, while using the past experiences of others, for he recognized that knowledge did not begin with him. We hope that in our times people will realize that what we embrace securely may seem foolish in future centuries.

If the Hippocratic method is used today, the physician can observe objectively, avoid rigid postures, foreswear arrogance, and shun abject adherence to doctrines. Furthermore, we are just beginning to learn once again the Hippocratic doctrine of attending to the whole person in his own environment.

"Life is short; and the art long; and the right time an instant; and treatment precarious; and the crisis grievous. It is necessary for the physician not only to provide the needed treatment but to provide for the patient himself, and for those beside him, and to provide for his outside affairs." (Translation by Dickinson Richards)

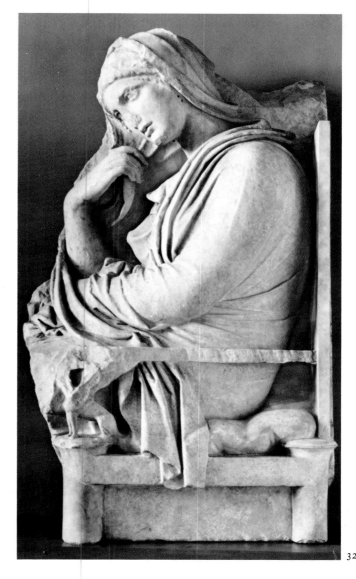

321

321 *Mourning woman on marble gravestone of about 400 B.C. The Hippocratic writings provided insight into mental illness, including anxiety and depression. Metropolitan Museum of Art, New York*

Medical Sects and
the Center at Alexandria

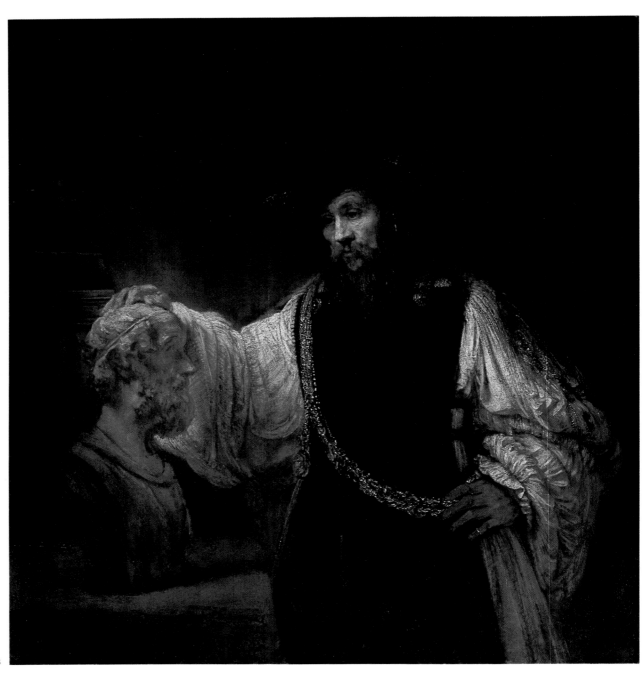

AFTER the time of Hippocrates, groups of teachers and practitioners split up into a variety of separate medical systems, or sects. The ideas of the philosophers Plato and Aristotle were among the important influences, for as Aristotle pointed out one might begin with philosophy but would end with medicine; or start with medicine and find oneself in philosophy.

Plato (c. 429–347 B.C.), a contemporary of Hippocrates, a student of Socrates, and the teacher of Aristotle, became one of the most influential thinkers in the history of the Western world. Some of his own heritage can be traced to Pythagorean doctrines, since mathematics, especially geometry, figured prominently in his philosophic system. Plato's interests lay mainly in the nature of the soul and matter, and his medical speculations—logical, but without direct experimentation—led to a number of faulty conclusions about the human body. However, several of these opinions were staunchly held beliefs of the time, and even some investigators of later centuries were unable to shake them. Plato's method of reasoning at a distance rather than at the dissecting table or the bedside was resurrected and perpetuated in the Middle Ages. Some of his teachings on the responsibilities of government even have a bearing on medical practice today, for Plato expected the ideal state to provide for the health of its citizens and to prevent poverty and overpopulation.

The physicians who rallied around his doctrines, particularly in the third century B.C. and after, were called Dogmatists. For them, reasoning superseded observation. Experience was indeed a means of testing, but mainly to prove the correctness of one's deduction. The Dogmatists classified all diseases according to the humors; for instance, they referred to an illness as mucous or bilious and used an appropriate remedy against the particular excess humor. They considered their practices based on Hippocrates, but except for looking to him as an authority they showed little evidence of following his spirit of objectivity or his principles of treatment. Most of the Dogmatists, and there were many, used extreme therapeutic measures, including drastic purgings and bleedings, and treated fevers with dehydrating regimens.

Praxagoras of Cos (fl. c. 340 B.C.) was among the first to separate the functions of arteries and veins, but he believed that both systems contained air. Praxagoras extended the number of humors to eleven and used bleeding extensively, but he placed emphasis on the pulse, showing that disease affected its characteristics—one of his most important contributions.

Diocles of Carystos (first half of fourth century B.C.), another famous Dogmatist, wrote many works on clinical subjects, drugs, dietetics, embryology, and anatomy. Called the Hippocrates of his time, Diocles perspicaciously distinguished between pleurisy (inflammation of the lining over the lung) and pneumonia (disease of the lung itself), between intestinal cramps and intestinal obstruction, and recognized fever as a symptom rather than a disease.

Aristotle (384–322 B.C.), son of a physician and pupil of Plato, also had profound influence on later medicine, especially among the Arabic authors. His writings illuminated an extraordinary number of fields: logic, metaphysics, psychology, politics, zoology, poetry, drama. He was also known as a great teacher and was hired by Philip of Macedonia to tutor his son Alexander.

Aristotle's methods were based on careful investigations of both animals and humans, and his studies—in which he was lavishly supported by Alexander—were milestones in science. In embryology he described the *punctum saliens* (the first sign of the embryo), the early development of the heart and great vessels, the beating of the embryo's heart (the first such observation), some differences between arteries and veins, the great arterial vessel the aorta (which he named), and the course of the ureter. Aristotle taught that the fetus did not breathe while in the uterus and that male and female embryos did not develop in different compartments. His writings on the anatomy of vertebrates and invertebrates were so extensive that they earned him recognition as the founder of comparative anatomy.

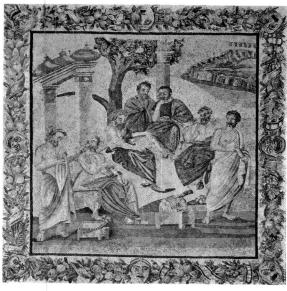

323

322 Aristotle Contemplating the Bust of Homer (1653), by Rembrandt van Rijn. The importance of Aristotle to Western thought—even some 2,000 years after his death—is honored in this painting, in which the great philosopher-scientist also acknowledges a debt to his forebears. Metropolitan Museum of Art, New York

323 Pompeian mosaic showing some of the greatest of the ancient Greek philosophers, including Plato, pointing to the globe, and, counterclockwise, Zeno, Aristotle, Pythagoras, Epicuros, Socrates, and Theophrastos. Museo Archeologico Nazionale, Naples

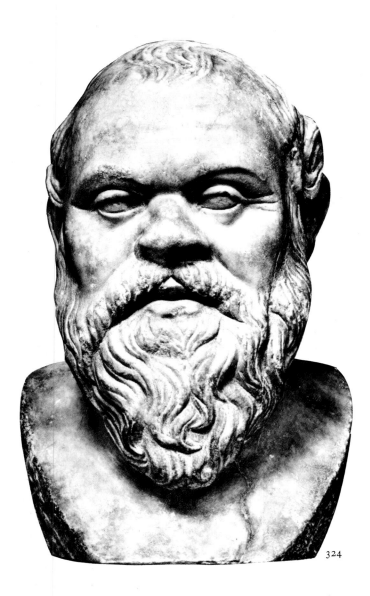

324

324 *Socrates, the great teacher of Plato, is seen in this Roman copy of a Greek bust, c. 380–360* B.C. *Museo Archeologico Nazionale, Naples*

325 *Plato, a contemporary of Hippocrates, is shown here in a Roman copy of a Greek original. The physicians in Alexandria who considered themselves followers of the doctrines of Plato and of Hippocrates were called Dogmatists. Vatican Museums, Rome*

326 *This Roman copy of a Greek sculpture is thought to represent Aristotle, who wrote in virtually every field of knowledge. A pupil of Plato's and father of comparative anatomy, his direct observations and experiments were detailed and exhaustive. Palazzo Spada, Rome*

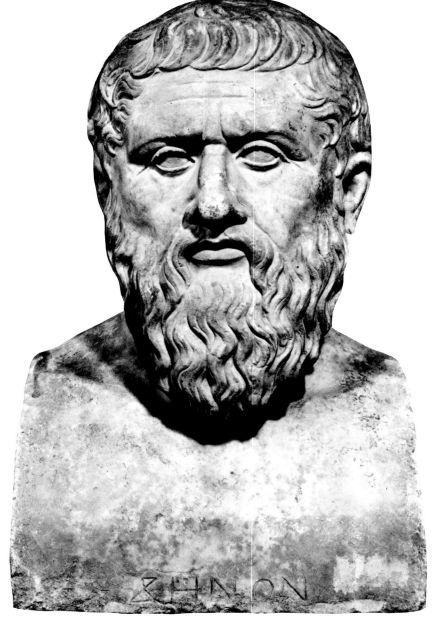

325

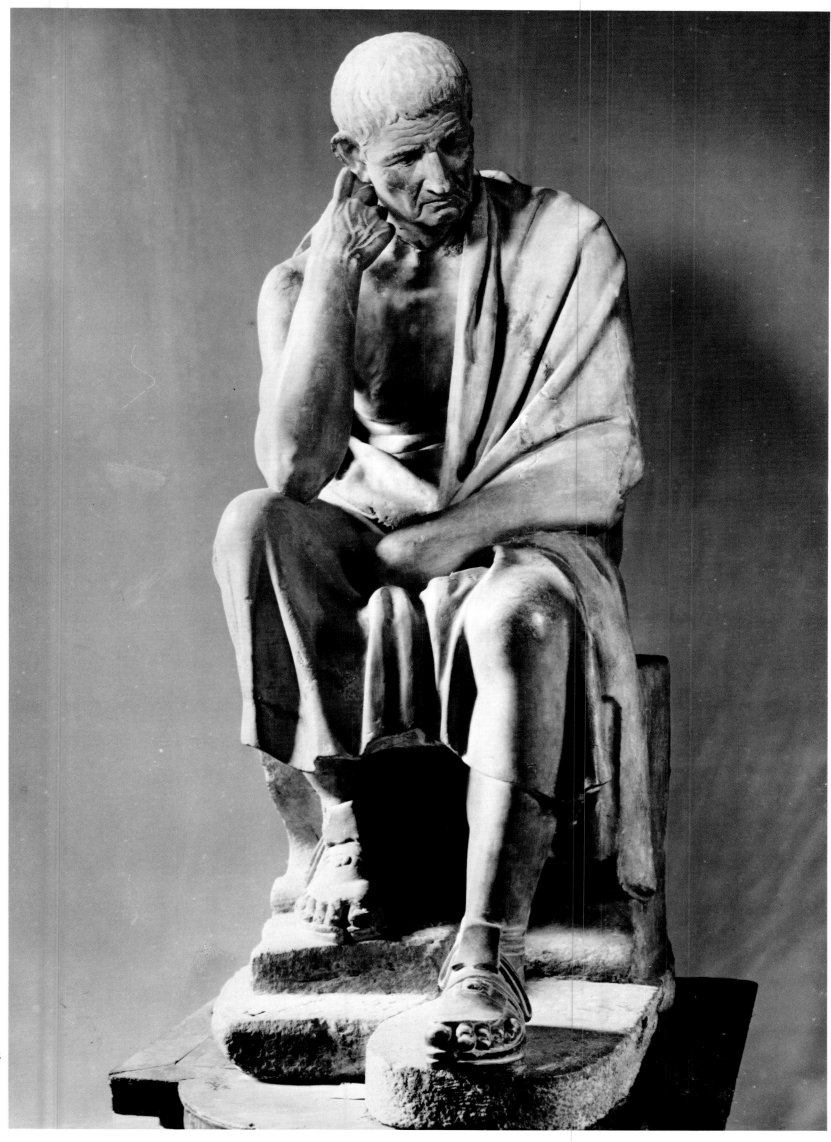

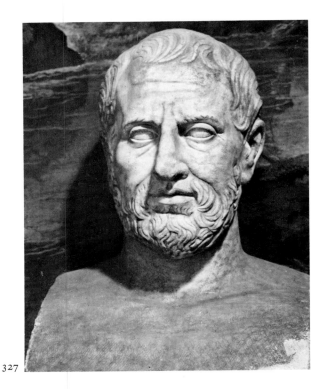

327

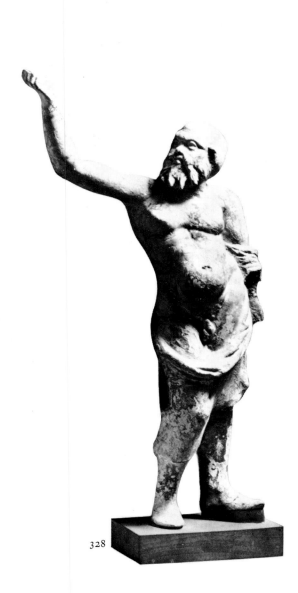

328

Yet Aristotle reflected the intellectual boundaries of his time. He believed that the doctrine of the humors had some foundation and placed the seat of intelligence in the heart. He confused nerves with ligaments and tendons (the Greeks used the same word for all three) and linked veins from the liver to the right arm and from the spleen to the left arm. Therefore, in treatment he advocated bloodletting on the side corresponding to the location of the diseased organ.

Aristotle also subscribed to dreams as portents of the future (as was typical of his time), but he was primarily an experimentalist, in contrast to Plato, whose teachings were more mystical and metaphysical. Their doctrines were to have profound influence on science and medicine in the Middle Ages and the Renaissance. Together with Hippocrates before them and Galen afterwards, they were the principal authorities of pagan, Christian, and Muslim medical thought.

Theophrastos (c. 370–285 B.C.) probably Aristotle's most famous disciple, continued the investigative and experimental approach, adding his own ideas to explain various symptoms such as fainting, dizziness, and sweating. Among his important studies on botany were descriptions of over five hundred plants, dealing with morphology, biological characteristics, and medical uses.

In addition to the Dogmatists, other systems of medicine arose. In the third century B.C., under the philosophical influence of the Skeptics, there emerged a group of physicians called Empiricists, for whom the effects of treatment were what mattered, not possible reasons for illness. One's previous experience with symptoms displayed by a patient should indicate the probable outcome and most effective treatment for a malady. In these views the Empiricists followed the Hippocratic principles of observation, experience, and prognosis, yet some Empiricists who wrote on Hippocrates were highly critical of his teachings, probably because of the humoral explanations in the Collection. Not seeking causes or reasons for results, they ended up rejecting inquiry into anatomy or physiological mechanisms. Even Philinos of Cos (third century B.C.) who studied under Herophilos, one of the great Alexandrian anatomists, did not consider human dissection of practical use. The outstanding Empiricist Heraclides (second century B.C.) wrote extensively on symptomatology and surgery. He also made many contributions to pharmacy.

In the first century B.C., the influence of Greek medicine received great impetus in Rome through the personality and teachings of Asclepiades (discussed in the next chapter). About 50 B.C., one of his followers, Themison, founded another medical system, Methodism, which abandoned the doctrines of the four humors that had dominated Greek pathologic thinking for centuries. In his system disease was caused by constriction or relaxation of the "pores," as judged by evacuations, secretions, and feverishness in the sick. All other information was useless. If the "pores" were contracted, the physician ordered a scant diet, warm baths, poultices, humid air, bleeding, and medications to produce evacuations. Against the opposite, a relaxed condition, he prescribed an increased food intake, cold baths and air, and styptic medications to induce constriction.

Another system, Pneumatism, was opposed to Dogmatism, Empiricism, and Methodism. Also Greek in origin, it had its principal influences in Rome in the first and second century A.D. Athenaeus of Cilicia, the founder of Pneumatism, applied the all-pervading cosmic principle of the ancient Stoics to a general physiologic view that people breathed in this spirit, the *pneuma*, which went first to the heart and then through the arteries to all parts of the body. Conceptions of disease involved complicated theoretical relationships among the *pneuma*, warmth, and moisture inside the body. Yet despite the abstruse wanderings of their theories and their employment of medicines combined from an extraordinary number of drugs (one remedy is said to have contained over six hundred substances), the practices of the Pneumatists were often pragmatic. For instance, bleedings were infrequent and limited. Furthermore, Athenaeus had concern for public health, including maintenance of unpolluted water and adequate housing.

A final sect, Eclecticism, arose from the Pneumatists. Adhering to no single, consistent system, the followers chose ideas according to their own needs to explain and treat illness. Even Galen considered himself an Eclectic.

One of the early Eclectics was Archigenes (c. A.D. 100), who was active principally in Rome. As we learn from Galen, his observations on symptomatology, physical diagnosis, and drug therapy were brilliant, but his contributions to surgery are remembered best. For instance, he described amputation with considerable perceptiveness: ligating the main vessel first; using temporary tight constriction above the level of incision to control bleeding; operating not just for established gangrene but also for extensive injuries that would result in gangrene. Furthermore, he counseled against surgery for people who might be too weak to withstand the trauma.

Among other Greek writers during the Roman hegemony over Greece was Aretaeus of Cappadocia (c. A.D. 120–180), whose writing, as translated by Francis Adams, was precise although sometimes pedantic. He gave vivid descriptions of many diseases, including a type of diabetes, and what might have been diphtheria, pneumonia, and migraine. In suggesting that jaundice was due to obstruction of the biliary ducts he indicated an advanced understanding over earlier times. Following Hippocrates he paid attention to the environment as well as the patient's makeup. He subscribed to the doctrine of the *pneuma*, but in treatment used all the methods of his period: regimens, diet, and drugs (some of which were drastic). However, he continued to minister to the sick even after it was hopeless, a practice not widely advocated. "When he can render no further aid, the physician alone can still mourn as a man with his incurable patient. This is the physician's sad lot."

The tenets of the various sects of medicine (Dogmatism, Empiricism, Methodism, Pneumatism, and Eclecticism) extended from the fourth century B.C. well into the Christian era. While these systems were developing, the most important locus of medical thought and practice was the great center of Greek learning at Alexandria, founded in 331 B.C. by Alexander the Great and governed by a dynasty stemming from his general Ptolemy. Indeed, most of the originators of the medical sects were students at one time at Alexandria. Scholars flocked there from all over the world, and the prestige of having studied at Alexandria, one of the greatest cities of the Hellenic world, was prized and recognized. The Ptolemaic rulers gave lavish financial support to the researchers in all fields, including philosophy, mathematics, astronomy, music, poetry, history, and especially the natural sciences. Ptolemy I Soter (r. 305–284 B.C.) and Ptolemy II Philadelphos (r. 285–246 B.C.) founded botanical and zoological gardens and also two building complexes, the Museum and the Serapeum, each with a vast library where the most renowned investigators and writers of many different racial and cultural backgrounds could assemble to study and to teach.

A contemporary rival center of learning existed in Pergamon, though only after c. 250 B.C., in the reign of Eumenes I. However, the Ptolemaic pharaoh jealously guarded the supremacy of Alexandria by forbidding the export of the papyrus plant or its products. It is said that because of this forced shortage of papyrus Pergamon developed a material derived from animal skin, subsequently called *Pergamos* (parchment).

The Alexandrian center eventually included among its savants Euclid (fl. c. 300 B.C.), who systematized previous works in geometry; probably Archimedes of Syracuse (c. 287–212 B.C.), the great physicist and expert on hydrostatics; Heron (fl. c. A.D. 62), who invented a primitive steam engine and other mechanical devices; Callimachos (c. 305–240 B.C.), the famous poet and librarian who catalogued the huge collection of scrolls; and Dionysos Thrax (c. 170–c. 90 B.C.), who laid the foundations of grammar as a discipline. Medical research in the Alexandrian Museum became famous; indeed, its reputation lasted long after

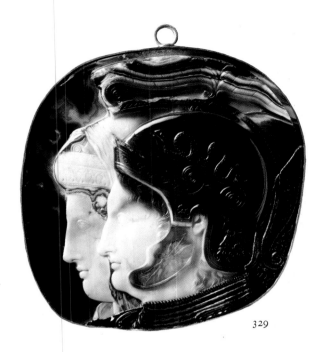

329

327 *This Greek herm of Theophrastos, a disciple of Aristotle's, was found in the Villa of Cassius, near Tivoli. The writings of Theophrastos on botany and medicinal plants were the basis for many subsequent works on pharmacy. Villa Albani, Rome*

328 *Papposilenos shown teaching, a clay figure said to have come from Centuripe, Sicily. Outstanding teachers of medicine were found in centers throughout the Hellenistic world. Collection Norbert Schimmel, New York*

329 *Alexander the Great and his foreign bride, the Bactrian princess Roxana, as seen on a Hellenistic cameo. Having conquered Persia, Alexander adopted Persian dress for state occasions. Kunsthistorisches Museum, Vienna*

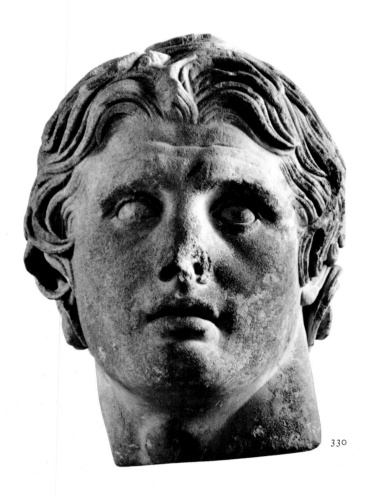

330

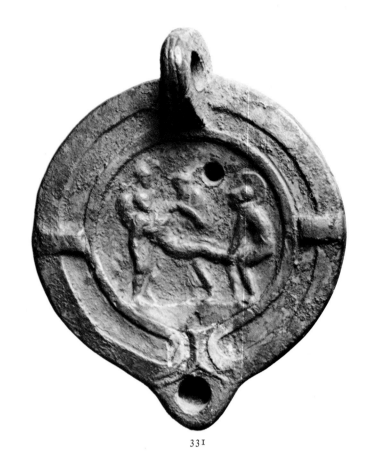

331

330 *Marble head of Alexander found at Pergamon (late 3d or 2d century* B.C.*), a rival center of learning to the famous one he founded at Alexandria in 331* B.C. *Archaeological Museum, Istanbul*

331 *Greek oil lamp in terra-cotta showing soldiers carrying a wounded man. Much as in the campaigns of Alexander, the soldiers had to look out for each other. Cabinet des Médailles, The Louvre, Paris*

332 *Bust of Marcus Modius Asiaticus, a leader of the Methodists, one of the principal medical sects in Alexandria and Rome. Among the other sects were the Dogmatists, Empiricists, Pneumatists, and Eclectics. Cabinet des Médailles, The Louvre, Paris*

333. *The death of Alexander, as shown in a 16th-century Persian miniature illustrating a copy of the* Shah-nama *(Book of Kings) begun by Firdausi in the 10th century. Alexander became a demigod hero among the very peoples whom he conquered. Gift of Alexander Smith Cochran, 1913, Metropolitan Museum of Art, New York*

334 *(Overleaf) In an Islamic text on hygiene, written over 1,500 years after his time, Aristotle is pictured showing disapproval of his pupil Alexander (known as Iskandar in Persia), who is about to take a cup of wine. Bibliothèque Nationale, Paris*

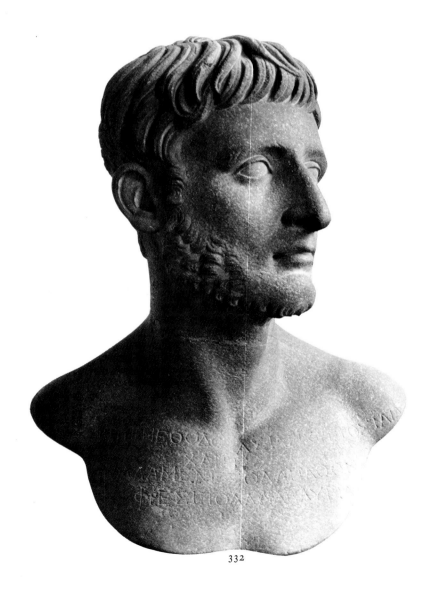

332

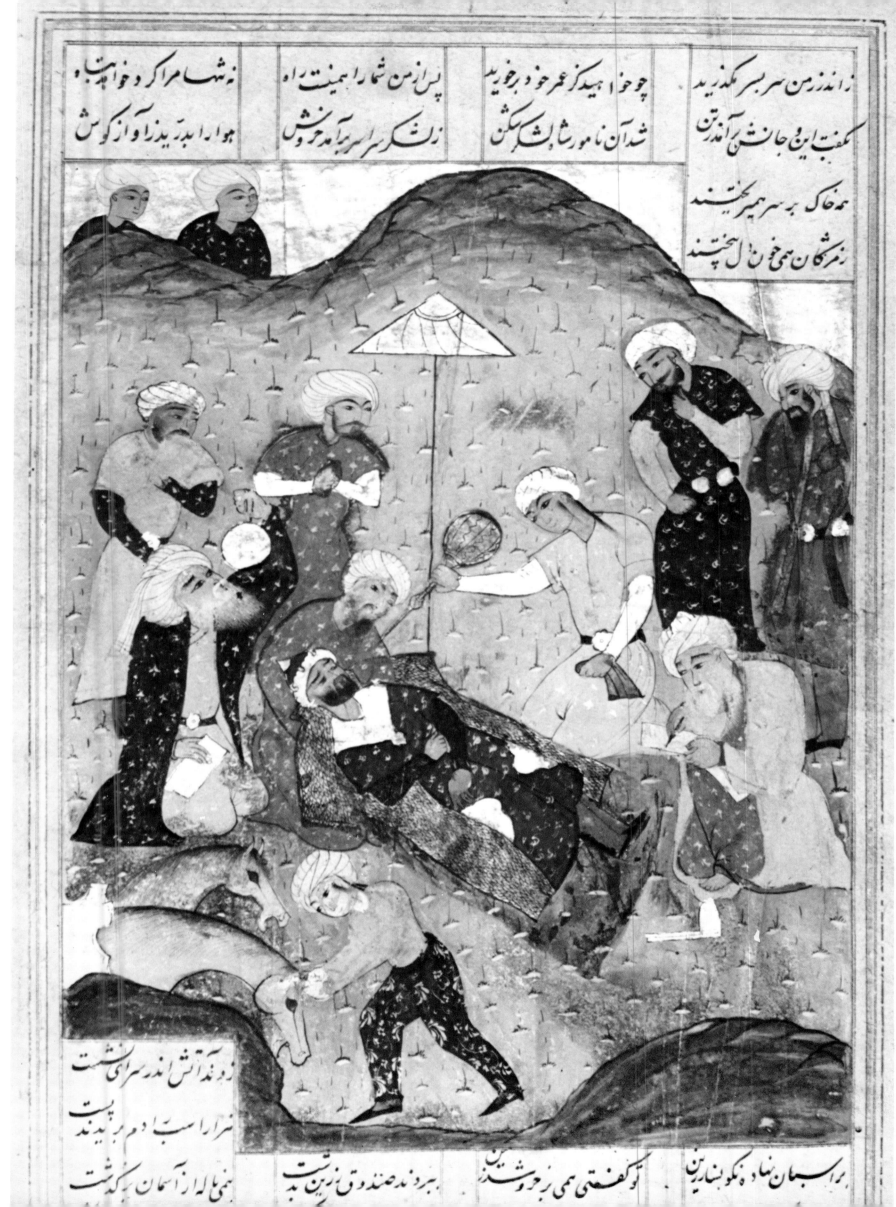

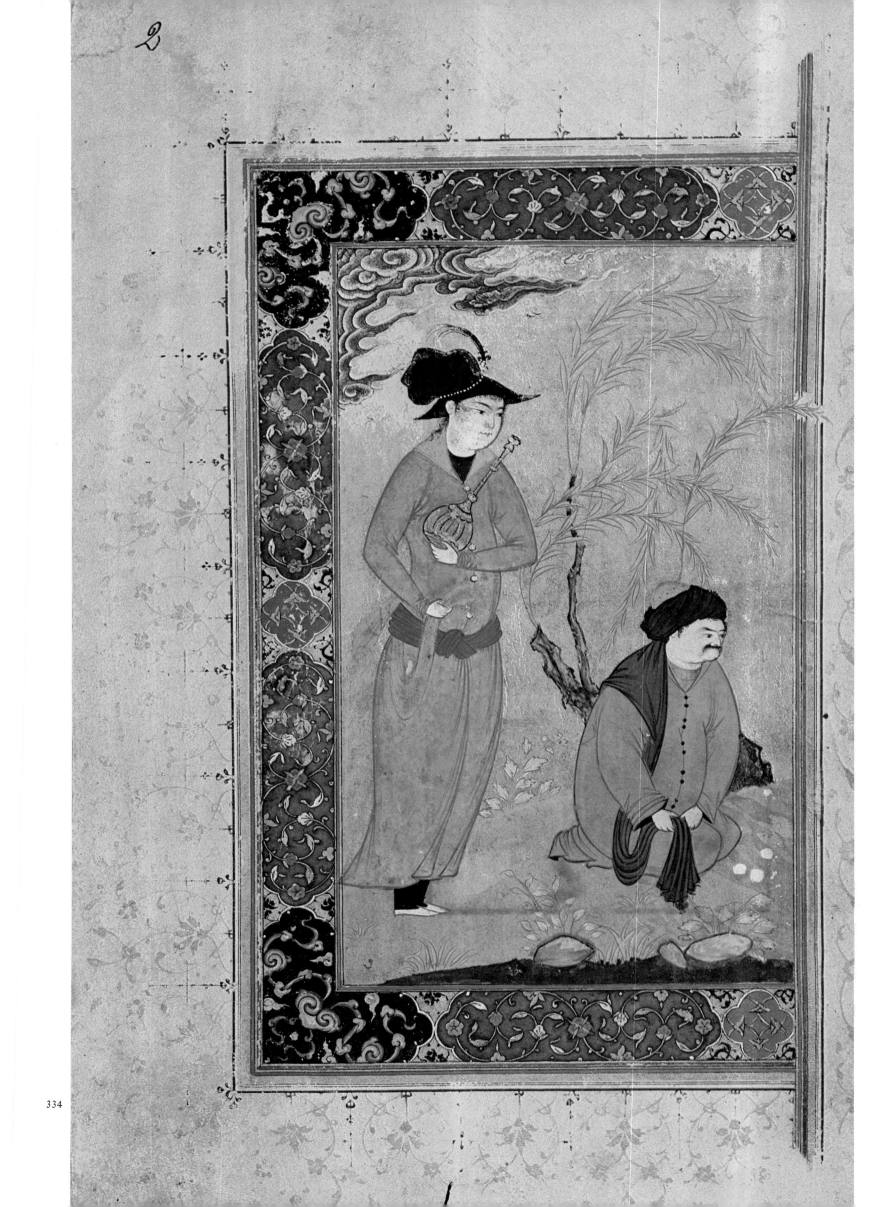

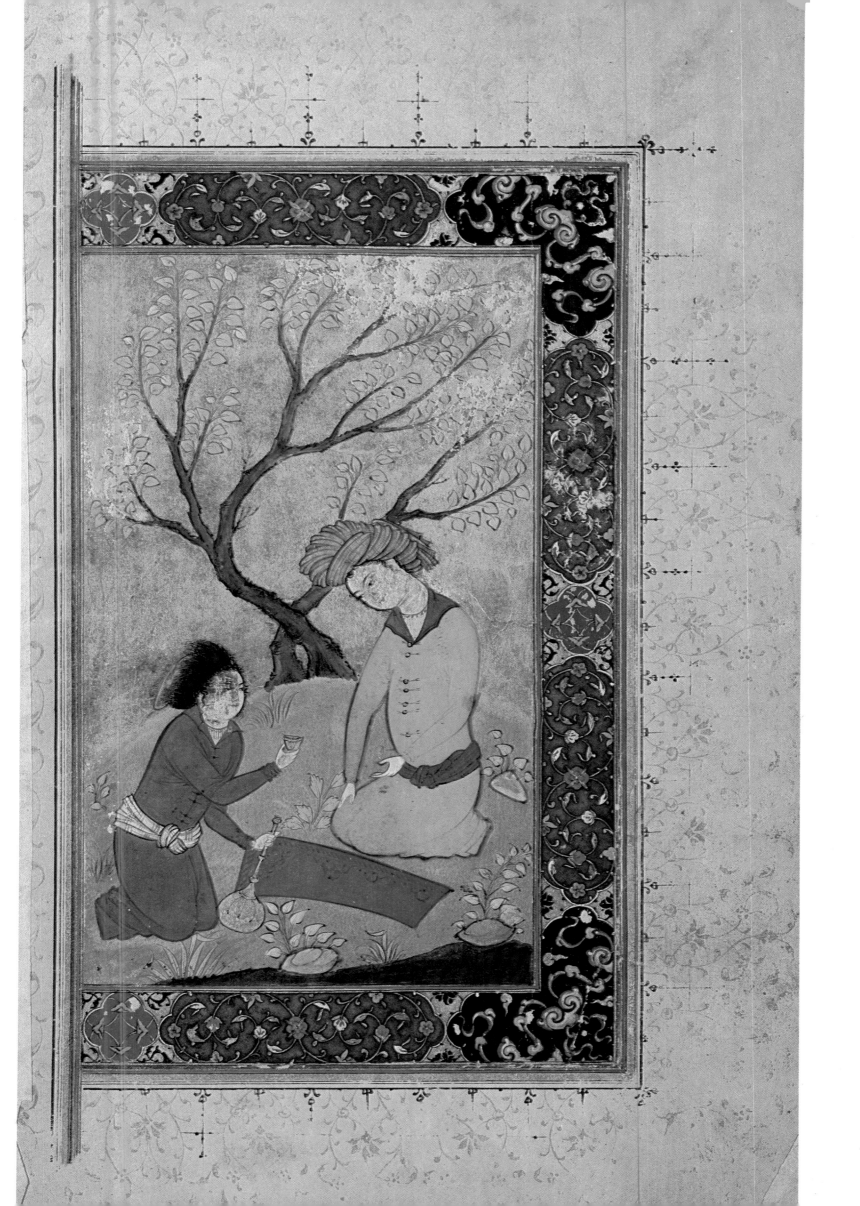

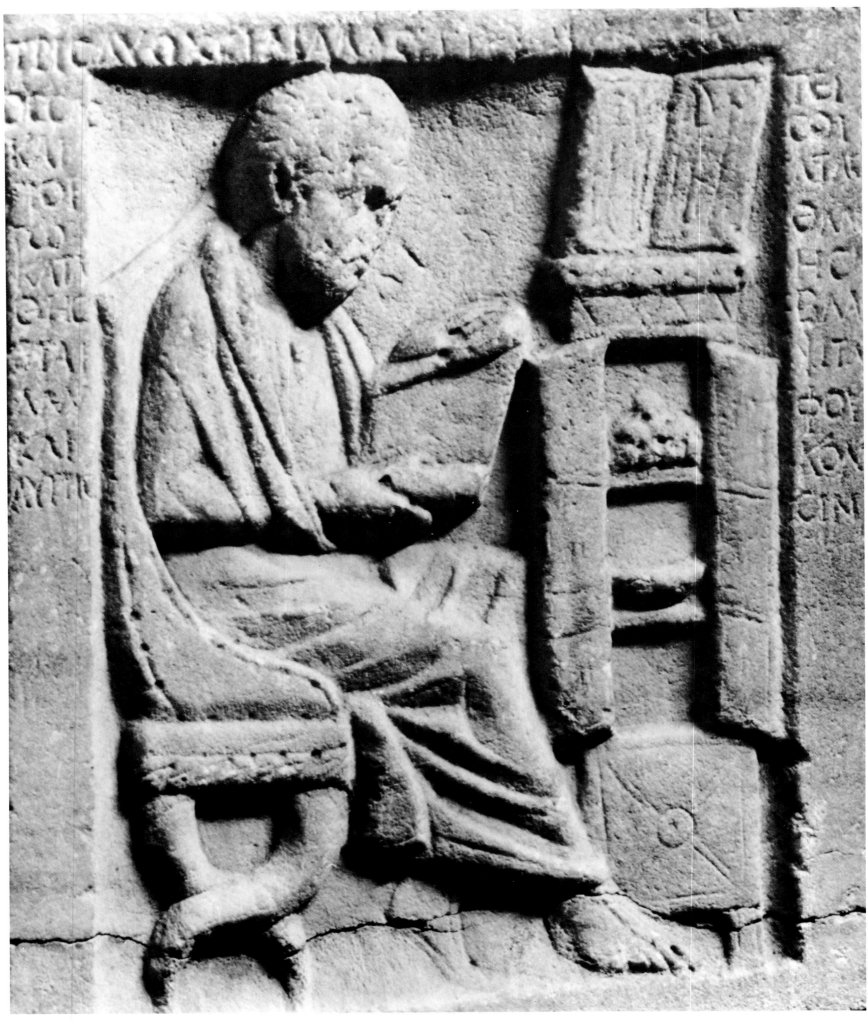

335

the Ptolemaic dynasty ended with the death of Cleopatra VII in 30 B.C.

The two outstanding medical investigators there were Herophilos (fl. c. 280 B.C.) and Erasistratos (fl. c. 250 B.C.). Most of our knowledge of these two is derived from later commentators, especially Celsus and Galen in the Roman period.

Herophilos had been a pupil of Praxagoras of Cos, a Dogmatist, and is especially remembered for his contributions to human anatomy. In keeping with the Alexandrian attitude of using every means to accumulate information, dissection of corpses was a regular practice, probably for the first time in history. Celsus reported the rumor that the anatomists used living people, such as criminals, in vivisection, but Galen made no mention of it.

Herophilos was responsible for a multitude of discoveries about human anatomy. He described various parts of the brain, the intestinal tract, the lymphatics, the liver, the genital organs, the eye, and the vascular system. He pointed out that the heart transmitted pulsation to the arteries and described extensive variations in the pulse. Furthermore, he stated that arteries were six times thicker than veins and had different structure. Along with brilliant, accurate, objective observations, Herophilos employed the ancient doctrine of the four humors in his treatment. He used bleedings and drastic drugs to evacuate the plethora of humors. However, in the fields of surgery and obstetrics he understood much of the mechanics and generally followed pragmatic methods.

Erasistratos has been particularly commended by historians for his emphasis on physiological experimentation, but he was also an original anatomical investigator as well. He differentiated between sensory and motor nerves although he also confused ligaments with nerves as others had before him. His accurate observations extended to the structure of the brain, the trachea (windpipe), the heart, and the vascular system, including the association of ascites (fluid in the abdomen) with a hard liver (probably cirrhosis). He also described the epiglottis and explained its function of blocking off the air passages during swallowing.

Turning away from the humoral pathology embraced by Herophilos, Erasistratos was a proponent of the idea that atoms were the basis of the body's structure. Thus the later solidistic theories of the Methodists (Asclepiades and Themison) had their origin in Alexandria. Erasistratos believed that atoms required *pneuma* from the inspired air to be activated and that they circulated in arteries which contained no blood. But whatever his theories, his practice was to use moderate measures: diet, mild drugs, and baths, without recourse to bleedings.

Followers of Herophilus and Erasistratos became embroiled in acrimonious debate for centuries. Galen in the second century A.D., for instance, considered himself part of the tradition of Herophilos because of his emphasis on anatomy and humoral pathology, and probably also because Herophilos looked to Hippocrates. On the other hand he reviled Erasistratos for his solidistic theories and his disagreement with Hippocrates on humoral doctrines.

In retrospect we can see that many of these acid controversies were based principally on theoretical concepts. Time has wiped out their foundations. The teachers propounded, the followers disputed, the practitioners wrangled, and the sick hoped. To the extent that the physician's treatment was based on unprejudiced observations of the patient's condition, honest evaluation of past results, and sincere concern for the welfare of the ill person, the patient received benefit no matter which theory, sect, or doctrine was espoused.

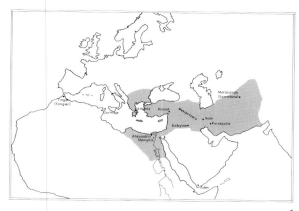

336

335 *Graeco-Roman bas-relief of the 1st century* A.D., *showing a physician at his desk and a case of surgical instruments on top of his cabinet. Metropolitan Museum of Art, New York*

336 *Map of the empire of Alexander the Great in 323* B.C.

Medicine
in Roman Times

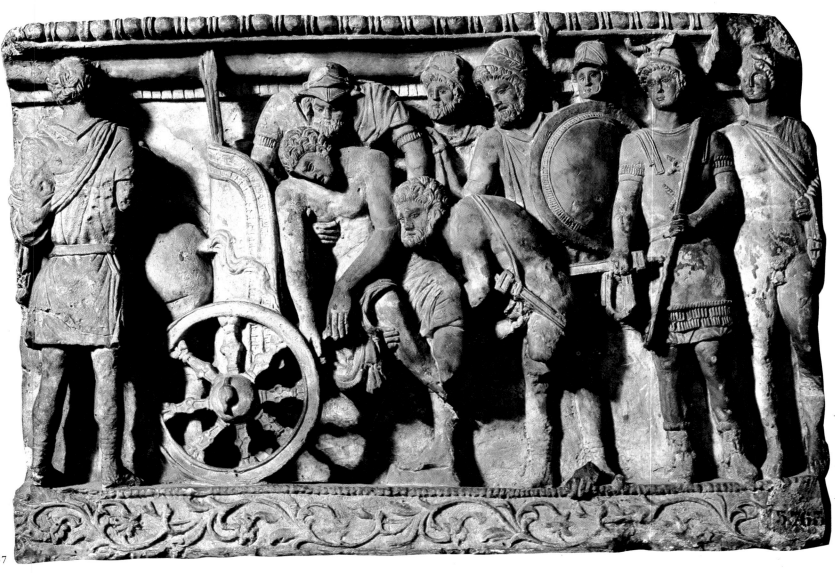

GREEK medicine after Hippocrates reached a peak in Alexandria and shortly afterward began to infiltrate Rome, which exercised hegemony over the Greek world after 146 B.C. The various medical sects growing out of developments in Alexandria were taken to Rome by Greek practitioners and subsequently underwent their principal development there.

Roman medicine had had a long history of its own, inherited from the Etruscans in both secular and religious aspects, but it was the religious healing that had the more lasting influence. The Etruscan inheritance is shown in the early Roman reliance on divination from the entrails of animals, the use of Etruscan prognostic charts, and the propitiation of the gods to stop epidemics (religious processions to ward off plague continued well into the Middle Ages). As early as the seventh century B.C. there was a College of Augurs, and for virtually each disease or symptom there was a special divinity. According to legend, the Greek medical deity Asclepios (Aesculapius in Latin) was introduced to Rome in 295 B.C. in the form of a snake sent from the temple of Epidaurus.

Over the years, theurgy and superstition gradually gave way to more rational attitudes. In the Roman Aesculapian temples the suppliants were bent on receiving more than just treatment by the god and his snakes; they often insisted on prescriptions for drugs to carry away with them. As Rome came more and more to dominate Greece politically, Greek culture ironically became the predominant force in the intellectual life of the Romans. Greek was the language of the rich and educated, who had their children taught by Greek tutors and derived their literature from Greek models. Especially in medicine the attitudes, methods, and practices were almost entirely Greek.

HEALERS AND THEIR METHODS

In the first century A.D., Pliny wrote, "The Roman people for more than six hundred years were not without medical art but were without physicians." However, the Aquilian Law of the third century B.C. made a medical practitioner liable for his neglect of a slave treated by operation, so at least someone was publicly practicing the healing arts. For the most part each family was ministered to by the head of the household himself, but no citizen would think of practicing outside his home. The Roman upper class had the same aversion to manual work as did the early Greeks and felt that practicing medicine was unworthy of cultured men. With the influx of Greek practitioners over an extended period, Roman contempt for Greeks in general and healers in particular varied with the political scene, internal changes in the profession, and the needs of rulers and the populace for medical attention.

Cato, the censor (234–149 B.C.), was especially incensed at the virtual control over Roman intellectual life of Greek ideas, which he considered effete and dishonest. According to Pliny, he railed particularly against the physicians, endeavoring to reinstitute what he considered pragmatic Roman methods. Cato advised the use of cabbage and wine for maintaining health and treating illness, but he accompanied his treatments with magic formulas and incantations.

An increasing number of Greeks and other foreigners continued to pour into the rich, exciting, and powerful city of Rome. In 46 B.C. Julius Caesar, in an attempt to limit a famine, temporarily banished all foreigners from the city except for physicians, to whom he granted citizenship. Many early healers were probably incompetent and unscrupulous, and their social status was low (most were slaves), but more and more freedmen and even citizens began to enter practice. Thus Greek and Roman attitudes and methods gradually merged.

The first well-known Greek physician to come to Rome was Archagathos of Sparta, about 219 B.C., and his career illustrates the swings in the Roman attitude toward physicians. Initially he was hailed by the populace and the Senate, receiving the honor of citizenship, and his brilliant surgical procedures earned him the

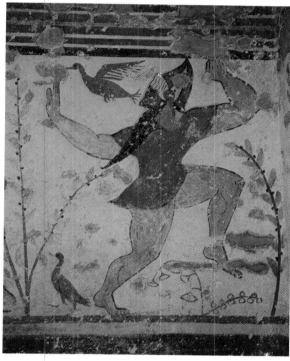

338

337 *Wounded man being lifted onto chariot for removal from the battlefield. Detail from an Etruscan urn that also shows the medically skilled Achilles caring for Patroclus. Museo Archeologico, Florence*

338 *Scene from the Tomb of the Augurs (540–530 B.C.) in the cemetery of Monterozzi, Tarquinia. Belief in augurs was an Etruscan inheritance that persisted well into Roman times.*

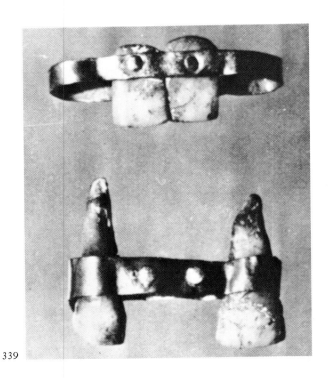

339

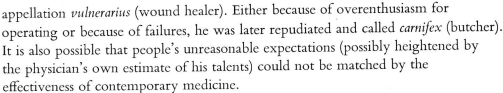

339 *Excavated examples of Etruscan dentistry, showing how extracted teeth—minus roots—were mounted on gold bridges between good teeth. Merseyside County Museums, Liverpool*

340 *Bronze model of a sheep's liver (3d century B.C.), used by the Etruscans in divination. Similar to clay models used by the ancient Mesopotamians in prognosticating disease. Museo Civico, Piacenza*

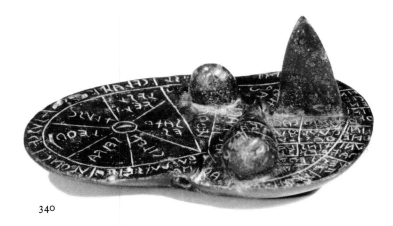

340

appellation *vulnerarius* (wound healer). Either because of overenthusiasm for operating or because of failures, he was later repudiated and called *carnifex* (butcher). It is also possible that people's unreasonable expectations (possibly heightened by the physician's own estimate of his talents) could not be matched by the effectiveness of contemporary medicine.

An important impetus to acceptance of Greek practitioners in the first century B.C. came from Asclepiades of Bithynia (c. 120–c. 70 B.C.), who was influenced by teachings originally advanced by Erasistratus in the third century B.C. He was apparently a man of immense personal charm and dynamism, with a brilliant mind. Some of his contemporaries and also later writers, notably Galen, counted him a near-charlatan, but a majority of people in high place and low considered him "a messenger from heaven." Probably the poet-scientist Lucretius and the political leader and orator Cicero were among his admiring close friends. The general populace was impressed by his personality, methods, and results, which he was quick to exploit, for Asclepiades sought to cure *tuto, celerites ac jucunde* (safely, quickly, and pleasantly). His reputation was also advanced by the report that he had restored a dead man to life.

His teachings were a deliberate repudiation of Hippocrates, for he believed that the physician, not nature, cured disease. He abandoned the doctrine of the four humors totally. Instead he erected an elaborate solidistic system (an extension of the earlier theories of Democritus and Heraclides) which regarded the body as composed of an almost infinite number of atoms of different sizes always in motion, between which flowed the body liquids. Health depended on the smooth activity of the atoms; sickness occurred when the motions were disordered. Themison, a pupil of Asclepiades, developed these ideas further in founding the system of Methodism, which became one of the most influential systems for centuries afterward.

In practice Asclepiades used mild methods, such as diet, exercise, massage, soothing medications, enemas, music, and singing. One of his most successful procedures was tracheostomy (making an opening in the windpipe) for obstruction to breathing. For "phrenitis," a term he applied to mental illness, he employed opium, wine, and hygienic measures. His principle was to avoid wherever possible drastic and weakening procedures. Yet he did employ bleeding and in fevers continued the debilitating and dehydrating custom of markedly restricting both food and drink.

The overthrow of authority, rejection of the four humors, avoidance of teleological explanations, and promulgation of a materialistic approach to body mechanisms were steps toward rationalism. However, over two hundred years later Galen railed at Asclepiades and also against the more ancient Erasistratus for repudiating Hippocrates and the four humors. He was particularly incensed at Asclepiades for rejecting the principle of assisting nature and for downplaying anatomy. Indeed so damning were Galen's writings that the name of Asclepiades almost disappeared during medieval times and was virtually forgotten until the Renaissance. Nevertheless, through his practices, principles, and reputation, Asclepiades improved the standing of physicians in Rome, especially that of the Greek doctors.

Although free citizens probably did eventually practice medicine, most Roman practitioners were mainly freedmen and slaves. Physicians were usually of Greek origin, but immigrant Egyptians and Jews also practiced. The upper-class Roman often had a private slave-physician for his own family, but sometimes he was hired out to others. There were also municipal or government slave-physicians to minister to sick slaves and slave-physicians who were assistants to free and freedmen physicians. These slaves could buy their freedom, but they were so valuable to their professional masters that a law had to be passed setting the manumission price according to the worth of the slave as an assistant rather than as a practicing physician.

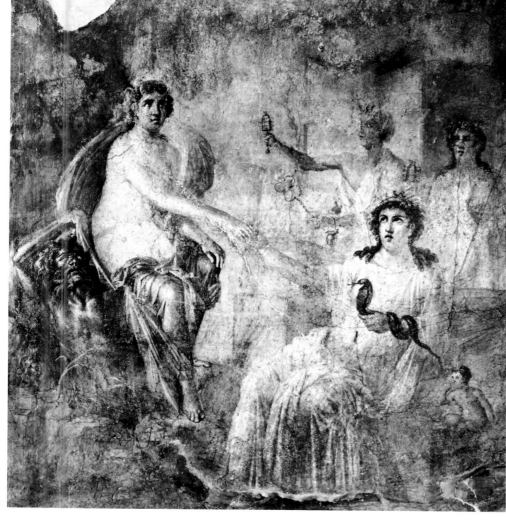

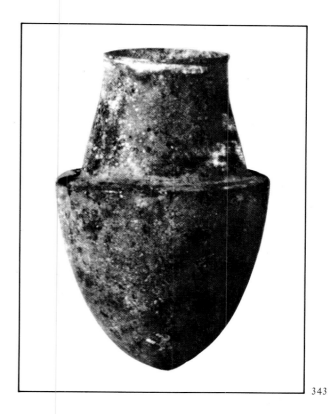

341 The Coming of Io into Egypt, *from the Temple of Isis in Pompeii, showing the nymph being welcomed by the goddess Isis–Hygeia, whom the Romans invoked against the evil eye. Roman and Egyptian deities were frequently merged. Museo Archeologico Nazionale, Naples*

342 Bronze and iron surgical and gynecological *instruments found in the House of the Surgeon (c. A.D. 62–79), Pompeii. Museo Archeologico Nazionale, Naples*

343 Bronze cupping vessel found on Corfu, similar *to the type used in Roman times. British Museum, London*

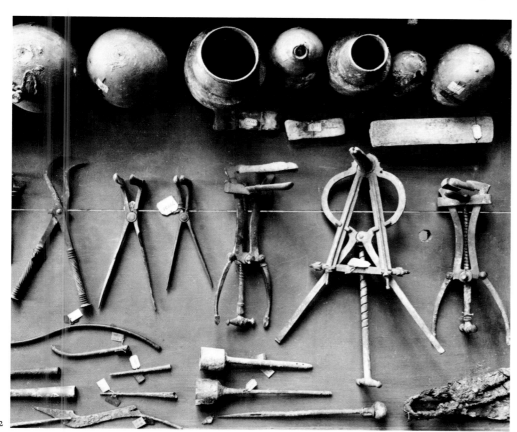

344 *Private bath in the House of the Menander (c. 2d century B.C.–A.D. 79), showing the type of bathing facilities the wealthy often provided for themselves.*

345 *Glass jars, possibly for ointments, made in the Rhineland in the 3d century, shown with bronze instruments used by Roman surgeons and coins showing scenes of healing. Semmelweis Medical Historical Museum, Budapest*

346 *Roman coin (A.D. 117/118) showing the Emperor Hadrian, who exempted doctors from military service and other public duties. Private collection*

347 *Bronze medallion (A.D. 159) showing the Roman Emperor Antoninus Pius, who restricted the number of those who could qualify as doctors and exercise their special privileges, which included exemption from taxes. Staatliche Münzkabinett, Berlin*

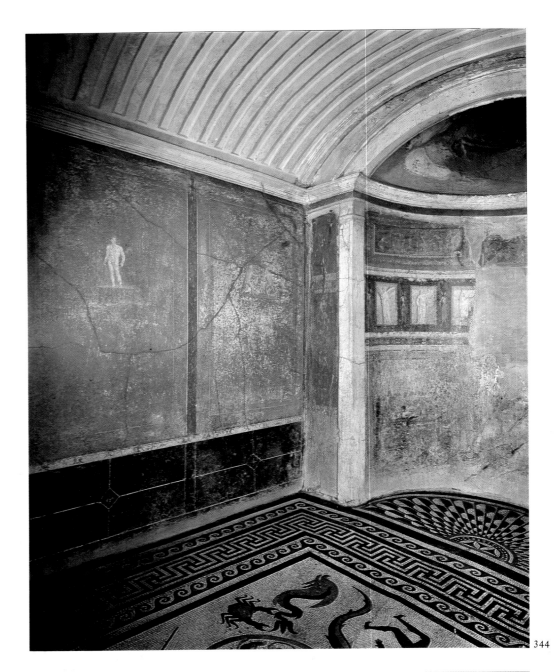

344

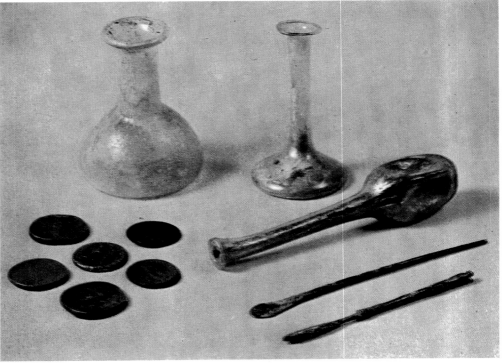

345

Many healers who were not considered physicians indulged in medical care, usually in special places, as for example in the baths, barber shops, and theaters. Again the problem of determining what was outright quackery and what merely empiric medicine is difficult to resolve. Thessalus of Tralles was an uneducated practitioner who achieved great popularity. He repudiated all teachings of the past, scorned science of any kind, and used showmanship to advance his reputation. Calling himself the "Conqueror of Physicians," Thessalus announced that he could impart the knowledge of all medicine in half a year. One wonders how far off he may have been.

Each military unit had a specific number of physicians according to the size of the force, who may have been but simple soldiers with special experience in medical lore. Even here foreigners (especially Greeks) rather than Roman freedmen may have been the medical practitioners.

As in earlier times in Greece, midwives actively practiced obstetrics. Their standing in Rome appears to have been much higher than in Greece, and some women were even looked upon as female doctors. But women in some respects found themselves in approximately the same position as in Greece, for the head of the household had total power of life and death over his daughter, and few women were included in the discussions and activities of men. On the other hand, women were better off legally in Roman society than in Greek, for increasingly they were able to marry and divorce independently.

The regulation of medical practice was at first nonexistent. Anyone could call himself a physician. Even under Augustus, who in A.D. 10 granted physicians exemption from taxes (in grateful recognition of the successful treatment of his rheumatism by Antoninus Musa), neither licensure nor definition determined who could practice. The privileges were further extended by Vespasian (A.D. 69–79) and Hadrian (A.D. 117–138) in relieving doctors of military service and other public duties. So desirable had the self-proclaimed position of physician become that Antoninus Pius (A.D. 138–161) restricted the privileged exemptions to a limited number and to those who remained in their native villages. Finally, Emperor Severus Alexander (A.D. 222–235) passed comprehensive laws regulating training, certification, and control.

The training of physicians changed from unregulated individual instruction for a fee to supervision by the *Collegium Archiatri* (a sort of guild) to salaried teachers in a school that included courses other than medicine. Bedside teaching was required, an activity not always popular among patients, as indicated by these lines from Martial:

> I was getting sick and you came at once,
> Together with a hundred students, O Symmachus;
> A hundred frosty fingers probed me;
> I had no fever, O Symmachus; now I have.

PUBLIC HEALTH AND HYGIENE

In some respects, Roman attitudes about health and disease were similar to the Greek. The hopelessly ill and deformed were little cared for. The same disdain extended to unwanted newborns and led to their disposal. The poor of both countries lived in mean, crowded housing, but Roman multiple dwellings, though they were still slums, seem to have been better constructed and better provided with drainage, water supply, and paved streets. Certainly the homes of the rich Romans were far more opulent than the houses of their counterparts in Greek times, and the Roman emphasis on agriculture led to a larger and more varied supply of food. Not that famine was unknown, but in general the sometimes elaborate Roman meals were a contrast to the frugal diet of the Greeks.

The greatest glories of Roman hygiene were the water supply and the

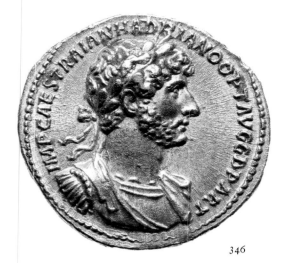

346

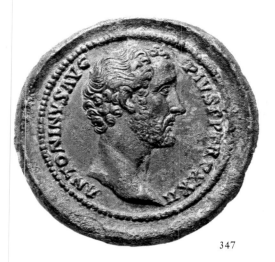

347

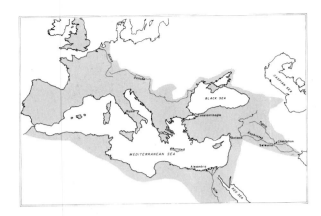

348 *Map of the Roman Empire in* A.D. *117*

349 *The doctor Iapyx shown removing an arrow from the thigh of Aeneas, hero of Troy, in a Pompeian fresco. Vergil tells how Aeneas's wound was then treated with dittany collected by Venus on Mt. Ida. Museo Archeologico Nazionale, Naples*

350 *Ruins of a Roman tenement (c. 2d century* A.D.*) in Ostia, typical of the kind of multiple dwelling in which the lower classes lived.*

351 *Bas-relief showing a woman pharmacist, possibly the goddess Meditrina. In Rome, women engaged in commerce, and probably also medicine, as well as pharmacy. Musée des Antiquités Nationales, St.-Germain-en-Laye*

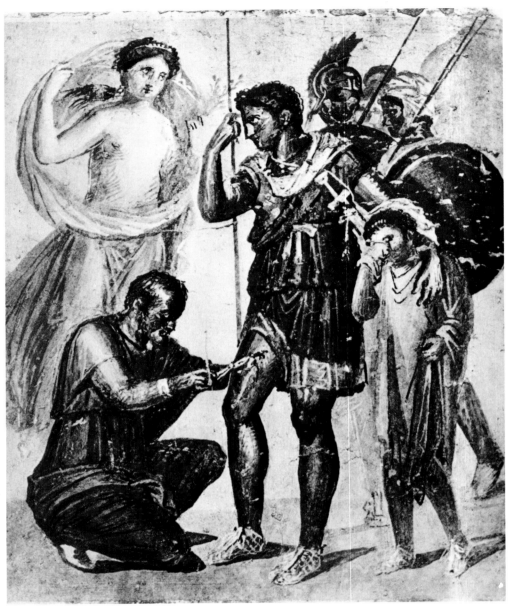

349

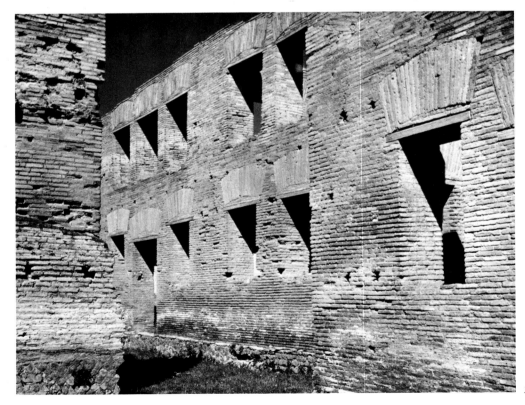

350

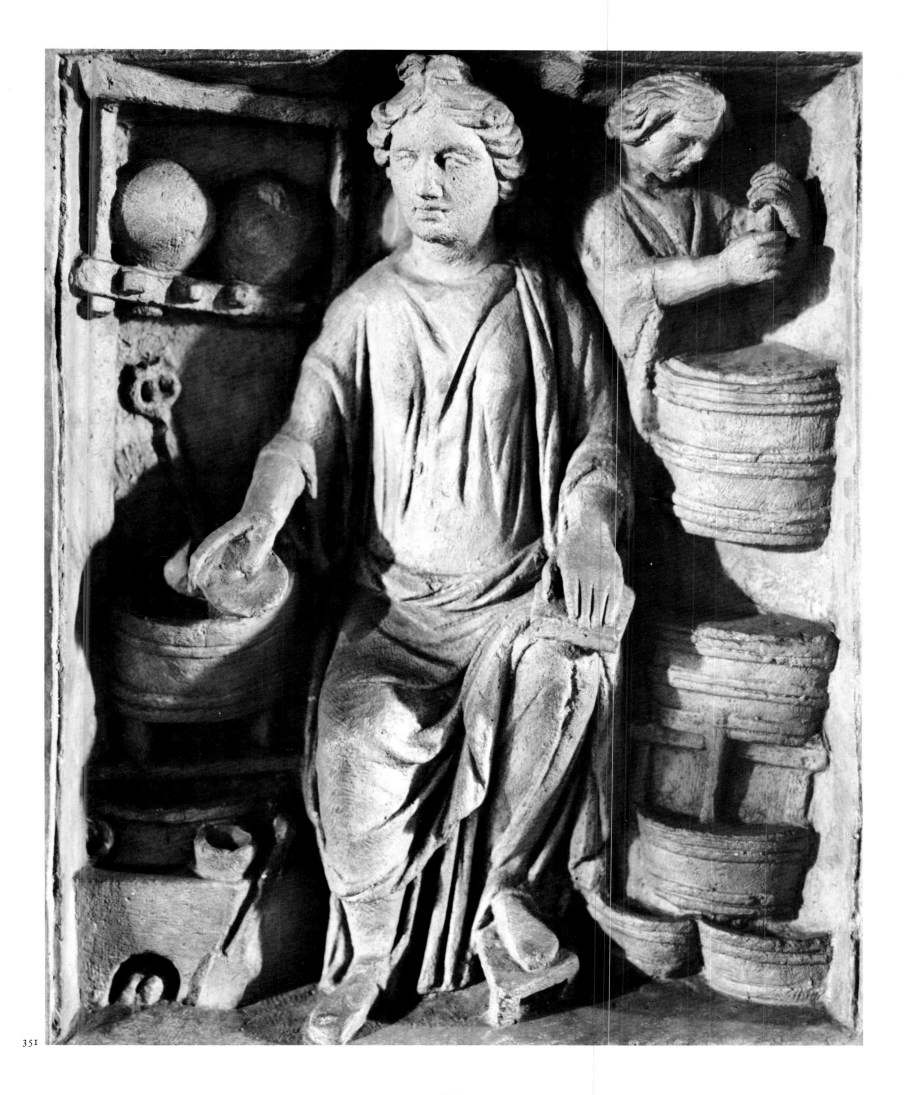

351

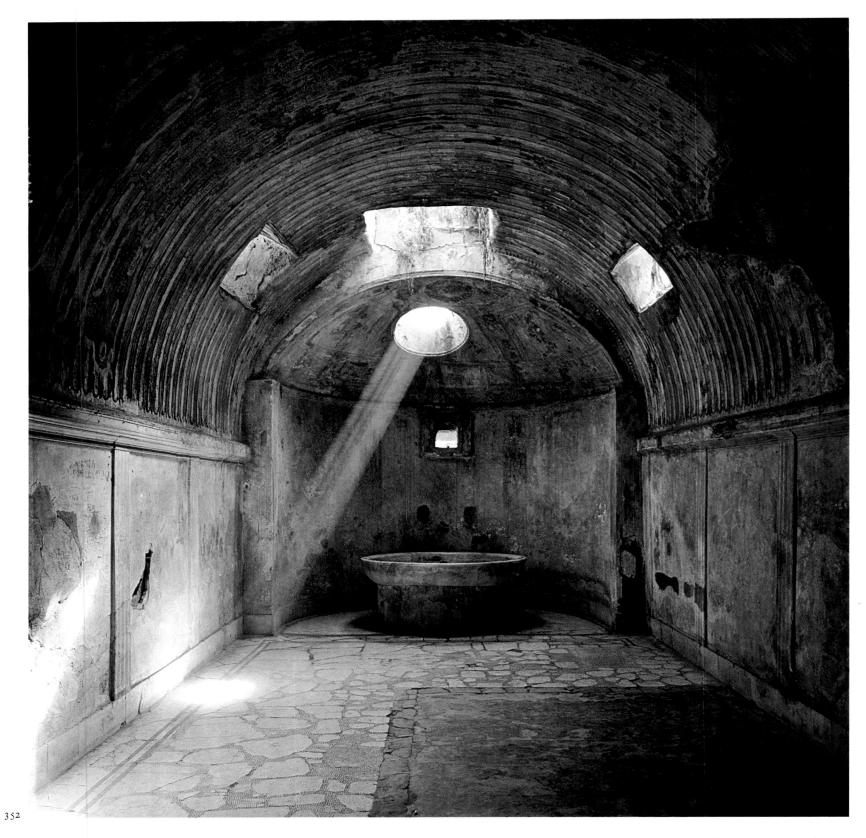

352

352 *Caldarium in the bathhouses in Pompeii known as Forum Thermae (c. early 1st century B.C.), where the atmosphere was kept warm by hot air circulating through pipes in the walls and floor.*

sanitation system. By the end of the first century A.D. nine aqueducts were channeling water to Rome, and later there were more. (Purification was achieved mainly through settling basins and intermediate reservoirs along the route, and drinking water was kept separate from the rest.) Destined principally for the public baths and fountains, water was available for private use at a fee, thus enabling the rich and influential to obtain as much as they desired. Although the less wealthy could also afford enough water, many of the poor still relied on wells and water carriers. In some far-flung Roman cities pure water was even more widely available to all classes of society than in Rome.

Along with supplying water into the city there was a system of draining used water and sewage out of the city (that is, into the Tiber). The famous *Cloaca Maxima* was only one part of a great complex of sewers and conduits running beneath buildings and streets. In some dwellings, people still emptied refuse and chamber pots directly into streets, but for the most part streets, roads, and alleys were kept clean, abundant pure water was available, and swamps and stagnant pools were regularly drained. The association of marshy land with disease was long recognized, and in the first century B.C. Marcus Varro had advised against building near swamps "because there are bred certain minute creatures which cannot be seen by the eyes, which float in the air and enter the body through the mouth and nose and there cause serious disease."

Apparently the Roman talent for organization did not extend as readily to institutional care of the sick and injured. Nevertheless, infirmaries for sick slaves were established, and Seneca said that even free Romans sometimes used them. There were really no other places except the offices and perhaps homes of physicians where the ill and wounded could be domiciled, treated, and cared for.

Only among the military legions was a system for hospitalization developed. At first wounded soldiers had been quartered in the homes of the rich, especially during a serious battle. Then field tents were set up separate from the barracks. Later, infirmaries (*valetudinaria*) were erected in all the garrisons along the frontiers. Apparently these stone and wooden structures were carefully planned and also stocked with instruments, supplies, and medications. However, it was not until the fourth century A.D. that hospitals for civilians appeared in the cities. The first was founded in Rome around the year 394 by the Christian benefactress Fabiola.

Pedanius Dioscorides (fl. c. 41–68) was probably a military physician who, traveling with the army to many lands, had the opportunity to study and record the medical uses of hundreds of plants and to write what is probably the first thorough, systematic materia medica. Diocles of Carystus in the fourth century B.C. was an earlier source of information on medicinal plants, and Aristotle's pupil Theophrastus presumably also made extensive contributions to botany and medicinal herbs. Cratevas in the first century B.C. had written the first illustrated herbal with colored plates, but from subsequent descriptions it is doubtful that the treatment was thorough or systematic. It was the work of Dioscorides which was to become the basis for all subsequent studies and writings on pharmacology and materia medica.

CELSUS AND PLINY

Much of the information on Alexandrian and on Roman medicine is based on the writings of two encyclopedists: Cornelius Celsus and Caius Pliny, the Elder, both of the first century A.D.

Celsus (fl. 14–37) was apparently a patrician layman who tried to summarize most of the knowledge available at the time, including agriculture, law, military science, philosophy, rhetoric, and medicine. Only the eight books comprising his *De Medicina* and a few additional fragments on the other subjects have survived. These extensive works had some influence in his own time, but were lost until the Renaissance, when reborn interest in the ancients led to their discovery by Pope Nicholas. Celsus was the first medical author to be printed (1478) in movable type

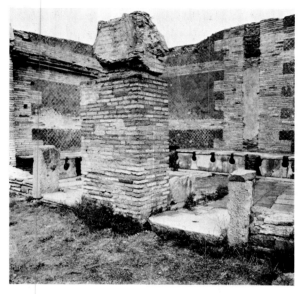

353

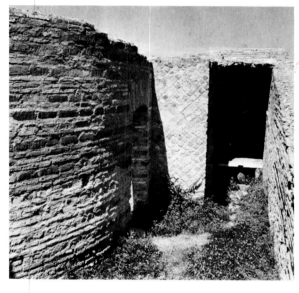

354

353 *Public lavatory on Via della Forica, Ostia, typical of the facilities available in most large Roman cities, where running water carried off the waste.*

354 *Lavatory in the House of the Fortuna Annonaria (late 2d century A.D.) in Ostia, which shows the kind of facility found in the privacy of wealthy homes.*

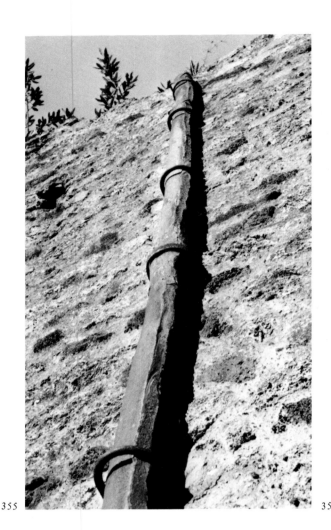

355

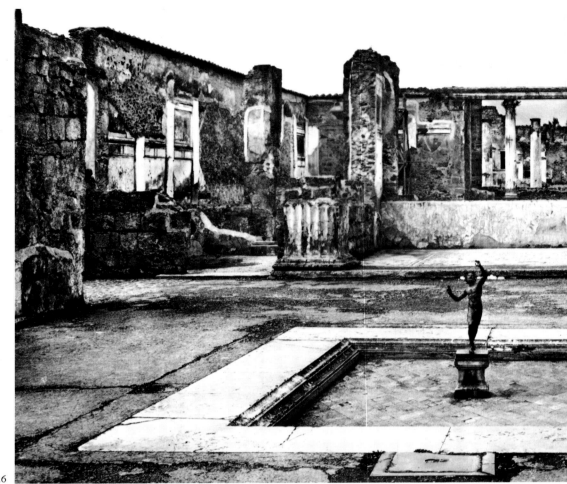

356

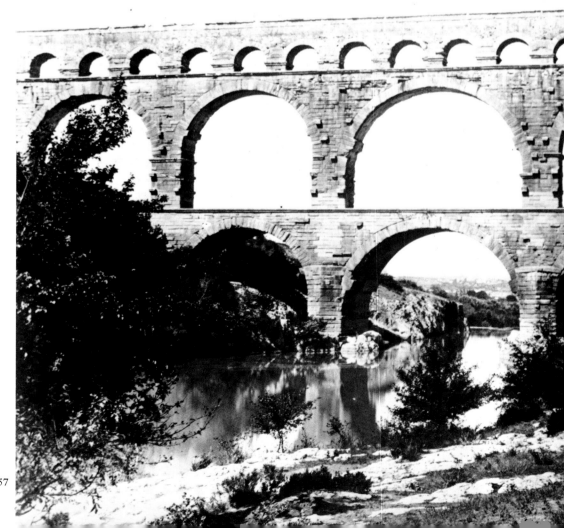

357

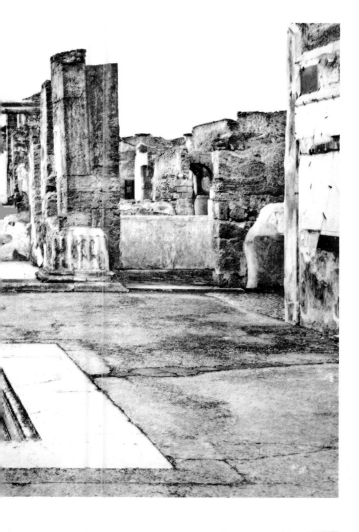

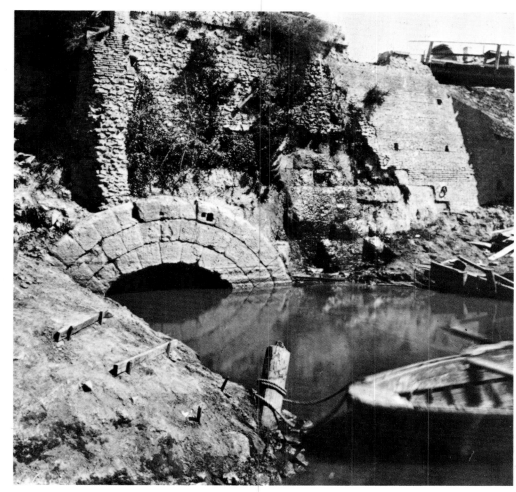

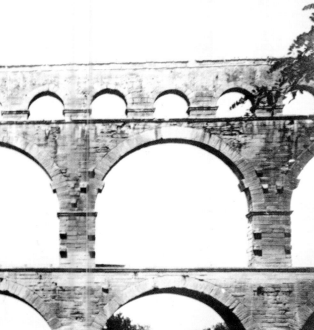

355 *Lead pipe on side of private house in Pompeii, which brought water into the dwelling—but at a hazard of lead poisoning only appreciated much later in history.*

356 *Interior courtyard of the House of the Faun (2d century B.C.), one of the most richly decorated houses in Pompeii.*

357 *Pont du Gard, Nîmes, an aqueduct built in the early 1st century A.D. by the Romans, who regularly used this system to bring abundant water to their cities throughout the empire.*

358 *The outlet into the Tiber of the Cloaca Maxima, the elaborate and extensive system of sewers beneath the streets of Rome, which may have originated with the Etruscans.*

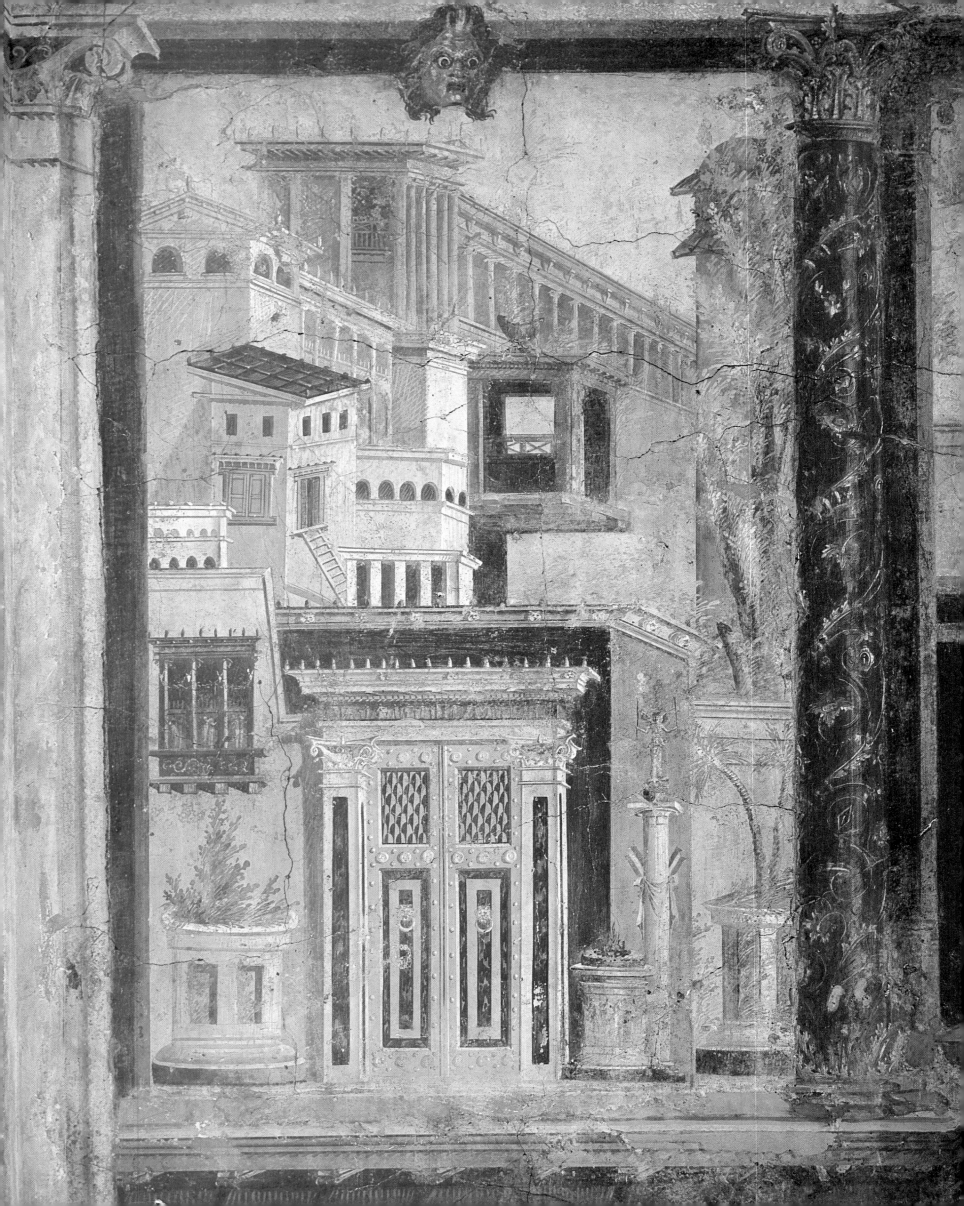

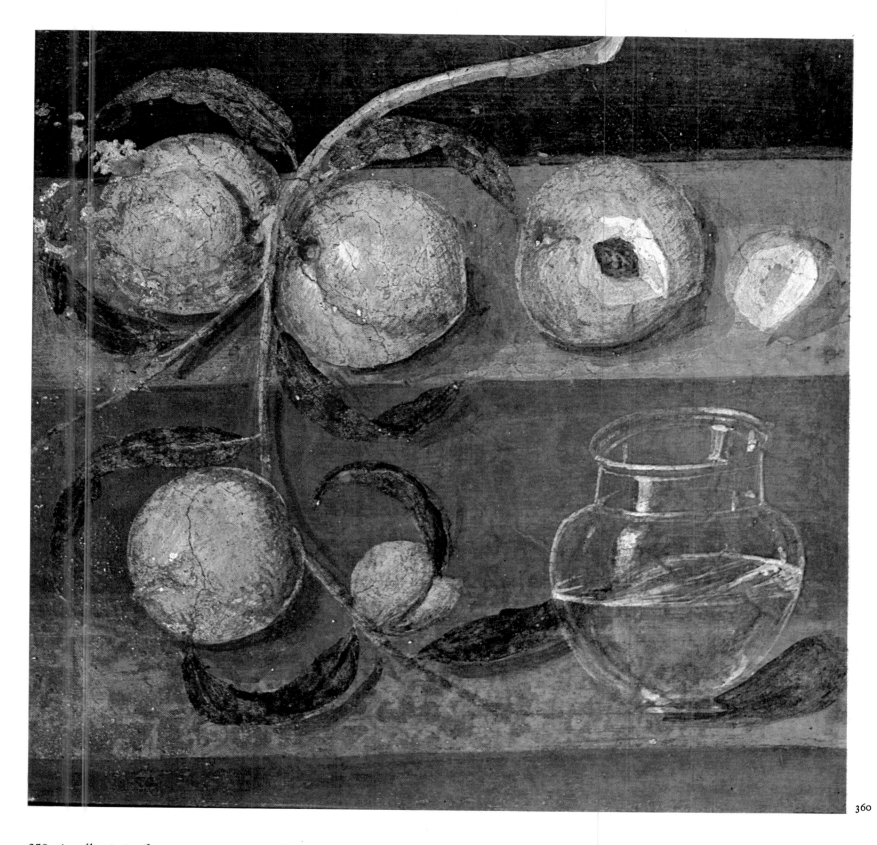

359 *A wall painting from a 1st-century* B.C. *villa at Boscoreale, near Pompeii, which gives a fine idea of what it must have been like in a Roman city of the period. Rogers Fund, 1903, Metropolitan Museum of Art, New York*

360 *A fresco (c.* A.D. *50) from Herculaneum, which was destroyed in the same Vesuvian eruption as Pompeii. Pliny the Elder, the great encyclopedist, lost his life during that disaster. Museo Archeologico Nazionale, Naples*

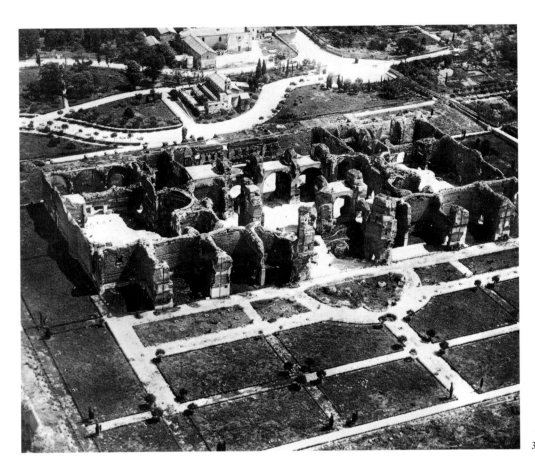

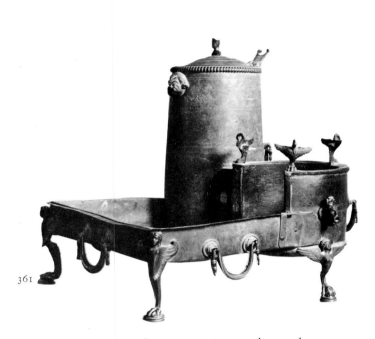

361 *Roman bronze vaporizer used to produce steam in treating various ailments. Museo Archeologico Nazionale, Naples*

362 *Ruins of the Baths of Caracalla (A.D. 211–17) in Rome. Housed in a building over 700 feet long, the Baths provided hot, cold, and tepid immersions and two large rooms for exercising.*

363 *Restoration drawing by G. Abel Blonet of the Tepidarium of the Baths of Caracalla. Thought to have stretched some 200 feet, the Tepidarium provided an elegant setting for socializing and the exchange of ideas.*

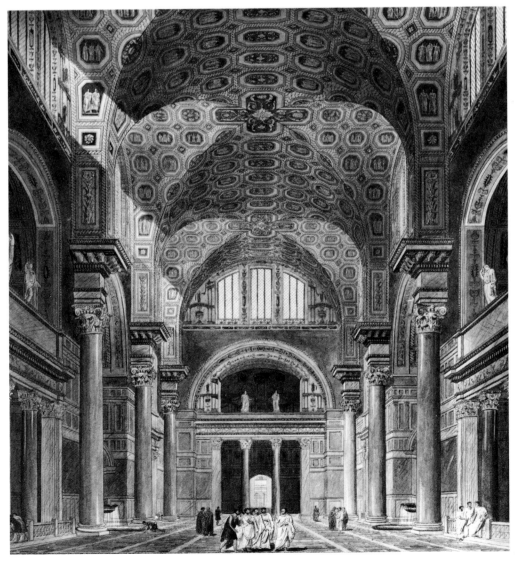

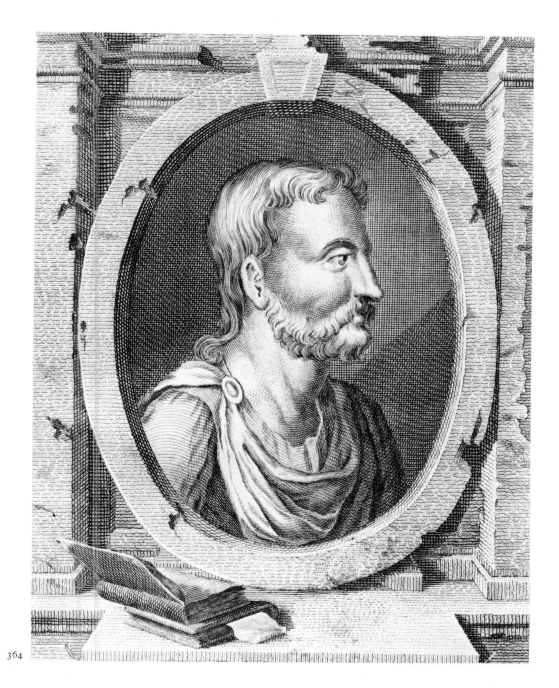

364

364 *Detail from a print dated 1765 showing a portrait of the medical encyclopedist Cornelius Celsus (53 B.C.–A.D. 7). Celsus presumably was not a doctor, but his detailed descriptions suggest firsthand acquaintance with surgical procedures. National Library of Medicine, Bethesda*

365 *Model constructed by R. Schultze of a Roman* valetudinarium, *the Legionary Hospital at Vetera, part of the system for hospitalization developed by the military legions. Rheinische Landesmuseum, Bonn*

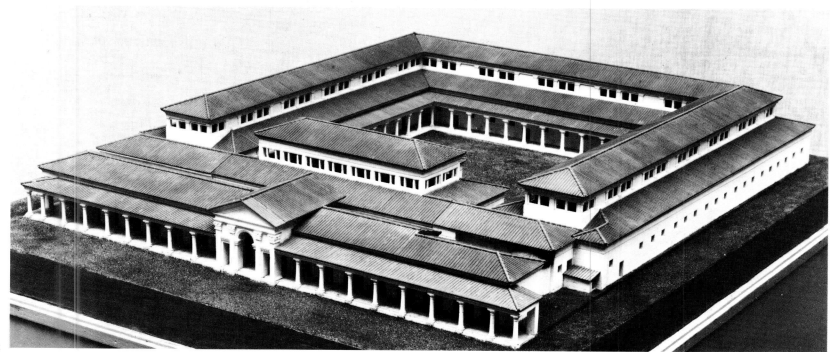

365

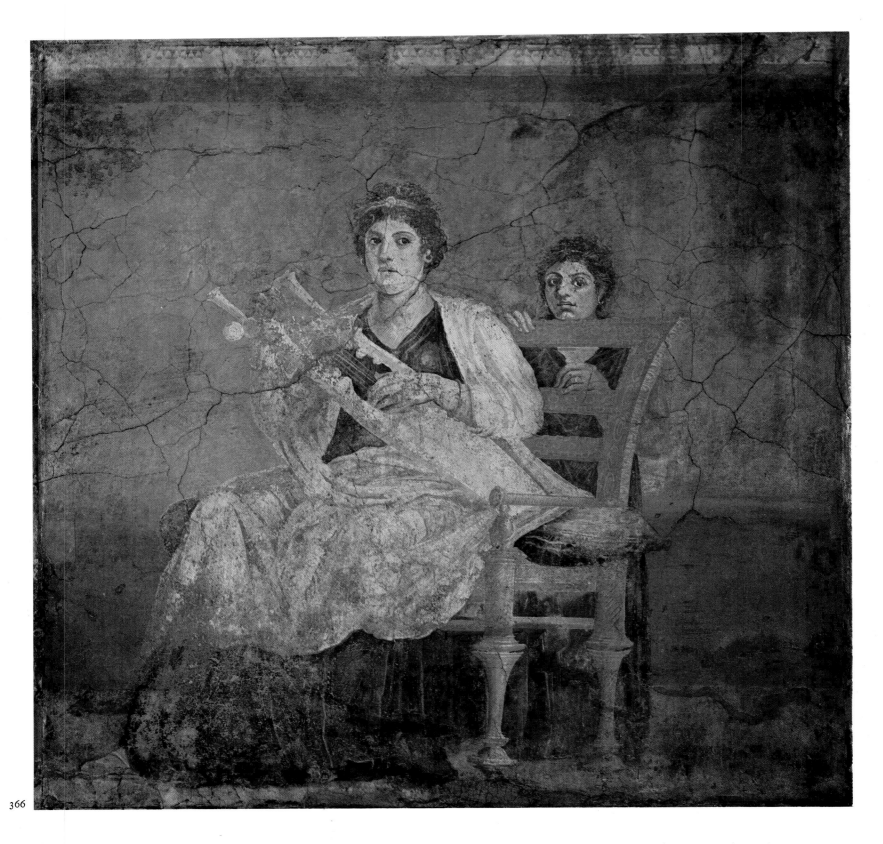

366

366 Woman Playing a Kithara, *fresco (c. 50 B.C.) from a villa at Boscoreale near Pompeii. Greek ideas of the therapeutic values of music, stemming from the Pythagoreans, persisted on into Roman times. Metropolitan Museum of Art, New York*

367 *Wild blackberry described and illustrated in an edition of De Materia Medica by Dioscorides, prepared for Juliana Anicia, daughter of Emperor Anicius Olybrius, in A.D. 512. Österreichische Nationalbibliothek, Vienna*

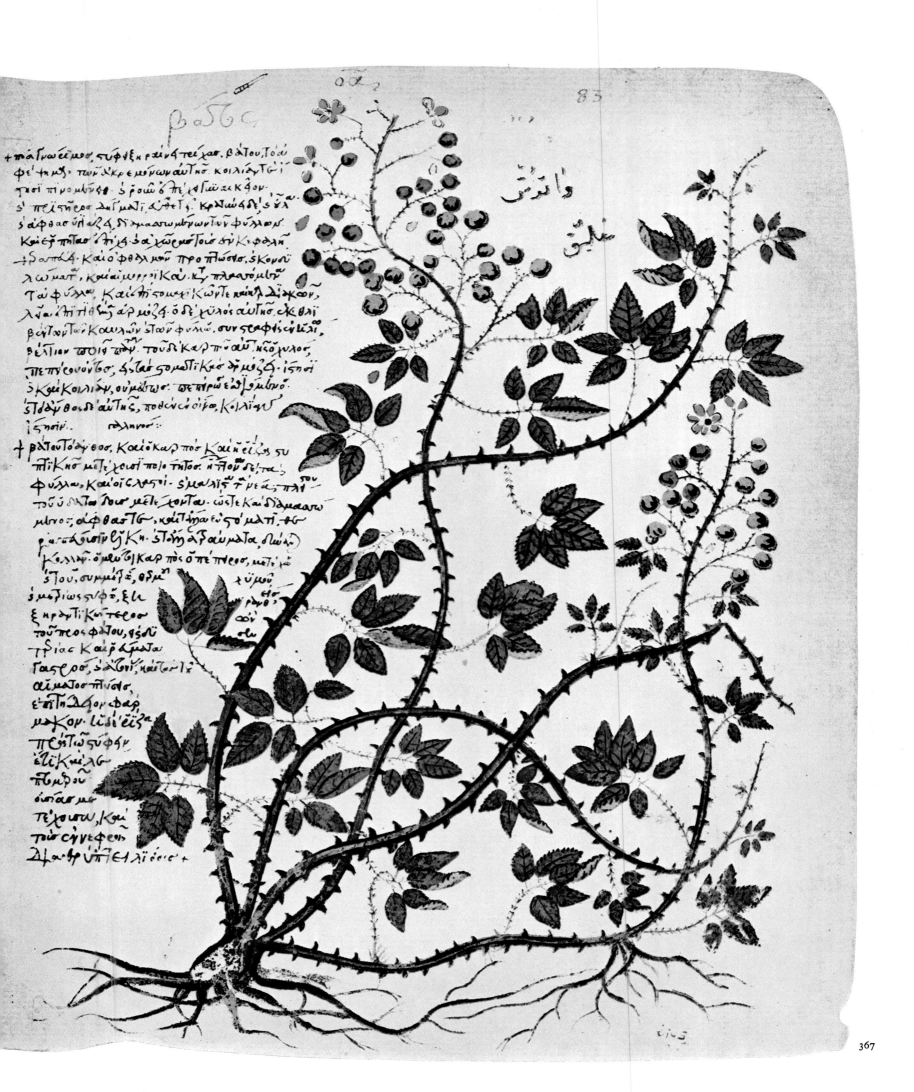

βάδος

πάλιν ἔμεος συφλεη ράενα τεῖχασ. βάτου, τοῦ
φείτιμη, τῶν ἀκρεμόνων αὐτῆσ, κοιλίαντ' ἔτι
ταιοι πιριομύθεσο· ὴ ρουῶ ὅ πεῖς ται ἐεκλόη·
ὁ πεῖσ ἥερο διμαλι, ἀσεις, κραλιωλδἐ·σ ἰλ
ὁ ἄφρας ὑηαλδ, διεμασωμοήντων φύλλων.
καιἐγ' πῖτασ· Ἀιχ·δ' ἀχωρεμοιουσ δικεφαλ
δασπλΔ· και ὀφθαλμῶν προ πλυοσο, ἐκοποῦ
λωματ᾽, και αἰμεργγ' και τῇ πλεασομεθ'
ταϊφυλλ', και πισομε ζ' κωῆτε νᾶνλ δικελου,
λ δ·λ πιθοθη ἀ μι ζ ὁ δε ζυλός αὐτῆσ δε θιι
βαΐτου ταϊ κοιλιῶν ἰσ τοῦ φύλω. συν σεαφισεικιλᾶ
βέλτιον ταοιο πῶλ' του δικ' καρπῶ αὐ ηεο ζυλοσ,
πεπυεἰ εουνϊρε, δ·ελαε ξομεσ τικι διμεξ· ισηοι
ὁ κρα κοιλιΔ, συμέωφ. πεπιρῶ εελεζ ελμμβ̄
ὁ ἰ δ' δ' βλθοσ δ' ἀϊ της, ποδενεο οικα, κοιλιω
ἰσ ηοικ·   ρληνοσ··

βάτου τ' ὁ ἀγγεοσ, και ὁ καρπος και ἥ εεζσ συ
πϊικῶ μεθ ἔχωϊ πολο τητοσ· ἡ πιοῦ δε ται
φυλλω, και οἰ ϊ ελεσδι· δ μελαϊσ ῖ τ μεας παι του
τοῦ υ δικ' τοισ μεζ ϊονται· ωστε και διδμεασω
μιλτος, αλφθας τε, και τήμαι ευϊ δ' ματι θο
ρα αλδ ιοτιυ λῖ κμ·ϊσ τόεη λ ραυματα, διλῶ
κολλῆ· ὁμεϊ ϊ καρ πὸς ὁ πεϊ πεεσσ, μετε ϊδ
ὁ του, συμμεϊ ζ, θδμᾶϊ
ὁ μελ δι ωσ συφ ᾶ, ελ
ξ ηραιτϊ και τεεσσ
τοῦ πεοσ φατου, ιεϊλῖ
τρϊας και ἀρμματα
γασεεσ, ὁ ἀλϊ νἥϊ, και τοι ε̄ζ
αἱμιλτοσ πλυοσ,
ε πϊτ δ αδιομεφασ
μεκορ ιῶ ει ει ζα
πεϊτῶ συφ δ ε τ
ελικ ελδε
πιμ δ οϊ
οιοιοισ με
τεχοιου, και
τοϊσ εϊνεφεω
δλ αλ ϕ υπεϊ ελι εειτ·

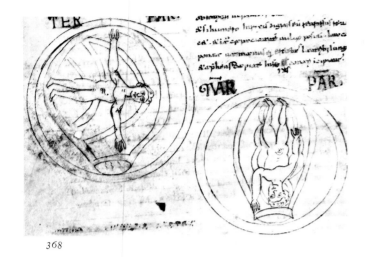

368

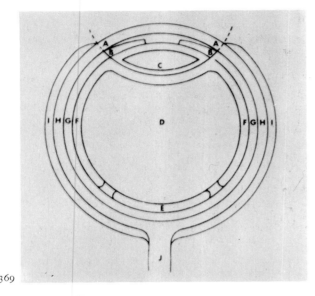

369

368 *Illustration of* fetus in utero, *from 12th-century manuscript based on writings of Soranus of Ephesus, 1st-century Roman doctor whose writings on obstetrics and the diseases of women were considered authoritative for many centuries.* Codex 1653, *Royal Library, Copenhagen*

369 *Drawing of the eye, based on descriptions by Rufus of Ephesus in the 2d century, who clearly understood the correct course of the optic nerves and the relationships of the parts of the eye. Courtesy John Scarborough, University of Kentucky, Lexington*

after Gutenberg's invention. Part of the reason for the earlier neglect of Celsus was probably his of Latin. Since scientific and medical treatises of his time were written in Greek, apparently no one would expect to find an intellectual contribution in Latin.

In the opinion of most scholars, Celsus was not a medical practitioner, but so perceptive are his detailed descriptions and judgments that surgeons will especially appreciate his writings on hernia, wounds, and amputations. "Now the laying open is to be done boldly, until the outer tunic, that of the scrotum itself, is cut through, and the middle tunic reached. When an incision has been made, an opening presents leading deeper. Into this the index finger of the left hand is introduced, in order that by the separation of the intervening little membranes the hernial sac may be freed."

He made a particularly outstanding, perhaps the first (Heliodorus may have preceded him), description of ligating and dividing bleeding vessels. "The blood vessels that are pouring out blood are to be grasped, and about the wounded spot they are to be tied in two places, and cut across in between, so that each may retract and yet have its opening closed."

The internist may also be impressed by his good sense. "The failings of those who practice medicine are not to be charged to the art itself. . . . The physician of experience is recognized by his not at once seizing the arm of his patient as soon as he comes to his side, but he looks upon him and as it were sifts him first with a serene look, to discover how he really is; and if the sick man manifests fear, he soothes him with suitable words before proceeding to a manual examination."

The *De Medicina* of Celsus covered a wide range of topics: the history of medicine, the preservation of health, and derangements of almost every organ system of the body. Celsus approached each therapeutic maneuver with understanding. His description of cosmetic surgery included restoration of the prepuce, for evidently some Jews in Rome sought to obtain positions and social acceptance by hiding their origins.

Celsus advised mild methods, relying much on exercise and rest, measures for which he gave credit to Asclepiades. Perhaps he has been best remembered for his description of the characteristics of inflammation: redness and swelling with heat and pain (*rubor et tumor cum calor et dolor*). Today these are still called the four cardinal signs of inflammation.

Whereas Celsus was selective in what he reported and approved, Caius Pliny (23–79) had a voracious and omnivorous intellectual appetite. His monumental *Historia Naturalis* contained every bit of information he could gather from the past or present. Virtually every waking hour for two years was devoted to collecting and recording. Indeed, Pliny is reported to have died satisfying his curiosity about volcanoes during the same eruption of Vesuvius that buried Pompeii and Herculaneum.

Owing to his extensive writings on history, physics, biology, chemistry, geography, food, philosophy, magic, folklore, plants, and medicine, subsequent generations were able to obtain voluminous information about the past—some of it fanciful. Pliny stated that light travels faster than sound and that the world rotates rapidly, but he also mistakenly concluded that every liquid becomes smaller when frozen. He recognized that some additives to wine were poisonous, but he was probably not aware that lead in water vessels and pipes was more noxious. Many of his descriptions of plants and drugs were correct, but others were superstitious and inaccurate. He had a horror of menstruation, reporting that dogs went mad if they licked the fluid, that even ants discarded their food if a menstruating woman came near.

Pliny did not believe in an afterlife. "I deem it a work of human weakness to seek to discover the shape and form of God. Whoever God is—provided there is a God—and wherever he is, he consists wholly of sense, sight, and hearing, wholly of soul, wholly of mind, wholly of himself." Yet he accepted as truth many fantastic marvels, such as one-footed people who used the giant foot to shelter themselves from the rain. Pliny also believed that there had been "rains of milk, blood, flesh, iron, sponges, wool, and baked bricks."

He reserved most of his ire for Greeks, especially the physicians. "And there is no doubt that they all busy themselves with our lives, in order by the discovery of some new thing or another to win reputations for themselves." "There is alas no law against incompetency; no striking example is made. They learn by our bodily jeopardy and make experiments until the death of the patients, and the doctor is the only person not punished for murder."

Despite their extraordinary variety of facts and opinions, Pliny's works were regarded as authoritative throughout the Middle Ages and are still a valuable source of information about the ideas and customs of antiquity.

There were a number of other outstanding contributors to medicine in Rome in the second century A.D., notably Soranus (fl. c. 98–138) who came from Ephesus in Asia Minor. Although he wrote on injuries and diseases, his principal field of work was obstetrics and the diseases of women. He was a popular practitioner, and his works served as a textbook in the Middle Ages. Soranus showed an understanding of menstruation and parturition and their difficulties, including the interference of genital tract inflammation with both menstruation and conception. He also noted the complications in delivery due to pelvic abnormalities and the improper presentation of the baby. His methods of correcting abnormal positions were sound, as were his measures to prevent tearing of the pelvic soft parts during delivery.

His instructions extended to the care of infants and the management of diseases of later childhood. Soranus clearly differentiated the uterus from the vagina, proved that the uterus could be removed without fatality, cautioned that manual removal of the placenta (afterbirth) could produce inversion of the uterus, advised emptying the bladder with a catheter before delivery, suggested psychological methods in difficult menstruation, and favored rupture of the membranes to hasten delivery in delayed labor. He also explained how to reduce the vagina to virginal size by inserting a tampon saturated with an astringent.

Rufus of Ephesus (c. 110–180) made important anatomical observations while in Rome. He described clearly the correct course of the optic nerves and the parts of the eye including the capsule of the lens. He confirmed some anatomical information earlier reported but not fully appreciated; for instance, that nerves originate from the brain, that some nerves direct movement and others sensation. He also recognized the heartbeat as the cause of the pulse and discussed its many properties. Rufus also subscribed to the theory of the *pneuma* (the Stoics' idea of a vital force borne in the air), as did most of his contemporaries, but he apparently belonged to no particular medical sect. Not only was Rufus an investigator but also a highly respected physician. His recognition of the psychological import of dreams is an example of his astuteness.

But of all the practitioners, contributors, medical writers, and teachers of Roman times, one gigantic personality, Galen, towered above all, not only in his own period but also in many succeeding centuries.

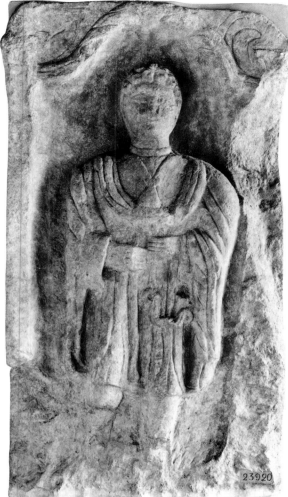

370

370 *Limestone relief of a veterinarian shown holding a farrier's knife in his left hand and a horseshoe of ancient type—leather shoe with metal bottom—in his right. Musée Historique Lorrain, Nancy*

371 *Handle of a farrier's knife that shows a groom leading a horse named Stratilates. Musée Dauphinois, Grenoble*

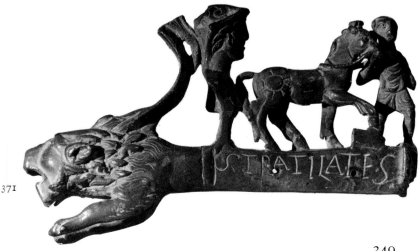

371

Galen

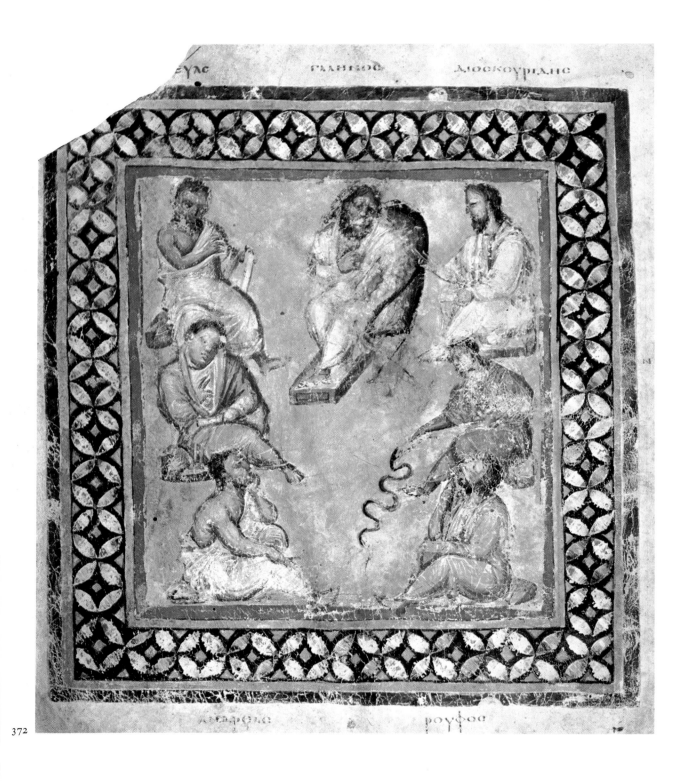

372

THE Greek physician Galen (c. 129–c. 200) was probably the most influential writer of all time on medical subjects. For nearly fifteen hundred years his works were the unimpeachable authority on medicine in many different lands. A bitter polemicist yet broad in view, Galen was both a careful, accurate observer and an uncritical believer, a dogmatic authoritarian and an original thinker.

Born in Pergamum to a father of wealth, position, and education, Galen received tender but intensive instruction from this parent, whom he called a man of "justice, modesty, and goodness." At the age of fourteen, he was further trained in philosophy, mathematics, and natural science by philosophers who exposed him to the importance of anatomy, empiricism, and the doctrines of Hippocrates. Galen reported that his father guided him in the direction of medicine on advice from Asclepios in a dream.

At the time, the city of Pergamum (Gr. Pergamon) was a great cultural center in Roman Asia Minor where Galen's medical studies could have continued with profit, but after his father's death Galen traveled widely. Wherever he went, he found anatomy repeatedly emphasized; in Smyrna, Corinth, and Alexandria he came under the influence of several famous teachers of anatomy. He found pharmacologic information about plants and minerals also widely available in each new region. Furthermore, Galen was able to observe many kinds of illness, treatments, and medical philosophies, especially in Alexandria where physicians from all over the Roman world gathered to study, teach, and practice. There he also had opportunities for direct clinical experience by participating in the care of patients.

When he returned to Pergamum after years of voyaging, he had already gained some renown from a few writings on anatomy and physiology and from displays of clinical acumen. Possibly because of his reputation and his family's standing, the chief of the local gladiatorial games appointed Galen physician to the gladiators. The need to keep these performers fit taught him the importance of hygienic regimens and preventive measures. Treating the severe injuries which were part of a gladiator's existence enabled him to observe living human anatomy, particularly of bones, joints, and muscles, and to develop skill in treating fractures as well as brutal chest and abdominal wounds.

When he again left Pergamum, to go to Rome for the first time, he was an experienced, skillful physician. Although he gave up surgical activities in Rome (the social pressures to avoid operations may have been too strong) his former association with surgery formed the basis for his extensive, detailed, and brilliant discussions of surgical treatment.

He left Rome but had the good fortune of being recalled by the emperor himself, Marcus Aurelius. He was evidently the most prestigious and successful practitioner in Rome, and royal favor added unmistakable luster to his star. Yet, he was not content to repose at the pinnacle; he mocked and ridiculed opinions and methods contrary to his own—whether contemporary or earlier.

In the midst of traveling, studying, practicing, dissecting, experimenting, debating, demonstrating, and absorbing all the medical knowledge of the time, Galen wrote voluminously in Greek, his native tongue and the language of science. Anatomy, physiology, pharmacology, pathology, therapy, hygiene, dietetics, and philosophy were all subjects for his keen mind and ceaseless pen.

Inherent in the entire body of his work are teleological explanations for everything. A view that the purpose of everything was predetermined sometimes deluded him into distorting what he saw or into presuming a function for an organ because Nature must have given it a clear purpose. These preconceptions (which led him on a path of error from today's vantage point) were the very characteristics in his teachings that were attractive to medieval Christian minds. Aristotle had said, "Nature does nothing without a purpose." Galen insisted that he could perceive the purpose.

A second characteristic was his use of the humoral theory inherited from early

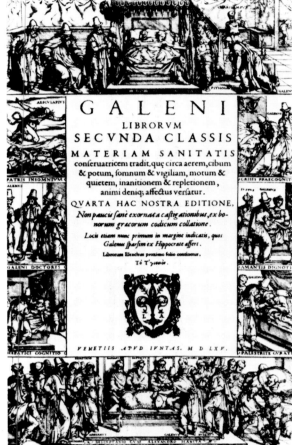

373

372 *Manuscript illustration from a 5th-century edition of Dioscorides showing Galen, in top center, conversing with the botanist Cratevas, Apollonius, Andreas de Caryste, Dioscorides, Nicandre of Colophon, and Rufus of Ephesus. Österreichische Nationalbibliothek, Vienna*

373 *Title page of an edition of the works of Galen printed in Venice in 1565. The voluminous writings of Galen were looked to as the ultimate medical authority for about 1,500 years. Collection Bertarelli, Milan*

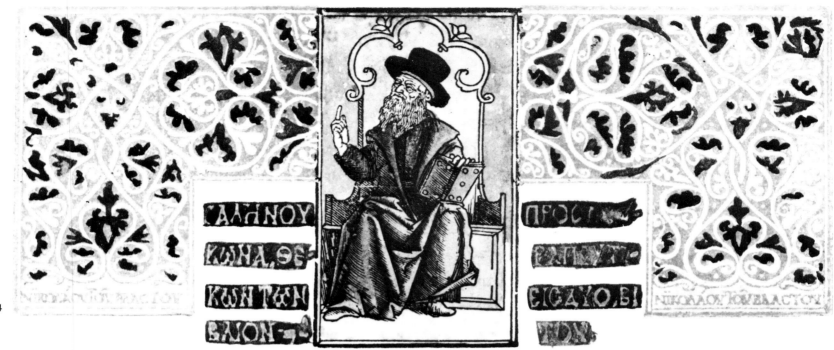

374

375

374 *Miniature in a medieval manuscript (c. 1500) showing Galen teaching. Virtually all scientific works were written in Greek during Roman times—and even into the Middle Ages. Wellcome Institute for the History of Medicine, London*

375 *Roman marble copy, long known as* Dying Gladiator *(c. 1st century* B.C.*), after a bronze sculpture (c. 230–220* B.C.*) from Pergamum, where Galen was physician to the gladiators. Museo Capitolino, Rome*

376 *Bronze equestrian statue (c.* A.D. *176) of the Emperor Marcus Aurelius, who, according to Galen, bestowed royal favor on him and solidified his position as foremost practitioner in Rome. Piazza del Campidoglio, Rome*

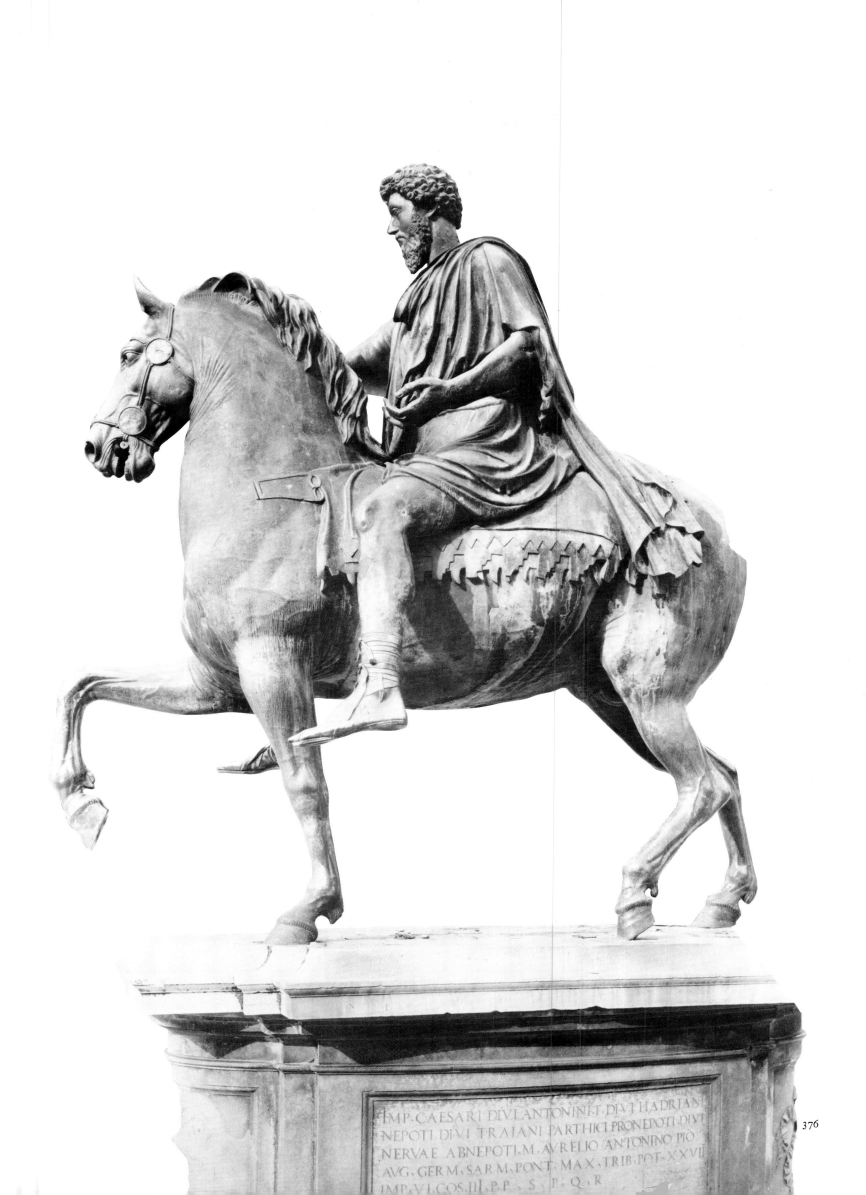

IMP. CAESARI. DIVI. ANTONINI. F. DIVI. HADRIANI
NEPOTI. DIVI. TRAIANI. PARTHICI. PRONEPOTI. DIVI
NERVAE. ABNEPOTI. M. AVRELIO. ANTONINO. PIO
AVG. GERM. SARM. PONT. MAX. TRIB. POT. XXVII
IMP. VI. COS. III. P. P. S. P. Q. R

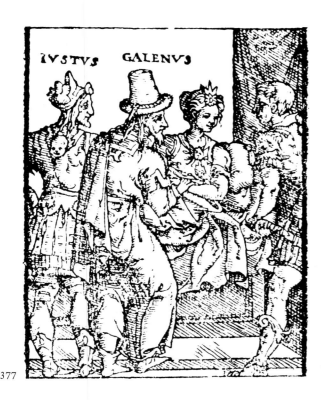

377

377 *Illustration from a 1586 edition of the works of Galen, showing the great doctor, whose diagnostic acumen enabled him to recognize that a lady's illness was due to unrequited love rather than physical causes. National Library of Medicine, Bethesda*

378, 379, 380, 381 *Galen's contribution to the ancient doctrine of the four humors, as illustrated in this medieval manuscript, was to tie them to four basic temperaments: sanguine, phlegmatic, choleric, and melancholic. Ms. C. 54, Zentralbibliothek, Zurich*

Greek times. The four fundamental humors (phlegm, blood, yellow bile, and black bile) were responsible for health and illness, and Galen elaborated this conception in classifying all personalities into four types: phlegmatic, sanguine, choleric, and melancholic, terms still used to characterize dispositions.

Another attribute of Galen's works is the concentration on anatomical details. Some of his studies were pioneering. For instance, he showed that veins are connected to the heart but that nerves arise from the central nervous system. He described the nerve to the voice box, the anatomy of the spinal cord, the ureters, the bones and their muscle attachments. Since direct dissection of the human body, which had earlier been the principle in Alexandria, was no longer practiced, Galen and other anatomists had to seek information in other ways: observing the chance exposure of organs in an injury; discovering fortuitously an abandoned corpse; dissecting animals and assuming their similarity to humans.

Because his knowledge was derived for the most part from animal (principally the Barbary ape) rather than human dissection, Galen made many mistakes, especially concerning the internal organs. For example, he incorrectly assumed that the *rete mirabile*, a plexus of blood vessels at the base of the brain of ungulate animals, was also present in humans. In addition, he sometimes postulated the presence of structures not there in order to fit his theories. Although normally there are no direct connections between the left and right heart chambers, Galen "found" openings in the dividing septum to fit his theoretical system in which blood had to pass from one side to the other.

In spite of Galen's mistakes and misconceptions, one is astonished at the wealth of accurate detail in his writings. Scholars of later centuries swallowed his descriptions whole—correct and incorrect—not even subjecting them to the scrutiny called for in Galen's principle of discovery by experiment. In actually testing animals he differentiated sensory and motor nerves, elucidated the effects of transection of the spinal cord, examined the physiological actions of the chest cavity, and proved that the heart could continue to beat without nerves. In stopping the squealing of a pig by cutting a particular nerve in the neck he demonstrated its function. He showed for the first time that arteries contained blood not air. Of course some of his contributions may have had antecedents which did not survive, but he has been referred to as the first experimentalist.

As a clinical observer, Galen was probably unequaled in his time. One has to say "probably," because most information about contemporary medical practice is obtained from Galen's own writings. Unlike Hippocrates, who reported good and bad results without bias or boast, Galen recounted mostly successes, often accompanied by expressions of self-satisfaction. But he did display great acumen. When the physicians of Marcus Aurelius concluded that the emperor's symptoms were the beginning of a severe febrile illness, Galen diagnosed a milder ailment (an "upset stomach"), from which the patient quickly recovered. The treatment, which consisted of applying to the abdomen wool soaked in medicaments, probably had little to do with the course of the sickness—a common circumstance in the practice of medicine in all times. He paid considerable attention to the pulse and developed a complicated lexicon of descriptive terms. In addition, Galen understood the uncertainties and fears of the sick, as well as the interrelations of emotions and bodily symptoms. Although he used bloodletting often on a basis related to the theory of the four humors, he advised caution in the amount of blood to be removed. Despite his recourse to purgings and cuppings, much of his treatment was in the tradition of Hippocrates—helping nature by gentle methods such as diet, rest, and exercise. Prevention of illness through hygienic regimens was also of special concern to him.

A particular characteristic attached to the name of Galen was the large-scale use of medications. He gathered medicinal plants and prepared his own prescriptions—out of mistrust for the rhizotomists and drug sellers. The many ingredients which he put together in a single preparation have sometimes been

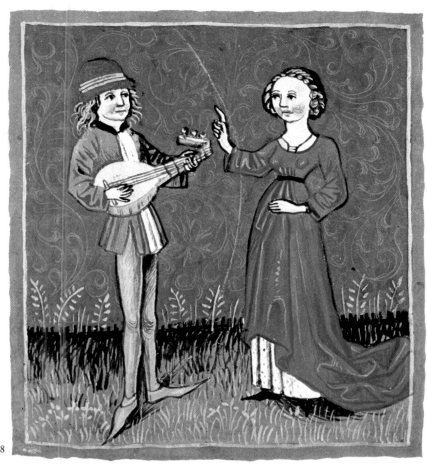

378

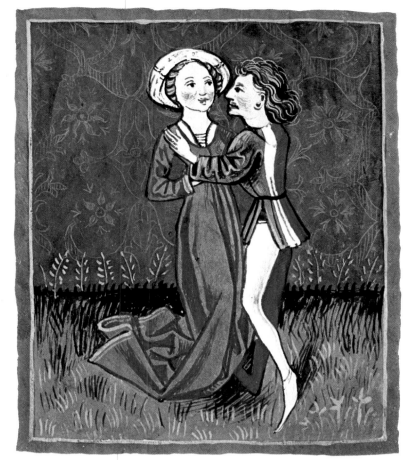

379

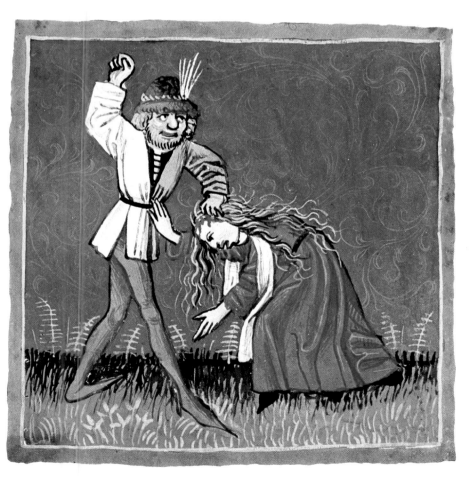

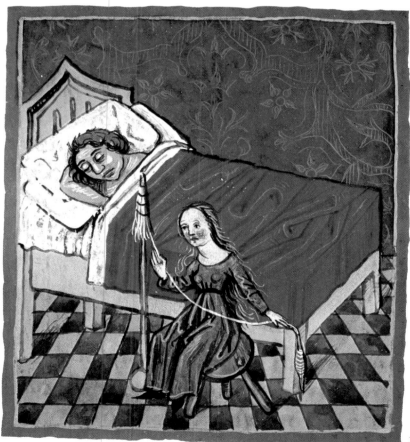

381

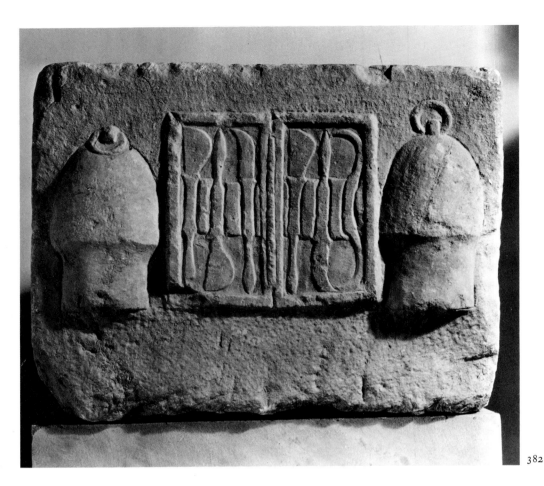

382

382 Bas-relief from the Temple of Asclepios, Athens, showing Greek surgical tools and cupping glasses. The Romans enlarged upon the variety of instruments available for surgery, and Galen wrote detailed instructions on their use. National Archaeological Museum, Athens

383 Galen shown dissecting a pig, detail from the frontispiece of a collection of Galen's works published in Venice, 1565. Most of his knowledge of anatomy came from animal rather than human dissection, which accounts for some of his errors. National Library of Medicine, Bethesda

384 Clinic scene, or Medicatrina, from Venetian edition of Galen's works published in 1550, showing surgical procedures described by Galen—on the head, eye, leg, mouth, bladder and genitals—still followed in the 16th century. Collection Bertarelli, Milan

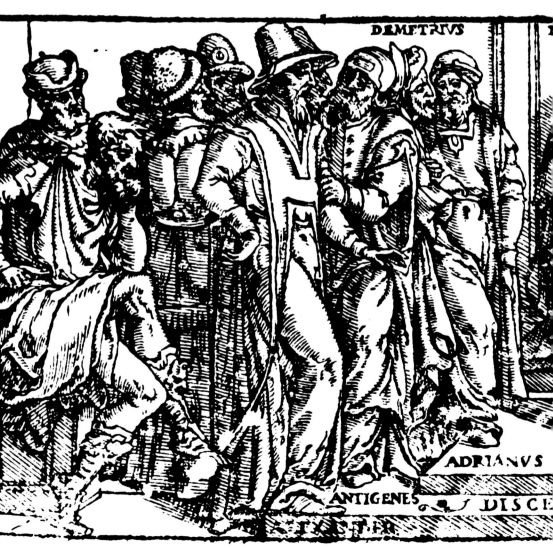

383

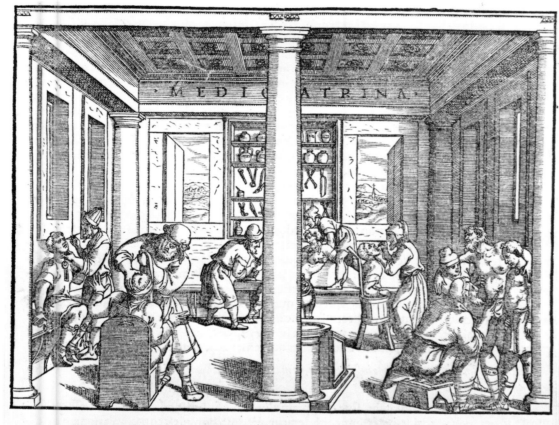

GALENI IN LIBRVM HIPPOCRATIS

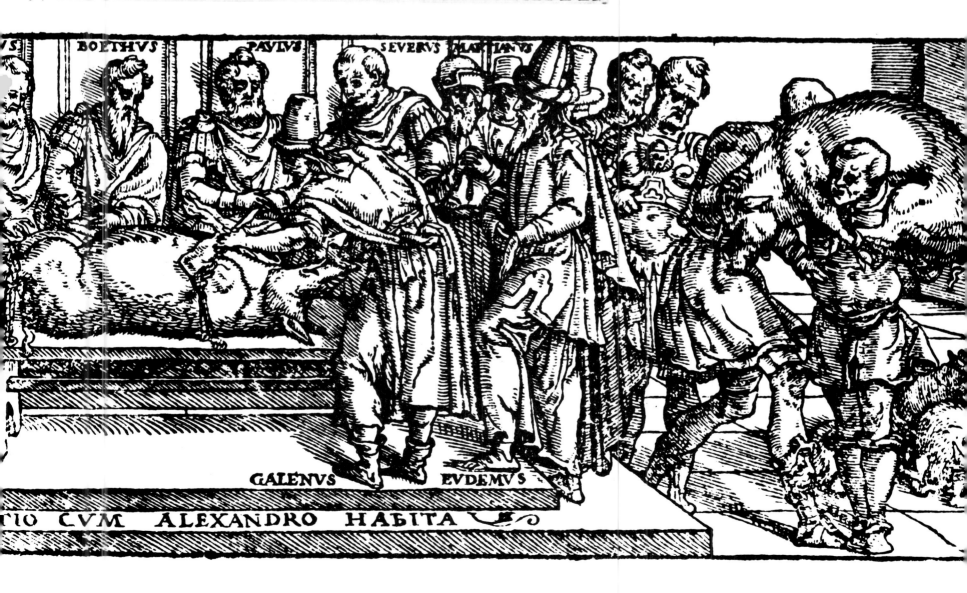

BOETHVS   PAVLVS   SEVERVS MARTIANVS

GALENVS   EVDEMVS

...TIO CVM ALEXANDRO HABITA

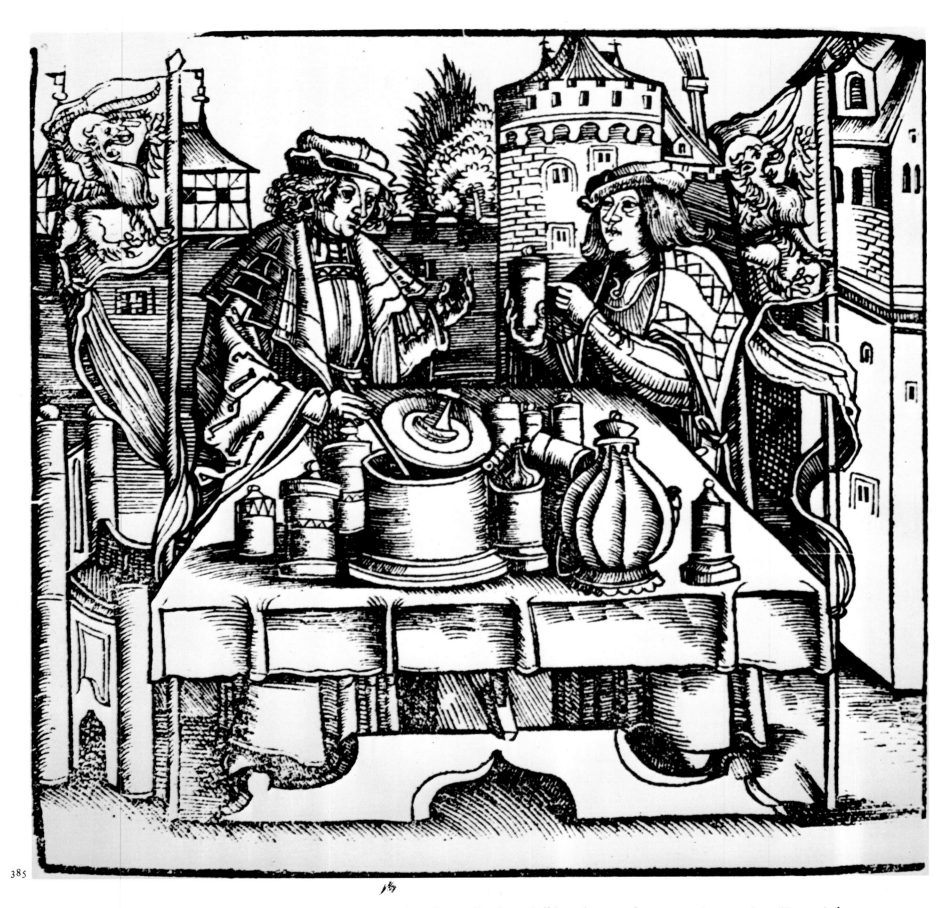

385

referred to as "Galenicals," but the term has no precise meaning. He carried polypharmacy to an extreme, mixing and blending agents whose properties he classified according to the humors and their qualities of hot, cold, dry, and moist. For example, an illness categorized as hot required a drug which was in the cold category—a classification system founded on speculative doctrines.

One extraordinary pharmaceutical combination which Galen elaborated even further was theriac. This ancient multi-ingredient preparation originated as an antidote against snakebite and eventually was used to combat all poisons and even pestilences. The legend is that Mithridates VI, King of Pontus (132–63 B.C.), experimented on slaves to find antidotes to poisons, of which he had a fanatical fear. His final combination was called *mithridatium*. In the first century A.D., after viper's flesh was added to the formula by Nero's physician Andromachus, the preparation was designated theriac, a word derived from the Greek for "wild beast."

More and more items were added to theriac over the years. Galen increased its ingredients beyond seventy, and in the Middle Ages the number exceeded a hundred. This universal antidote, after a production process lasting months, was supposed to be aged for years like vintage wine before use, although it appears to have been more solid than liquid. So important was theriac in medical practice and thinking that its use persisted throughout the Middle Ages and Renaissance into recent centuries. The most important and effective criticism of it came in the eighteenth century from William Heberden, but even then it took decades before it was dropped in England. Indeed pharmacopoeias in France, Spain, and Germany were still listing theriac in the last quarter of the nineteenth century.

The educated and ignorant, the sensible and foolish, all seemed to rely on theriac ("treacle" comes from the same root) to prevent illness, to treat inflammations, to ward off the Black Death, to cure venomous bites of all kinds—including that of humans (the exceptional danger of which was recognized by Celsus, Pliny, Galen, and others). At least some of its popularity may have been due to the presence of opium among its many elements. Galen, like others of his day, thought so highly of theriac that he compounded it personally for the several emperors he served.

The many studies of Galen's investigative, clinical, and pharmacologic activities have sometimes obscured his talents and incisive observations on surgical practice. "All the operations in surgery fall under two heads, separation and approximation. Approximation has to do with the reduction and dressing of fractures, reduction of dislocation of the joints, reductions of prolapsed intestines, uterus, or rectum, suture of the abdomen and restoration of tissue deficiencies, as in the nose, lips, and ears. Division is concerned with simple incisions, circumcisions, elevations of skin, scalping, excision of veins, amputation, cauterization, scraping, smoothing, excisions with the saw."

He gave sensible suggestions on the use of instruments, of which the Romans had a wide variety, including knives of different sizes, scissors, forceps, splints, and retractors to hold operative incisions open. His advice on placing incisions and closing them, on the management of the open abdominal cavity, and on the draining of abscesses was astute. He boldly excised tumors and infected bone but was not reckless. Even allowing for his tendency to boast, he wrote descriptions which reflect a surgeon of skill and pragmatism.

In summing up the complexities of Galen's writings, one is prompted to ask why his works were so durable, exercising a profound influence virtually unchallenged for fifteen hundred years. In the first place, the unsettled conditions of the Middle Ages produced a longing for certainty and authority, an attitude prevalent in the Muslim East as well as the Christian West. Galen's dogmatic, didactic, even pedantic style met the desire for absolutes, and Galen left no questions unanswered. Furthermore, his repeated insertions of teleological reasoning made his ideas easy for the Christian Church to embrace. Also, his encyclopedic codifications which integrated all earlier knowledge made them ready sources of medical information. Indeed, an important reason for their influence lay in the fact that of his five hundred known works eighty-three medical treatises survived. Finally, the early compilers and commentators after him enshrined his name. Oribasius, Aetius, Alexander of Tralles, Paul of Aegina, themselves authorities in high repute, spoke of Galen as the fountainhead of all medical knowledge.

No one equaled him or challenged him effectively until the sixteenth century, when Vesalius, anatomist of the Renaissance, shook the foundations of authority.

385 *Sixteenth-century woodcut showing the preparation of theriac, the ancient universal panacea that Galen further elaborated by increasing the number of its ingredients beyond 70. From H. Brunschwig,* Das Neu Distiller Buch, *Strassburg, 1537. National Library of Medicine, Bethesda*

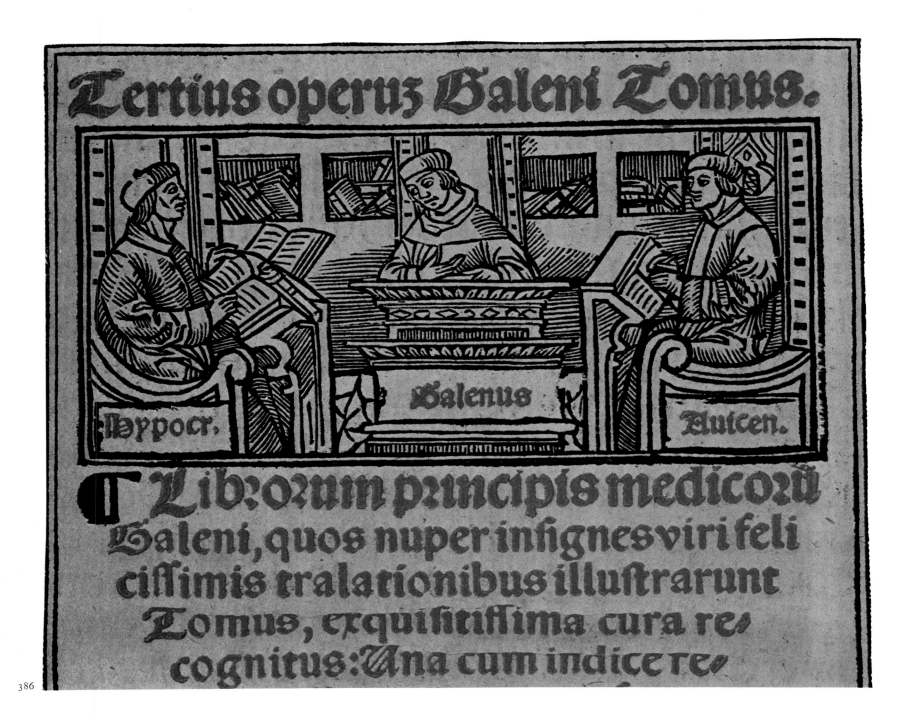

386

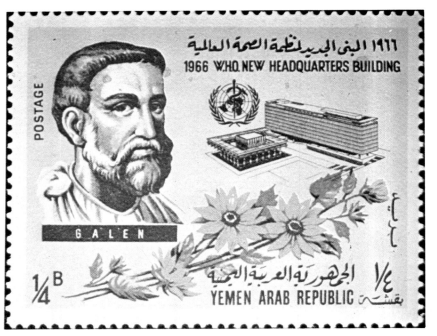

387

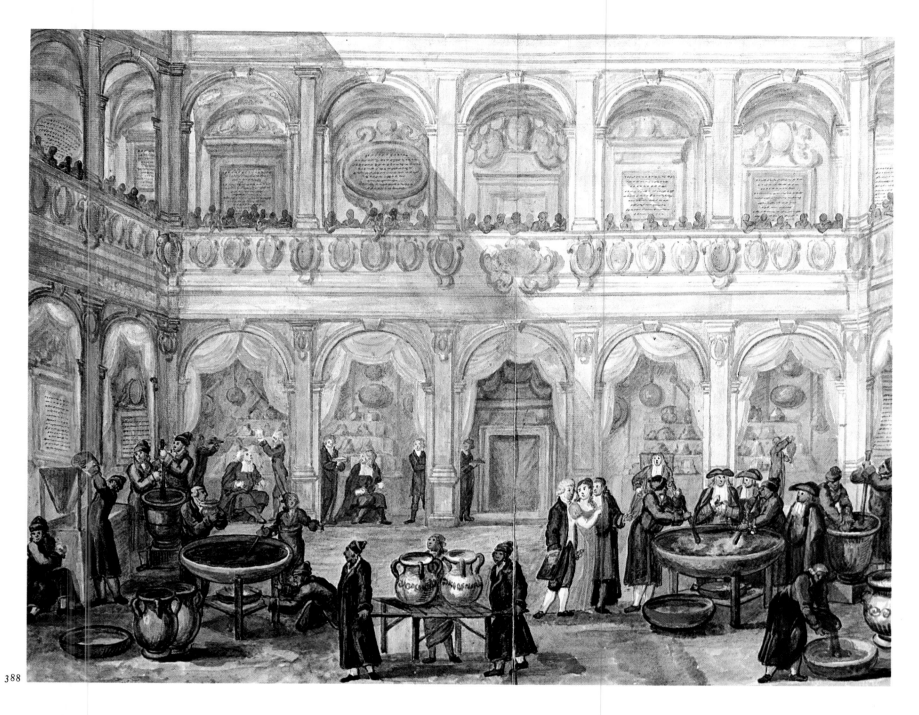

388

386 *Manuscript illustration showing Galen flanked
by Hippocrates and Avicenna, from an edition of
the works of Galen published in Lyons in 1528.
As Galen looked back to Hippocrates as his authority,
Avicenna looked to Galen. National Library of
Medicine, Bethesda*

387 *The presence of Galen on a postage stamp of
the People's Democratic Republic of Yemen testifies
to the lasting influence of the great doctor's writings.
Courtesy the author*

388 *Communal preparation in the late 18th century
of sufficient batches of theriac for an entire city's
use is shown in this illustration from Giuseppe
Guidicini,* Vestiari, usi, costumi di Bologna, *1818.
Biblioteca Communale dell'Archiginnasio, Bologna*

MEDIEVAL
MEDICINE

The Rise of Christianity

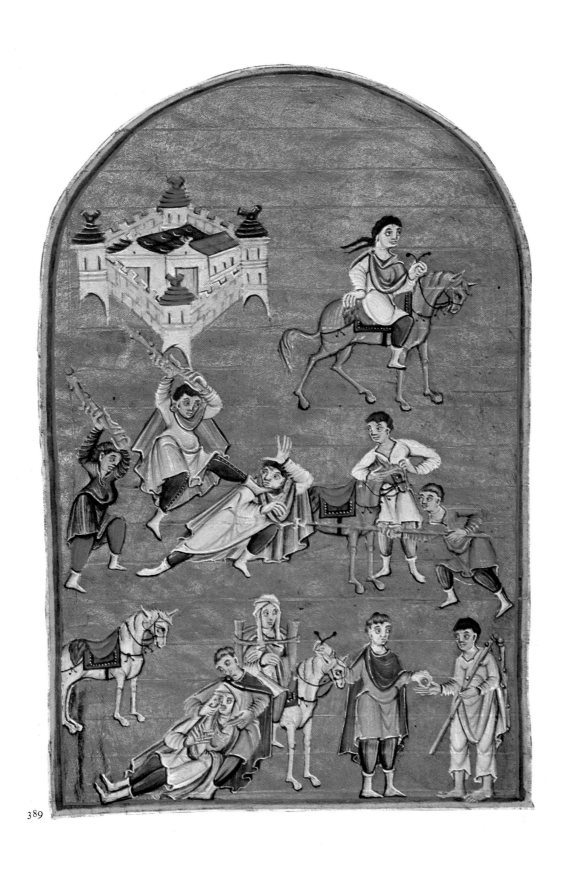

389

THE early followers of the crucified Jesus Christ of Nazareth were convinced of the imminence of his Second Coming, the Day of Judgment, and the resulting end of the "here and now." Not unexpectedly, such an otherworldly attitude toward the present did not promote concern with man's mundane physical afflictions—the starting point for any system of medicine.

ORIGIN OF DISEASE AND ITS TREATMENT

In Judaic thought disease had long been equated with sin's punishment or with divine disfavor. The early Christian Church did little to discourage popular acceptance of this relationship, and gradually sickness began to be equated with a kind of sin for which the sole appropriate response was to suffer (as Job did) and from which the only possible cure was through Grace, that undeserved and unpredictable intervention of God. This interpretation of the cause and cure of disease was to be fully developed by Gregory of Tours in the sixth century, but it exerted considerable influence before that time. As the end of the world proved less than imminent—and thereby less certain—concern for the problems of everyday life returned. Prime among these, to be sure, were considerations of health and disease.

Among the earliest followers of Christ one found a radically different, though ultimately related, interpretation of divinity and disease which was given considerable development in the Gospels. This was the "Healing Mission of Christ." In each of the Gospels by Matthew, Mark, John, and Luke (who was himself a physician), many instances of Christ's acting as a healer were cited in curing the paralytic and lame, the dumb and the blind, the leprous and the febrile. St. Mark's first reference to Christ's healing (1:23–27) was to the "tearing out" of an unclean spirit, but it was followed shortly by similar cures of physical complaints. St. John and St. Luke the physician also cited numerous instances in which Christ's healing of obviously physical infirmities was quite similar to the casting out of devils and other spirits. The modern reader of the Gospels might feel a certain disappointemnt that the writers failed to differentiate among faith healing, exorcism, and miracle, but the "treatment" was the same, whether for physical infirmity, mental instability, or outright death. Throughout, the means of healing were supernatural (what later medieval philosophers would call *praeter naturam*—beyond nature—by which it was implied that all rules covering the here and now were suspended).

Although at times Christ's mere presence was sufficient to provide cure, generally more was required. Touching was extremely important, be it Christ's reaching out or the afflicted's being able to touch even the hem of his garment. This miraculous aspect of Christ's nature, at least by the time of the writing of the Gospels, was stressed as one of the strong points in preaching the Christian story. Centuries later, the miraculous attributes of candidates for sainthood were utilized in dual fashion—both "proving" sanctity and making it desirable to revere the saint involved.

In the Gospels a somewhat different exemplar for the Christian virtue of healing is found in Christ's parable of the Good Samaritan, told in answer to the question: "And who is my neighbor?" This model of the benevolent person performing good works out of compassion for his fellow man has been a strong influence on the development of the concept of "Christian charity." Its relationship to the treatment of disease helped establish a nexus between the developing Church and concern for the sick.

DEVELOPMENT OF THE CHURCH

The early Christian church, in spite of adversity, not only flourished but saw its character and organization change within a short period after Christ's death.

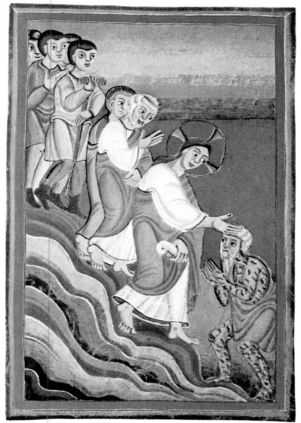

390

389 *Parable of the Good Samaritan illustrated in the Gospel Book of the Emperor Otto III (late 10th century). This lesson of compassion for one's fellow man strongly influenced the concept of Christian charity. Ms. 4453, fol. 167 v., Bayerisches Staatsbibliothek, Munich*

390 *Christ shown healing a leper in the Echternach Gospels Lectionary (mid 11th century). One of many treatments of the Healing Mission of Christ. Ms. 9428, fol. 23, Bibliothèque Royale Albert 1er, Brussels*

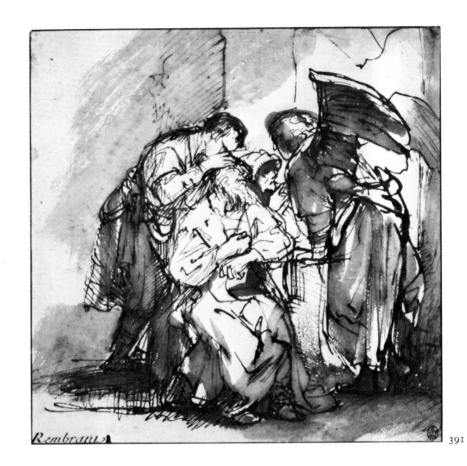

391 *In* The Healing of Tobit (*c. 1649–50*), *Rembrandt presents an example from the Old Testament of the power of faith in God to cure illness. As in the story of Job, sickness was thought to result from divine displeasure. Staatliche Museen, Berlin*

392 *Christ is shown healing the sick in Rembrandt's* Hundred Guilder Print (*c. 1645*). *Rijksmuseum, Amsterdam*

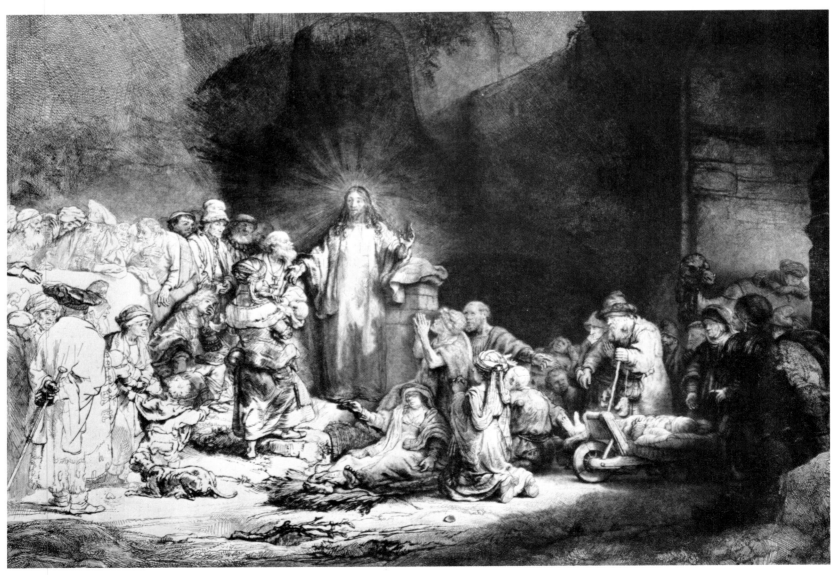

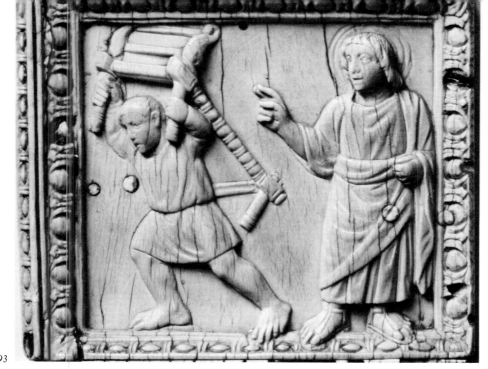

393

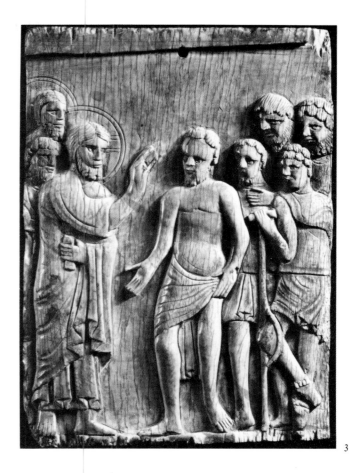

396

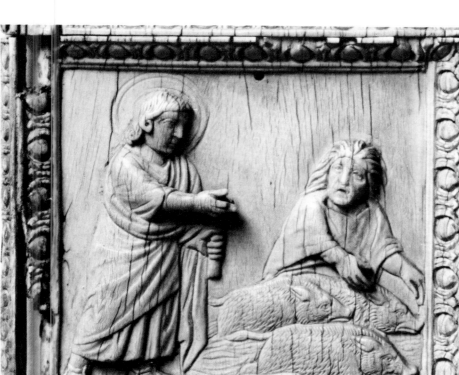

394

393, 394, 395 *Ivory plaques from Italy (late 5th century) illustrating miraculous cures by Jesus. Top: Christ commands the paralytic to pick up his bed and walk. Middle: Christ casts out the demons of a man possessed. Bottom: A woman hemorrhaging is healed through faith by reaching out to touch Christ's garment. The Louvre, Paris*

396 *Ivory plaque of the 11th century, from southern Italy, showing sick people being brought to Christ, whose mere presence was thought to cure illness. Museum of Fine Arts, Boston*

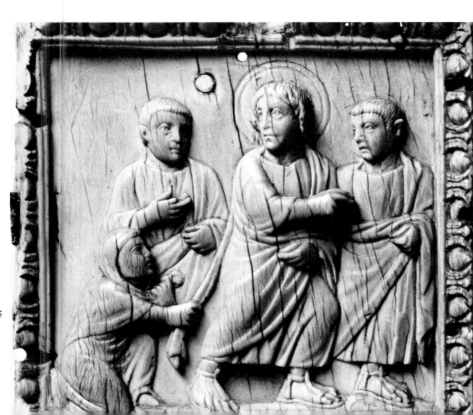

395

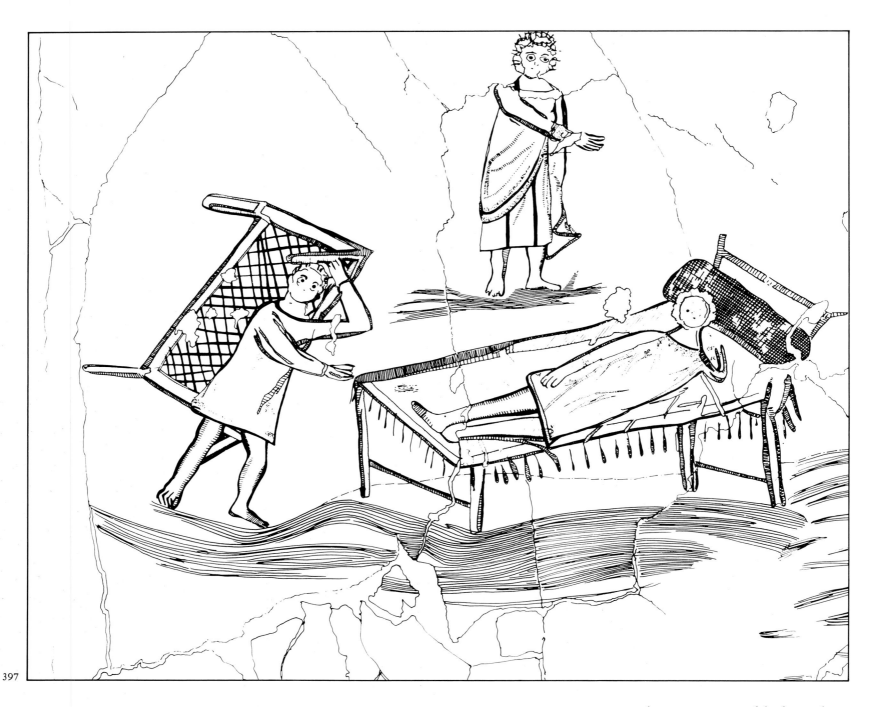

397

397 *Drawing by Henry Pearson of the fresco* Christ Healing the Paralytic (*early 3d century*), *from the Christian house-church at Dura-Europos, Syria. This is the earliest-known representation of the miraculous cures of Jesus. Yale University Art Gallery, New Haven*

398 *The power of Jesus to heal also went beyond the grave, as shown by Rembrandt in* The Raising of Lazarus (*c. 1630*). *Collection Howard Ahmanson, Los Angeles County Museum of Art*

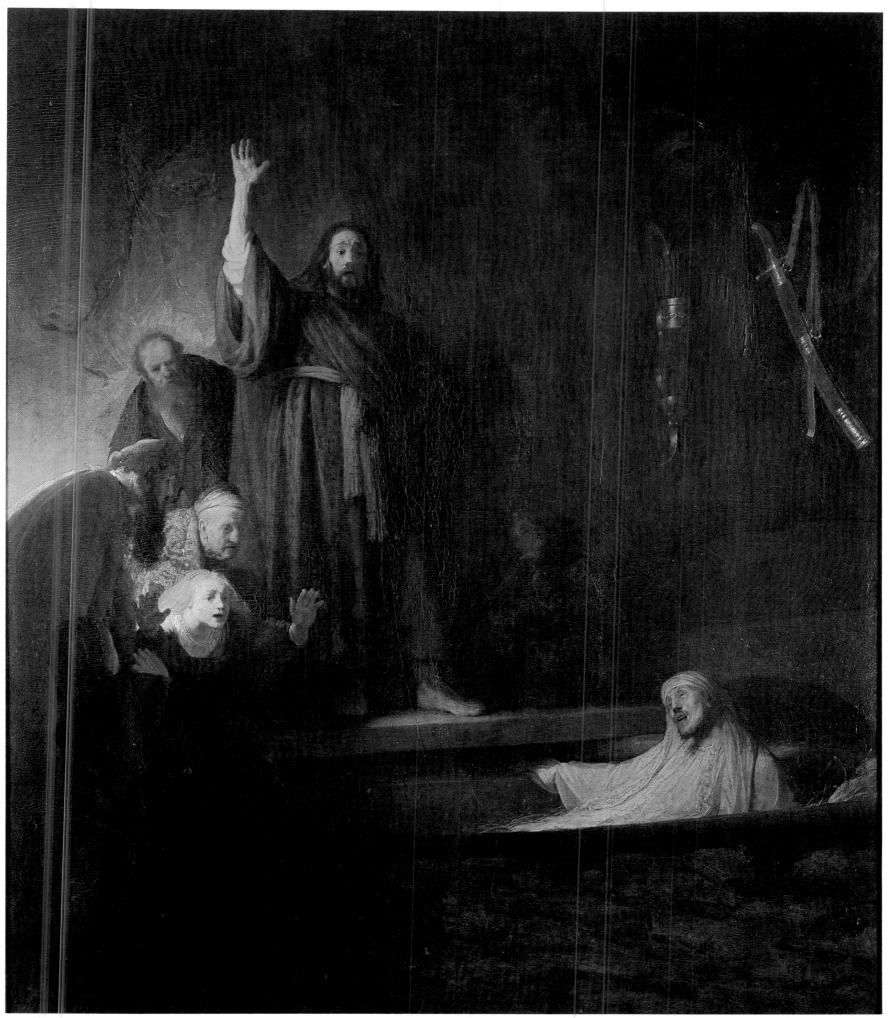

398

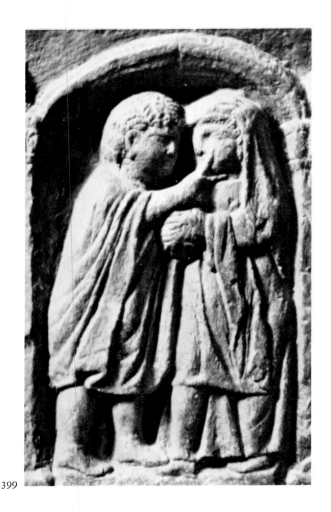

399

399 *Funerary stele (c. A.D. 300–400) showing a doctor examining a woman's eye, probably to see what treatment he can properly apply. Musée Barrois, Bar-le-Duc*

400 *Detail from an ivory sculpture (6th century), showing a scene of the miraculous restoration of sight to a blind person. Vatican Museums, Rome*

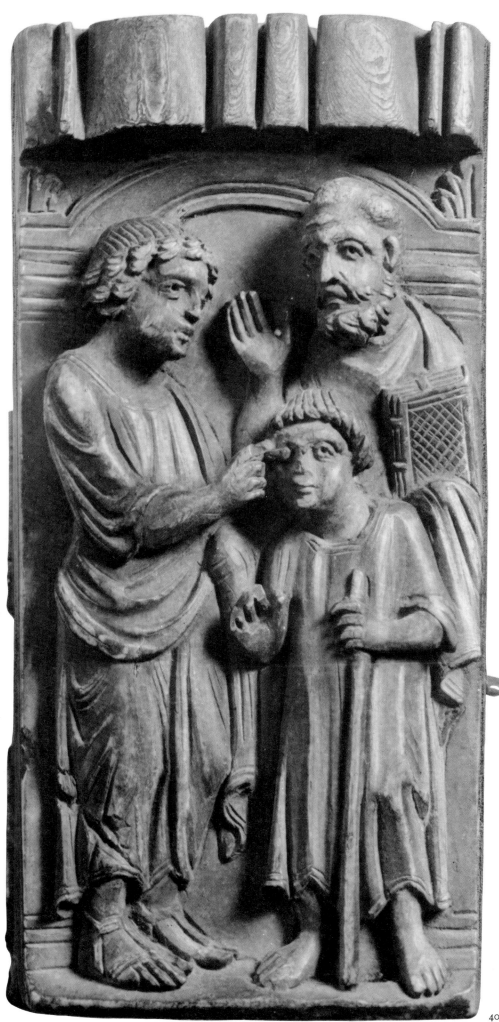

400

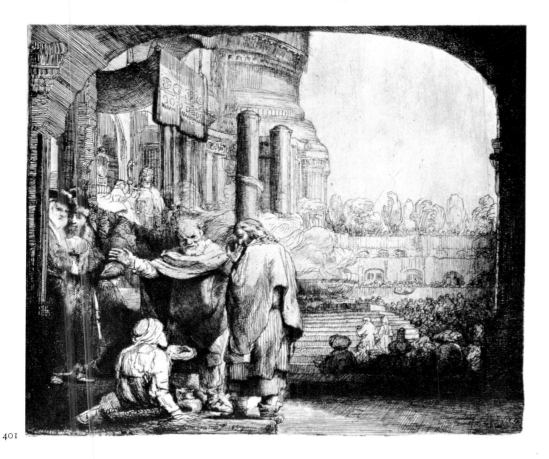

401

401 *Etching by Rembrandt,* Peter and John Healing the Cripple at the Gate of the Temple *(1659),* illustrating that Christ's healing power was shared by his disciples, of whom only Luke was a physician. *British Museum, London*

402 *Detail from a predella (c. 1316 ?) by Pietro Lorenzetti, in which St. Humilitas miraculously heals a nun as the doctor leaves, feeling that he has done everything he can for the patient. Gemälde- galerie, Berlin*

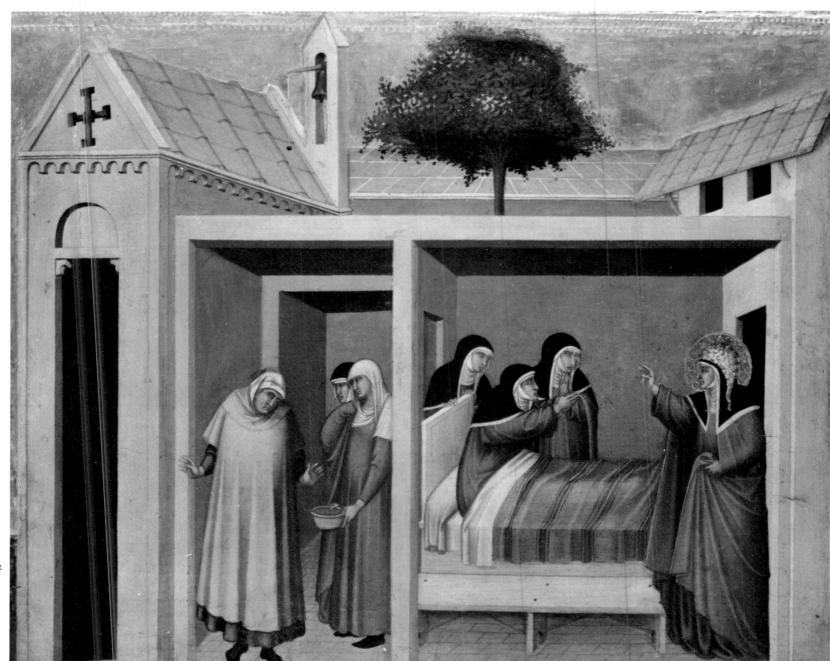

402

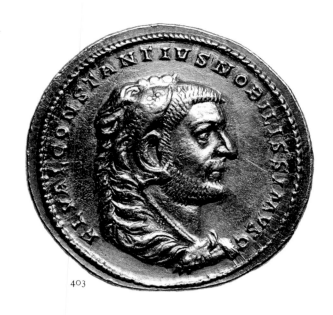

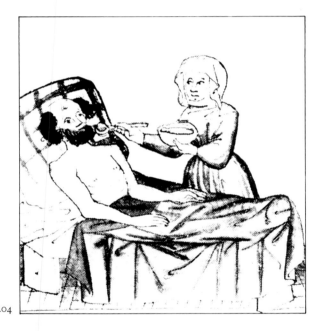

403 Gold medallion (A.D. 296–99) with a portrait of Roman Emperor Constantine I, who, in granting universal religious freedom, gave Christianity equal footing with other religions in the Roman Empire. British Museum, London

404 Nurse shown feeding a sick man, from a Saxon Work of Charity (c. 1450). The role of Christian charity in motivating women to do "good works" was important in the development of hospitals. New York Academy of Medicine

Originally a minor Judaic sect in the Roman province of Palestine, Christianity was soon given a decidedly Greek and Hellenistic cast by St. Paul. As time passed and the Day of Judgment seemed less, rather than more, imminent, the early Church was less able to rely upon a theology dependent solely on that event, and the Second Coming was given a less certain definition.

The development in the Roman world of an antirational, though practical, system of medicine with a strong overlay of religious mysticism had preceded the influence of Christianity. The increasingly mystical and magical beliefs of the later Empire created fertile ground for the establishment of an otherworldly religion which would overcome feelings of loss of control, security, and dominion as Romans saw their former power slipping ineluctably away, and plague and famine added insult to injury.

The Church itself underwent considerable change as its governance was given an increasingly ordered structure; orthodoxy became a greater concern than preparation for an imminent salvation, especially in the churches of the Eastern Roman Empire, a permanent division after the death of Theodosius in 395, the last ruler of the united Empire. Unlike the pagan religions which tended to abandon those individuals thought to have incurred the disfavor of the gods, the developing Christian church emphasized a need for reenactment of Christ's healing mission, even if this were done more for the salvation of the caretaker than for the patient. In this way, there was little conflict with the common belief that disease was a reflection of sin. Only the Grace of God could provide a cure, and so those providing care were relieved of that responsibility.

These feelings led to the establishment of numerous kinds of facilities for the care of the diseased and the oppressed: *ptochia* for the poor; *gerontochia* for the elderly; *xenodochia* for strangers; *brephotrophia* for foundlings; *orphanotrophia* for orphans; and *nosocomia* for the sick and downfallen. St. Helena, mother of the Roman emperor Constantine (who, in granting universal religious tolerance, gave Christianity equal footing with other state religions), founded a hospital about 330, the year Constantine moved the capital of the Roman Empire to ancient Byzantium and renamed it Constantinople. In the year 369, St. Basil established a hospital for the sick poor at Caesarea, capital of Cappadocia. A plague hospital was built at Edessa by St. Ephraem (c. 306–373), and, before the year 394, Fabiola, a wealthy Roman matron who later became a pupil of St. Jerome (c. 343–420) in Bethlehem, founded the first Christian public hospital in Europe.

Although these hospitals may have been modeled on the military hospitals of the Roman Empire, there were significant innovations in the Christian institutions. First aid and time for convalescence had been provided in the Roman military hospitals, but since their prime, if not sole, mission was the return to the army of troops capable of resuming battle, extensive treatment or nursing care was never considered. In marked contrast, the Christian hospices were the first ever to be devoted to long-term support of the diseased, poor, and downtrodden. Enthusiasm, charity, and good cheer sustained those in charge, often women of "good birth," in their provision of the simplest forms of care, hardly ever above the level of nursing support. Nevertheless, Emperor Julian, the Apostate, (331?–363) in attempting to return the Empire to the ancient religion, credited in part these women and their hospitals for the tenacious hold the early Church had on the masses, and he suggested setting up pagan hospitals to serve as counterforce.

The three centuries following Constantine's recognition of Christianity saw an intense struggle over the development of an orthodoxy which did much to establish for the succeeding millennium the interrelationships of man and God through Church and State. The drastically different solutions of the Eastern and the Western churches created opposing climates of opinion which were directly responsible for differences in both Christian iconography and medical practice. Before the imperial acceptance of Christianity in the fourth century, the areas of strongest Christian influence were in the eastern provinces of Syria, Palestine, and Egypt, the lands of the Bible. Local and even external influences were crucial.

Not without difficulty, the commandment of the Decalogue (Exodus, 20:4)

272

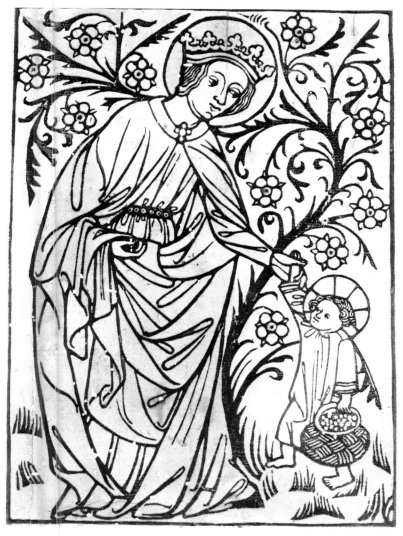

405

405 *Early-15th-century woodcut of the 4th-century martyr St. Dorothea. A type of holy image thought to possess some of the healing or intercessionary power of the saint pictured. Staatliche Graphische Sammlung, Munich*

406 *Emperor Constantine, struck with leprosy, rejects pagan advice to cure it by bathing in the blood of 3,000 children—whose mothers are shown appealing to him in this 13th-century fresco. Rewarded with a vision to call for St. Sylvester, he is cured and converted to Christianity. Quattro Santi Coronati, Rome*

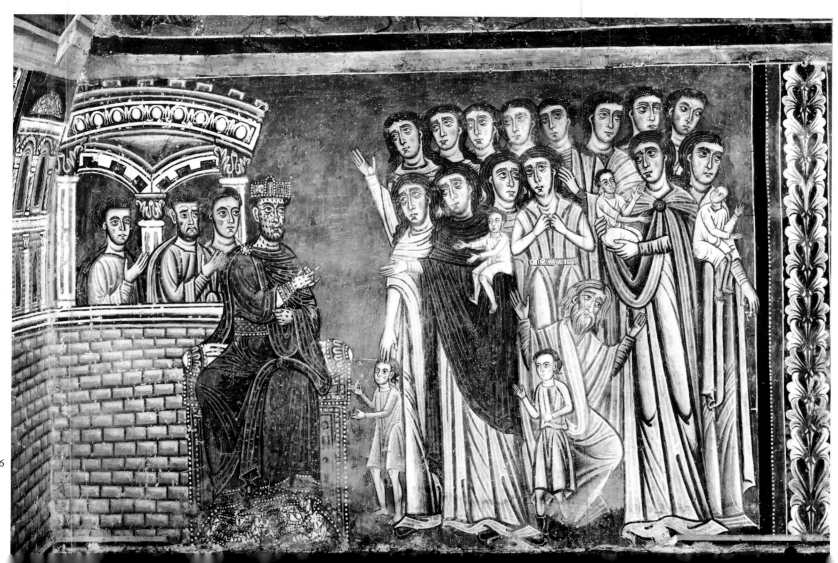

406

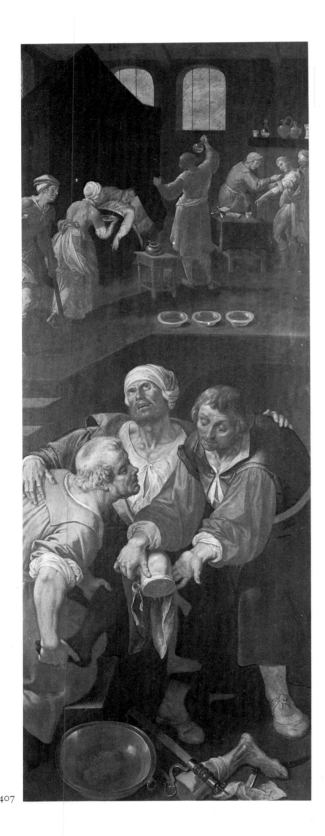

407

forbidding graven images was put aside and two iconographic styles developed for the portrayal of Christ: the bearded Jesus with shoulder-length hair was derived from portrayals of the Parthian kings, whereas the presentation as beardless young man came directly from that of the Egyptian god Horus. Plotinus (205–270), the founder of neoplatonism, developed a theory whereby a representation of divinity could partake of its divine essence. According to the doctrine of emanation, divine substance flows from the Godhead, or prime principle, into an image, instilling something of the divine power of the figure represented—be it Christ, Mary, or a saint. Therefore, early in the Church's history, a means of incorporating divine substance into sacred representations for direct and personal use was justified, and the veneration of icons, especially in the Eastern Church, has remained integral to this day. The early tradition of the Healing Mission of Christ and the advantage of utilizing curative miracles in the proselytization of Christianity rapidly led to the creation of numerous icons, at first of Christ, and later of the saints in the act of healing. The doctrine of emanation made these illustrations of even greater value in their becoming instruments of healing themselves. Though never inclined to the veneration of icons, the Western Church nevertheless developed a veneration of relics of saints, deriving ultimately from the Greek tradition of hero worship—as brought to Gaul and Italy by emigrants from Asia Minor.

Other aspects of earlier Oriental religions found in Eastern Christianity were adopted by Western Christians, and some were critical in the ultimate schism of East and West in the year 1054. The cult of Mary developed in Egypt from the Isis-Horus (mother-son) relationship and in Syria where a virgin was said to have given birth to the sun god. Both of these gods were thought to have been born on December 25th, the date early appropriated by the Christian Church for its founder's birth. Christ assumed not only the birthdate of earlier gods but also many of their attributes, iconographically exemplified in the extensive use of the nimbus, or halo. Soon extended to the saints, this tradition was quickly taken over by the emperors of Byzantium.

As the Roman Empire waned in the West, Christianity was rapidly made crucial to the self-justification of the Eastern Empire—the religio-cultural nexus of Christianity and its claims of universality were essential. Orthodoxy thereby was established, and the earlier tradition of Roman tolerance was abandoned. The predictable conflict of Eastern emperor and Roman pope, however, was to lead inevitably to a schism in Christendom. Even in the East a monolithic church-state orthodoxy could not be maintained for long, and church councils were called both to define and to impose orthodoxy. Irreversible splits were common, and one of them had a special influence on the history of medicine.

In Egypt and Asia Minor, where Artemis, Cybele the Earth Mother, and the mother goddess Atargatis were still being worshiped, it was felt that Mary should be venerated as the Mother of God. Nestorius (d. 451?), Patriarch of Constantinople, objected, saying that Mary was only the mother of the human person of Christ, son of God. However, at the Council of Ephesus in the year 431, his opponents won their case by declaring that Nestorius was denying the true Godhead of Christ since he divided the one Christ into two persons. Nestorius was deposed as patriarch and forced to emigrate with his followers to Antioch, Arabia, and finally Egypt. His cause was also supported in Assyria and Mesopotamia, where at Edessa a medical school was founded, soon to rival the famous center at Alexandria. In 489, however, Bishop Cyril had the Byzantine emperor Zeno condemn the school and expel its heretical founders from the empire. The Nestorians went to Persia and founded the medical school at Gundishapur which flourished for many centuries.

407 Sts. Cosmas and Damian, seen caring for an amputee in this late-16th-century painting by Ambrosius Francken, had numerous miraculous cures attributed to them and later became patron saints of the healing professions. Koninklijk Museum voor Schone Kunsten, Antwerp

408 St. Lucy, as envisaged in the 15th century by Francesco del Cossa, was popularly invoked for protection from eye diseases. National Gallery of Art, Washington, D.C.

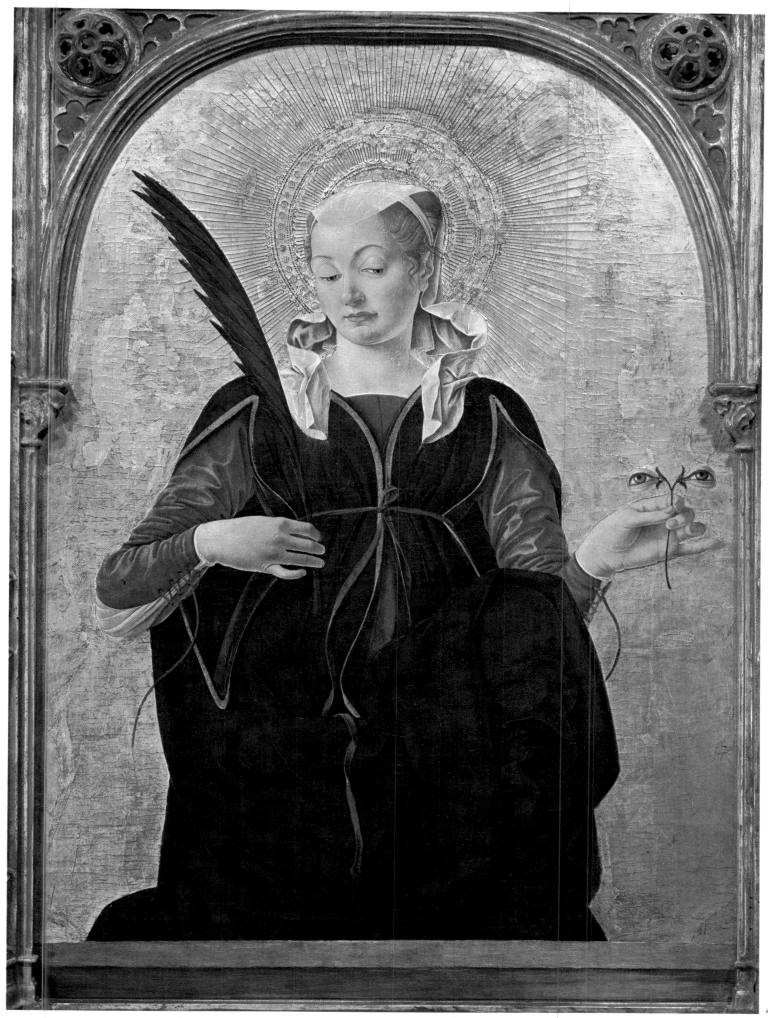

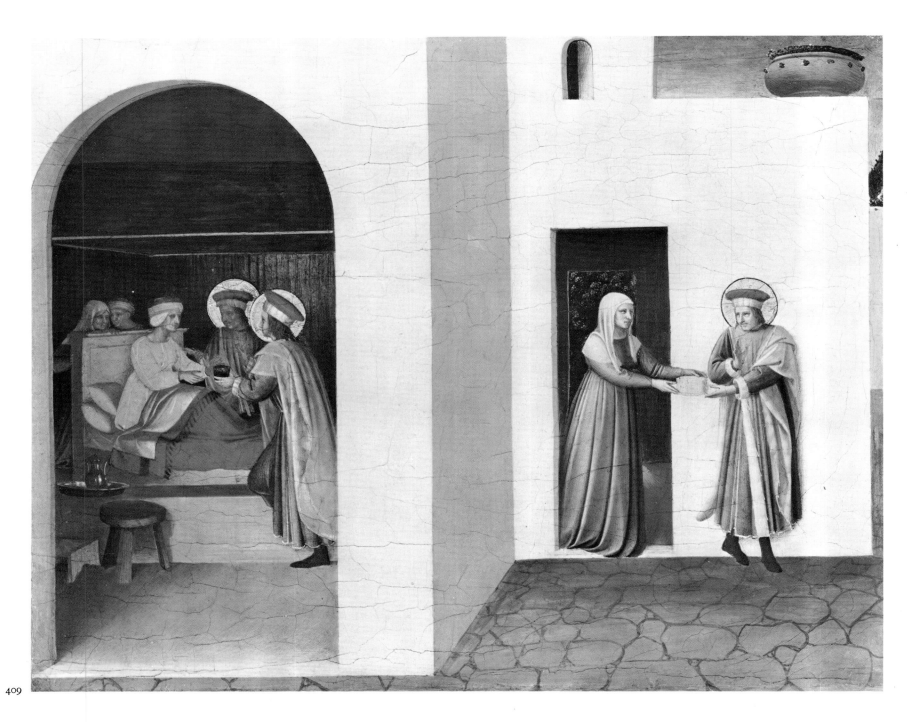

409

Monasticism

The final institution of the early Eastern Church to have a significant influence upon both Eastern and Western civilization in general and medicine in particular was monasticism. Following the hermitic tradition of withdrawal from worldly society in preparation for the world-to-come, the earliest Christian monks individually had left society to lead an isolated existence of ascetic mysticism in the desert. Monks began to band together, however, under the leadership of Pachomius (d. 348), a hermit who later devised the first set of monastic rules for a cenobitic house.

In the West, things were somewhat different. St. Benedict of Nursia (480–554) knew the Rule of Pachomius, but when he established his own monastery at Monte Cassino, unlike his Eastern brethren, he accentuated a religious community over an anchoritic association of hermits. Intellectually, however, the first Benedictines were of the same bent as the Byzantines, maintaining and copying old manuscripts. It was only the chance association of the early Christian charity hospital and the developing monastic orders that allowed for the monasteries' assumption of organized medical care in the West for more than five hundred years.

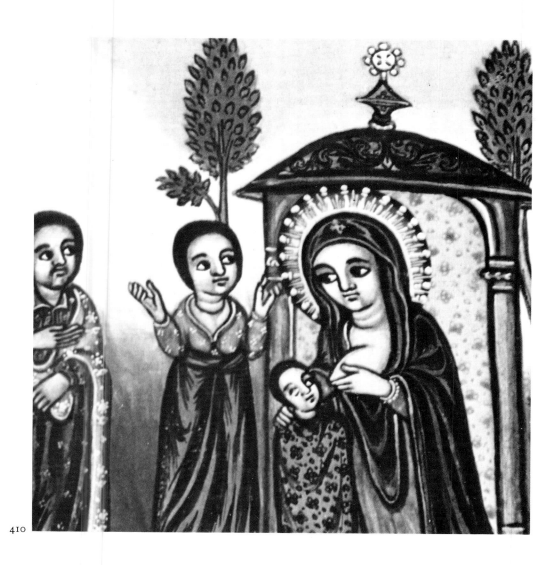

410

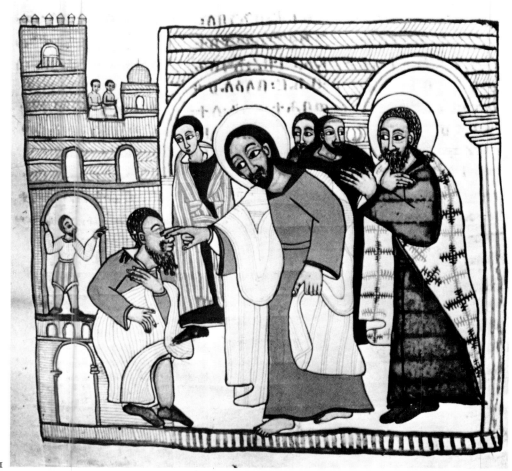

411

409 *Fra Angelico, in the mid 15th century, depicts another miraculous cure by the martyred twin physicians in* The Healing of Palladia by Sts. Cosmas and Damian. *National Gallery of Art, Washington, D.C.*

410 *Illuminated Ethiopian Coptic Church prayer book, showing St. Mary sprinkling a maiden's eyes with the milk of healing and mercy in a treatment for blindness. World Health Organization, Geneva*

411 *Fourteenth-century miniature from Ethiopia, illustrating the healing touch, as Christ cures a suppliant of blindness. World Health Organization, Geneva*

The Dark Ages

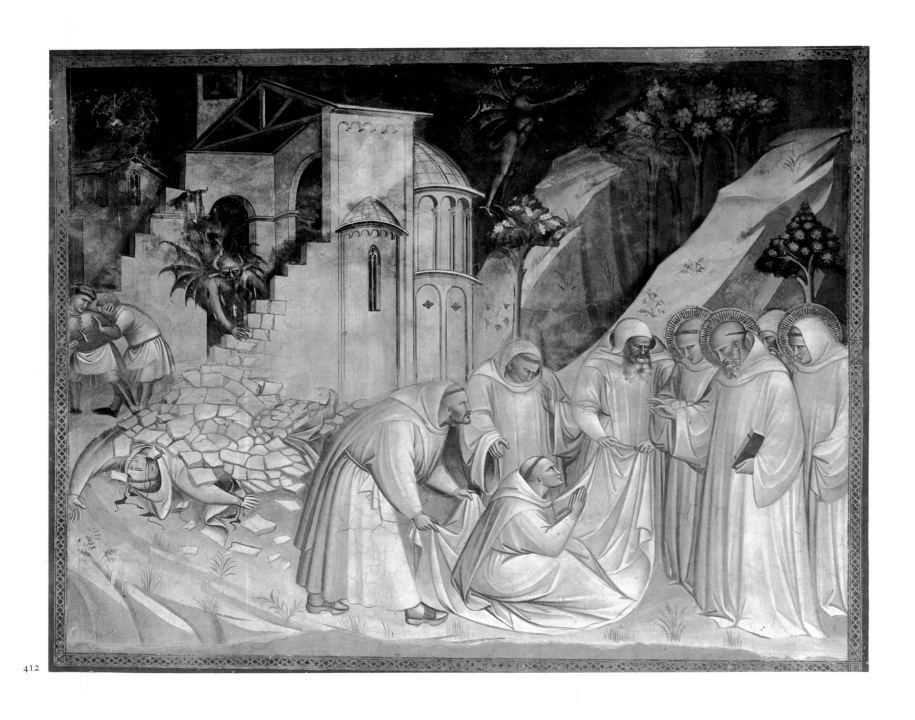

THE Fall of Rome to the Goths in 476 and the Fall of Constantinople in 1453 to the Turks are often cited as marking the beginning and end of the Middle Ages. The common characterization of this period as the "Age of Faith" reflects a dramatic loss of confidence in the individual, but ultimately it does not provide an understanding of why man felt no longer capable of learning from his own observations and took life "on faith."

In any of the sciences, one must be able to believe in a constancy of cause and effect which is not subject to the whims of forces beyond nature. Precisely this belief was wanting in the medieval period, and its lack was of prime significance to the static—even at times declining—nature of the sciences and to an increased interest in magic and other distinctly unnatural phenomena. Less important, though more commonly noted, was the unsettling influence on the period of marauding conquerors: the Muslim descendants of bedouin tribesmen of the East, and the Germanic invaders of the West. Although the intellectual impact of Arabic science on Western Europe did not become significant before the tenth or eleventh century, a common characteristic of many of the Germanic tribes, especially in Italy, Spain, and Gaul, was their ready acceptance of the cultural and intellectual milieu of the peoples they had conquered. Latin civilization, though at times forced to go underground, persisted.

BARBARIAN INVASIONS

The strong frontier north of Constantinople necessitated a more western migration for the Germanic peoples forced out of their territories by the tide of Slavs more to the east. As the Goths and Lombards poured into northern Italy, the Slavs completed the separation of East and West by occupying Dacia, the region through which land contact between Rome and Constantinople had been maintained.

In spite of the dissolution of the Western Empire, immediately following the Fall of Rome to the Goths, a transient period of relative stability was found in northern Italy and Gaul through establishment of the Frankish, Lombard, and Gothic kingdoms, especially under Theodoric (c. 454–526). Many Roman institutions appear to have survived, even if no longer under the authority of Rome. During the fifth to the seventh centuries, the Germanic peoples—Ostrogoths, Lombards, Franks, Visigoths—who had conquered the northern perimeter of the Western Empire easily adapted the sophisticated Roman system of jurisprudence to the development of practical codes regulating personal interactions within their communities. Issues of public health and concern with physicians were prime in all these codes. Probably physicians were still exclusively nonclerical. Fees were almost always defined by ordinance, and these were often high, but punishment for malpractice, or misfortune, was also severe. The physician's rights and penalties were more commonly defined by the rank of the patient, and physicians themselves were probably of low status (certainly not among the "learned," having little formal training). Hospitals under nonclerical administration existed in the sixth century at Lyons and Merida.

Other Germanic peoples, occupying lands to the north of the former empire where vestiges of Latin civilization quickly evaporated, had contact with neither Roman law nor Roman medicine. Among them the belief that supernatural forces engendered disease prevailed. The sick were cured by the word in exorcism and by the administering, internally and externally, of healing plant substances. Teutonic women were very important as healers, especially in battle, by bloodsucking. The Celtic peoples to the north and west of the Franks were under the general leadership of the Druids, who combined both priestly and curative functions. Even the tribes settling the Russian steppes had practitioners of folk medicine, the *volkhava* or wolfmen, who relied heavily on magical powers.

A major exception in northern Europe to this return to a folk medicine

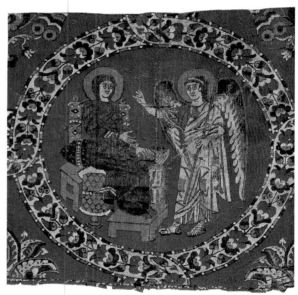

413

412 *St. Benedict, founder of the Benedictine Order (c. 529), shown reviving a monk in a fresco (c. 1387) by Spinello Aretino. St. Benedict encouraged his monks to care for the sick, but forbade the study of medicine because he believed cures were possible only through divine intervention. San Miniato al Monte, Florence*

413 *Silk twill medallion (7th–8th century), with the Annunciation in purple, brown, and green on red ground, illustrates, in its Syrian iconography and Byzantine style affinities, the influence of Eastern Christendom on the West. Sancta Sanctorum, Vatican, Rome*

414 *Scythian gold figure (c. 6th century* B.C.*), typical of the artifacts of marauding barbarians, who confined their cultural interests to what was portable. They also transported ideas that supernatural forces caused disease, which they treated through exorcism and plant medicine. The Hermitage, Leningrad*

415 *Remains of Hadrian's Wall (*A.D. *122–30) mark the border between England and Scotland and the northernmost limit of the Roman Empire. To the north and west lay the lands of the Celts, whose leaders, the Druids, combined priestly and healing functions.*

416 *Detail of richly carved wooden headpost (c.* A.D. *825) found in a Viking ship burial at Oseberg, Norway. The head's menacing stare reflects the reputation for fierceness of the far-northern peoples and their respect for supernatural forces. Universitetets Samling av Nordiske Oldsaker, Oslo*

417 *Relief on a column capital (c. 1160) showing devil taking possession of a woman. From earliest times, it was common for illness to be attributed to possession and for exorcism to be practiced in treatment. Cathedral of the Annunciation, Nazareth*

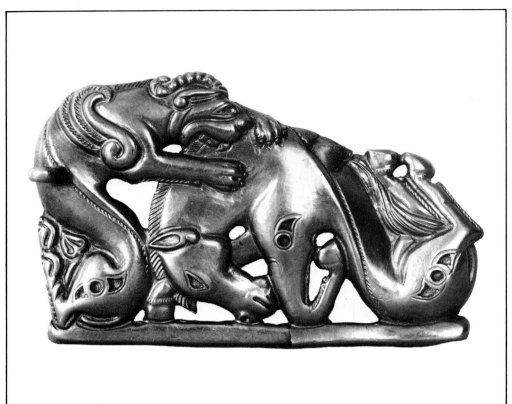

414

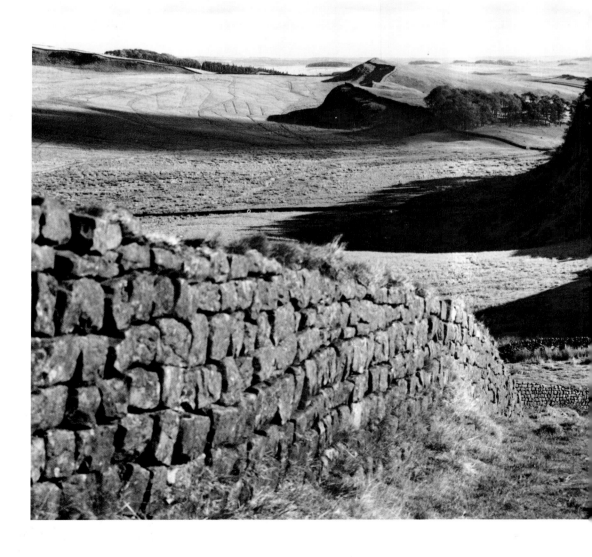

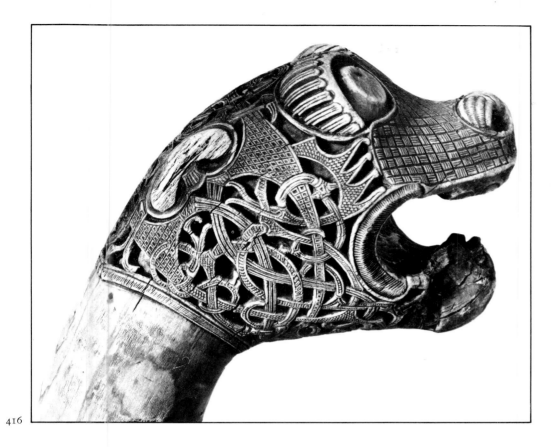

416

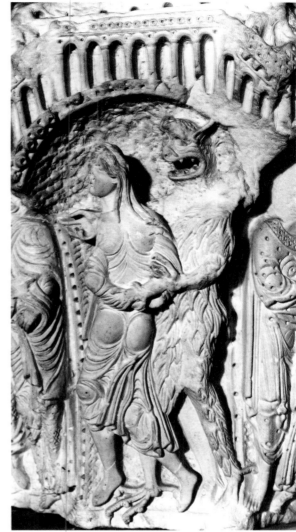

417

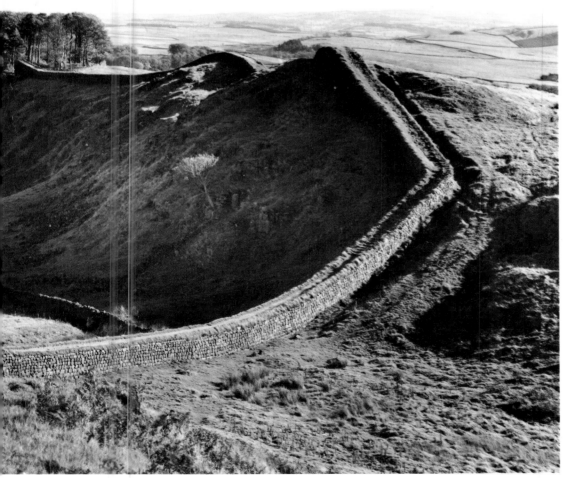

415

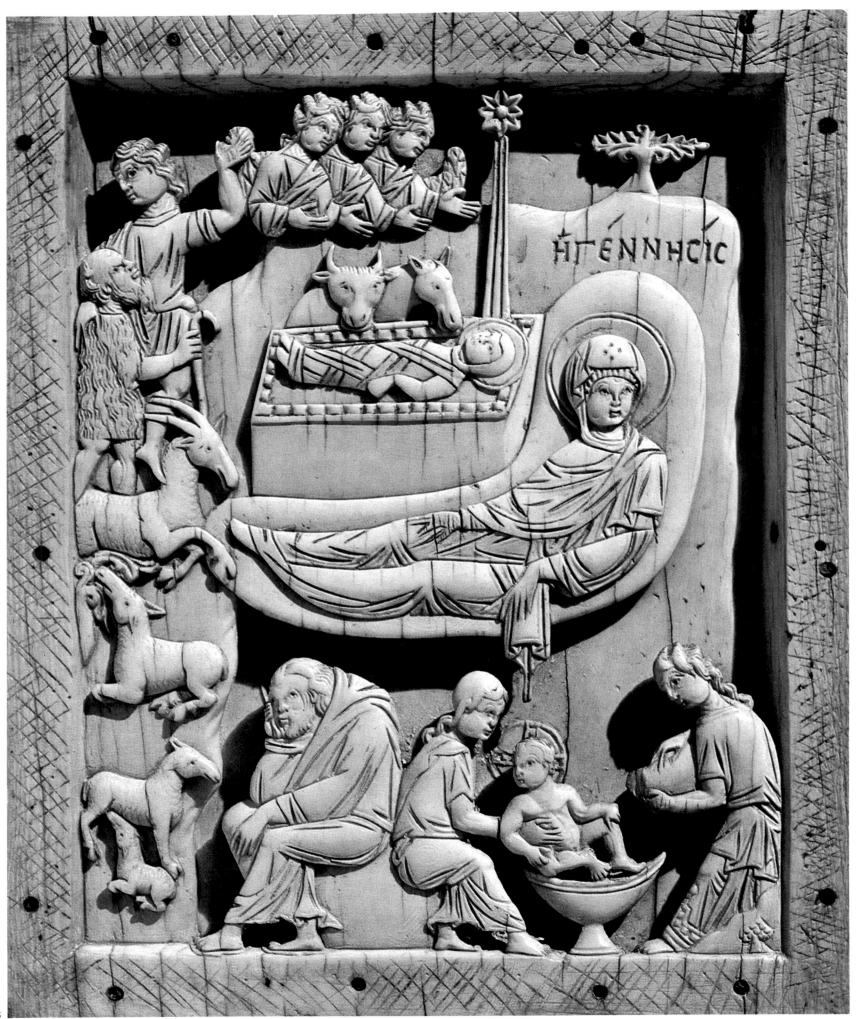

intertwining religious and medical functions was found in the British Isles, part of which had been brought into the Empire by Julius Caesar himself, where several centuries later Christianity was to follow. As the Roman Empire underwent its death throes, St. Patrick (c. 385–461), a native Briton, brought Christianity to the Celtic peoples of Ireland, and the spirit of monasticism became deeply rooted. In part because of the end of Roman influence in the British Isles, the Irish monks rapidly developed a tradition of firm independence while maintaining strong contact with the monastic communities of both Italy and the East. Later these monks, as missionaries, were to convert to Christianity and introduce Latin civilization to large numbers of Frankish and Teutonic conquerors of Europe who had had no direct contact with Mediterranean peoples.

The stability of northern Italy during the reign of Theodoric in the early sixth century was short-lived. Only so long as the conquering Goths and Lombards were able to remain aloof were they able to remain in charge. Unlike other migrators, they allowed the native Italian population to remain, and within a century the conquerors submitted culturally to the conquered. Although the adaptation of Roman institutions early served a general good, within a short time alliances among the various conquering peoples based on ties of blood and marriage disintegrated. Rivalry ensued. Isolationist anarchy was encouraged by the nearly total suppression of trade and a return of city-dwellers to the land.

Among the first Roman institutions to be dispensed with were those of law and medicine. Might increasingly made right, and doctors and patients each had to fend for himself. Ultimately, for reasons not entirely clear, nonclerical physicians just ceased to exist. One influence, however, was the ascendancy of the Church in Rome—especially the papacy—in the vacuum created by the moving of the capital of the Western Roman Empire to Ravenna. The Church maintained the strongest link to the past, and this was reinforced by its continued contact with the Eastern Church. The deference of the conquerors, especially important in northern Italy and Gaul, to the traditions of the culturally superior conquered peoples, became more and more a deference to the Church of Rome, as the legal, social, and intellectual carry-overs of the imperial period were successively lost or even suppressed by the anarchic conditions surrounding the Goths' squabbling and attempts to reestablish society.

MONASTERIES, MEDICINE, AND MIRACLES

St. Benedict of Nursia encouraged the care of the sick in the statutes founding his order at the monastery of Monte Cassino on the site of an ancient temple of Apollo. However, because the cure of disease was possible only through prayer and divine intervention, St. Benedict forbade the study of medicine. Thus, the Healing Mission of Christ was institutionalized in a fashion that was to control medical care almost completely for the next five hundred years.

Aurelius Cassiodorus (480–573), after serving as private secretary to Theodoric the Great, entered the Benedictine order and recommended the study of Latin translations of Hippocrates, Galen, and Dioscorides, as well as the works of Caelius Aurelianus. Within a short period, the provision of medical care had become integral to the Benedictine order. In an age where literacy was most uncommon, the Benedictines also made a conscious effort to preserve the literary tradition of the Latin world. Though by no means confined to medical tracts, many were thereby preserved, even if these treatises had little or no influence upon the kind of medicine that was being practiced within the monasteries housing them.

Many well-developed ancient medical procedures, especially surgical, were lost, and cauterization replaced many techniques of surgery. Pharmacology abandoned all experimental aspects and regressed to a simplified herbalism characteristic of many types of folk medicine. But as the Benedictine and other orders expanded and extended themselves across Western Europe, an herb garden,

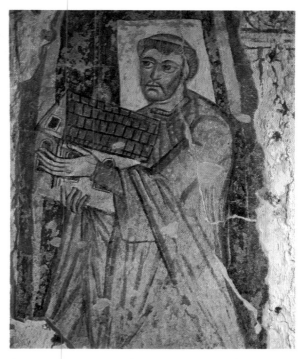

419

418 *Ivory book cover (10th–11th century) showing Nativity scene with infant Jesus wrapped in swaddling clothes, an ancient practice that persists even today in certain Eastern countries. Vatican Museum, Rome*

419 *Ninth-century fresco portrait of St. Benedict of Nursia, whose Order not only provided medical care for 500 years but copied and preserved Latin texts, including medical tracts. Chiesa di San Benedetto, Malles Venosta*

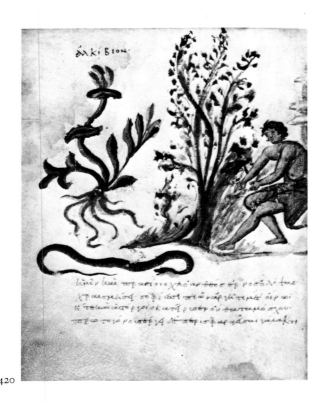

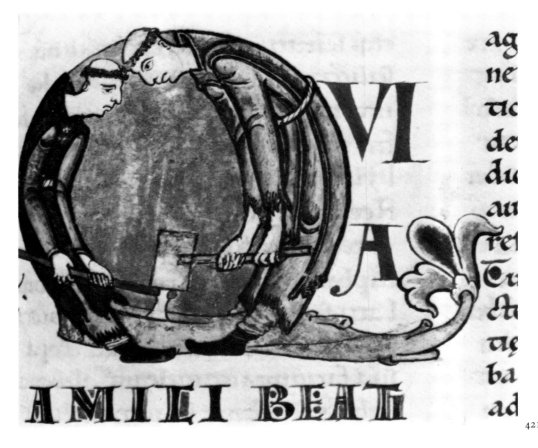

420 *Manuscript page from the 11th-century* Theriaca *of Nicander, after Dioscorides, showing peasant cutting* alkibios (Echium rubrum) *used in curing snakebite. Ms. suppl. gr. 247, fol. 16 v., Bibliothèque Nationale, Paris*

421 *Monks shown splitting firewood in initial* Q *from St. Gregory's* Moralia in Job (c. 1111). *In addition to caring for the sick, monks performed all tasks necessary to running a monastery. Ms. 170, fol. 75 v., Bibliothèque Municipale, Dijon*

422 *Dedication page of 6th-century copy of Dioscorides,* De Materia Medica *ordered by Juliana Ancia (shown here between allegorical figures Magnanimity and Prudence). Daughter of a Roman emperor, she recognized the medical value of this herbal. Österreichische Nationalbibliothek, Vienna*

423 *The four humors—phlegm, blood, black bile, and yellow bile—of classical medicine presented, with their characteristics, as a fourfold schema in this 8th-century manuscript. Ms. lat. Monac. 14300, Bayerisches Staatsbibliothek, Munich*

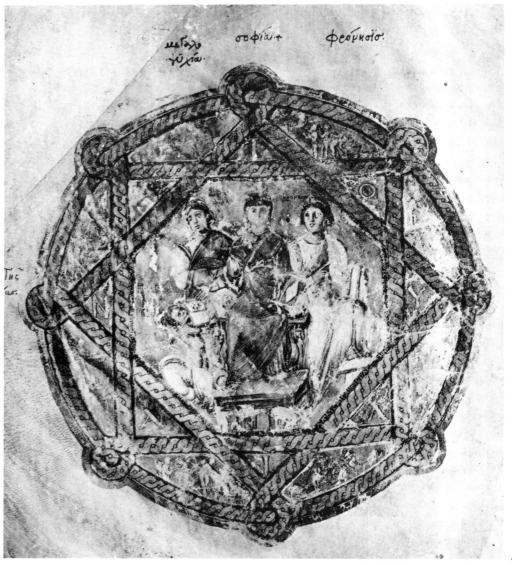

frigido quidem terra aerem humido ipsequoque aer meli
ur inter duo conpugnantia pxturam hoc e. inter aquam
& igne inr̄u que illud elimentum sibi conciliat quia aqu r
humore & igni calore coniungitur. igir quoque cūsit cali
dus & siccus calore aeri adnectitur. siccitate uū incon
munionem terrae sociatur adq̄ per taxibi ph unc circui
ui quasi p quendā corū concordita cietate coniuguntur.
unde & grece oena dicuntur. quae latine elementa
uocantur eo q̄d sibi conueniunt & conentiant quorū dirunc
tā conmunem subiecti circuli figura declarat.

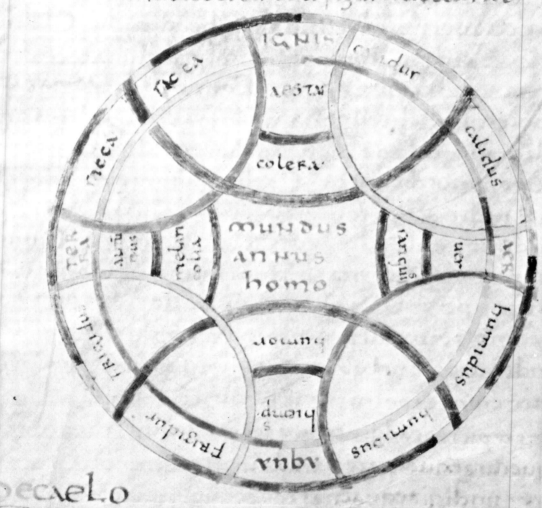

DE CAELO

Caelum spiritaliter ecclesiā quae inhuius uitae noc
te sc̄orū uirtutib; quasi claritate siderū fulget. plura
liter autem caeli nomine sc̄i omnes uel angeli intelle
guntur. si quidē caelos etiā pphetas & apostolos.
accipere debemur de quib; scriptū e. Caeli enarrant
gloriā di utiq; quia ipsi aduentū & mortem ipsi quoq; resur

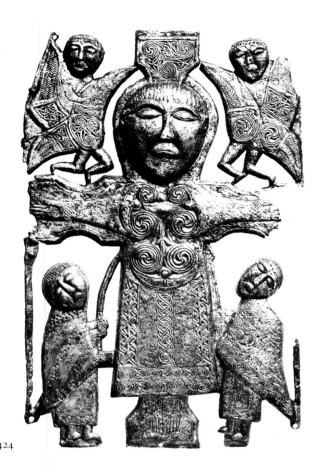

424

424 *Celtic cast-bronze Crucifixion (c. 8th century),
possibly from a book cover. Converted to Christianity
by St. Patrick, the Celts of Ireland, in turn, sent
missionaries to convert the Frankish and Teutonic
conquerors of Europe. National Museum of Ireland,
Dublin*

425 *Golden, jewel-studded reliquary of St. Foy
(c. 980), one of many artifacts made to house relics
of saints for veneration and direct appeal for cure of
illness. Cathedral Treasury, Conques*

a library with scribes to do copying, and an infirmary were almost always the essential elements of a monastery.

The Celtic peoples of Britain and Ireland were early to adopt the monastic way of life and even maintained better and longer contact with the Eastern orders than did the Italian monasteries. Fired by a new religion and culture totally alien to their Druidic past, they not only incorporated the Benedictine penchant for the preservation of Latin civilization but also, in the seventh century, began to transport this back to the European continent, where as missionaries under St. Columbanus (d. 615) in Gaul, St. Gall (d. 646) in Switzerland, and St. Willibrord (d. 739) in the Frankish domains, the Benedictines converted many Frankish and Germanic tribes and established monasteries, the most notable of which were St. Gall and Fulda. All were more or less modeled after the Benedictine monasteries of Italy, and the ascendancy of clerical medicine was assured.

Monasteries founded near centers of medical learning in the old Empire were often able to establish a connection with whatever had survived the disruption of the Empire, as at Ravenna in Italy, Lyons in Gaul, and Merida in Spain. When Charlemagne had unified under single rule many of the Frankish and Germanic tribes at the end of the eighth century, he not only was anxious to attain legitimacy by being crowned Holy Roman Emperor by the Pope but also sought to extend Latin civilization through schools associated with church and crown. Not only at the *Schola Palatii*, where famous Englishmen taught the sons of Charlemagne and other nobles, but also throughout the system of cathedral schools medicine was expected to be taught in addition to classical studies and politics based upon the economy of the Roman Empire and the papacy.

The character and quality of medical practice during this period—almost totally dominated by the Church—left much to be desired, at least to the modern eye. Although physicians had become so much a part of the medieval monastic environment that many monasteries had entire divisions for the *medici* (those members of both higher and lower orders whose major occupation was medicine), much of their labor was devoted to such unscientific techniques as prayer, the laying on of hands, exorcisings, use of amulets with sacred engravings, holy oil, relics of the saints, and other elements of supernaturalism and superstition.

Reliance upon the quasi-magical was not restricted to medicine in the Middle Ages, but it must be granted that the supernatural was called upon to do more in that field than was common for other human endeavors—even in the "Age of Faith." The origins of this situation lay only partly in the Healing Mission of Christ. Much of the appeal of Jesus derived from his miracles, the vast majority of which were of a healing nature. Also, as the expected Day of Judgment failed to arrive and problems on earth seemed magnified by plague, war, and economic and political anarchy, people in general felt powerless to help themselves. At first, God was beseeched directly for assistance. The early Church, especially before it became an established church, had little formal organization; and though, of course, there were always leaders, no priestly caste with extraordinary functions appears to have existed. However, even after the Crucifixion, miracles continued to be a mainstay of the Church's development and growth. Although the Grace of God remained the mediator of these miracles, particular holy individuals began to be thought of as intercessors for these actions, and as had been true in the development of the concept of Christ's divinity, the newer miracles began to be regarded as evidence of the sanctity of the people through whom they were performed. Thus, the substantiation of sainthood progressively required the performance of miracles, which then led to the expectation of further miraculous intervention, even after the death of the individual saint.

The Christian priest's assumption of many of the roles of the imperial Roman priest after the Church became an established religion accelerated the development of his function of intercessor with God. (The adjective "pontifical" was derived from *pontifex maximus*, chief priest of pagan Rome.) The process of increasing the

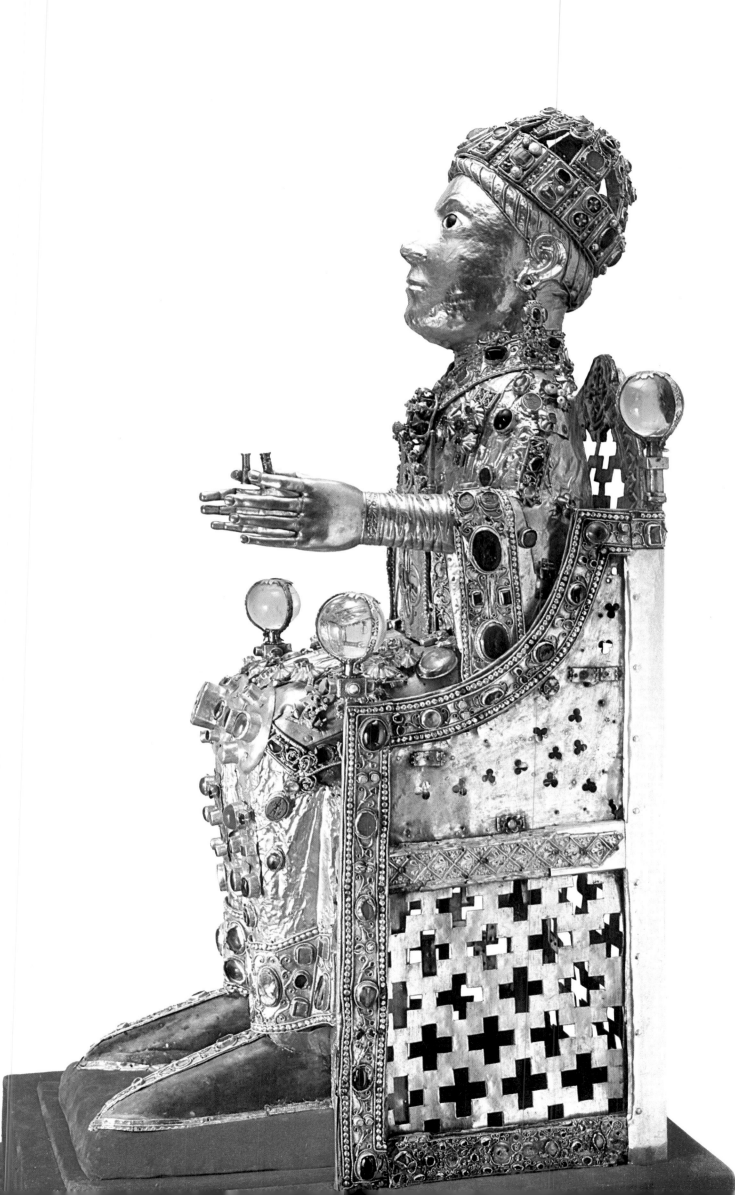

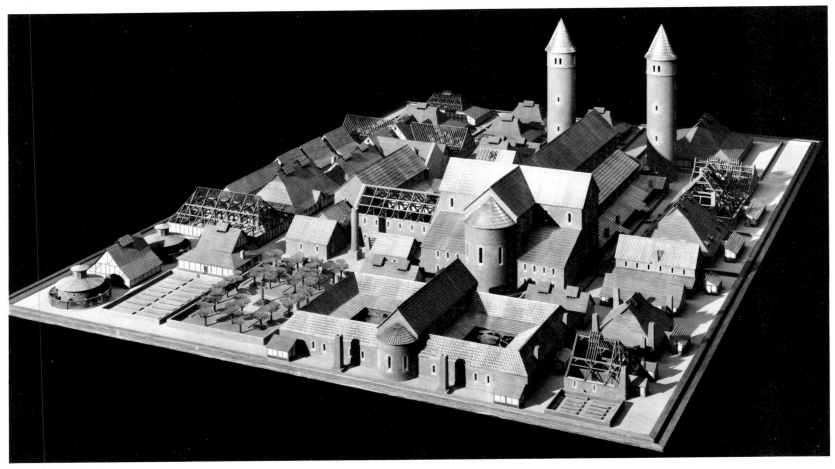

426

426 *Model by Walter Horn and Ernest Born of the*
St. Gall plan (before 830) for an ideal monastery.
Never actually carried out, the plan illustrated in its
extensive medical facilities the importance attached
to the monasteries' role in caring for the sick.

427 *Thirteenth-century manuscript illustration show-*
ing reception and treatment of the impoverished sick
in a monastery infirmary, where housing, food, and
prayer were freely available. Ms. lat. 8846, fol. 106,
Bibliothèque Nationale, Paris

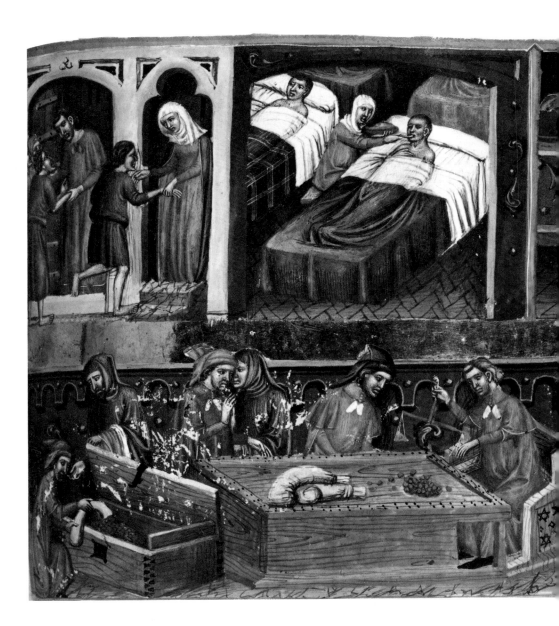

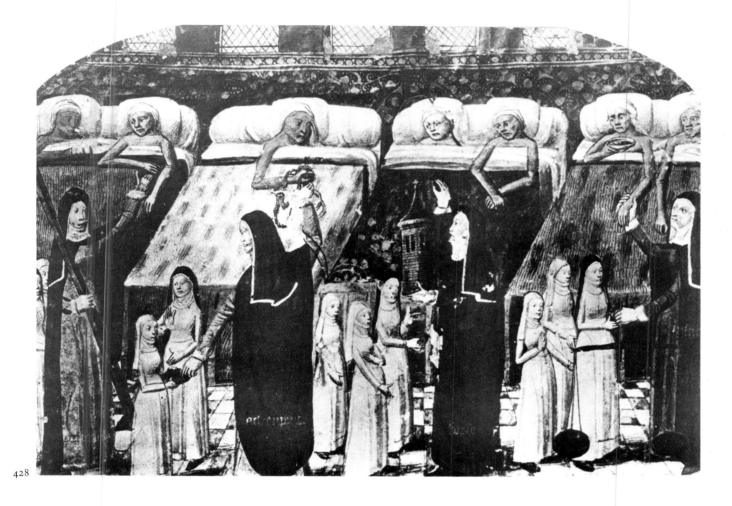

428

428 *Medieval book illustration showing monks and nuns caring for patients (two to a bed) in a monastery hospital. World Health Organization, Geneva*

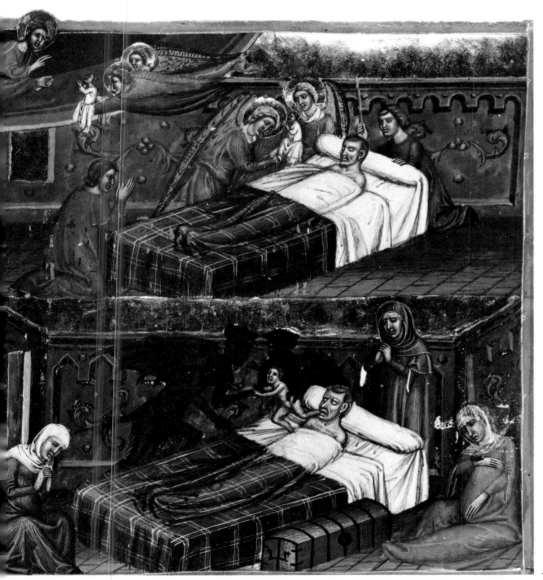

427

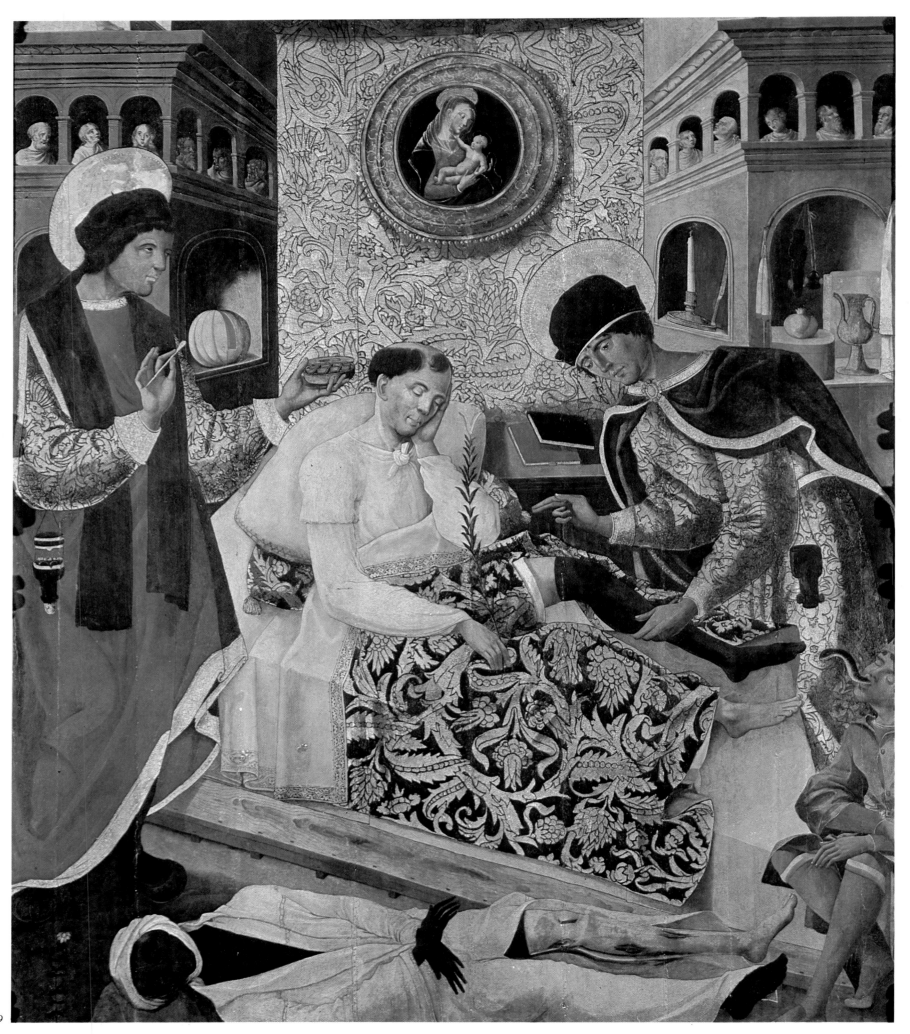

distance between the ordinary individual and God accelerated in both East and West. In the Eastern Church during the most sacred portion of the Mass, a screen was (and still is) placed between the congregation and the celebrants.

As the medieval Church relied more heavily on the intercession of saints, the saints themselves gained increased significance and consideration in Church writings, liturgy, and iconography. Although the evangelist St. Luke was himself a physician, the first saints whose intercession was sought almost exclusively for relief from disease were the twins Cosmas and Damian. Born in Cilicia in the third century, they were physicians who in the hope of gaining converts to Christianity provided their services without fee. They suffered a grotesque martyrdom in the year 278 during the reign of Diocletian but soon gained a following, at first in the East and later in the West, for numerous miraculous cures both in life and after death. Furthermore, under the patronage of Emperor Justinian (483–565), the church of their name in Constantinople, modeled on the temples of Asclepios, was open day and night for the cure of the sick by *incubatio*. Their most famous miracle occurred at a church named after them in a formerly pagan temple at the edge of the Forum in Rome, where they appeared posthumously to replace the gangrenous leg of the church's sacristan with the leg of a Negro who had died of old age. Their popularity in the West expanded quickly, and they soon gained importance iconographically not only for physicians and surgeons but also for closely related apothecaries and barbers.

Another Eastern saint to gain popularity in both East and West as a patron of medicine was Pantaleon of Nicomedia (d. c. 305). Like Saints Luke, Cosmas, and Damian, Pantaleon practiced medicine among the sick poor without accepting fees. In doing this, and because he was a Christian, he gained the enmity of his pagan colleagues and was put to death. His cult was early established in the East and later spread to Rome and Western Europe. (Ironically, Pantaleon was later associated in Venetian commedia dell'arte with the image of the comic, which slowly supplanted, at least in the West, the concept of the healing saint, and his name even provided the term "pantaloon" for men's trousers.)

The utilization of saints as intercessors with the divine developed during the period 500–1000 but became even more "specialized" thereafter. The growing belief in the intercessory powers of the Virgin (so-called Mariolatry), especially encouraged by the French troubadors' cult of chivalry, also supported belief in the efficacy of saints. As we shall see, medicine and the devotion to various saints were to become more intertwined when miraculous cures were to be sought not only of Christian physician martyrs but also of individual saints associated with specific diseases or even parts of the body.

The growing significance of superstition and magic in medieval Europe is often attributed to the anarchy following the fall of the Western Empire, but such a view is overly simplistic, especially as this antirationalism was strongest in the later Middle Ages, after the year 1300. Moreover, similar superstitious developments can be found in Constantinople and the East. Alexander of Tralles (525–605) was a skilled physician and independent scientist with excellent powers of observation. He bound himself to neither Hippocrates nor Galen (nor to any of the schools in between) and traveled extensively in Spain, Gaul, Italy, and Greece before settling down in Rome. Though he made many independent observations and startlingly accurate deductions about many diseases—such as the origin of epilepsy in the brain (an association reported by Hippocrates in the fifth century B.C.), the use of finger pressure in edema (fluid under the skin) and ascites (fluid in the abdomen), and the detection of an enlarged spleen by palpation—he was also capable of advising rather obviously magical cures. For intermittent fever, he advised carrying an olive upon which were written the mystical but meaningless syllables "ka, ra, a." Many another physician trained in the Byzantine Empire was able to combine the concepts of a rationally derived Hellenistic medicine with chants and potions, dung-filled amulets, and chants.

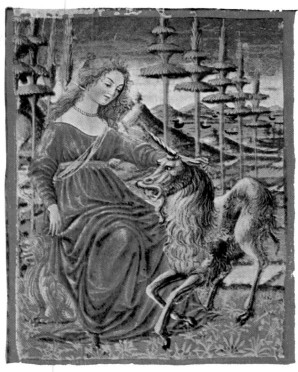

430

429 *Sts. Cosmas and Damian, the martyred twin physicians, shown in this 16th-century painting attributed to Fernando del Rincòn performing their most famous posthumous miracle: the replacement of a sacristan's gangrenous leg with that of a dead Negro. The Prado, Madrid*

430 *Detail of an "allegory of chastity" from St. Albertus Magnus, Commentary on Aristotle's "De Animalibus" (1463), showing a unicorn, the mythological creature whose powdered horn was prescribed for epilepsy, impotence, barrenness, plague, smallpox, worms, and many other ills. Museo Aurelio Castelli, Siena*

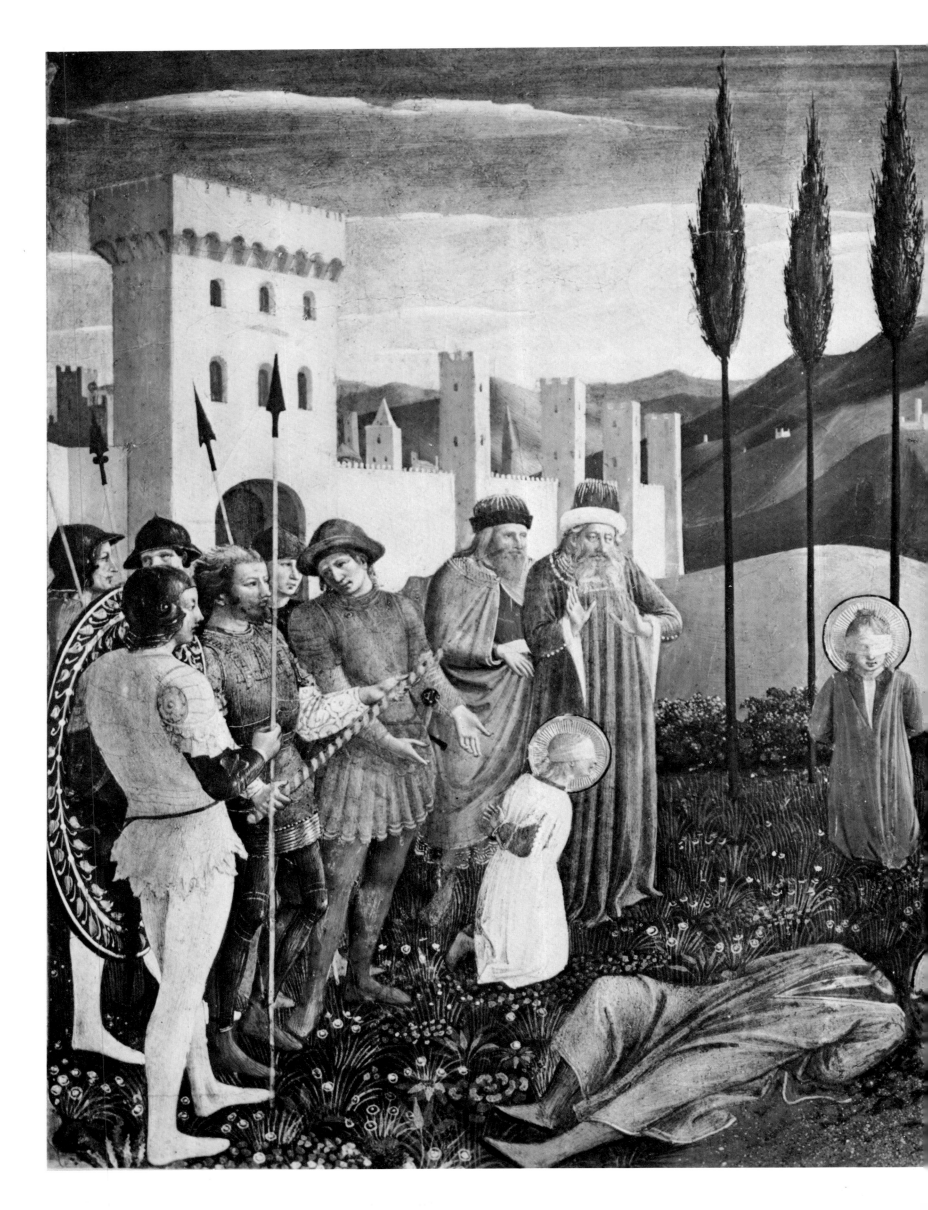

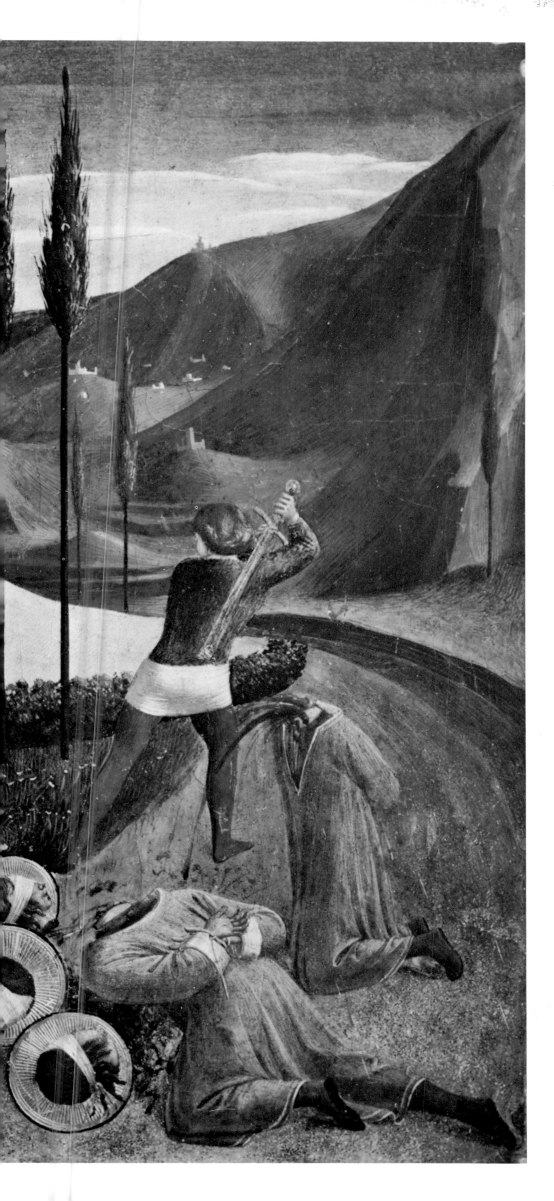

431 *The martyrdom of the sainted physicians Cosmas and Damian, as envisioned by Fra Angelico in a painting from the predella of the San Marco altarpiece (c. 1438–40). The Louvre, Paris*

Medicine under Islam

Arabic Medicine

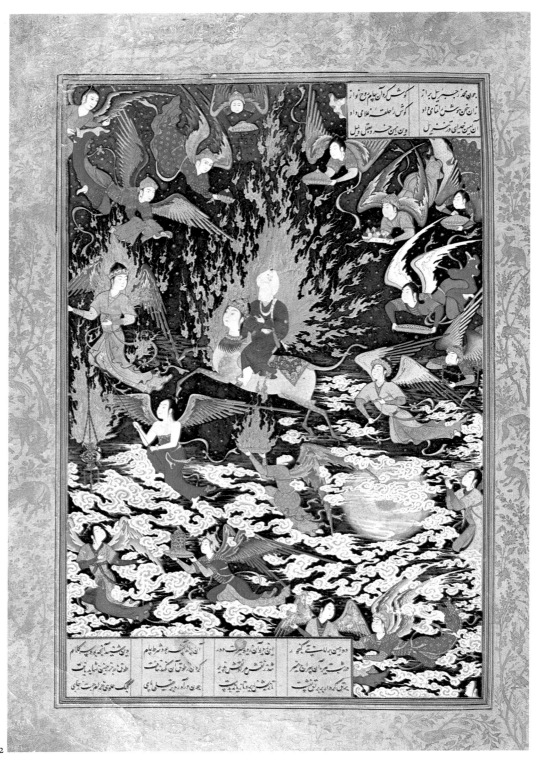

During the first five centuries of the Christian era, barbarian invasions of the West, recurrent disasters and pestilences, and the zealous anti-Hellenism of the Christian Church led to the physical loss of much of the Greek and Roman writings that were the basis of Western civilization. However, in the seventh century the new evangelical religion of Islam was moved to preserve the classical learning still extant and later to yield it back to the European world.

Based on the role of Islam, many have characterized Arabic contributions to medicine as principally preservation and compilation. As one historian commented, "Certainly they contributed no original or novel ideas to develop Hippocratic thought, but in a period of unrest they were preservers of tradition; they disseminated lay medical culture, they gave medical studies an honored place in their civilization, and they were intermediaries from whom the Western world retrieved a precious heritage." But this sweeping statement fails to recognize the lasting, original contributions of the Islamic thinkers and the Christians, Persians, Jews, and others who resided in Muslim countries. Together they are sometimes called "Arabists," for their writings were mostly in Arabic.

It was their respect for learning that caused the Arab conquerors to become the fountainhead of Greco-Roman knowledge during those many centuries that Latin Europe had little contact with ancient writings. Through translations, studies, and elaborations of Greek and Roman works, the world of Islam assembled an enormous body of information in virtually all fields of endeavor, especially philosophy, mathematics, and science—on which the intellectual development of the West depended.

The Arabic world had had previous contact with Greek culture, including medical theory, well before Muhammad's founding of Islam. In the year 489, Nestorian Christians (supporters of the Patriarch Nestorius who had been expelled from Constantinople for heresy in 431) were in turn driven away from Edessa in Mesopotamia (where St. Ephraem had established a hospital) and subsequently founded another hospital at Gundishapur in Persia. There they had also found Greek physicians whose forebears had been in the East since the time of Alexander's empire in the fourth century B.C. Greek philosophers had also gone to Gundishapur when Justinian closed the Academy in Athens in the fifth century A.D. Even earlier, when Jerusalem was destroyed by the Romans in A.D. 76, Jews had fled to Arabia bringing with them much Greco-Roman knowledge. Thus by the time of Muhammad (570–632), Greek ideas were not unknown among the Arabs.

THE SPREAD OF ISLAM

Over the next hundred years, Islam swept through the Near and Middle East into Africa, Spain, and part of France. The extent of this dispersion led to the emergence of three principal dynastic caliphates: in Persian Baghdad, the Abbasids (750–1258); in the Spanish West, particularly at Cordova, the Umayyads (756–1031); in Egyptian Cairo, the Fatimids (909–1171).

The earliest dominant center of Islam was Baghdad, where two of the most famous Muslim leaders reigned, al-Mansur (712?–75) and Harun al-Rashid (764?–809), caliph of the *Arabian Nights*. With encouragement and support from the caliphs, cultural richness rivaled the magnificent buildings and general opulence. Greek and Roman writings were rendered into Arabic from earlier translations into the Syriac of the Nestorians and the Hebrew of the Jews; in later centuries these works were translated again, this time into Latin by compilers in the West. In medicine and science the works of Aristotle, Hippocrates, and Galen were the most frequently translated. Some treatises, including several by Galen, had been completely lost in the original Greek and came down to subsequent generations only in Arabic. Among the early well-known translators were Hunain ibn-Is-haq (d. 767?) and al-Kindi (796–c.874). Philosopher-commentators of influence were al-Farabi (870?–950) and al-Biruni (973–1048). Rhazes (850–932) and Avicenna (980–1037) became the most famous of the Persian Muslim writers.

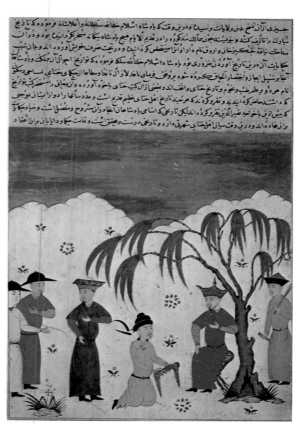

433

432 *The Ascension of Muhammad, 7th-century founder of Islam, as seen in a 16th-century Persian manuscript. British Library, London*

433 *Ghazan Khan, Mongol ruler of Iran, accepting books from Chinese sages, symbolic of cultural exchanges among countries which led to the spread of medical knowledge. From Rashid al-Din's* Universal History *(c. 1425), British Museum, London*

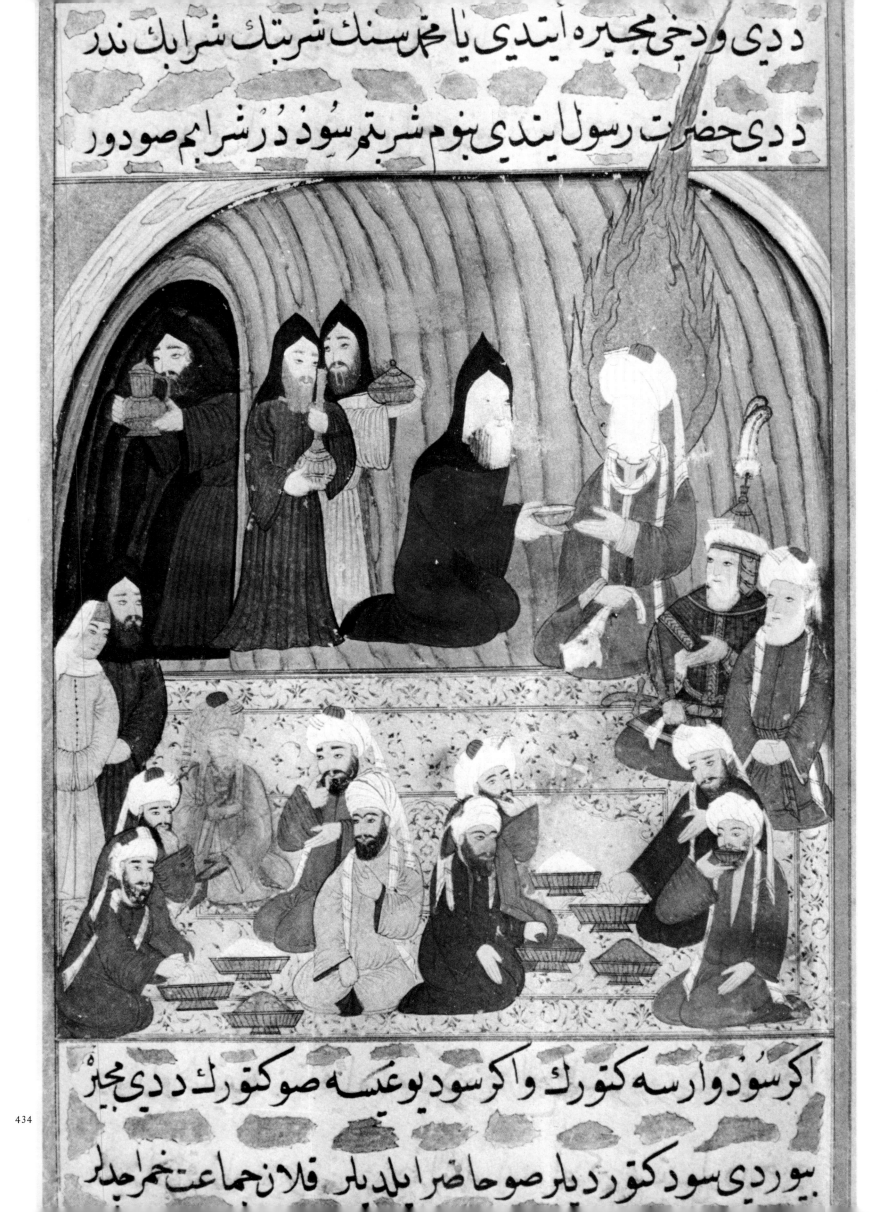

دديى ودخى مجيره أيندى يا محمد سنك شربتك شرابك ندر

دديى حضرت رسول ايندى بنوم شربتم سود درشرابم صودور

اكرسود وارسه كتورك واكرسود يوعسه صوكتورك دديى مجير

بيوردى سود كتوردى لرصو حاضر ايلديلر فلان جماعت خمر جددر

434

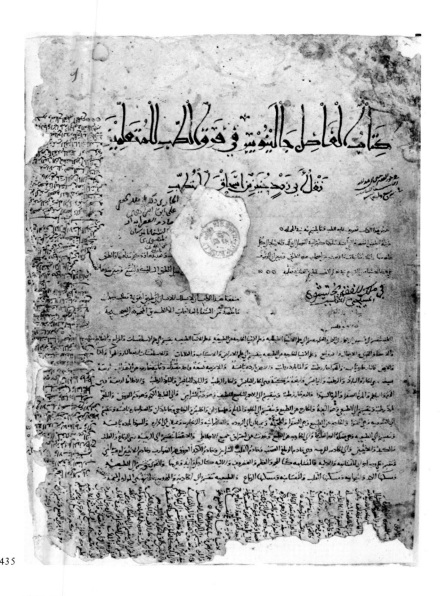

435

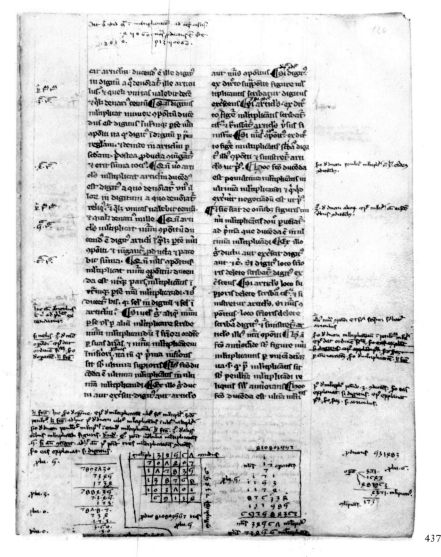

437

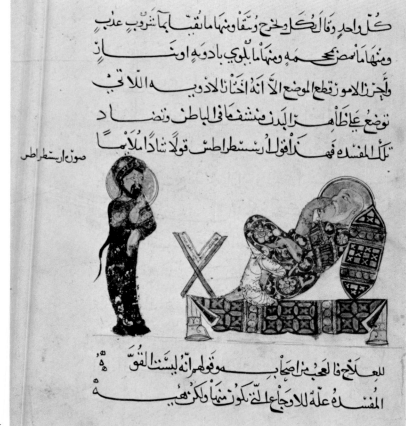

436

434 *Muhammad (veiled and nimbused in flame) in discourse with Christian monks, illustrating his precept to seek knowledge everywhere. From* Siyar e Nabi *by Mustafa Tarik (c. 1594–95), Topkapi Sarayi Museum, Istanbul*

435 *Leaf from 11th-century Arabic translation of Galen bearing Avicenna's autograph. Galen was a favorite authority of Arabic medical writers. Ms. arabe 2859, fol. 1, Bibliothèque Nationale, Paris*

436 *Greek physician Erasistratos, shown with an assistant, had been an important teacher in 4th-century B.C. Alexandria. Arabic physicians looked back to Greek authorities as a basis for their own medicine. Arabic Ms., Baghdad school (1224), Freer Gallery of Art, Washington, D.C.*

437 *Manuscript page showing computations in Arabic numerals, probably derived from India, a great improvement over cumbersome Roman numerals and a major contribution to mathematics and science. Garret Ms. 99, fol. 120, Princeton University Library*

Nave of Abd-er-Raman I, Mosque of Cordova, begun in A.D. 785. Along with Baghdad and Cairo, Cordova was one of the principal centers of Islam, and its intellectual ferment nurtured the talents of the outstanding physician-philosophers Averroës, Avenzoar, and Maimonides.

Cordova in the West became more prominent in Islam as the caliphate in Baghdad lost influence. The same intellectual ferment that had been shown in the East was also a characteristic of the western caliphate, where Averroës (1126–98), Avenzoar (1091?–1162), and Maimonides (1135–1204) were outstanding physician-philosophers.

In the sultanate of Egypt, where science was an important concern, the hospital in Cairo was a jewel in the crown of Muslim medical care; it was probably far better developed, more efficient, and more progressive than any similar institution elsewhere in the Christian or Muslim worlds. The cultured ruler Saladin (1138–93) held court in Cairo, impressing the West with his learning and the Crusaders with his military skill.

THE ARABISTS

The Arabists (which included Nestorian Christians, Persians, and Jews, who were not ethnic Arabs) did much more than merely hold safe the traditions of the past. They were also responsible for the establishment of pharmacy and chemistry as sciences. Many drugs heretofore unknown or little appreciated became part of the materia medica. Methods of extracting and preparing medicines were brought to a high art, and Arabist techniques of distillation, crystallization, solution, sublimation, reduction, and calcination were to become the essential processes of pharmacy and chemistry. Although physicians often continued to prepare their own medications, pharmacy as a separate profession became established under Arabic rulers. The important role of the Arabists in developing modern chemistry is memorialized in the significant number of current chemical terms derived from Arabic: alkali, alcohol, alembic, and elixir, among others, not to mention syrup and julep.

There was a strong emphasis on clinical instruction, and some Arabic physicians contributed brilliant observations that have stood the test of time. They described diseases that had hardly been perceived as such by the Greeks, among them scabies (itch-mite skin disease) and abscess of the mediastinum (a central area of the chest). They understood tuberculosis and pericarditis (inflammation of the membrane surrounding the heart) better than their predecessors. Avicenna even suggested the communicable nature of tuberculosis.

The development of efficient hospitals was an outstanding Arabic contribution to medicine. The Roman military *valetudinaria* and the occasional Christian hospital, such as the one founded by the benefactress Fabiola, were but crude prototypes compared to the number, organization, and excellence of the Arabic hospitals after the time of Muhammad. The medical center at Gundishapur in Sassanian Persia founded by Nestorian Christians in the fifth century A.D. may have been a model, but even that complex reached its zenith under Muslim rule.

DISEASE

In some respects the attitude of Islam toward the origin of disease was similar to the Judaeo-Christian idea in that Allah caused illness as punishment for a person's sins, or for reasons beyond man's ken, but sickness was usually borne without moral stigma. Although one might hope for curative miracles through prayer, one could also seek divine help through the agency of a physician. Giving aid and succor to the sick was good work—counting toward self-redemption, as in the Christian world—but Muslims also valued compassion for its own sake.

The Islamic religion held that there was an afterlife: the vital spark that remained in the human body after death was reawakened and rewarded appropriately in paradise. So as not to interfere with this, dissection of the human body was forbidden. Speculation on the nature of the internal organs and on blood flow led to perceptive reasonings. For example, al-Quff suspected a connection between the smaller arteries and veins through small pores, and ibn-Nafis

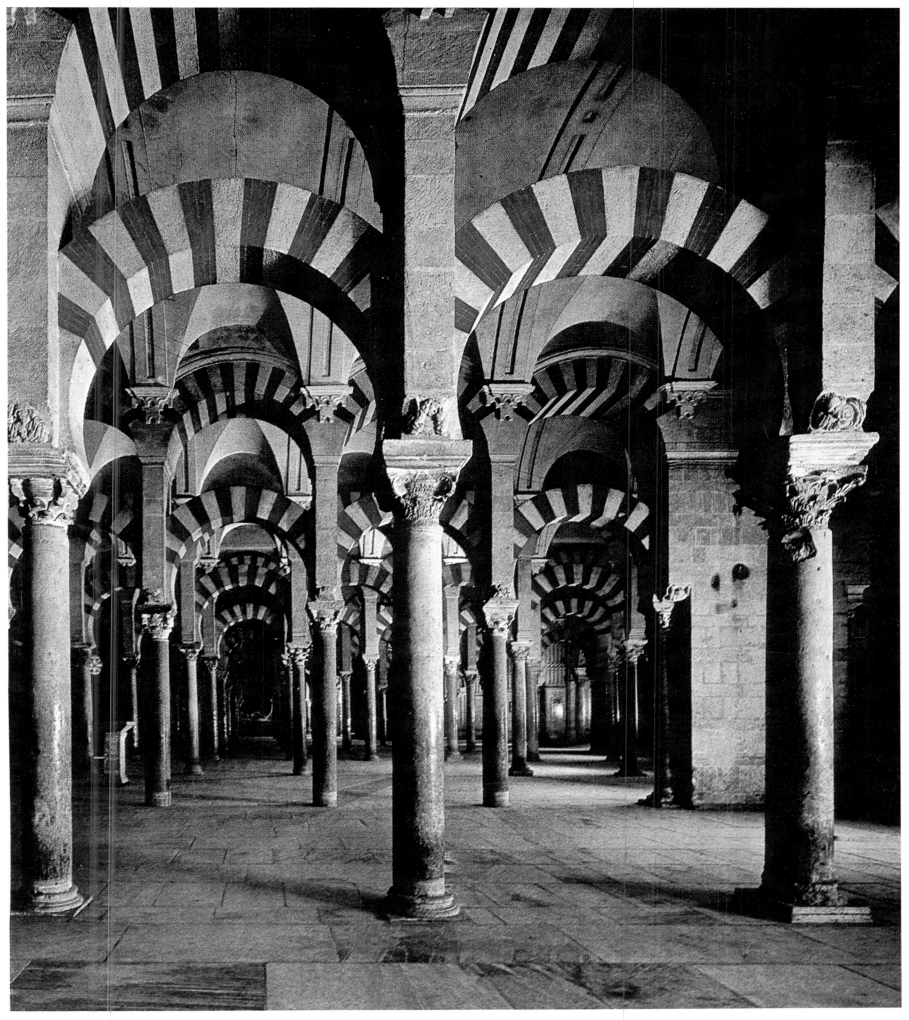

438

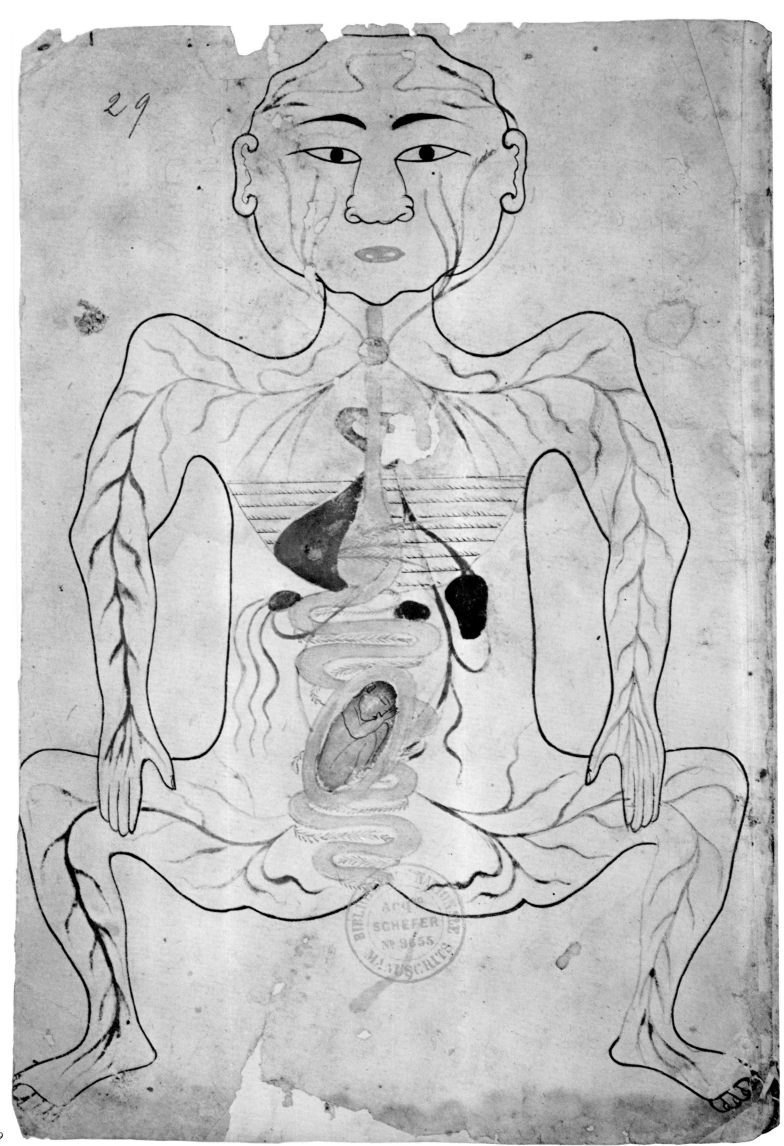

439

hypothesized such a connection in the lungs. But since there were no attempts to verify these theories through dissection, Arabic physicians relied on Galen for their anatomical knowledge.

METHODOLOGY AND TREATMENT

Arabist practitioners used essentially the same methods as the Greeks and Romans. Diagnosis was based on six criteria: the patient's behavior; the excreta; the other effluvia from the body; swellings; the character of pain; and the location of pain. The properties of the pulse were also carefully noted. Even astrology had a role, for the influence of the stars over health and disease was considered a part of natural science. Because of the emphasis placed on examining urine (uroscopy), the half-filled urine flask became a symbol of the physician. The urine's color, consistency, sediment, smell, and taste helped to determine what was wrong with a patient, to predict his prognosis, and to guide treatment.

Since surgery was held in low regard, much of the cutting, cauterizing, bandaging, bleeding, and cupping was done by untrained folk doctors, laymen, and charlatans. Nevertheless some outstanding physicians practiced surgery and wrote about it. Lithotomy (removal of stones from the urinary bladder) continued to be condemned as it had in Greco-Roman times, probably because of bad results.

The most common surgical technique of the Arabic physician was cauterization, which he used for both internal and external diseases. Anesthesia by means of a sponge saturated in a narcotic acid (or other soporific drug) held to the nose and mouth was widespread enough to have been imparted to Theodoric (454–526) in the Latin West. Galen's writings were interpreted to advocate formation of pus in wounds in order to induce healing, and salves were therefore commonly applied. This unfortunate doctrine of "laudable pus" influenced surgical thinking throughout all areas of Christendom as well as Islam.

The special characteristic of Arabist therapy was the wide employment of drugs of all kinds. The herbal *De Materia Medica* of Dioscorides (1st century A.D.) was studied closely. New medications, including mineral as well as vegetable and animal substances, were added to make up a voluminous Arabist materia medica. Ambergris, camphor, cloves, myrrh, and senna were introduced, and also preparations of syrups, juleps, elixirs, and many other concoctions of the apothecary. Some of these substances may have originated in China or India.

THE PRACTITIONERS

In the early years of Islam, medical practice was still carried on by Christian and Jewish physicians. There was little prejudice against non-Muslims, and Muhammad himself was treated by a nonbeliever. Muslim physicians came upon the scene when Alexandria, Gundishapur, and other cities became centers of Muslim intellectual life.

A physician acquired his training in a teaching center or unaffiliated hospital, and he received certification from his teachers. However, untrained and self-proclaimed healers practiced unmolested until the early tenth century when the caliph of Baghdad required all who wished to practice, except those of unchallenged reputation, to take an examination. The western caliphate later followed suit.

Although women occupied a secondary place in Muslim society, midwives were permitted to practice. The reluctance of Arabic physicians to violate social taboo and touch the genitals of female strangers ceded much of obstetrics and gynecologic practice to midwives. As in Greek and Roman times, however, the seriously ill were treated by physicians.

Academies, schools, and libraries as separate institutions or attached to mosques or to hospitals were found throughout the world of Islam. Medicine was usually only one of the disciplines taught. Philosophy and the sciences were combined.

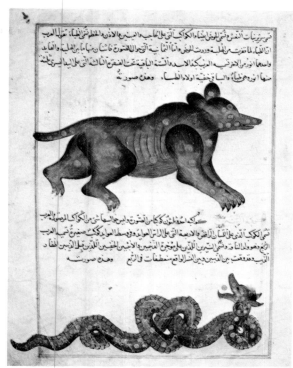

440

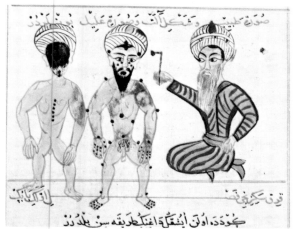

441

439 *Figure of a pregnant woman, from the* Treatise of Anatomy *done by Mansour ibn Ahmed for the Timorad prince Ziga el Hakk wa' I Soultaneh. Ms. pers. 1555, fol. 29, Bibliothèque Nationale, Paris*

440 *Constellations Ursa Major and Draco in astrology manuscript with information on using the stars for medical management of illness. From Ajaib al-Makblukat by al-Kazwini Irak (late 14th century), Freer Gallery of Art, Washington, D.C.*

441 *Miniature showing cauterization of leprosy lesions in 15th-century Turkish translation of* Imperial Surgery, *a 12th-century Persian manuscript. Ms. turc 693, fol. 46 v., Bibliothèque Nationale, Paris*

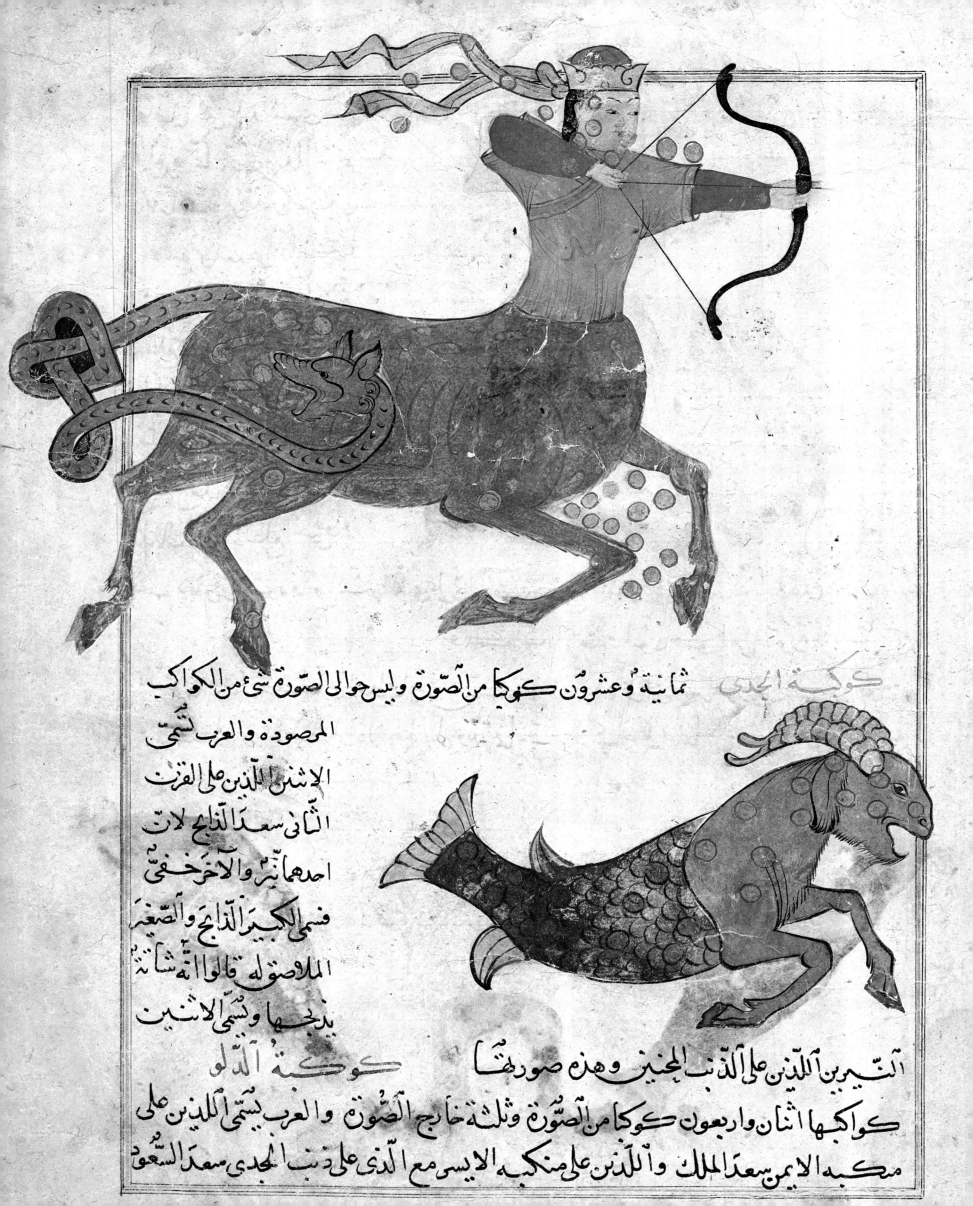

كوكبة الجدي

ثمانية وعشرون كوكبا من الصورة وليس حوالي الصورة شئ من الكواكب المرصودة والعرب تسمى الاثنين اللذين على القرن الثانى سعدا الذابح لات احدهما نير والآخر خفى فسمى الكبير الذابح والصغير الملاصق له قالوا وانه شاة يذبحها ويسمى الاثنين

النيرين اللذين على الذنب المحنيين وهن صورتها

كوكبة الدلو

كواكبها اثنان واربعون كوكبا من الصورة وثلثة خارج الصورة والعرب يسمى اللذين على منكبه الايمن سعد الملك واللذين على منكبه الايسر مع الذى على ذنب الجدى سعد السعود

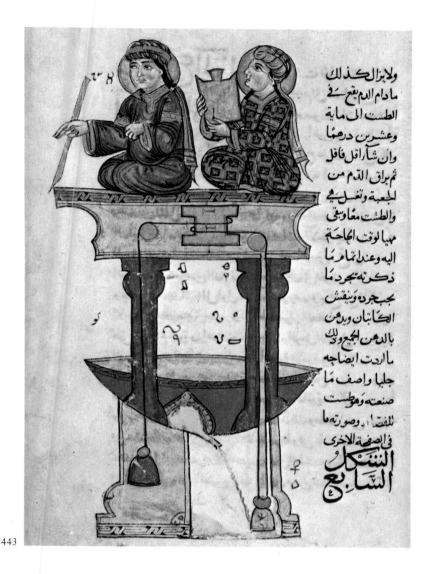

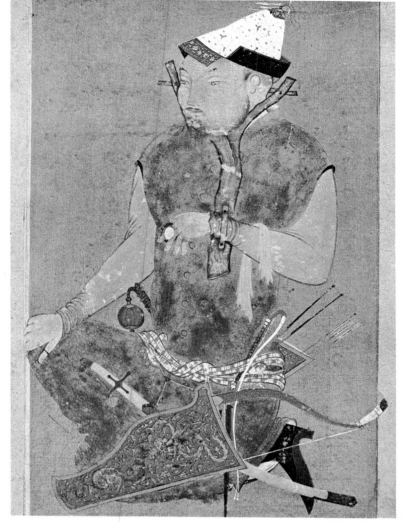

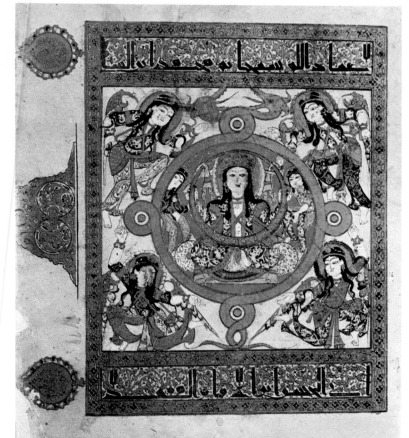

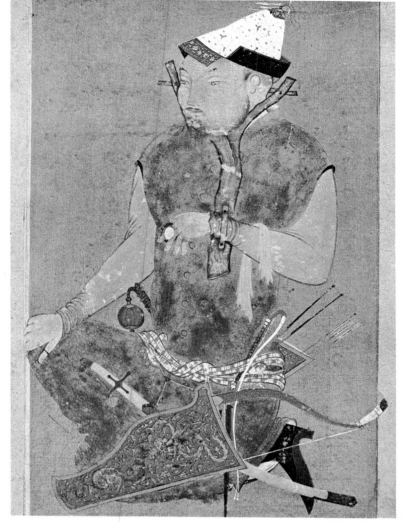

442 *Constellations Sagittarius and Capricorn in astrology manuscript concerned with use of stars in diagnosis and treatment of illness. From Ajaib al-Makblukat by al-Kazwini Irak (late 14th century), Freer Gallery of Art, Washington, D.C.*

443 *Two scribes atop imaginary device designed for collection and measurement during bloodletting, a popular Arabic medical practice. From the Automata of Al-Jazari, copied by Farruk ibn al-Latif (1315), Freer Gallery of Art, Washington, D.C.*

444 *Frontispiece of Book of Antidotes or Theriac (Kitab al-Diryaq) (c. 1200), an early example of the beginnings of Muslim painting in the ornamenting of scientific works. Ms. arabe 2964, fol. 37, Bibliothèque Nationale, Paris*

445 *Fifteenth-century military officer shown with wounded arm in wooden "sling." Collection Marquis de Ganay, Paris*

443

445

442

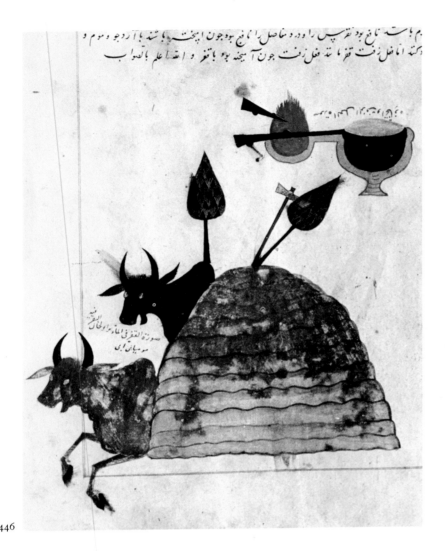

446

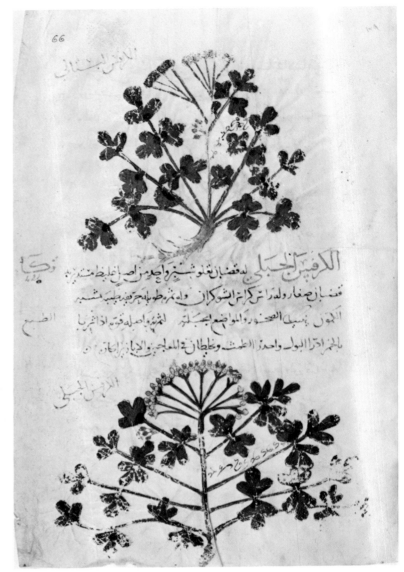

448

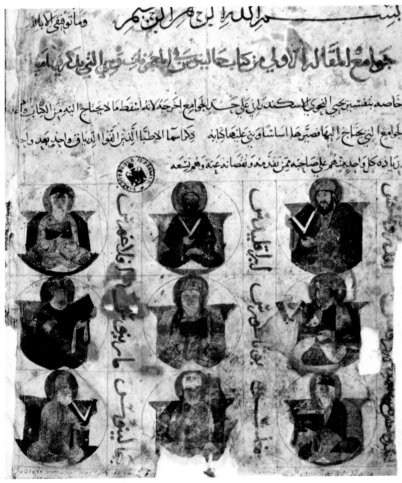

447

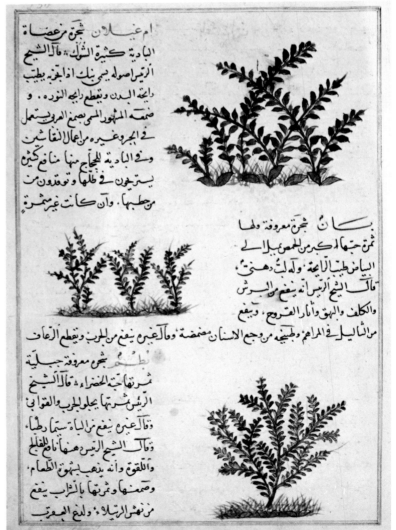

449

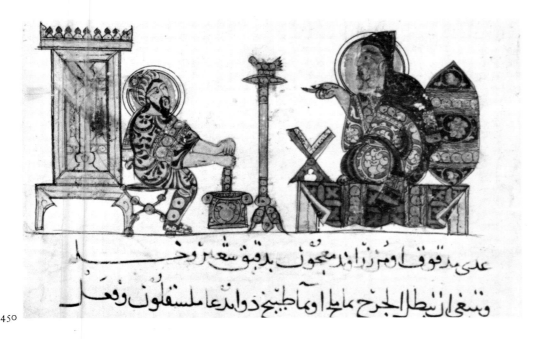

عدى مدقوق أومزرزا أند مجون بدقو شعبرزخ طمل
وشغلى انبطل الجرح ماياأ أو مآطبنخ دواندعا ملسفلون وفعل

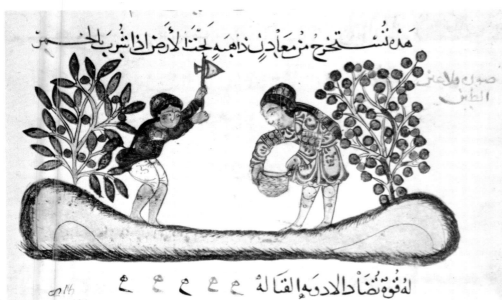

هذا نسخ تخرخ من معادن ذهبه بحتا لأرض اذا شرب بالخمر

صون ولاعن الطين

له قوة تضا دالادو به القاله

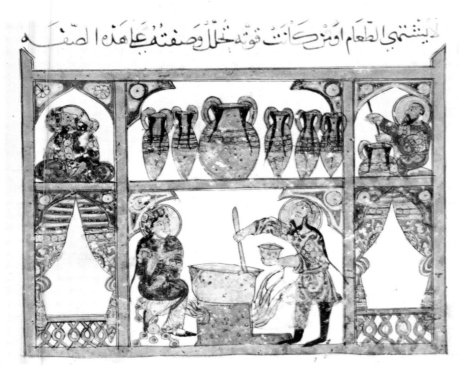

لينتهبي الطعام أومزركانت قوته دخل وصفته علي هذا الصفه

446 *Cows shown being fumigated by burning incense in a 15th-century Persian translation of Dioscorides. In Arabic medicine, animals were treated by the same methods as used on humans. Topkapi Sarayi Museum, Istanbul*

447 *Andromachus, inventor of the famous panacea theriac, shown with eight Greek physicians who expanded and embroidered the formula for this concoction, later used by Arabists and others for 17 centuries. From a 13th-century Dioscorides, Codex A.F. 10, Österreichische Nationalbibliothek, Vienna*

448 *Page of herbal by Dioscorides translated into Arabic at end of 10th century by Bahnam ibn-Mousa ibn-Yousouf, a Christian doctor. Ms. arabe 4947, fol. 66, Bibliothèque Nationale, Paris*

449 *Manuscript page showing Egyptian thora, ben, and turpentine trees, used in making many medicaments. From Ajaib al-Makblukat by al-Kazwini Irak (late 14th century), Freer Gallery of Art, Washington, D.C.*

450 *Arabic physician instructing assistant in method of making poultice set forth by Dioscorides in* De Materia Medica, *copied by Abdallah ibn al-Fadl Irak (1224), Freer Gallery of Art, Washington, D.C.*

451 *Two men shown digging Lemnian Clay, thought by the Greeks to have great curative powers for wounds and ulcers. From the Dioscorides copied by Abdallah ibn al-Fadl Irak (1224), Freer Gallery of Art, Washington, D.C.*

452 *Arabic pharmacist seen preparing medicine with a honey base, a technique learned from the Greeks, in this copy by Abdallah ibn al-Fadl Irak of the* De Materia Medica *by Dioscorides (1224). Bequest of Cora Timken Burnett, 1957, Metropolitan Museum of Art, New York*

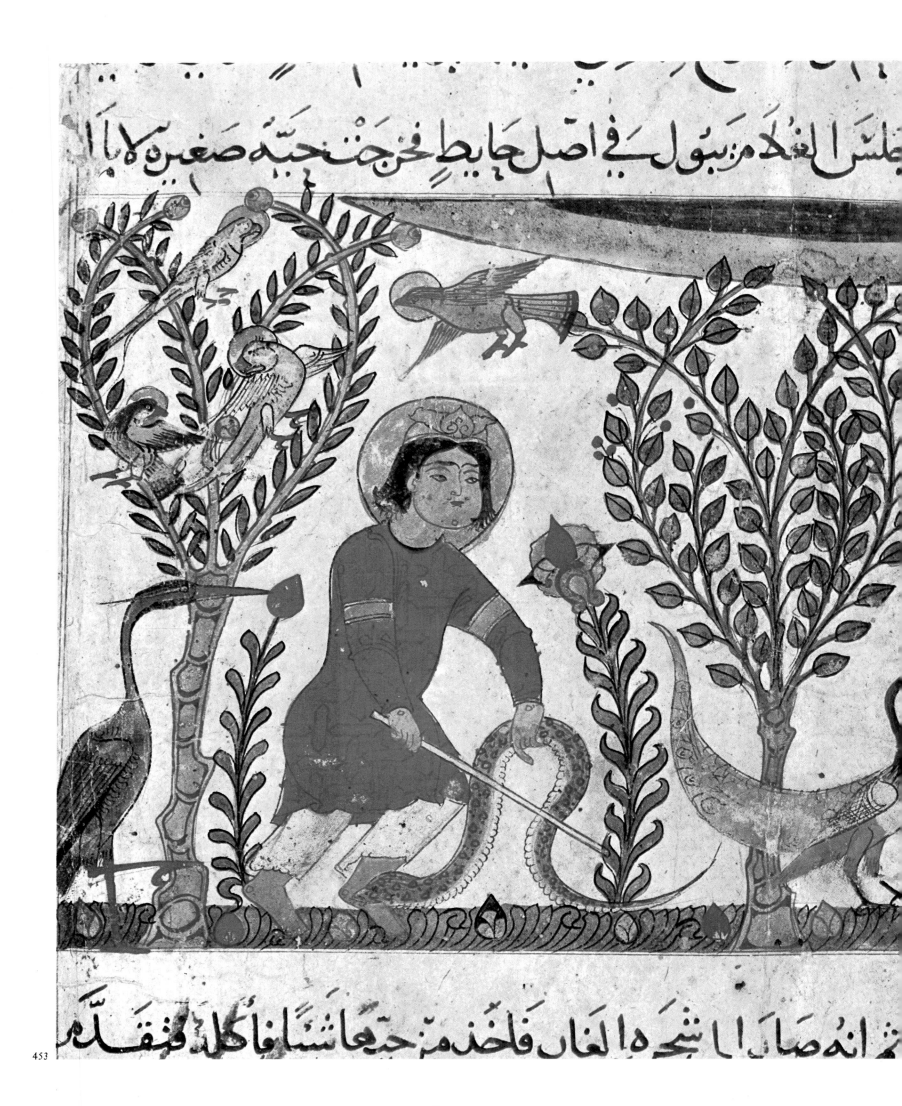

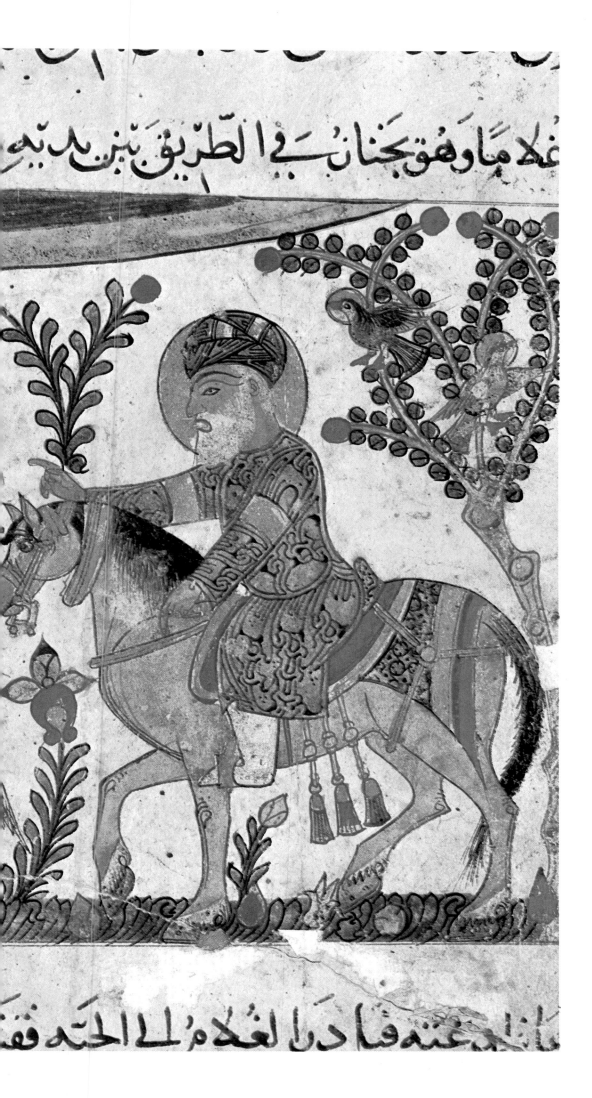

غلا ما وفوق بخنان بے الطريق نين بديه

عنه فما د را لغلا م لا الجنه فقه

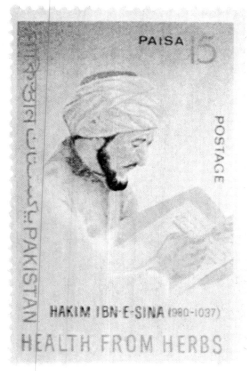

PAISA 15
POSTAGE

PAKISTAN

HAKIM IBN-E-SINA (980-1037)

HEALTH FROM HERBS

454

453 *Doctor shown arriving on horseback with plant antidote for snakebite, perhaps required by the man holding dead snake. Ms. Codex A.F. 10 (13th century), Österreichische Nationalbibliothek, Vienna*

454 *Avicenna (Hakim ibn-e-Sina) commemorated on Pakistani stamp. His Canon became one of the most influential medical works in both East and West!*

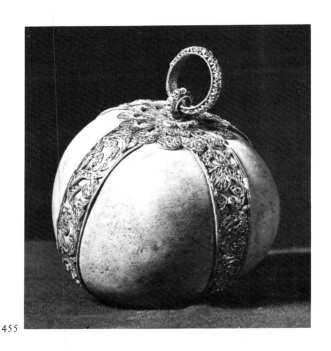

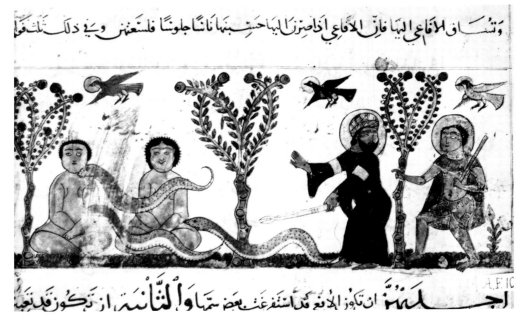

455 *Bezoar stone, a concretion found in stomachs of ruminants—especially goats—considered to have miraculous powers against poisons. Collection Archduke Ferdinand, Schloss Ambras, Kunsthistorisches Museum, Vienna*

456 *Manuscript illustration showing physician going to the aid of a man bitten by serpents. Ms. Codex A.F. 10 (13th century), Österreichische Nationalbibliothek, Vienna*

457 *Map of the Arab Empire,* A.D. *750*

458 *Arabic physician shown performing ancient type of cataract operation called couching, by displacing the opaque lens down from line of vision. World Health Organization, Geneva*

459 *Manuscript illustration from* The Makomad of Hairiri Neshki *showing a woman delivering in the ancient seated posture, while, above, the prospective father is also being cared for. Ms. arabe 5847, fol. 122 v., Bibliothèque Nationale, Paris*

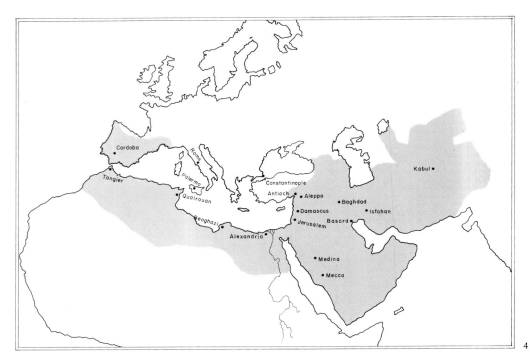

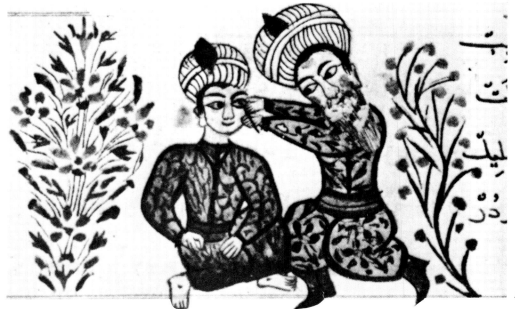

وَسَنَّى الإِمَامُ إِلَى عُمَانَ فَاكْتُنِي أَبُو زَيْدٍ بِالنَّحْلَةِ وَاهَبَ لِلرِّحْلَةِ فَلَمْ يَسْمَحِ الوَالِي

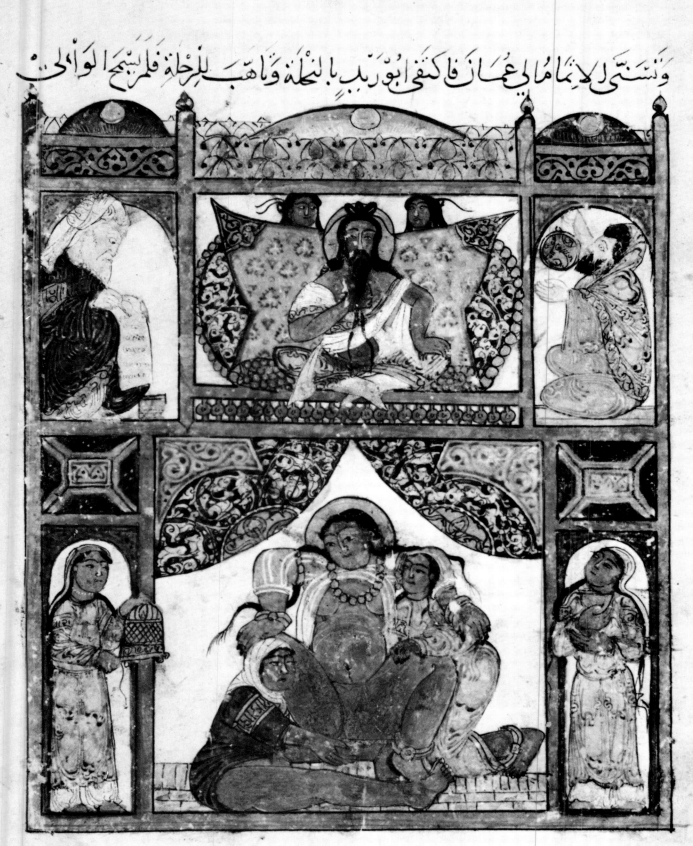

بَحَرَكَتِهِ بَعْدَ تَخْرِيبِهِ بَرَكَتِهِ بَلْ أُوعَدَ بِصَمِّهِ إِلَى خِزَانَتِهِ وَأَنْ يَطْلُقَ يَدَهُ فِي خِزَانَتِهِ

459

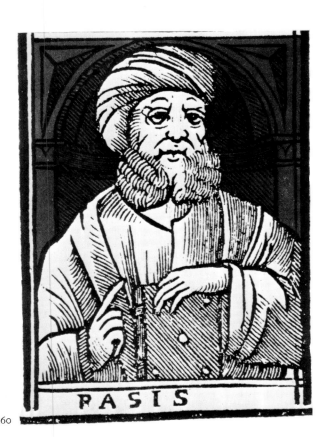

460

460 *Woodcut portrait of the Persian doctor Razi,
known as Rhazes in the West. Brilliant author of
more than 200 books and treatises on a variety of
subjects, he was also exceedingly generous in treating
the poor. New York Academy of Medicine*

461 *Physician taking patient's pulse in Persian
garden while assistants prepare medications. From
Canon of Avicenna (1632), Wellcome Institute for
the History of Medicine, London*

462 *Rwanda stamp showing cassia plant, the source
of senna, a widely used laxative drug. Arabic medicine employed exceptionally numerous and varied
medications, administered in virtually every possible
form.*

463 *Seventeenth-century Arabic anatomical drawing,
based on Avicenna's Canon of medicine and the more
ancient Galenic descriptions rather than on firsthand
dissection, which Muslims avoided. Ms. WMS Or.
155, courtesy of the Wellcome Trustees*

Gundishapur was a fusion of Arabic, Nestorian, Byzantine, Indian, and Jewish
medicine. There, in the eighth century A.D., the Bachtishua family, who were
Nestorian Christians, became prominent physicians. Other influential Nestorians
were translators and teachers, among them Ben Mesuë the Elder (also called Janus
Damascenus) and Johannitus (Hunain ibn-Is-haq).

FAMOUS HEALERS

Among the many outstanding physicians we can single out a few. In the eastern
caliphate were Rhazes, Avicenna, Haly Abbas, and Isaac Judaeus (850–950). In the
western, Spanish area of Islam were Abul Qasim (Albucasis in Latin), Avenzoar,
and Maimonides.

One of the most appealing healers from a modern vantage point was the
Persian Rāzi, called Rhazes in the West (abu-Bakr Muhammad ibn-Zakarīyā al-
Rāzi, 850–c. 923). He was outstanding in his generosity and always willing to treat
and help the poor. Students and practitioners thronged to his lectures, and
apparently he was also a brilliant bedside teacher. A man of his time, he revered
learning and based his knowledge on the books of authorities. But he was also an
independent thinker, not afraid to rely on his own observations when they
contradicted the past; he counseled others that "all that is written in books is worth
much less than the experience of a wise doctor."

Rhazes became blind in his last years (some say as the result of a brutal beating
ordered by a caliph angered by his candor). Despite the large fees and honors he
received, his generosity to the less fortunate left him poor at the time of his death.
Of his 237 books on many subjects—including alchemy, anatomy, physiology, and
ethics—much has been lost. A large part of his work was a compilation of the
theories of Hippocrates, Galen, and others. Through the clarity of his writing and his
influence over students and contemporary physicians he brought much of Greek
medicine to the Arabic world. His most celebrated work, *Al-Hawi (Liber Continens)*,
summarized the medical and surgical knowledge of his time.

Rhazes's fame rested on clear-cut clinical descriptions of illness, original
observations, and a pragmatic approach to treatment. However, he followed Galen's
humoral pathology, practiced bloodletting, saw a place for precious stones in
medication, and believed that the wrinkles of a pregnant woman could foretell the
number of her children. On the other hand, he gave the first accurate descriptions
of smallpox and measles, advised proper food in preference to drugs in treatment,
opposed employment of the abstruse mathematical formulas of al-Kindi in
therapy, and recommended simple rather than complex remedies.

The most widely influential Arabic contributor to medicine was Avicenna
(abu-Ali al-Husayn ibn-Sīna, 980–1037), whose standing in both Islam and
Christendom was equal to that of Galen. Born near Bokhara, Persia, he was a boy
prodigy and is said to have mastered the Koran by the age of ten. Aristotle's ideas
intrigued him, and he also studied the commentators, such as al-Farabi. The
Nestorians at Baghdad were Avicenna's principal teachers, and the entire gamut of
human knowledge was within his purview: grammar, poetry, geometry,
astronomy, anatomy, physiology, materia medica, surgery. When only twenty-one,
he wrote a scientific encyclopedia.

Although he may at times have practiced medicine, his principal contribution
was as a compiler and commentator. The most renowned of his approximately one
hundred books was *The Canon (Al-Qanun)*, upon which untold numbers of
translators, teachers, students, and practitioners based their medical ideas and
procedures for hundreds of years. In fact, until the mid-seventeenth century, the
medical curriculum of the Christian universities, including those in the British
Isles, was based on Avicenna's writings.

Haly Abbas (Ali ibn' ul-Abbas, d. 994), also from the eastern caliphate, in the
late tenth century wrote highly popular and perceptive commentaries on

310

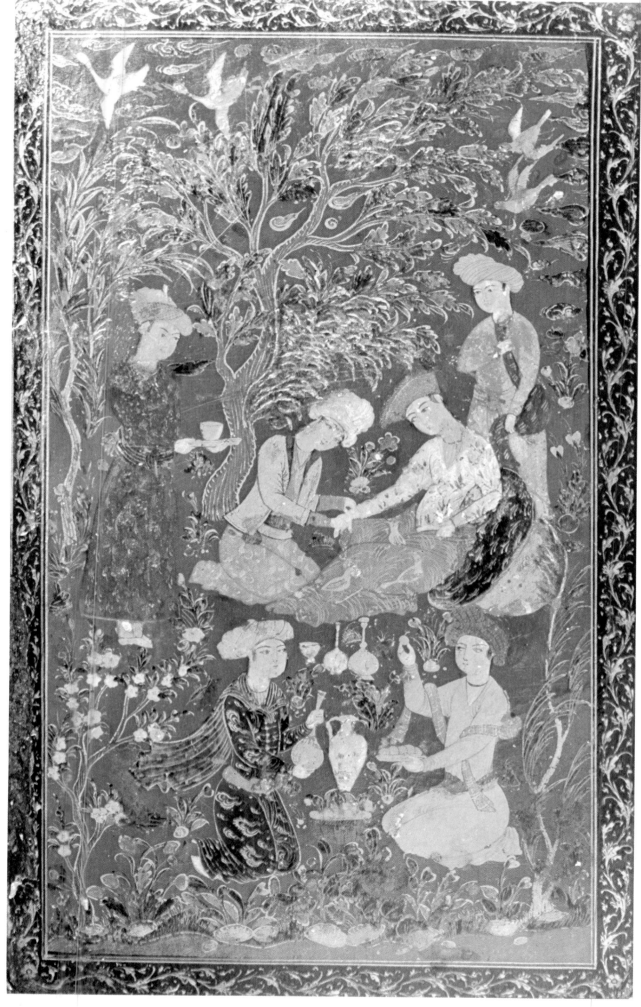

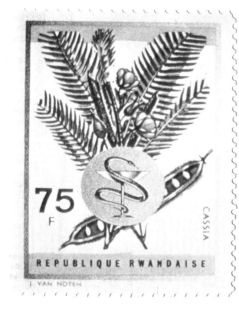

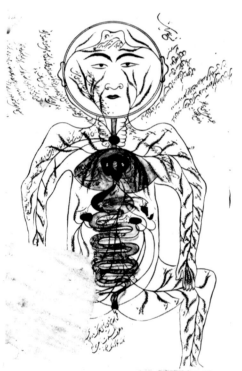

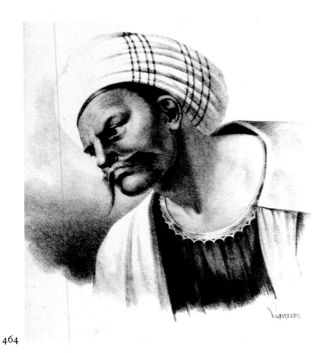

464

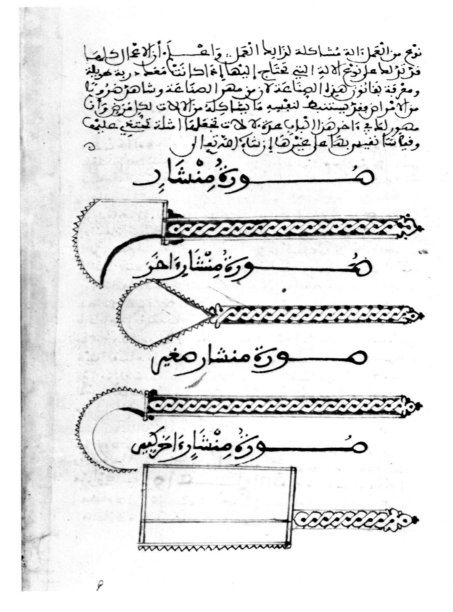

465

464 *Twelfth-century Moorish philosopher Averroës, learned in philosophy, medicine, and law, offended political and religious authorities and had to hide out among the Jews. Lithograph by Vigneron, courtesy of the Wellcome Trustees*

465 *Arabic surgical saws illustrated in 16th-century Moroccan copy of text by Albucasis, the leader of Arabic surgery. Ms. arabe 2953, fol. 79 v., Bibliothèque Nationale, Paris*

466 *Imagined meeting between the philosophers Averroës and Porphyry in the 14th-century herbal* De Herbis et Plantis *by Manfredus. Arabic philosophers and scientists placed emphasis on Aristotle's teachings. Ms. lat. 6823, fol. 2 v., Bibliothèque Nationale, Paris*

467, 468, 469 *Illustrations from a 15th-century Turkish translation of* Imperial Surgery, *a 12th-century Persian manuscript. Top, woman supposed to be operating on a hermaphrodite. Middle, treatment for a fracture. Bottom, castration being performed. Ms. turc 693, fols. 110 v., 197 r., 110 r., Bibliothèque Nationale, Paris*

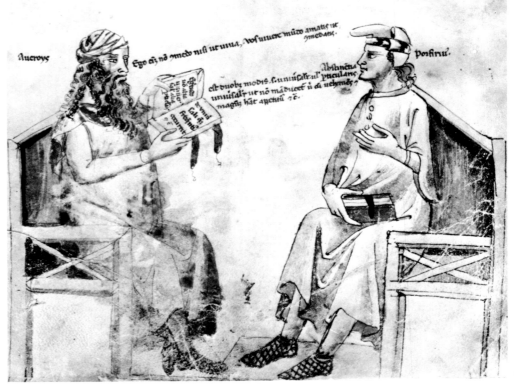

466

Hippocrates, Galen, Oribasius, Paul of Aegina, and Rhazes, which were standard Arabic texts before Avicenna's *Canon* came upon the scene. Early Christian translators introduced Haly Abbas's works to the West, especially his surgical writings.

The name of Isaac Judaeus (Abu Ya'qub Is-haq Sulayman al-Israili) is linked with Haly Abbas because the translator Constantinus Africanus erroneously attributed to Isaac Judaeus some texts that may have been written by Haly Abbas. Among the genuine contributions of Judaeus, a physician of high repute in Egypt, was a collection of aphorisms in Hebrew, some of which were probably inspired by Rhazes. Examples are worth repeating:

> Most illnesses are cured without the physician's help through the aid of Nature.
>
> If you can cure the patient by dietary means, do not turn to drugs.
>
> Do not rely on cure-alls, for they mostly rest on ignorance and superstition.
>
> Always make the patient feel he will be cured when you are not convinced of it, for it aids the healing effort of Nature.

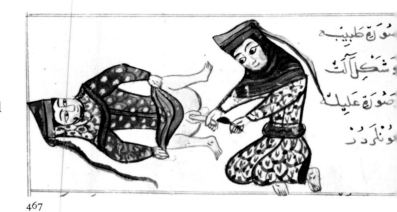

467

Albucasis (Abul Qasim al-Zahrawi, 936–1013), the major Muslim writer on surgery, greatly influenced the Christian West. His *al-Tasrif* contained a section on surgery which was the first illustrated, systematic text on this subject. Most of the content was a repetition with modifications of the earlier contributions of Paul of Aegina and others, but Albucasis's careful descriptions and pragmatic advice revealed a cautious, ethical, thoughtful approach. The Arabic reliance on the cautery, cupping, and bleeding was part of his practice too, but his embrace of surgery as a worthy art and his emphasis on anatomy (even though it was based on Galen) were in contradiction to the tendency of Arabic medicine to relegate both surgery and anatomy to an inferior position.

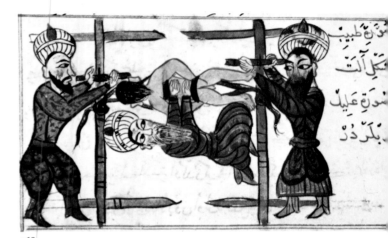

468

Avenzoar (abū-Marwān ibn-Zohr, 1091?–1162) was an Arabist physician born in Seville. The son of a Jewish physician, he rejected much of Aristotle and Avicenna, condemned astrology and mysticism in medicine, and disagreed strongly with some of Galen's teachings. His clinical acumen led to accurate descriptions of scabies and pericarditis, a disease from which he himself suffered. He wrote on the preparation of drugs, on the practical uses of diet, and on alchemy. His reports on tracheotomy (cutting into the windpipe) suggest that he may have practiced surgery. Avenzoar recommended reliance on one's own experience rather than traditional doctrines. Through translations of his works into Hebrew and Latin he exercised great influence over the medical and alchemical teachings of medieval Europe.

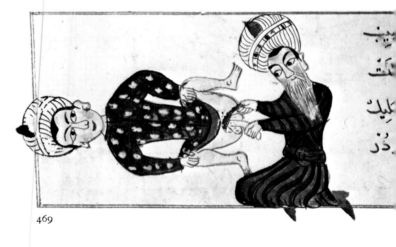

469

Averroës (abul-al-Walid Muḥammad ibn-Aḥmad ibn-Rushd, 1126–98), a pupil of Avenzoar, was primarily a philosopher, but he also studied law and medicine. He wrote a medical compendium based on Aristotelian theory, but he is best known for his criticism of established religion and authority. Both Avicenna and Averroës were admirers and followers of Aristotle. But while Avicenna reconciled Aristotelianism with accepted religious views, Averroës held that religion should not be a branch of knowledge and that there was no personal immortality but rather a merging of the soul with nature and the universe. This interpretation of Aristotle was condemned by both Islam and the Christian Church.

Averroës held high political positions in Cordova and Morocco for many years, but eventually his pantheistic, irreverent views forced him to drop out of sight. Aided by his pupil Maimonides, he went into hiding among the Jews. His philosophy was spread throughout Europe by Jewish intellectuals after their expulsion from Spain.

The most famous Jewish physician in Arabic medicine was Maimonides (Moses ben Maimon, 1135–1204). Born in Cordova, he fled in 1160 with other Jews to Fez in Morocco when the strictly orthodox Muslim dynasty of the Almohades began to harass nonbelievers. He later migrated to Palestine and then to Cairo, where

313

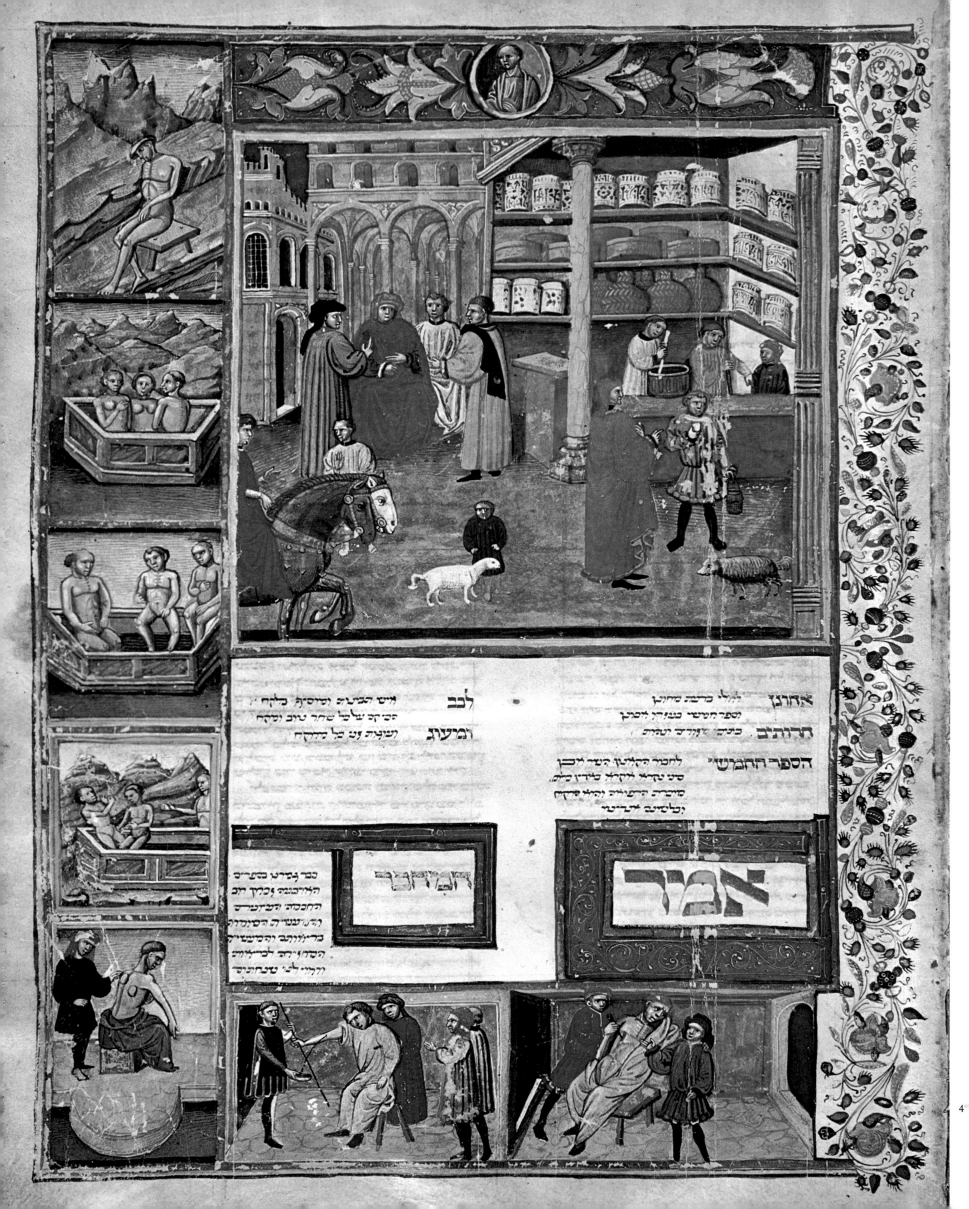

financial needs prompted him to enter medicine as a career. He rose rapidly, finally becoming physician to the sultan Saladin.

Maimonides's writings contained sage advice on diet, hygiene, first aid, poisons, and general medical problems, but his primary focus was on philosophy. He tried to reconcile scientific reasoning and religious faith, and he advanced the "heresies" of Averroës. Orthodox Jews of his time were sometimes hostile to his views, and wholehearted acceptance of Maimonides by Jewish intellectuals as a great medical and philosophical sage came only after his death.

Although he was a proponent of the ancient Galenic doctrine of the four humors and followed the general methods of Arabic medicine, Maimonides aimed at practical therapeutics. He translated the voluminous *Canon* of Avicenna into Hebrew, but his collection of the aphorisms of Hippocrates and Galen was written in Arabic, as was his popular *Book of Precepts*, which was composed as a collection of letters to Saladin. Translations of the writings of Maimonides into Hebrew and Latin were widely read throughout Christian Europe. Although the Morning Prayer of the Physician is attributed to him by some, he was probably not the author. However, the principles expressed in this prayer were in keeping with his philosophy and behavior. A section of one of the many versions is often quoted:

> O God, let my mind be ever clear and enlightened. By the bedside of the patient let no alien thought deflect it. Let everything that experience and scholarship have taught it be present in it and hinder it not in its tranquil work. For great and noble are those scientific judgments that serve the purpose of preserving the health and lives of Thy creatures.
>
> Keep far from me the delusion that I can accomplish all things. Give me the strength, the will, and the opportunity to amplify my knowledge more and more. Today I can disclose things in my knowledge which yesterday I would not yet have dreamt of, for the Art is great, but the human mind presses on untiringly.
>
> In the patient let me ever see only the man. Thou, All-Bountiful One, hast chosen me to watch over the life and death of Thy creatures. I prepare myself now for my calling. Stand Thou by me in this great task, so that it may prosper. For without Thine aid man prospers not even in the smallest things.

PUBLIC HEALTH AND HOSPITALS

In medieval times, the general health of the populace and its hygienic conditions probably were essentially the same in Latin Europe and in the Muslim world. Medical treatises of the era reveal a concern with the same diseases, acute and chronic. A special interest in eye treatments suggests that ocular afflictions were common. The excellent Arabic descriptions of epidemics marked by skin eruptions may indicate that such pestilences were as prevalent in the world of Islam as in Christian lands. Orthodox Muslims apparently accepted epidemics as inherent in the lot of man.

The streets and homes doubtless were as filthy in Islam as in Christendom. In some cities sewers probably existed, but they often emptied into the local streams from which people got their drinking water. The rich frequently chose to live upstream from the city; in Cairo, for example, relatively unpolluted water was available above the point where the Nile entered the city and became sullied with sewage and garbage.

Medical care by reputable physicians was mainly limited to the rich and noble. The repeated praises of kindly Rhazes who treated the sick poor free of charge makes one suspect that such generosity was not a common practice. Hosts of lay healers, mountebanks, and magicians plied their trades. But even when

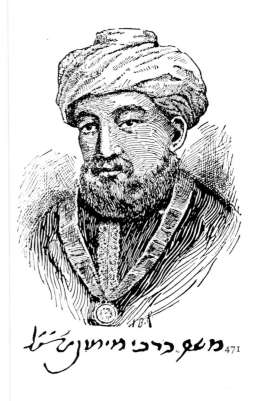

470 *Manuscript page of 15th-century copy of* Canon of Avicenna *in Hebrew, indicative of role Jews played as translators in preservation and spread of medical knowledge between East and West. Codex 2197, fol. 492a-38b, Biblioteca Universitaria, Bologna*

471 *Engraved portrait of Maimonides, as he was thought to look, with his autograph in facsimile. A Jewish philosopher and physician, his writings and practices achieved renown in Muslim Spain and Egypt. New York Academy of Medicine*

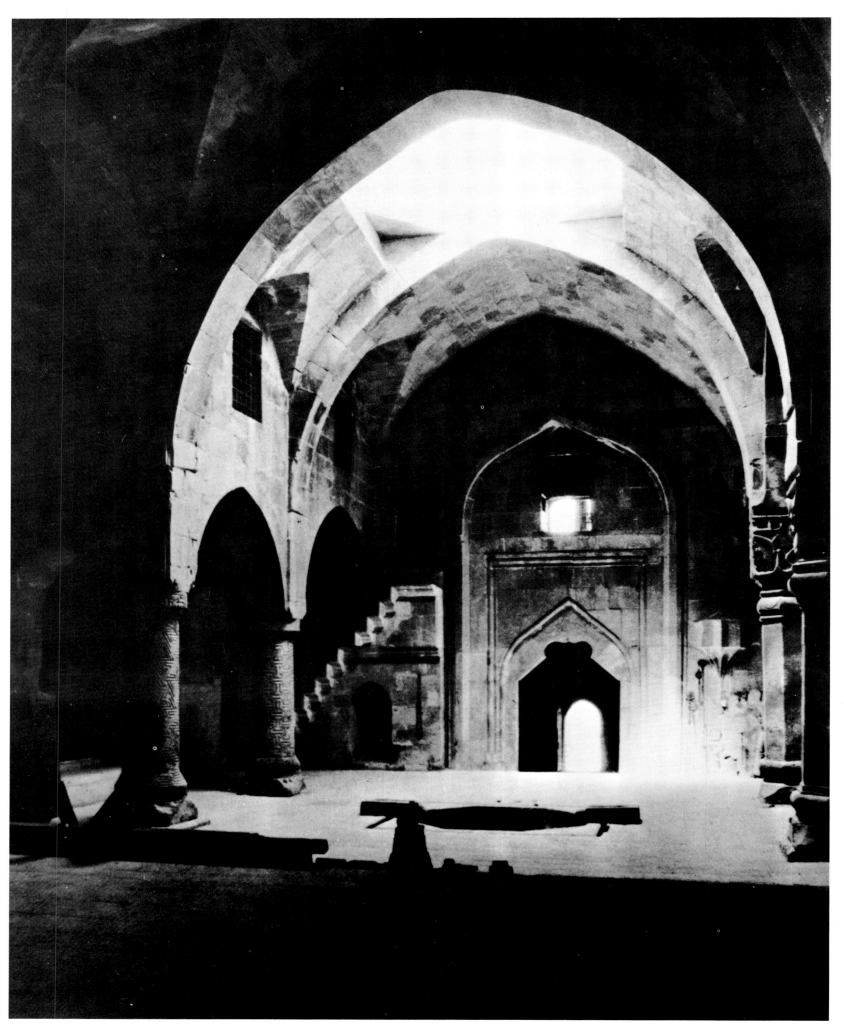

472

medical care was available, the deeply devout often resented the ministrations of physicians as an infringement on the province of Allah.

General health care under Islam outshone Christian society in at least one respect—the hospital system. Although Christian hospitals existed in the West, they were few, rudimentary, and greatly inferior in terms of sanitation, care, facilities, and medication to the centers in Muslim cities. Moreover Christians emphasized salvation of the soul rather than restoration of the body. Although the famous school and hospital at Gundishapur had been established by Nestorian Christians, its later support by Muslim rulers stamped it as a hospital of Arabic medicine.

The best-known of the great hospitals in the Middle Ages were at Baghdad, Damascus, and Cairo. Although hospitals had existed in Baghdad in the ninth century, the most ambitious was founded in the tenth century. In keeping with the principles enunciated by Rhazes, who taught and practiced there, clinical reports of cases were collected and preserved for teaching. The hospital and medical school at Damascus had elegant rooms and an extensive library. Healthy people are said to have feigned illness in order to enjoy its cuisine. Probably the largest and most magnificent was the Mansur Hospital in Cairo, founded in the thirteenth century and built by workers and artisans who were ordered by the sultan to give all their time to its construction. Even the sultan himself took a physical part in the project. Separate wards were set aside for different diseases, such as fevers, eye conditions, diarrhea, wounds, and female disorders. Convalescents had separate sections within them. On discharge, each patient received five gold pieces to support himself until he could return to work.

JEWS AS TRANSLATORS

Jewish translators occupied a special place in bridging Arabic and Latin learning. The open atmosphere of tolerance fostered by Islamic rulers (with a few exceptions) permitted and even encouraged scholars of all races and religions to pursue their studies. The contributions of non-Muslims to learning were eagerly absorbed and incorporated into the rich cultural heritage of Islam.

There was always some interchange between the Muslim and Christian worlds—during the supremacy of Muslim civilization and also during its decline. The familiarity of the Jews with Syriac, Hebrew, and Arabic gave them the opportunity to bring Greek writings (much of which had been translated into Syriac by the Nestorian Christians) into the Arabic orbit. And, later, Jewish writers were instrumental in returning Greek works to the Christian West through their translations. Especially in Spain, contacts between the Muslim and Christian cultures occurred. When Jews at the time of Maimonides fled persecution by the Almohades dynasty in Cordova, they dispersed to European centers of learning, among them Salerno and Montpellier, to which they brought Arabic science and medicine.

472 *Interior of the hospital for the insane (1228–29), founded by Malikaturan Malik, wife of Ahmet Shah, and attached to the Great Mosque at Divrig, Turkey. Under Islam, some hospitals were highly developed, outshining those of the Christian West.*

The Rise of
the Universities

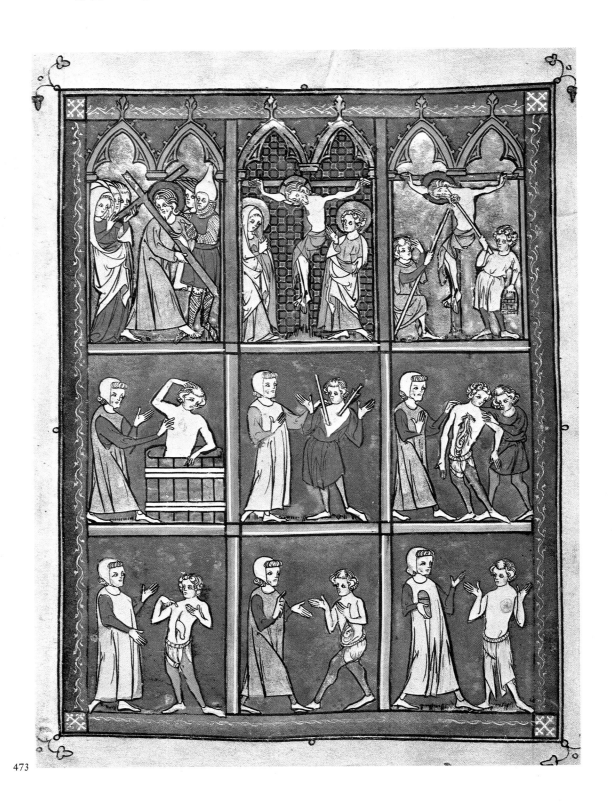

MEDICAL education was truly established in neither the monastic communities of orders such as the Benedictines nor the cathedral schools of the renascent Holy Roman Empire but in the newly established universities, among which Salerno in southern Italy was the most prominent. Although the legend of the school's founding in the ninth century by four physicians, one Greek, one Latin, one Hebrew, and one Arab, is certainly apocryphal, it does convey much of the innovative spirit of the new school.

By the second century B.C., Salerno, on the Gulf of Paestum, near Naples, was already a popular health spa and remained so during the Roman Empire. After the Fall of Rome to the Goths in 476, southern Italy and Sicily were initially part of the Eastern Empire, and for a time Sicily was even under Arab rule. As Islam spread westward in the eighth century, Christian descendants of the Hellenistic world of Egypt and Syria, especially the intellectuals and monastics, found themselves second-class citizens, and many chose to emigrate to the Greek West of southern Italy and Sicily.

SALERNO

Upon this palimpsest of Greek, Latin, and Islamic civilizations, the medical school of Salerno had its beginnings. Although the Benedictine monastery of Monte Cassino was nearby, Salernitan physicians remained remarkably free of clerical control. The school of Salerno was also open to female practitioners, and the most famous was the legendary Trotula, presumed author of a treatise on obstetrics. Throughout the early medieval period in Europe, midwifery was generally the province of women while other medical concerns save nursing care were mostly forbidden to them.

By the year 904, the school was so highly regarded that a Salernitan physician was welcomed at the royal court of France, and, in 984, Alberone, bishop of Verdun, went to Salerno seeking medical advice. Twelfth- and thirteenth-century manuscript copies of much earlier texts used in the school (entitled *Antrorarium* and *Antidotarium*) reveal a concern for the practical and a disdain for the philosophical, which were to be characteristic of Salerno's empiricism.

In the eleventh century, Garipontus of Salerno composed his *Passionarius*, which drew heavily on the ancients, especially Galen. Modified by generations of later writers, this work remained extremely popular throughout the medieval period. Another compilation of ancient texts, the *Practica* of Petroncellus, was also influential in reestablishing a practical bent to the study of medicine.

Constantinus Africanus (c. 1010–87) was crucial to the establishment of the spirit of Hippocrates and Galen in Salerno and, like Cassiodorus and St. Isidore of Seville before him, maintained a continuity with the ancient world. Born in Carthage about the year 1010, Constantinus traveled for four decades in Syria, India, Egypt, and Ethiopia accumulating medical manuscripts. Knowing Greek, Arabic, and Latin, he was uniquely qualified to study and translate the medicine of the Eastern (Islamic) world. Accused of practicing magic upon his return to Carthage, he fled to Salerno and then to Monte Cassino in 1076, where he died in 1087. Constantinus was most important for his translations into Latin of ancient Greek medical texts (often done from their Arabic renderings), but also of Arabic works such as the *Liber Regalis* of Haly Abbas.

A beautiful manuscript found at Breslau contains thirty-five treatises from Salerno written in the eleventh and twelfth centuries. The most famous, *De aegritudiorum curatione*, has two parts: the first, probably the work of a single author, deals with fevers; the second deals with all diseases *ab capite ad calcem*. In contrast to the mystical medicine being taught throughout Europe at the time, here even epilepsy and psychoses were given somatic causes and treatments. However, Salernitan anatomy derived almost exclusively from Galen, and physicians dissected animals, especially pigs whose internal anatomy was thought most to resemble humans'.

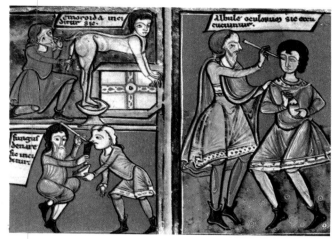

474

473 *Manuscript page from a 13th-century French translation of Roger of Salerno's* Chirurgia, *showing illustrations of various treatments for wounds. The School of Salerno had great influence throughout Europe. Ms. Sloane 1977, British Library, London*

474 *Eleventh-century manuscript illustration from the School of Salerno showing surgery for hemorrhoids and nose polyps and the technique for cataract couching. Ms. Sloane 1975, fol. 93, British Library, London*

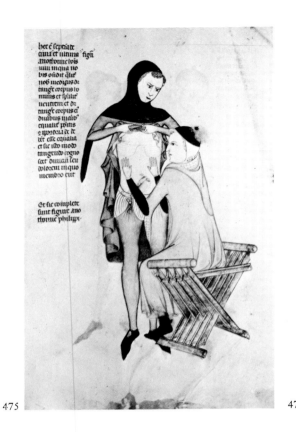

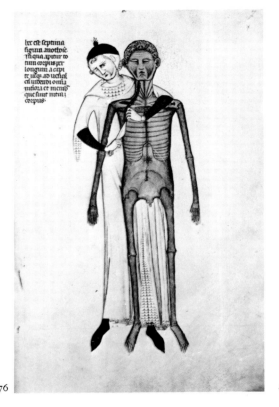

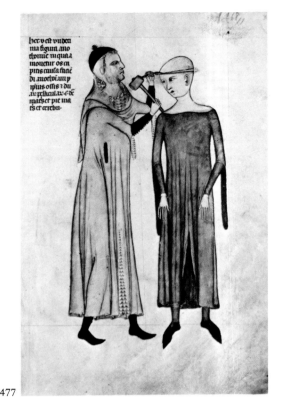

475

476

477

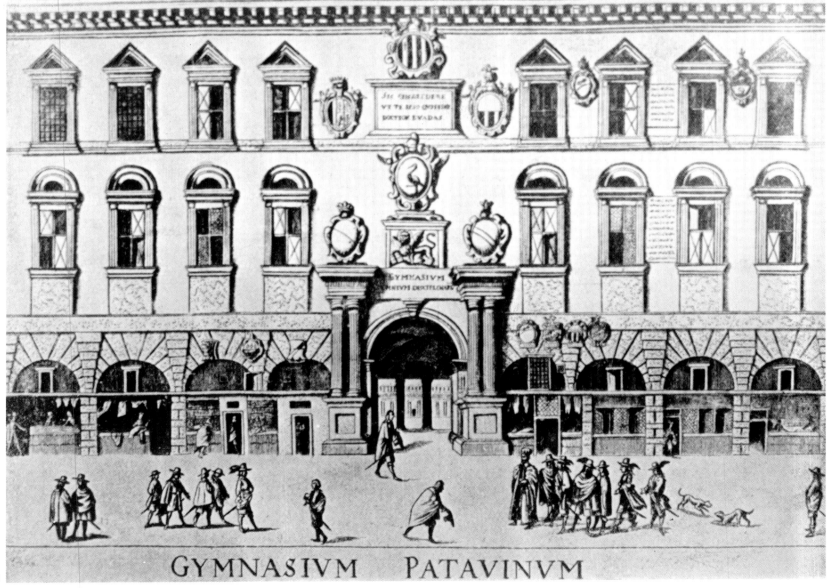

GYMNASIVM   PATAVINVM

478

The most famous work of the Salernitan school, a Latin poem of rational dietetic and hygienic precepts called *Regimen Sanitatis Salernitanum* (at times *Flor Medicinae*), derives from the last half of the thirteenth century. Its many versions, the earliest with as few as 362 verses and others with as many as 3,520, were certainly the result of many authors. More than three hundred editions, following the initial printing at Pisa in 1480, were made throughout Europe, and the work was a standard accompaniment of practicing physicians throughout the sixteenth and seventeenth centuries.

Roger II of Sicily in 1140 forbade anyone from practicing medicine without passing an examination. In 1224 his grandson the Hohenstaufen Emperor Frederich II specified that all candidates for medical licensure be publicly examined by the masters at Salerno after studying logic for three years, medicine and surgery for five years, and after practicing under the direction of an experienced physician for one year. The Salernitan school not only influenced the practice of medicine in the Kingdom of the Two Sicilies but also the development of the universities of Bologna, Padua, and Naples in Italy and of Montpellier in southern France.

MONTPELLIER

The university at Montpellier rivaled Salerno not only in its return to Western medicine based on Greek concepts but also in its contributions to the development of medical education. Like Salerno, Montpellier existed on the border between the Islamic and Latin worlds. Founded in the eighth or ninth century, Montpellier soon possessed a rabbinical school of Spanish origin which taught grammar and later medicine. By 1137 the school was called in official documents a *studium generale* with a *universitas scholarium et magistrorum*, and authorization in 1180 to admit Jews and Arabs was evidence of greater freedom from episcopal control than was generally found in other French schools. Although fifteen universities were to be established in France in the medieval period, the study of medicine was restricted to the *Douze médecins* of Montpellier and, later, to the University of Paris. In 1220, Cardinal Conrad, the papal legate, in concert with the bishops of France issued precise statutes for the university, continuing the somewhat remarkable acceptance of non-Christian teachers and students.

The Catalan Arnold of Villanova (c. 1235–1316), a doctor of medicine, theology, law, and philosophy at Montpellier, translated Avicenna on the heart and Avenzoar on diet and wrote one of the best of the medieval handbooks on medical practice.

UNIVERSITY OF PARIS AND OTHERS

The University of Paris, as might be expected, was more directly supervised by the French kings and the Church. In contrast, the inferior Collège de St. Côme (Cosmas), which concentrated on surgery, retained greater independence from Church and State, perhaps as a direct result of its less-academic pretensions. During the period from 1100 to 1400, many universities developed in France, England, Germany, and even in the Lowlands and Scandinavia. Two influences were almost universally found in the developing medical schools of these universities: the assignment of greater status to the practice of medicine over surgery, and a mandatory supremacy of Christian theology and philosophy over natural science.

SURGERY

During the so-called Dark Ages, many of the technical advances of Greco-Roman surgery had been entirely lost because of increasing ignorance of them through disuse. The Christian belief in the mediation of the Holy Ghost as the only possibility for cure led to the gradual abandonment of all save the simplest surgical

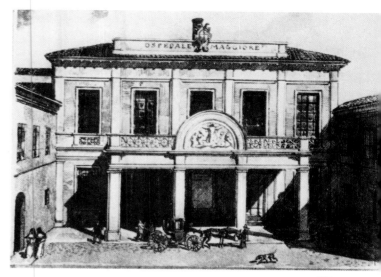

479

475, 476, 477 *Illustrations from the* Anathomia *of Guido da Vigevano (1345), showing a physician examining a patient by listening to the chest, and two examples of dissection, all suggesting an increasing importance to anatomical knowledge. Musée Condé, Chantilly*

478 *Engraving of the University of Padua (1623), an important medical center that stressed the teachings of past authorities.*

479 *Hospital at the University of Bologna, where, in the Middle Ages, Hugo of Lucca and Guglielmo Salicetti were among the outstanding teachers, including the pioneer anatomist Mondino de Luzzi. New York Academy of Medicine*

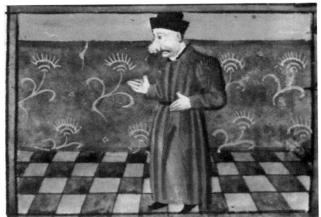

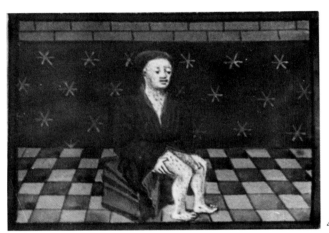

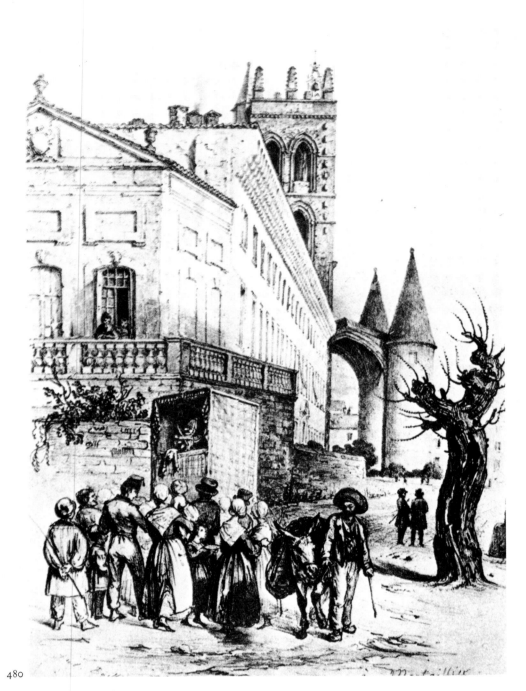

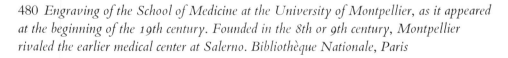

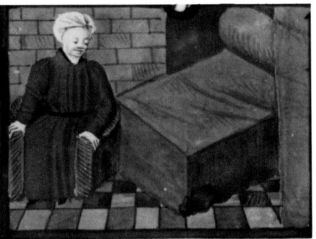

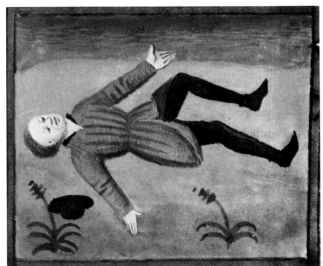

480

480 *Engraving of the School of Medicine at the University of Montpellier, as it appeared at the beginning of the 19th century. Founded in the 8th or 9th century, Montpellier rivaled the earlier medical center at Salerno. Bibliothèque Nationale, Paris*

481, 482, 483, 484 *Miniatures from a manuscript of the* De Proprietatibus Rerum, *in which descriptions of states of health and disease were carefully developed. From top to bottom,* the ailments are polyps, rash, dysentery, and epilepsy. *Ms. fr. 22532, Bibliothèque Nationale, Paris*

485 *Bernard de Gordon, professor at Montpellier from 1282 to 1318, shown evoking before his class the spirits of Hippocrates, Galen, and Avicenna. Ms. lat. 6966, fol. 4 v., Bibliothèque Nationale, Paris*

481

482

483

484

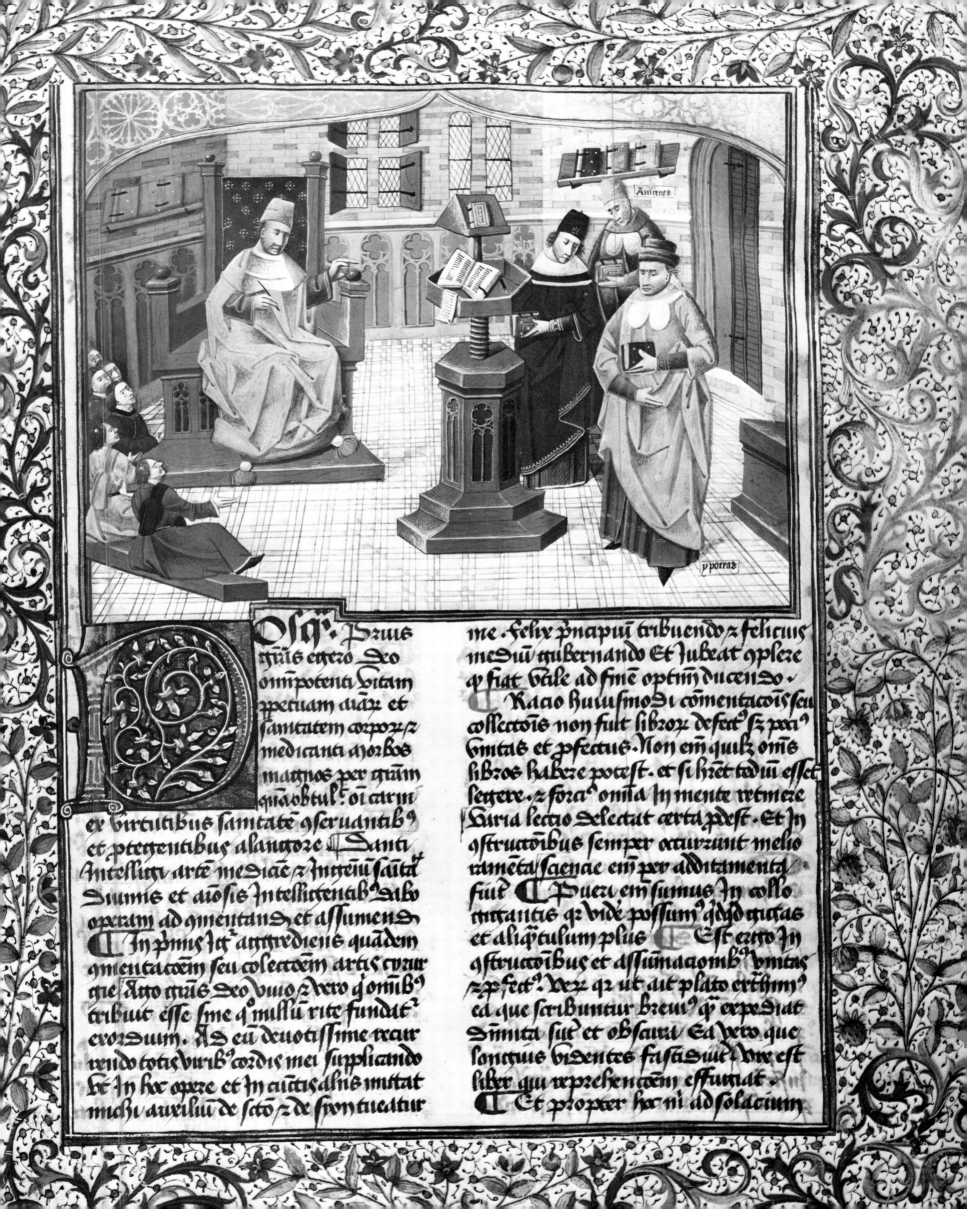

Oratio. Primus
actus est circa Deo
omnipotenti vitam
appetiam dare et
sanitatem corpore et
medicant morbos
maximos per quam
quia obtuli omni circa
ex virtutibus sanitate conservantib
et ptertenentibus alanctore Sancti
Intelligi arte mediate et intretum sautal
siumis et aliosis intelligentia Aib
operam ad inventantis et assumens
In primis sic intredicens quadam
inventatione seu colectone artis cyrur
gie Auto trius Deo unio et vero q omnib
tribuit esse sine q nullu rite fundat
exordium Ad eu deuotissime trahit
rendo totis viribus cordis mei supplicando
ut in hoc opere et in cunctis alius mittat
michi auxilium de seto et de spon tueatur

me felix principium tribuendo et felicius
medium gubernando Et iubeat q pleze
q fiat vale ad finem optimum ducendo
Ratio huiusmodi comentationis seu
collectonis non fuit libros defert sz pxi
unitatis et perfectus Non em quilz omes
libros habere potest et si hret tedium esset
legere et forum omnia in mente retinere
Curia lectio delectat certa prodest Et in
astructoribus semper occurrunt melio
ramenta scientie em per additamenta
fuit Quem em sumus in collo
enitantis q vide possumus quod quidem veritas
et aliquantulum plus Est certo in
astructoibus et assumationb unitas
z p fecit Ver q ut aut plato erthim
ea que scribuntur breuis q expediat
sunt sit et obscura ea vero que
sonetus videntes fasas sunt unde est
liber qui reprehensionem effumat
Et propter hoc ni ad solacium

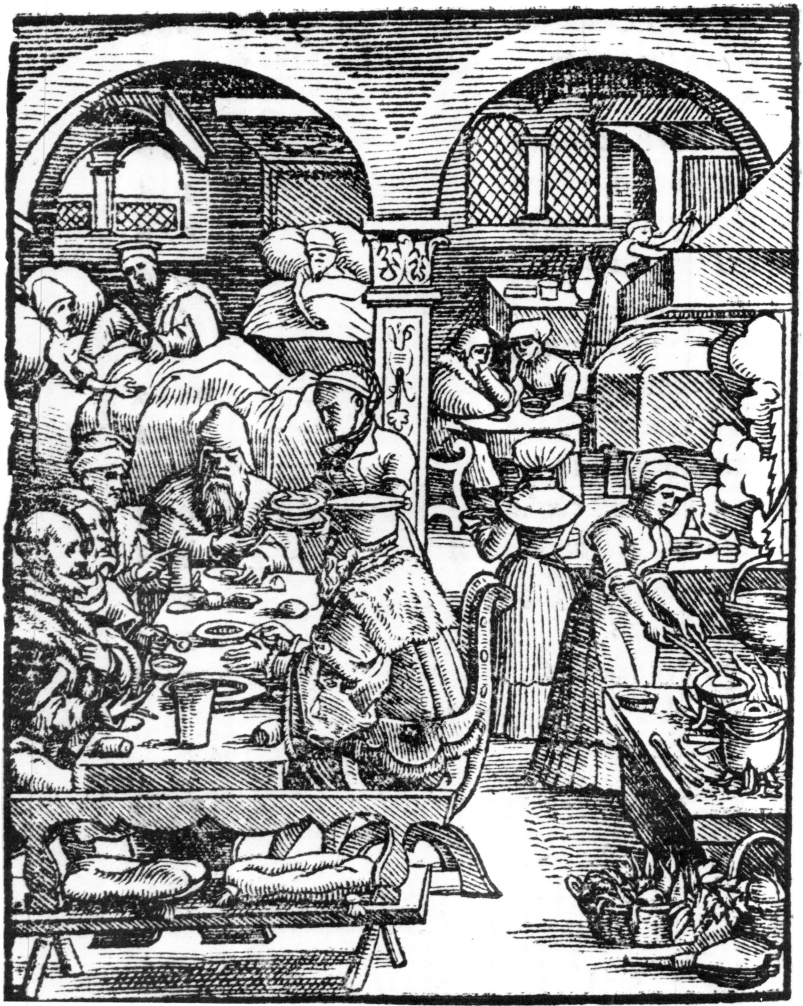

486

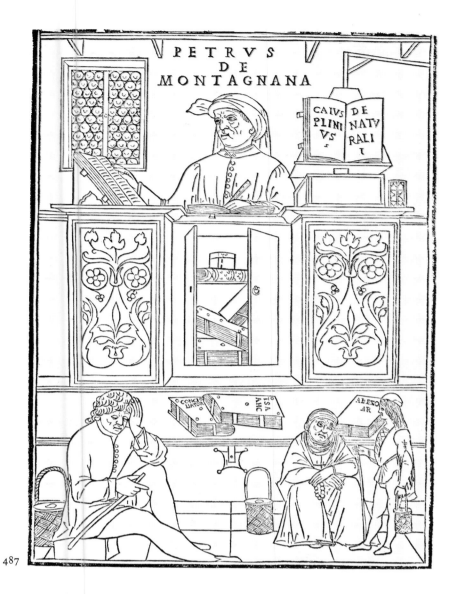

487

486 *Woodcut from a German edition of* Regimen Sanitatis Salerni-tatum *published in Frankfurt (1553), showing the doctors of Salerno dining, with their patients in the background. National Library of Medicine, Bethesda*

487 *Petrus de Montagnana, a teacher of Arabic medicine, was drawn by Gentile Bellini in his lecture chair surrounded by the works of Avenzoar, Pliny, Peter of Abano, and Isaac Judaeus. National Library of Medicine, Bethesda*

488 *Library of the University of Göttingen, as seen in an 18th-century engraving by Georg-Daniel Heumann, done shortly after the univer-sity was founded in 1737. Germanisches Nationalmuseum, Nuremberg*

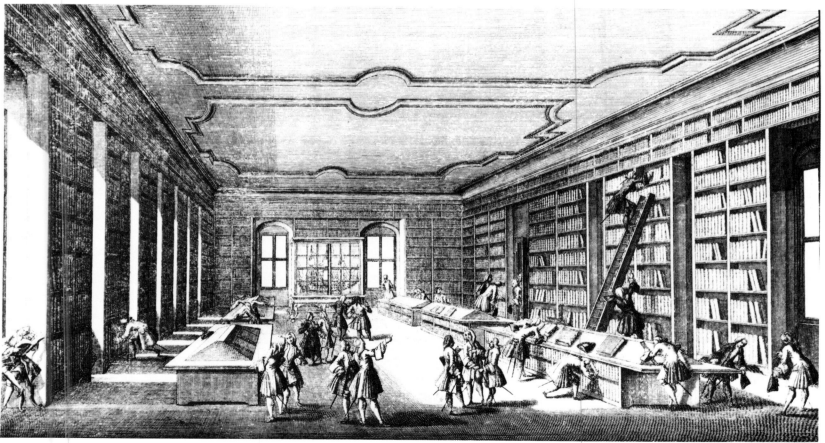

488

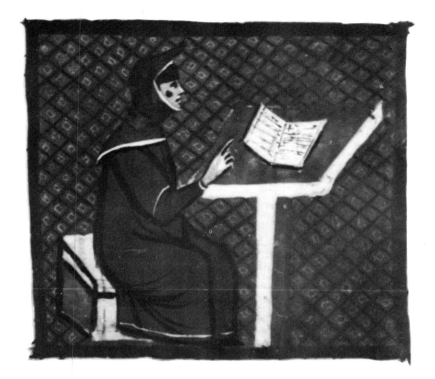

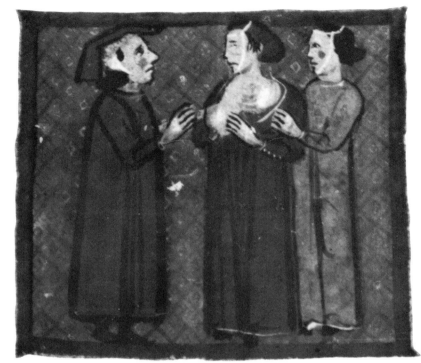

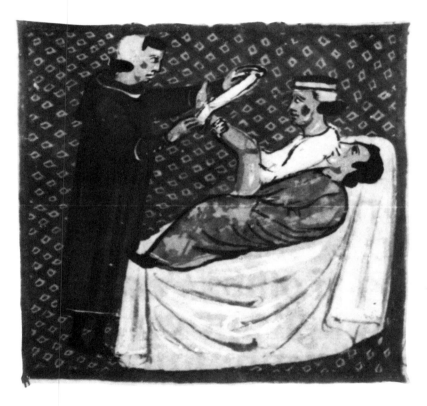

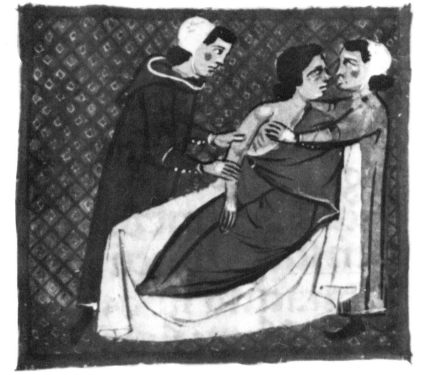

489, 490, 491, 492, 493 *Illustrations from the late-13th-century* **Cyrurgia** *of Theodoric Borgognone, detailing his own and his father's experience in surgery.* Left to right, top to bottom: *teaching; examination for breast abscess; bandaging the ankle; examining the arm; treatment of arm wound. Bibliotheek der Rijksuniversiteit, Leiden*

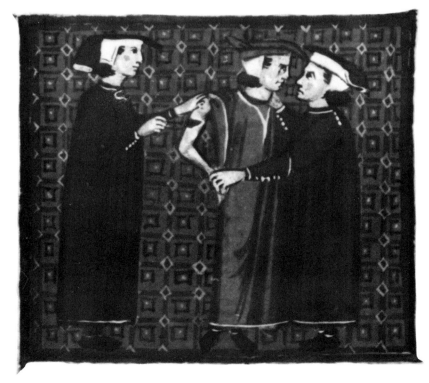

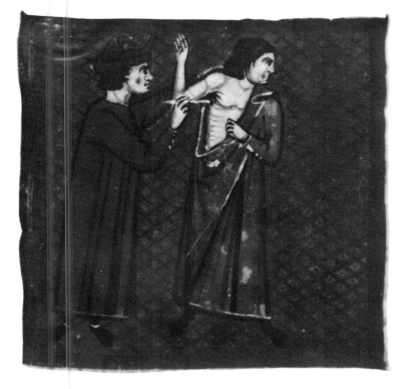

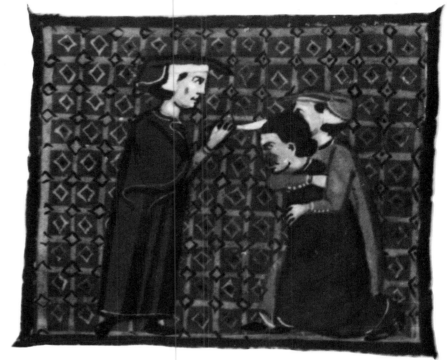

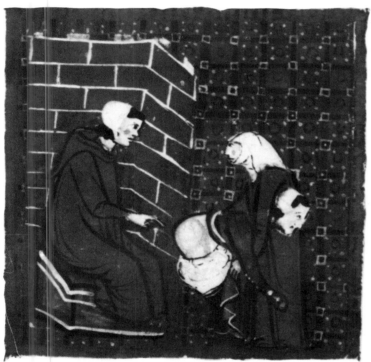

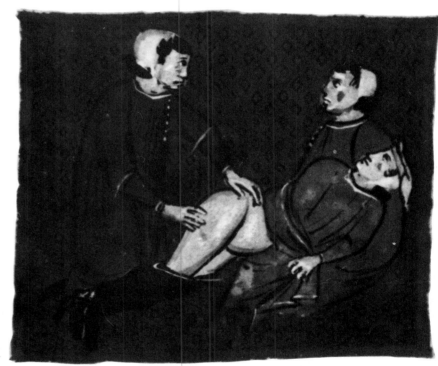

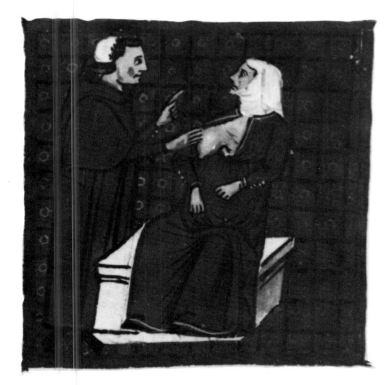

494, 495, 496, 497, 498 *More illustrations from the* Cyrurgia *of Theodoric Borgognone. Left to right, top to bottom: probing with an instrument; operation on the scalp; rectal examinations; examination for breast abscess. Bibliotheek der Rijksuniversiteit, Leiden*

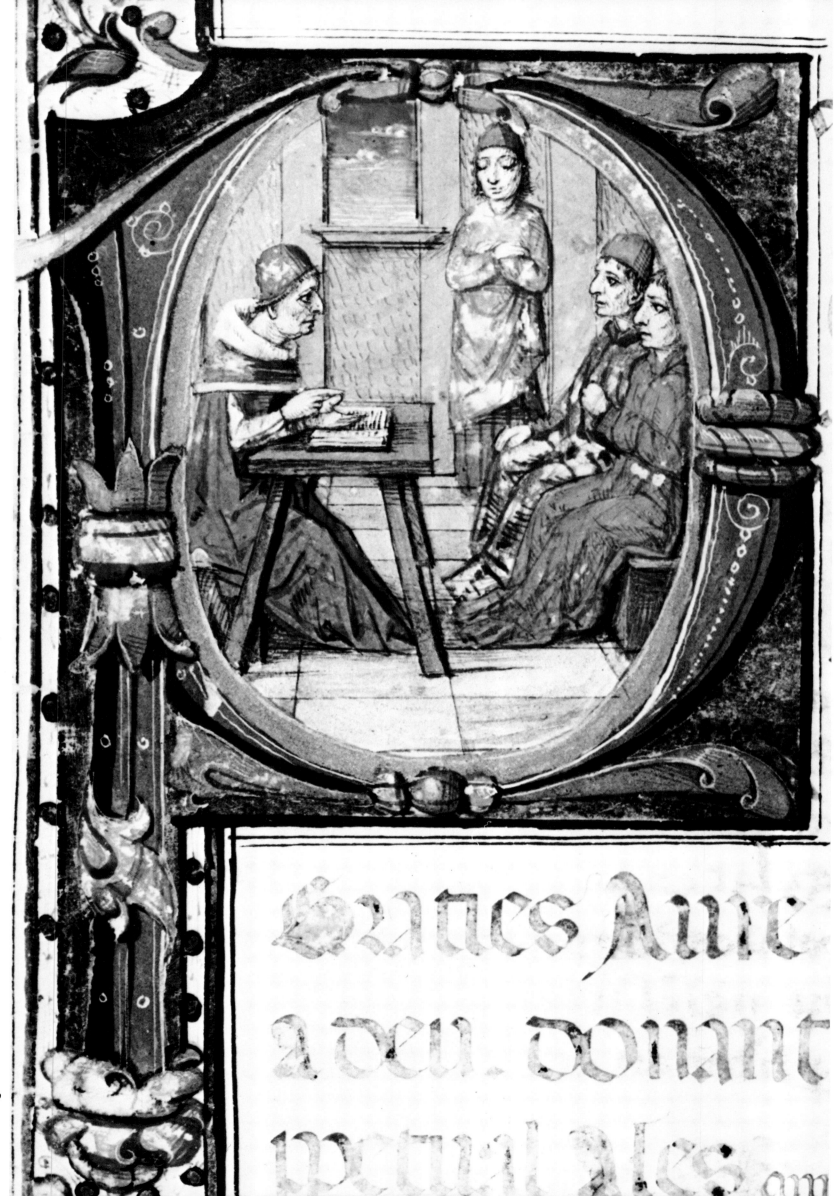

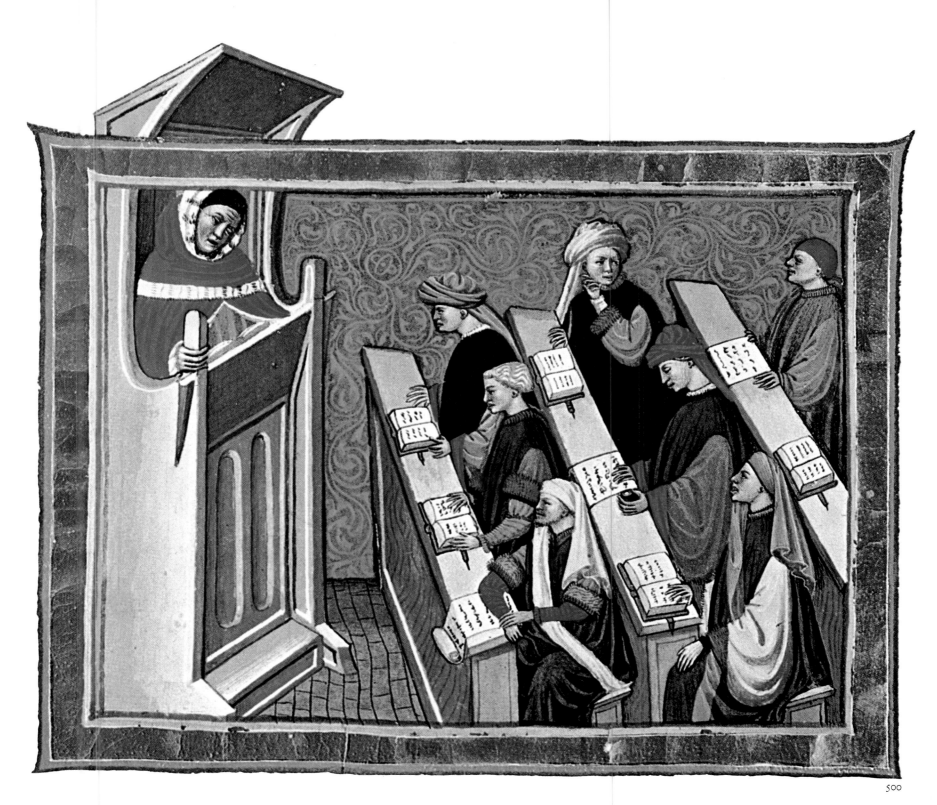

500

499 *Catalan edition of the* Grande Chirurgie *by Guy de Chauliac, the best-educated surgeon of the 14th century and one of the most influential teachers. Ms. lat. 4804, fol. 1, Biblioteca Apostolica Vaticana, Rome*

500 *Antonio da Budrio, early-15th-century teacher at Bologna, shown with pupils in his* Commentary on Decretals, *book 2. Salernitan teaching was rapidly taken over in Italy by Bologna, which then became a magnet for the best physicians and medical students throughout Europe. Ms. 596, fol. 1, Biblioteca Angelica, Rome*

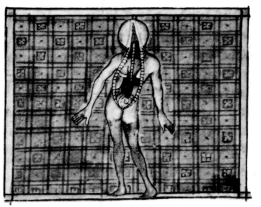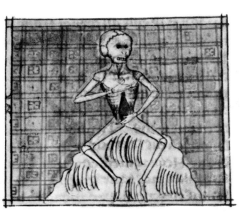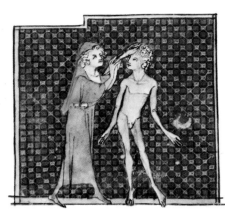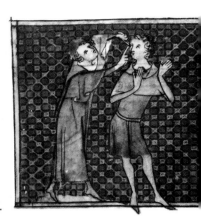

501—507

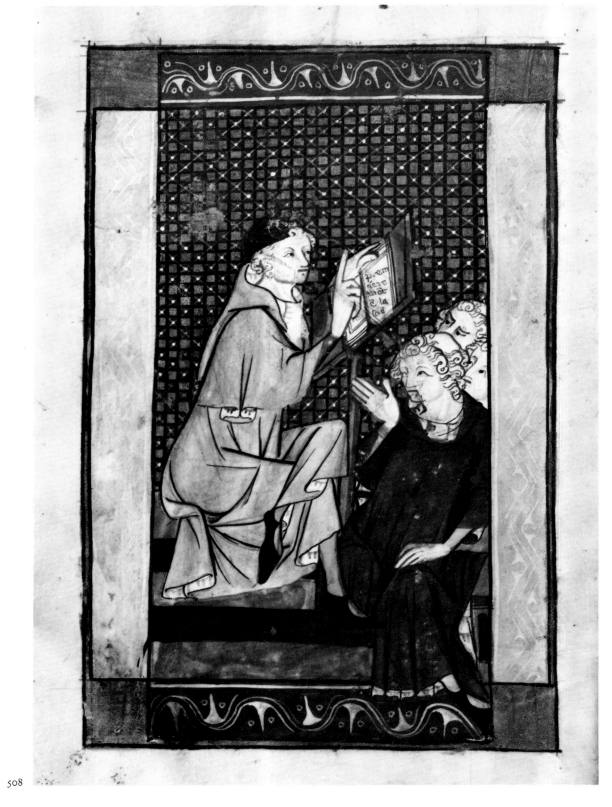

508

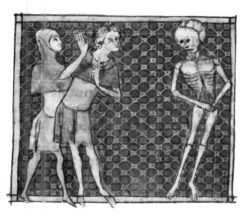 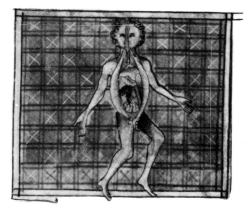 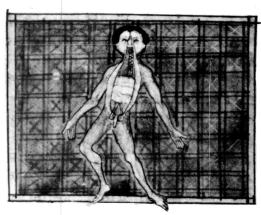

procedures, such as bloodletting, amputation, and tooth extraction. The Muslim schools (with a few notable exceptions—for example, followers of Albucasis) also abandoned many surgical procedures, except the setting of fractures and the favored use of the cautery. As a consequence, only a limited knowledge of anatomy was needed, and even the grossly distorted translators' versions of Galenic porcine anatomy provided sufficient guidance.

Europe again had to look to the Mediterranean schools for guidance, since surgery had long been thought a worthy discipline by the physicians of Salerno, who maintained a greater interest in practical matters (to the point of empiricism) than in philosophical explanations or a teleology derived from religion.

Typical of the best surgeons of the thirteenth century was Guglielmo Salicetti, or Salicet (c. 1210–77), who was professor at Bologna, city physician at Verona, and author of works on internal medicine and surgery. Salicetti preferred to use the knife rather than the cautery in most procedures, and he wrote the first known treatise on regional surgical anatomy, which quite graphically presented remedies by surgery for numerous traumatic and spontaneous conditions. His pupil Guido Lanfranchi of Milan was forced out of his native city for political reasons and journeyed to France, first to Lyons and later, in 1295, to Paris, where he did much to establish surgical practice on French soil. In his *Cyrurgia magna*, finished in 1296, he attempted a reconciliation between internal medicine and surgery. Henri de Mondeville (1260–1320) was surgeon to Philip the Fair and later professor of anatomy at Montpellier. Consistent with the teachings of Hippocrates, he advocated simple cleanliness in the treatment of wounds and the avoidance of pus, laudable or otherwise. Guy de Chauliac (1300–68) studied in France at Toulouse, Montpellier, and Paris and in Italy at Bologna. He was without doubt the best-educated surgeon of his time and encouraged a strong foundation in anatomy.

ANATOMY AND DISSECTION

Along with the development of surgery in the medieval period there was increased attention paid to anatomy. Whereas the Salernitans had earlier confined their studies to animal dissection and the Arabists had relied on anatomy lessons compiled from ancient works, especially of Galen, there was a revival of dissecting human cadavers in the fourteenth century. Although a desire for greater knowledge of anatomy was responsible for the revival of human dissection, rather different forces led to social sanction since the earliest dissections in the Middle Ages appear to have had an entirely medicolegal purpose, such as determining the cause of death in suspicious cases or attempting to learn about the nature of diseases, especially contagious, from pathological findings. The best of medieval dissectors was Mondino de Luzzi of the university at Bologna whose *Anathomia* was completed in 1316. However, his treatise was more an instruction book in dissecting techniques than a study of gross anatomy. First published in Padua in 1487, it went through nearly forty editions and remained the standard text (in spite of numerous Galenical errors) until the time of Vesalius.

501, 502, 503, 504, 505, 506, 507, 508 *Miniatures from the 14th-century* Cyrurgia *by Henri de Mondeville, showing various surgical procedures and conditions. In addition, Mondeville's writings dealt with cosmetic surgery of the breasts, the care of the face and hair, and techniques of plastic surgery. Ms. fr. 2030, fols. 170, 23 v., 8, 17, 15, and 11 v., Bibliothèque Nationale, Paris*

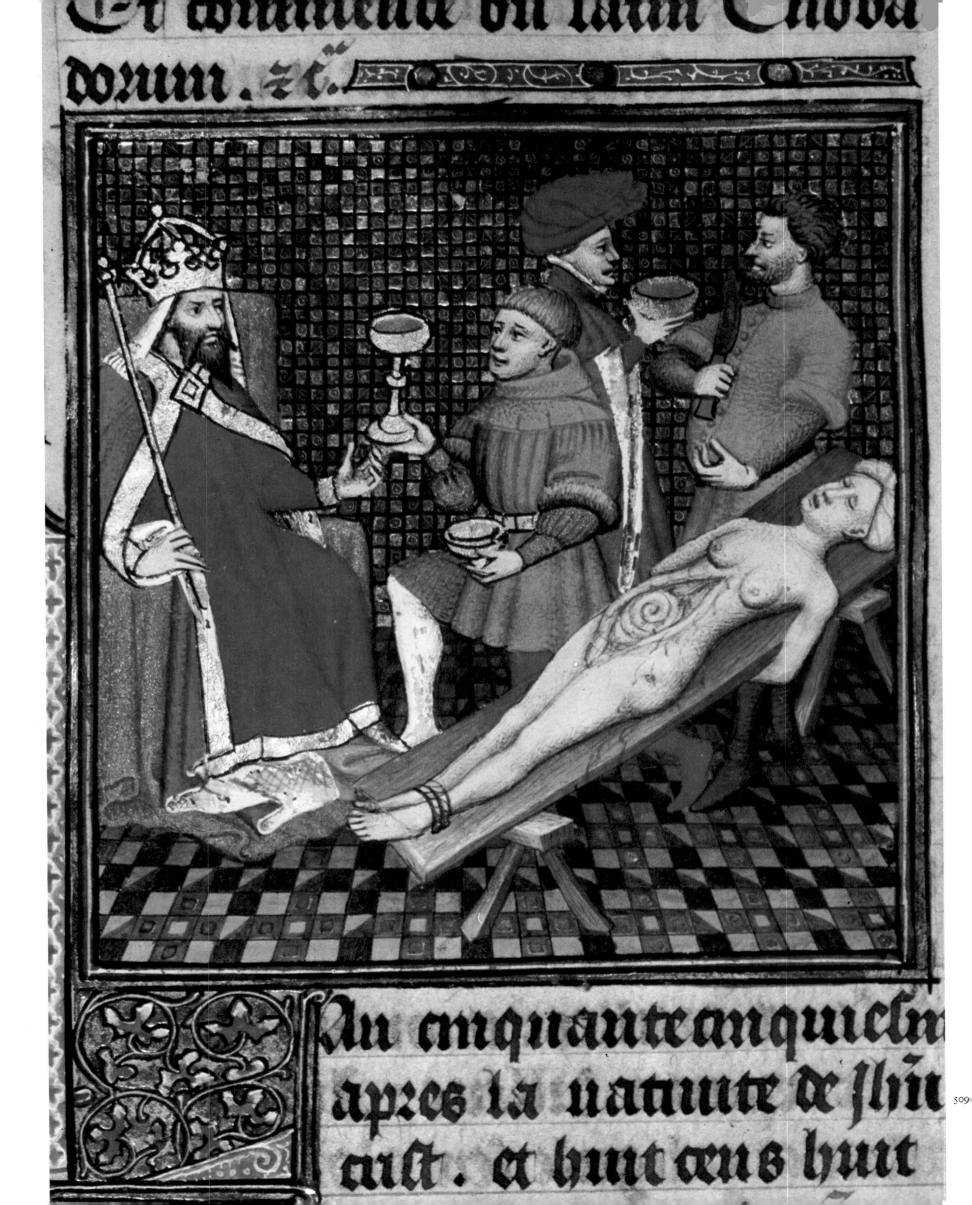

An cinquante cinq que l'en
apres la nativite de nostre
st. et huit cens huit

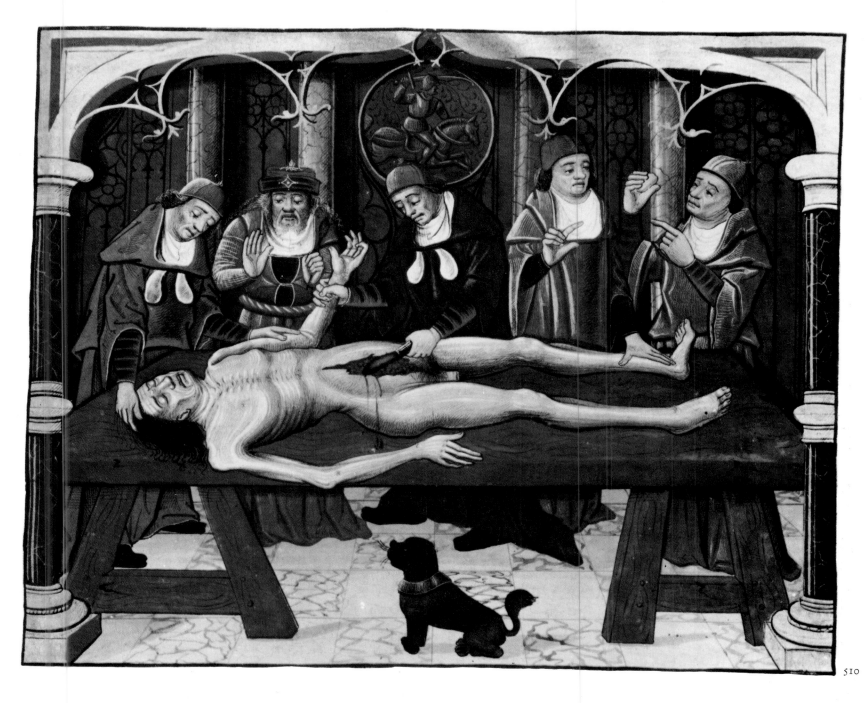

510

509 *Miniature from* Le Cas des Nobles et Femmes
*(c. 1410) by Boccaccio, showing Nero at the autopsy
of his mother Agrippina, whom he had put to death
in* A.D. *59. In the Middle Ages, autopsy was used
to determine cause of death in suspicious cases. Bibliothèque de l'Arsenal, Paris*

510 *Teaching at the dissection table, as seen in this
15th-century manuscript, became more frequent during the 14th century, but the descriptions of Galen
were accepted even if firsthand observation seemed to
contradict. Ms. fr. 218, fol. 56, Bibliothèque
Nationale, Paris*

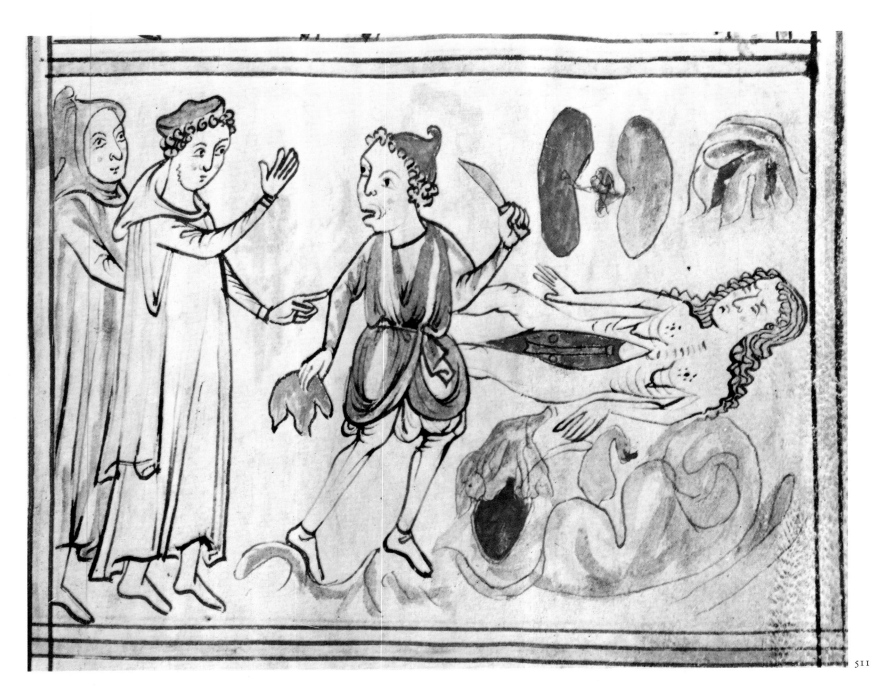

511 *Manuscript illustration presumably showing student caught while doing an illegal dissection, but not before having removed the kidneys, intestines, liver, gallbladder, heart, and lungs. Ms. Ashmole 399, fol. 34, Bodleian Library, Oxford*

512 *The great anatomist Mondino de Luzzi, in this engraving from* Fasciculus Medicinae *(1493) by Johannes de Ketham, is shown lecturing while an assistant dissects the cadaver as students watch. Collection Putti, Istituto Rizzoli, Bologna*

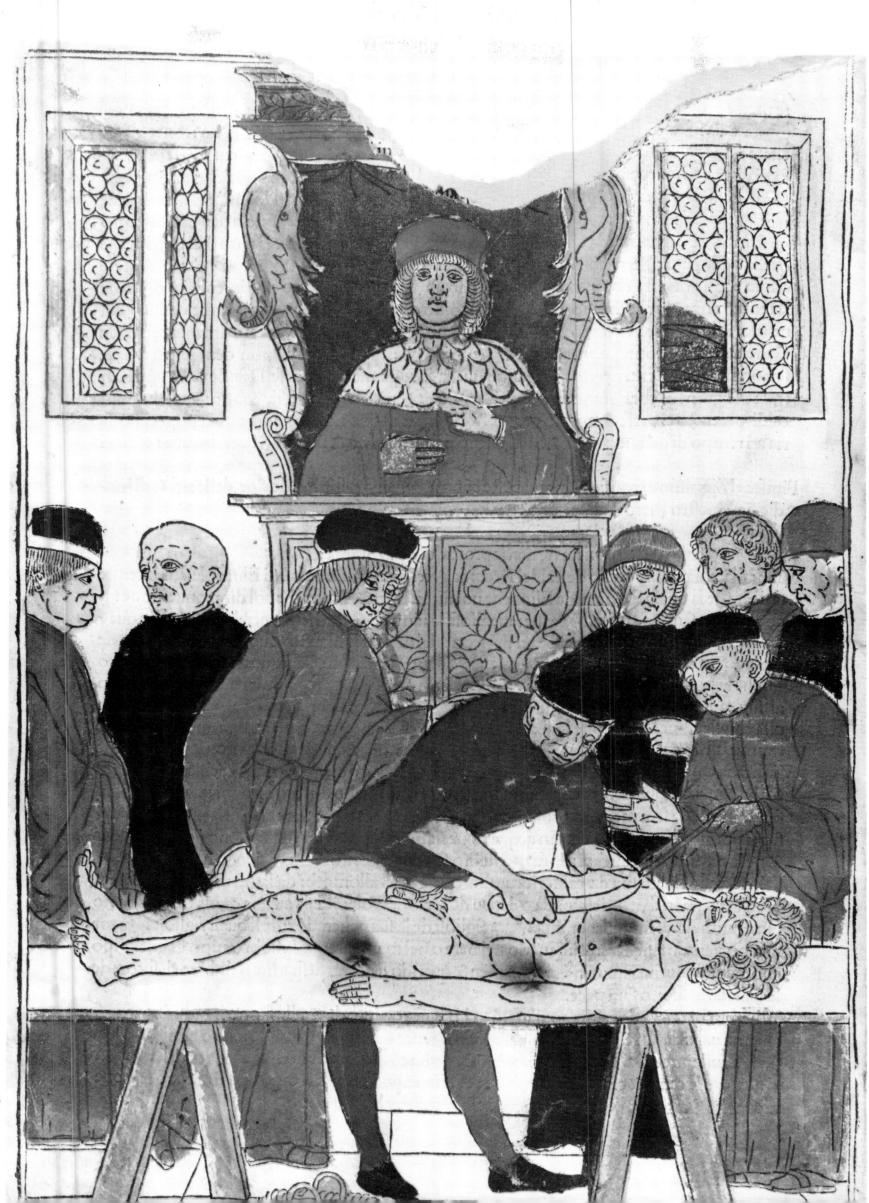

The Middle Ages

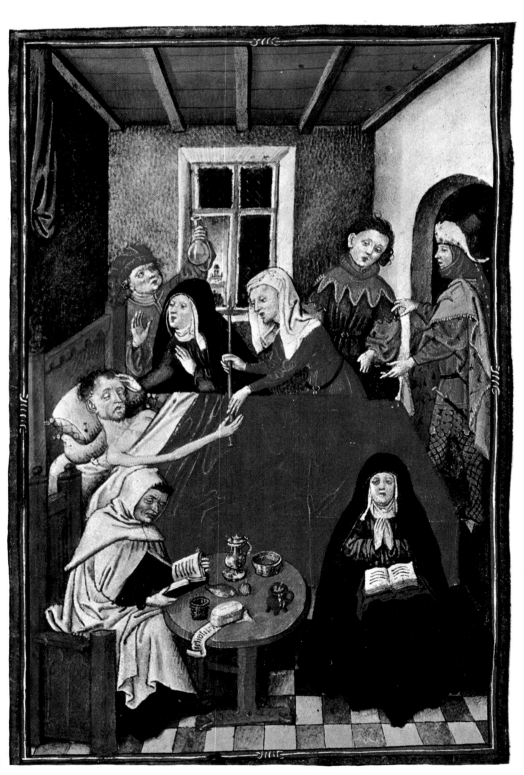

Western Europe emerged from the Dark Ages about the year 1000 in a spirit of enthusiasm, optimism, and cultural unity difficult for us to understand today, given our knowledge of the horrors, plagues, famine, war, and instability with which the Middle Ages came to an end nearly five centuries later. But in the year 1000 the future appeared bright. French culture, with its combination of faith, feudalism, and chivalry, progressively gave forth a model upon which European civilization was to be patterned, while the Mediterranean world was in temporary disarray.

Medieval philosophers, after a period of oscillation between Platonic concepts of transcendent universals (such as "Good" and "Beauty") and Aristotelian denials of their existence, ultimately sided with Aristotle, especially as interpreted by the Arabists. To them the only reality was individual reality, and the world was a pluralistic collection of individuals and particulars. Drawing upon Boethius (the Roman philosopher and translator of Aristotle through whose work Greek philosophy was transmitted to the early Middle Ages), the medieval philosopher encouraged all to "be yourself—for your personality belongs only to you!" Partly because of this strong tendency toward individuality, the rigid social stratification of a feudal society gained support, for each person had his appropriate function and position.

THE ROLE OF THE CHURCH

By the year 1200 the mendicant teaching orders of the Dominicans and Franciscans had assumed control of the intellectual life of Paris, and, as before, the Church remained a conduit for personal advancement, even in a feudal society. The first great thinker belonging to the *regulares* (members of a holy order living by a Rule; in contrast to the *seculares*) was St. Albertus Magnus (1193?-1280), who assimilated much of the Aristotelian thought imported from the borderlands of Western Christendom: Spain, Sicily, and Byzantium. The traces of neoplatonism which had survived among the Byzantine and Islamic successors of Hellenistic civilization fared poorly in Western Europe, where, nevertheless, virtually all intellectual activity remained deductive.

Near the end of the thirteenth century, Albertus Magnus's pupil St. Thomas Aquinas (1225-74) had formulated Aristotelian thought so thoroughly that it was impregnable throughout the remainder of the Middle Ages. His refusal to believe that nature abounds in unnecessary things anticipated the pronouncement of William of Occam (1300?-49) that the simplest explanation should be applied to observed natural phenomena. Having based his strongest reliance upon the eternal nature of being (*essentia*), Aquinas was forced to utilize a sophisticated system to explain the changes often observed in the natural world. In the same way that an acorn's nature is to become an oak, many substances have inherent potency to become something else; thus their essence would not really change but merely be fulfilled. Since no being could will itself a change for which it had no potential, all other changes must derive from some outside influence. It was here that Aquinas fell back on theology: God was the prime mover who became the ultimate source of all change in the natural world—other than the above inherently potential becoming. This doctrine of efficient causation—which became the cornerstone of Aquinas's system, known as Thomism or Scholasticism—gave the supernatural supremacy over the natural, but by implication the natural and supernatural worlds were separate if not independent. Although the brilliant synthesis of Scholasticism was to stultify independent thought during the Middle Ages, by the time Renaissance thinkers came to deny at least ordinary supernatural intervention in the natural world the foundations for the architecture of modern science had already been laid.

The earlier philosophical oscillation between a pluralistic world and one of transcendent universals also had relevance to medieval man, so that the idea of

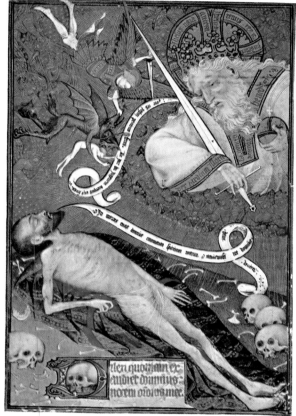

514

513 *Fifteenth-century deathbed scene from the* Heures de Catherine de Cleves, *showing doctor checking urine specimen of patient even while preparations are made for the Last Rites. Pierpont Morgan Library, New York*

514 *Dead man face-to-face with his Judge, as seen in the* Heures de Rohan *(c. 1418–25). Medieval man, constantly exposed to sudden and unexplained death, was warned by the Church to prepare for Judgment Day. Ms. lat. S471, fol. 159, Bibliothèque Nationale, Paris*

individual nation-states stood in marked contrast for him to the universality of Christendom. This discord was felt most devastatingly in Germany and Italy, where the confrontation of Holy Roman Emperor and Pope ultimately damaged both. Only on the periphery of the continent, and most notably in France, England, and Spain, was the king (or nation) able to assert authority over the Church, though only after long and bitter struggle. Individual loyalties were horizontal as well as vertical, and, in the face of an expanding Islamic world, Europe had to assume a common identity in Western Christendom. In spite of growing nationalism and the development of national languages, kings addressed each other in Latin as "brother," and the rules of chivalry maintained a common bond among the nobility of different countries. However, the Church of Rome was even more capable of crossing state lines, retaining sole authority over all who had taken holy vows. The growing power of the monastic orders led more directly to Rome than the legendary roads of the ancient Empire.

PHYSICIANS AND THE GUILDS

In spite of a more ordered system of trade during most of the medieval period, European society remained isolated and rural, based largely on a local agricultural economy. Only the royal and noble courts were mobile, of necessity to maintain control over their vassals. Physicians trained in the universities were available only to the higher ranks of society, and for them entrance into holy orders and celibacy were generally mandatory, although, ironically, Jewish physicians (with freer access to Arabic medicine) became increasingly popular among heads of state and even popes. The masses, however, continued to rely on folk-healers, as well as barber-surgeons and teeth-pullers. Childbirth, a dangerous time for all women until the recent past, remained in the hands of midwives. Even when serious problems arose and doctors were called in, women still remained as intermediaries.

In contrast to the complex medicinal formulations of trained physicians, folk-healers relied on simpler concoctions and rudimentary magic. With the growth of cities in the twelfth and thirteenth centuries, there was an increase in the number of apothecaries setting up shop and preparing medications on their own as well as under direction of physicians. Their shops at times were meeting places for doctor and patient, but perhaps were frequented as often for astrological consultation and alchemy.

During the Middle Ages, throughout Europe, men in the same crafts and professions banded together for mutual support and to promote high standards. The old separation of surgeons from other medical practitioners was reinforced and extended by the formation of guilds which were mutually exclusive. This custom was not solely a result of the academics' disdain for surgery but derived from the medieval tendency for crafts to be drawn together by the similarity of their tools and materials rather than the purpose for which they were used. Thus, surgeons' guilds admitted barbers, and physicians were allied to apothecaries and, surprisingly, to artists because of their common use of powders (as pigments for the latter in water-, egg-, and, much later, oil-based paints). The common guild of artists and physicians may have been a significant factor during the early Renaissance in the great advances in knowledge of human anatomy, a subject of great interest to both groups.

Even though the Church retained control of the universities throughout the Middle Ages, monastic medicine declined rapidly, but only in part because of people's growing interest in receiving earthly rather than heavenly rewards. In the twelfth and thirteenth centuries, control of hospitals and infirmaries was transferred from the Church to municipalities by mutual agreement. From this time date the origins of some of the great hospitals in Europe: the Hôtel-Dieu in Paris, Santo Spirito in Rome, and St. Thomas's and St. Bartholomew's in England.

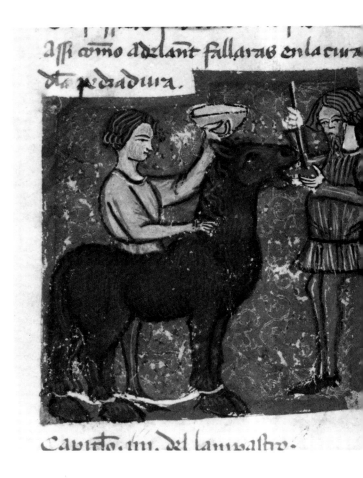

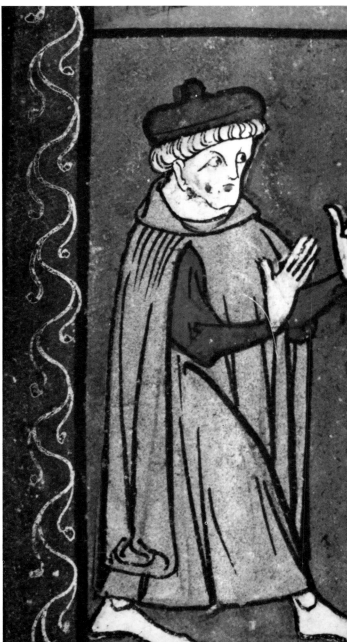

338

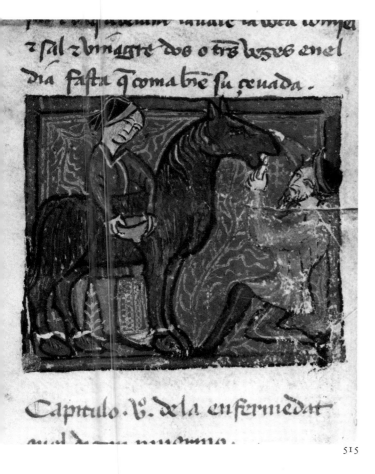

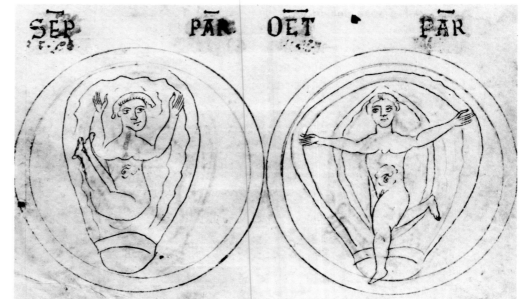

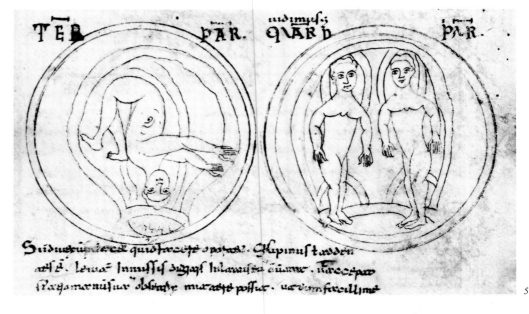

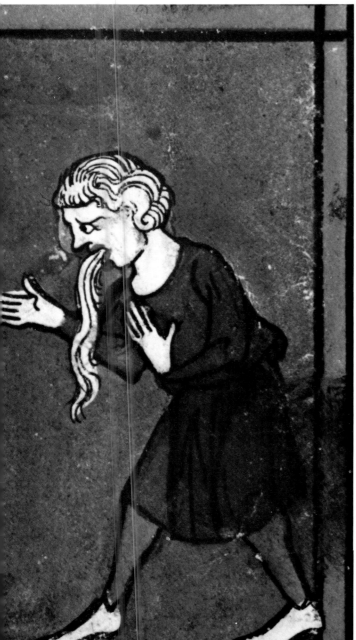

515 Illustrations from a manuscript in Spanish by
Juan Alvares of Salamelks on the proper care of
animals, an early volume of veterinary medicine. Ms.
Sp. 214, Bibliothèque Nationale, Paris

516 Person shown vomiting, probably following a
dose of purgative prescribed to relieve an illness
thought to result from an excess of one of the four
humors. Ms. Sloane 1977, fol. 50 v., British Library,
London

517, 518 Twelfth-century manuscript, based on the
work of Soranus, 1st-century forefather of obstetrics,
showing various fetal presentations—including twins
—and warning of complications. Codex 1653, Det
Kongelige Bibliotek, Copenhagen

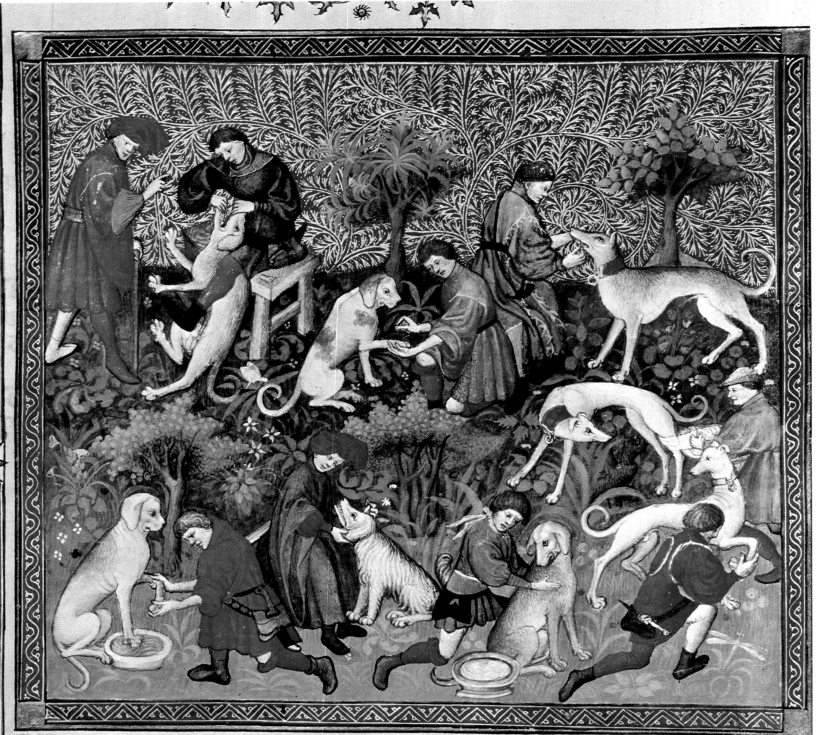

Cy deuise des maladies des chies
et de leurs curacions.

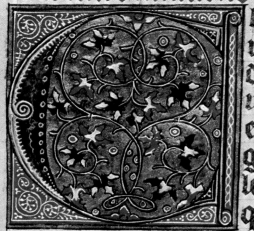 hiens ont
moult de
diuerses
maladies
et la plus
grant cest
la rage. de
quoy il y
a de ix. manieres desquelies ie
diray vne partie. La premier

rage curent et villent a voy cel
se. et non pas telement come
ilz souloient crier quant ilz
estoient sains. Quant ilz peu
eschaper. ilz vont tous ptout
mordant hommes et bestes. et
quant quilz treuuent deuant
eulx. et est moult perilleuse le
morsure. car ce que ilz mordu
de quoy ilz truuent sang. a
grant poine sera quil ne soit

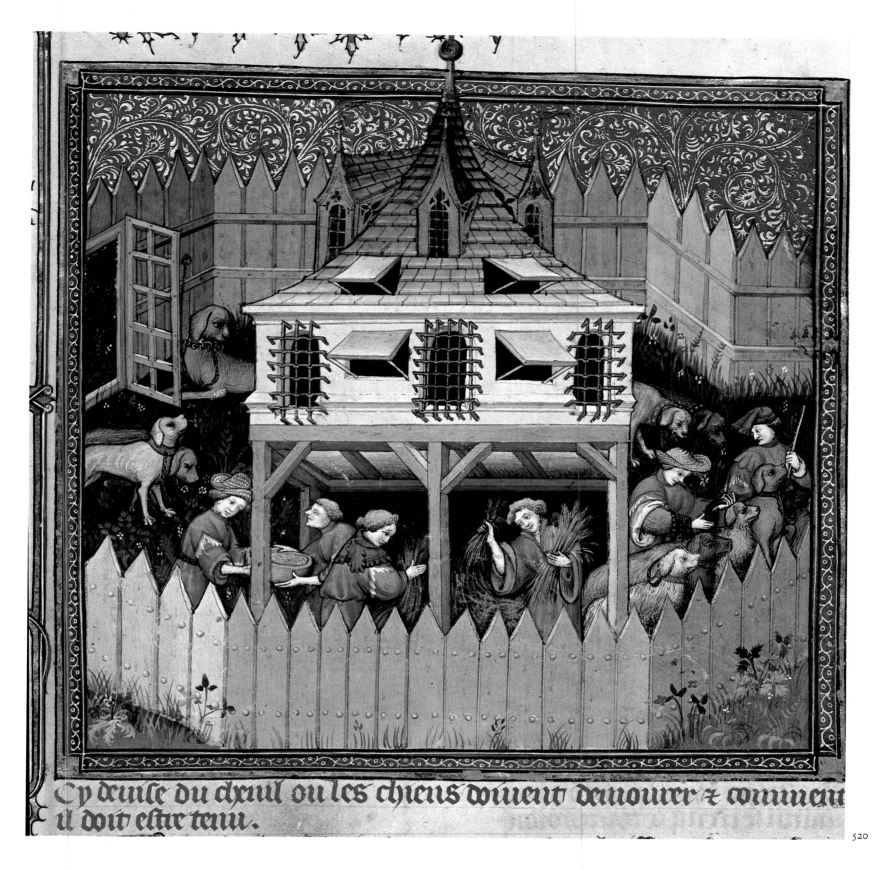

Cy deuise du chenil ou les chiens doiuent demourer τ comment il doit estre tenu.

519, 520 *Scenes typical of manor life in feudal France, which presented itself as a model of European civilization. Dogs played an important role in the hunt and required careful attention. Facing page,* "The maladies of dogs being treated," *and, above,* "Proper kennel for dogs," *from Gaston Phoebus,* Livre de la Chasse, Ms. fr. 616, fols. 40 v., 52 v., *Bibliothèque Nationale, Paris*

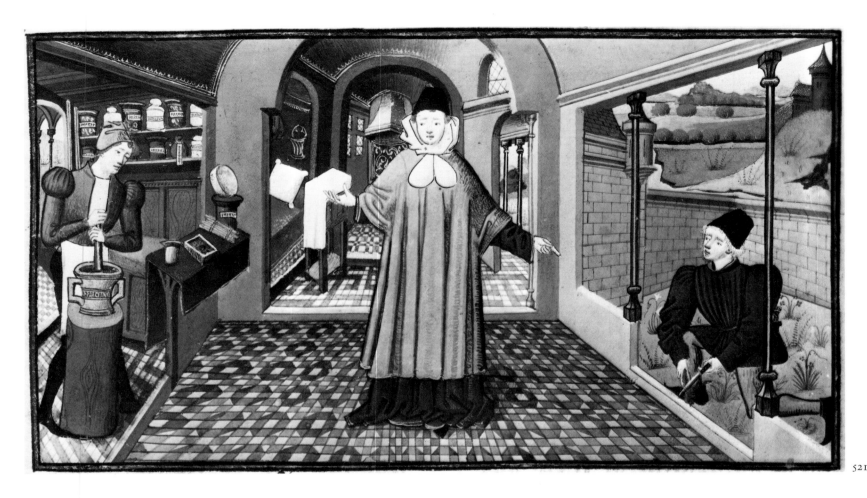

521 *Illustration from Guy de Chauliac's* Chirurgia, *showing the pharmacy in a 14th-century surgeon's office, with one assistant cutting herbs from the garden and another grinding them in a mortar under the doctor's direction. Ms. 6966, fol. 154 v., Bibliothèque Nationale, Paris*

522 *Medieval uroscopy chart, showing urine samples in various gradations of color and condition, with suggestions to the examining doctor of what maladies are responsible. Ms. anon. Ashmole 391v, fol. 10, Bodleian Library, Oxford*

523 *Birth scene from the Uttenheimer Altar (1480), with midwives swaddling the Christ Child and warming receiving blanket, indicative of the role of women in obstetrics and the care taken in a period of high infant mortality. Germanisches Nationalmuseum, Nuremberg*

524 *Engraving of the interior of the Hôtel-Dieu, Paris, about 1500, showing the crowded conditions and a familiarity with death, as corpses are routinely sewn into shrouds in full view of the patients. Ms. Ea 17 rés., Bibliothèque Nationale, Paris*

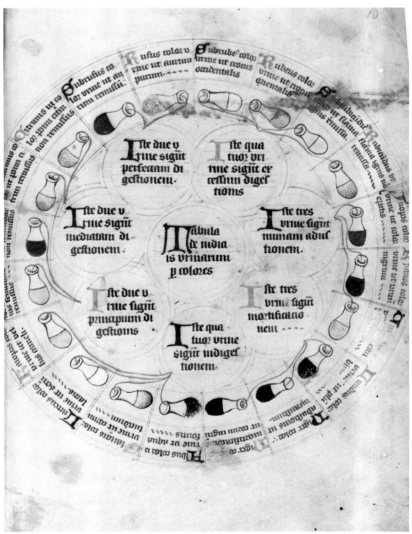

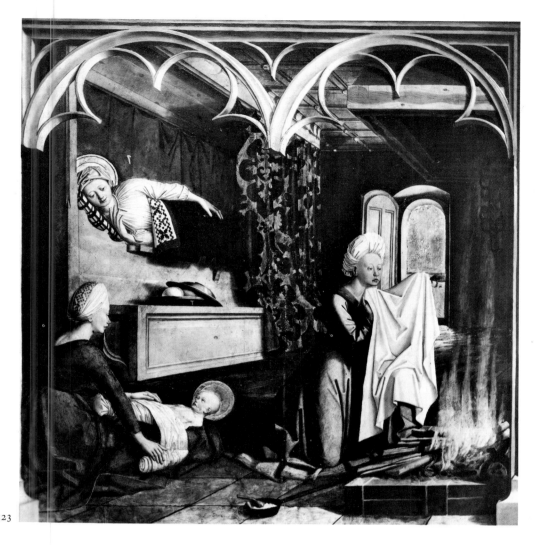

523

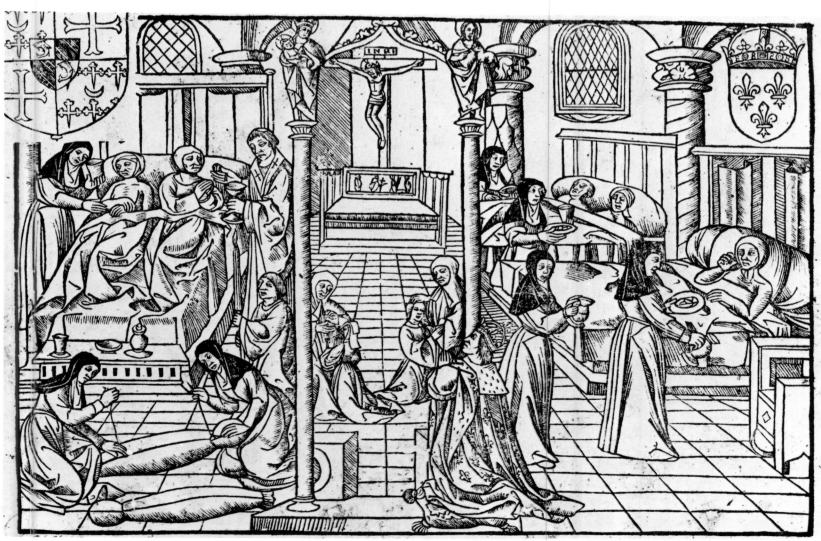

524

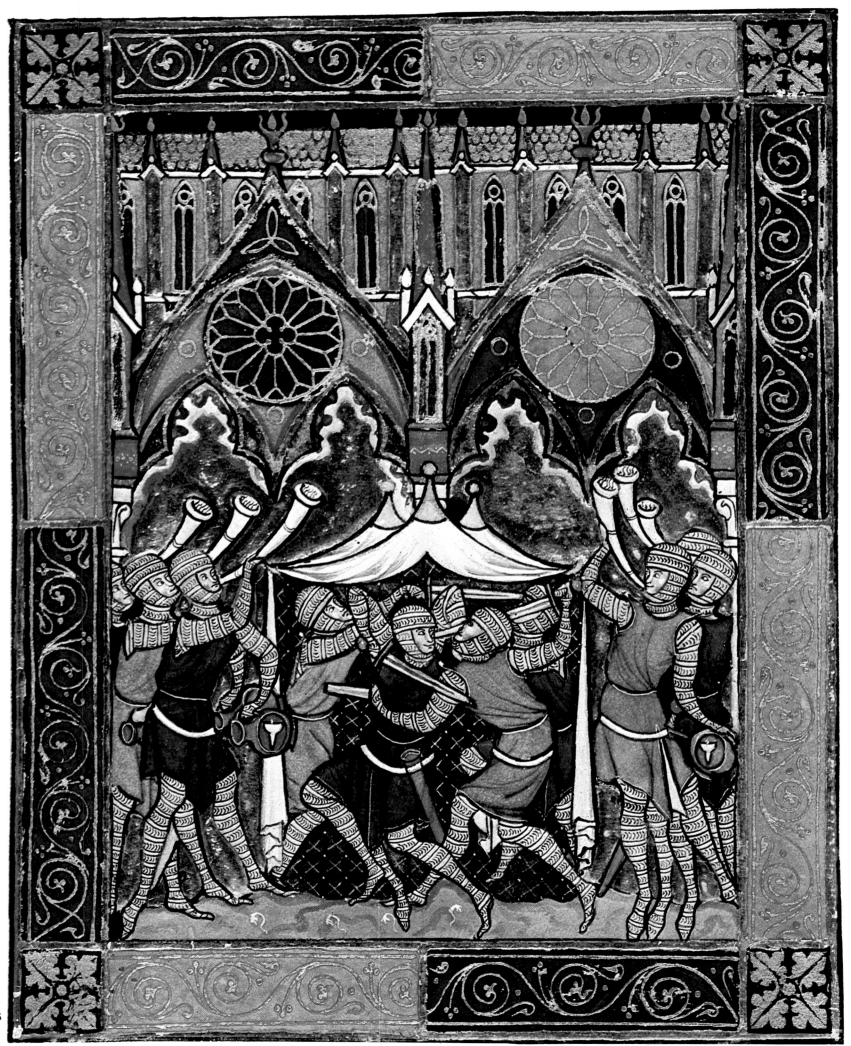

525

THE CRUSADES

Ironically, at the same time that church councils were forbidding the practice of medicine to those monastic orders once the mainstay of Europe, newer nursing and hospital orders were developing. The stimulus to the founding of these orders was not the need for medical care by indigenous populations but, rather, the Crusades, which ostensibly attempted the return of the Holy Land to Christian control. The Order of the Knights of the Hospital of St. John of Jerusalem, or Hospitalers, was founded in 1099. The order of the Knights of the Temple of Solomon (or Templars) and the Order of Lazarus (which was devoted to the care of lepers) were founded at the start of the twelfth century, while the Order of Teutonic Knights and the Order of the Holy Ghost were established somewhat later. These are only the most famous of a large complement of orders associated with the Crusades, and their later histories diverged widely. The Hospitalers looked after victims of the many epidemics which, we shall see, resulted in no small part from diseases brought home by returning Crusaders. The Templars, which became an increasingly military order, were ultimately subdued by the French state. The Teutonic Order, begun as a field hospital during the siege of Acre in the Third Crusade and approved by Pope Clement III in 1191, was influential in the establishment of formalized medical care in the German lands. Papal approval of the Order of the Holy Ghost (Santo Spirito) led to the founding of a hospital not only in Rome but in nearly every city of Europe. Many other Catholic hospitals were founded throughout Europe, but, unlike their monastic forebears, were almost never independent of the municipalities they were intended to serve.

The Crusaders brought home many things in addition to hospital orders. Exposure, especially of common soldiers, to the sophisticated and sensuous East created a material demand which simple piety was unable to squelch, and a flourishing trade with the East, mostly via Venice and Genoa, was quickly established. Nor did the more elaborate pharmacology of the Islamic East go unnoticed; new medical concoctions and sugar-based syrups began to appear in Europe for the first time.

LEPROSY AND THE PLAGUE

Disease, however, was the most significant import to Europe resulting from the Crusades. Throughout the period of the declining Roman Empire and the Dark Ages, leprosy was endemic at low levels in Western Europe, but after the Crusaders began streaming back home the number of lepers increased tremendously. During the Middle Ages, the stigma of leprosy was not restricted to the disease as we know it today but was applied to a variety of dermatologic diseases, only some of which had any degree of contagiousness. Nevertheless, all individuals called lepers were subjected to total ostracism from society, which was stringently enforced by governmental and ecclesiastical authorities, as in Biblical times. Distinctive clothing was mandatory, as was segregation in places of public assembly, even worship. However, the Order of Lazarus was so sympathetic to the care of lepers that Lazarhouse quickly connoted *leprosarium*, and thousands were soon built throughout Europe.

Many other contagious diseases were introduced into Europe by returning Crusaders. In spite of an elaborate system of hospices, travel in the medieval period remained arduous and risky; shipwreck, marauding brigands, and poor food added to the physical rigors. Epidemics of typhus, smallpox, and other diseases can be directly traced to returning Crusaders, but by far the most notorious epidemic to be imported from the East was that of the Black Death or bubonic plague.

Although plague had been known intermittently in Western Europe since ancient times, its reappearance in the mid-fourteenth century was dramatic and devastating. In the year 1347, the plague rapidly moved westward across India and

525 *The soldiers of Gideon and the Midianites are pictured as Crusaders in the mid-13th-century Psalter of St. Louis. B 50/278, Bibliothèque Nationale, Paris*

526 *Nun in the habit of the Knights Hospitalers, a nurse in the Hospital of St. John of Jerusalem during the Crusades. New York Academy of Medicine*

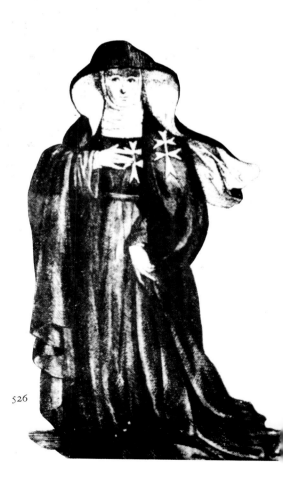

526

345

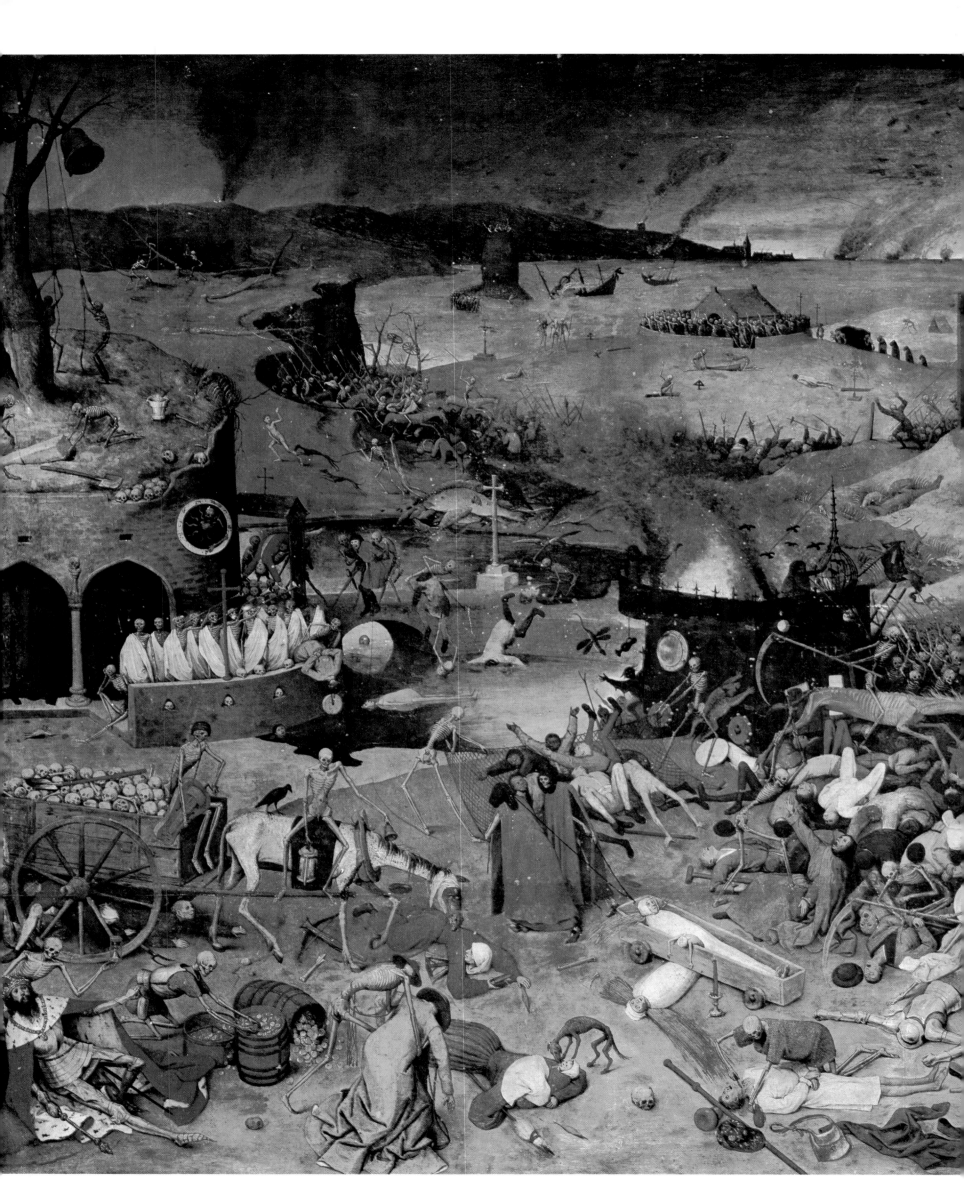

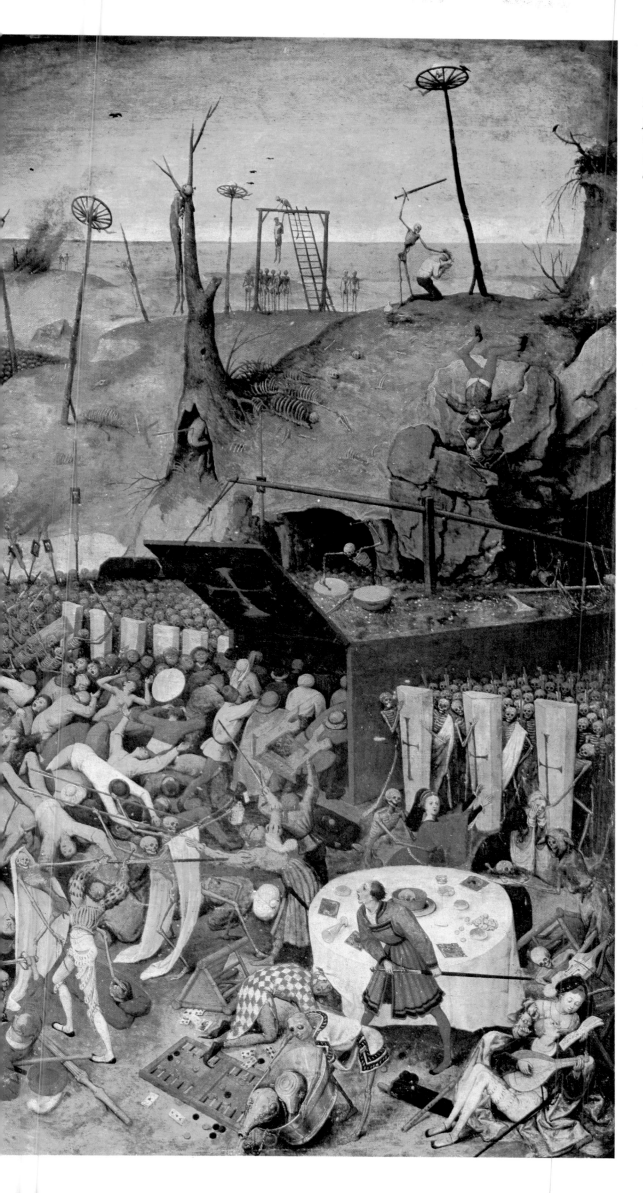

527 *The Black Death of 1347, which felled perhaps one-quarter of Europe's population, was seen in Bruegel's* Triumph of Death *(c. 1556) as a horrible loosening of the forces of darkness on mankind. The Prado, Madrid*

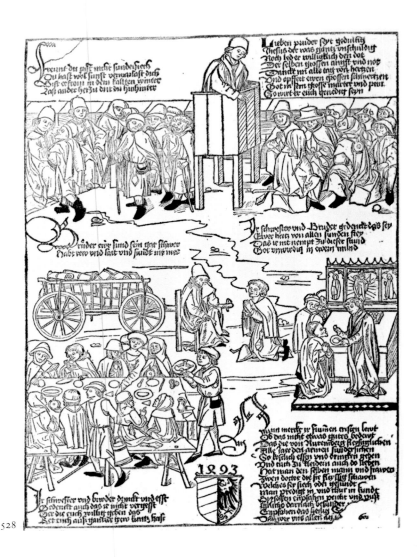

528

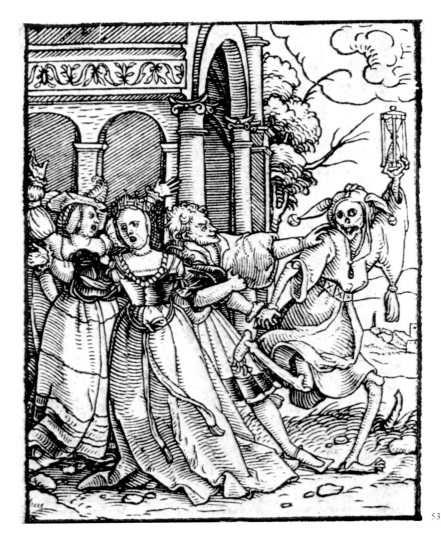

530

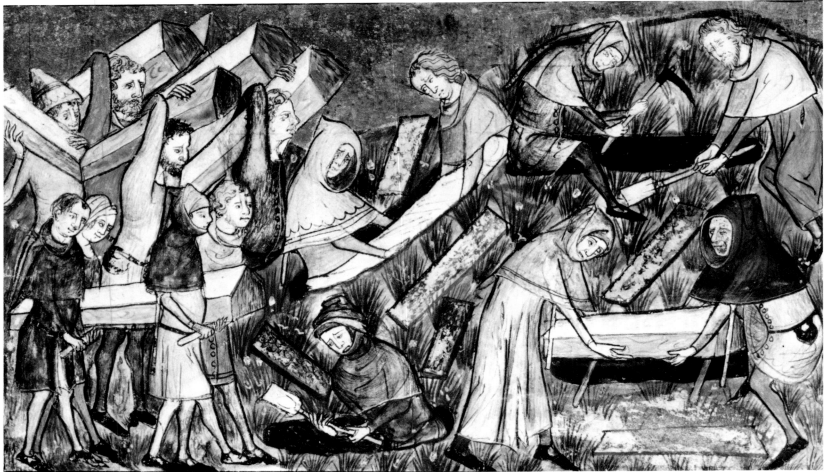

529

southwest Russia. The city of Caffa (present-day Feodosiya), in the southeast Crimea, was besieged by fierce Tartars and appeared to have been saved when the invaders were slaughtered by the plague. However, to disastrous effect, the departing Tartars catapulted corpses of soldiers who had died of plague into the city. (They, too, seemed to understand the meaning of contagion). The Christian defenders may have won the day, but in traveling home nearly all died at sea. Those who did reach Italy started an epidemic which quickly spread throughout Europe (as far away as Greenland), and within a year as much as a quarter of the population of all Europe was stricken. In Marseilles, four-fifths of the inhabitants were claimed within months. Ten years after the plague struck Florence, a superb description was given by Giovanni Boccaccio, author of the *Decameron*:

> In the year of our lord 1348, in Florence, the finest city of all Italy, there occurred a most terrible plague: *either because of the influence of the planets or sent from God as a just punishment for our sins*, it had broken out some years earlier in the East, and after passing from place to place and wreaking incredible havoc along the way had now reached the West where, in spite of all the means that art and human foresight could suggest, such as *keeping the city clear from filth*, and *excluding all suspected people. . . . Different from what it had been in the East, where bleeding from the nose suggests a fatal outcome, here there appeared tumors* in the groins or under the armpits, some as big as a small apple, others like an egg. Afterwards purple spots appeared in most parts of the body . . . the usual messengers of death. To the cure of this disease, *neither the knowledge of medicine nor the power of drugs was of any effect*, whether because the disease was itself fatal or because the physicians, whose number was increased by quacks and woman pretenders, could discover neither cause nor cure, and so few escaped. They generally died the third day after the appearance without fever. . . . The disease grew daily by *being communicated from the sick to the well.* . . . Nor was it [necessary] to converse or even to come near the sick; *even touching their clothes or anything they had touched was sufficient.* . . . The events and similar others caused various fears among those people who survived, all tending to the same cruel and uncharitable end which was to avoid the sick and everything that had been near them. . . . Some felt it best to live temperately . . . but others maintained free living and would deny no passion or appetite they wished to gratify. . . . And the public distress was such that all laws, whether human or divine, were ignored . . . [emphasis added].

Although in typical medieval fashion Boccaccio could not decide between astrological events or divine displeasure as the root evil, he and his society recognized the contagious nature of plague. He obviously also knew that in the East plague was primarily confined to the lungs (pneumonic) and not the lymph glands (bubonic) as in the West.

The general dissolution of societal restraints that resulted from total frustration and impotence in the face of forces beyond control is obvious. Throughout Europe, physicians, when available, protected themselves in elaborate garb and masks with pointed beaks in which they kept vinegar and sweet-smelling potions to counteract the stench of draining buboes and decaying bodies. In Ragusa (modern Dubrovnik), across the Adriatic from Venice, all immigrants were obliged to stay in isolation for thirty and later forty days, giving rise to the term quarantine (from "quaranta," Italian for forty).

Though by all standards the worst, the Black Death was only one of many severe epidemics to traverse Europe in the fourteenth and fifteenth centuries. In 1485 a new disease characterized by severe sweating appeared in England. Known as *sudor anglicus*, it brought death within days. Ironically, it was strong men who were struck down while old women and children were generally spared. A short

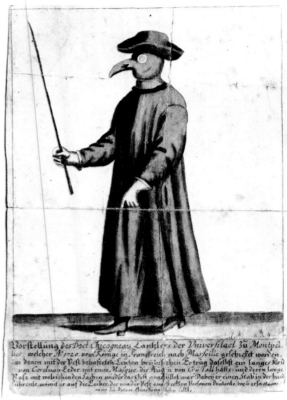

531

528 *German popular print called* Lepers' Banquet at Nuremberg (1493), *reflects the condition of lepers, who were permitted to enter the city only on certain holidays, when they attended Mass, said Confession, took Communion, and feasted before returning to everyday isolation. National Library of Medicine, Bethesda*

529 *Burying plague victims in coffins at Tournai in 1349, before mass burial became the only way to keep up with the deaths, as seen in Gilles le Muisit,* The Plague at Tournai. *Ms. 13076, fol. 24 v., Bibliothèque Royale Albert 1er, Brussels*

530 *The* danse macabre, *a frequent subject of art in the Middle Ages, is done here by Hans Holbein the Younger,* The Dance of Death—The Queen (c. 1540), *as an engraving. Metropolitan Museum of Art, New York*

531 *Doctor shown in this colored engraving (1725) in the distinctive outfit—with sweet-smelling substances carried in the "beak" to combat stench—that was developed to protect against the plague during the Middle Ages. HB 13157, Germanisches National-museum, Nuremberg*

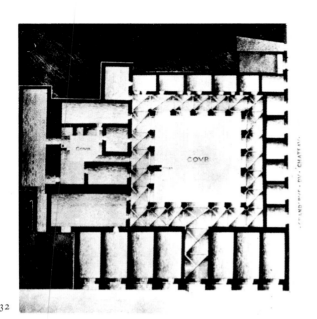

532

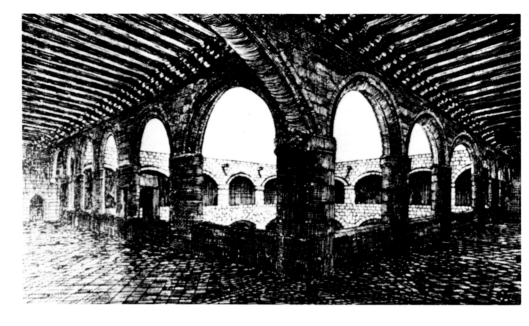

533

532, 533 *Ground-floor plan—showing division into separate rooms for isolation—and engraving of the first-floor gallery and court of the Hospital of the Knights of St. John at Rhodes, as seen in Albert Gabriel's* La Cité de Rhodes, 1310–1522 *(1923). New York Academy of Medicine*

534 *Fourteenth-century manuscript illumination of a Knight Hospitaler, whose order was founded in 1099 to care for epidemic victims during the Crusades. San Spirito 1, fol. 58 v., Archivio Centrale dello Stato, Rome*

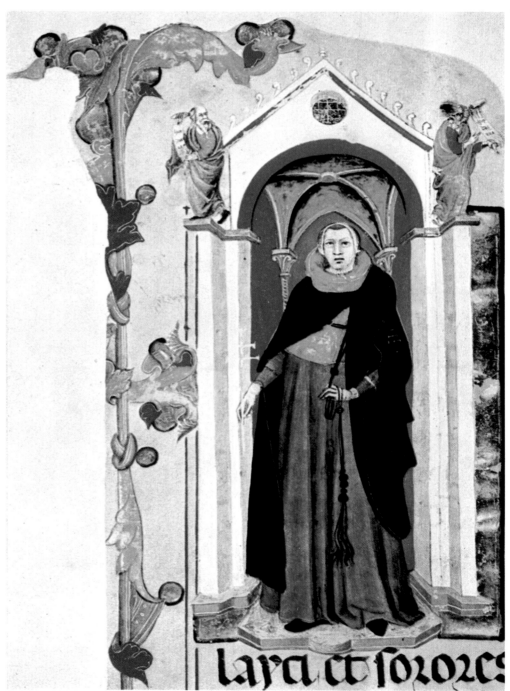

534

time later, outbreaks of the "sweating sickness" appeared in northern Europe, killing many, and, surprisingly, it suddenly vanished forever.

Had contagion been the only affliction to hit Europe at the end of the Middle Ages, things would have been bad enough, but as a result of the Crusades, a growing nationalism, and an influx into the cities, societal controls were already loosening when the Black Death struck. Boccaccio's description of the total collapse of society at the height of the plague eloquently speaks for itself. Afterward, as a markedly reduced population attempted to reconstruct itself, despair and dissolution could hardly be dispelled overnight.

Famines were unusually common, and a malnourished populace was subject not only to decreased resistance to disease but also to social unrest. The tremendous strains upon nearly all the people of Europe at the close of the Middle Ages were more severe on the general population than we can easily imagine. Lacking faith in all institutions, governmental or ecclesiastic, and lacking a tradition of individual closeness with their God, many people, often in desperation, gave up entirely or thrust their futures into the hands of new intercessors. Quacks abounded. Astrology and black magic, always popular, became even more necessary to the confused and terrified masses. Pilgrimages crisscrossed Europe in hopes that certain saintly relics or special blessings of holy water might be the particular mediator of salvation. And yet, could anyone be certain of salvation?

THE SAINTS

God, whose wrath was only too obviously expressed in disease, pestilence, famine, and civil strife, reassumed the stern visage of the Old Testament Jehovah. As the *danse macabre* became a subject of artistic presentation (especially in the countries north of the Alps), even Christ was depicted more often at the Last Judgment than as the Gentle Shepherd looking after his flock. Cults of the Virgin sprang up in hopes of gaining intercession with her son. Whereas in the Dark Ages intercession had been sought from those saints who were physician-martyrs of the early Church, in the Middle Ages there was a virtual explosion of cults devoted to all kinds of saints who might help cure diseases. Some, like St. Elizabeth and St. Roch, were famous for establishing healing centers or for providing medical care during their lifetimes. The popularity of these two wellborn saints was reinforced not only by the many miraculous cures attributed to them but also by their rejection of exalted station for an ascetic life of devotion to the poor and downtrodden. Elizabeth dared to treat lepers, and Roch (or Rocco, as he is known in Italy) cared for the even more dreaded victims of the plague. There are many other examples.

Most saints gained popularity during the decline of the medieval period. In contrast to physician-martyrs like Cosmas and Damian, the newer saints were increasingly associated with relief from a single disease or condition. A high degree of localism existed, and the connection of a saint to a given disease or part of the body often seems tenuous: St. Teresa of Avila was the protector of cardiac victims because an angel had shot an arrow into her heart.

At times even the individual solace offered by the Church was insufficient, and loss of emotional balance among the people of the Middle Ages led to mass panic, frenzy, and hysteria. Processions of flagellants traversed Europe with the firm conviction that their lashings reflected punishments decreed by God and foretold not only the dissolution of society but even the end of the world in the dread Day of Judgment. Another form of mass hysteria was a dancing madness called St. Vitus's dance, especially common in the German countries: men and women, generally peasants, would form circles and dance round and round frantically as if possessed until they fell to the ground, senseless and foaming at the mouth. Some historians consider the two disastrous "Children's Crusades" as further examples of mass hysteria.

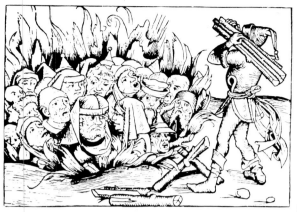

535

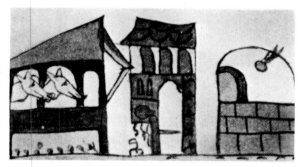

536

535 *Fifteenth-century woodcut from the* Woxo-chronicle *depicting the burning of Jews as scapegoats for the plague.*

536 *Illustrated hygienic precept from the 13th-century* Sachsenspiegel (Heidelberg manuscript), *indicating an awareness of contagion:* "The cattle stall, the baking oven, and the privy should be three feet away from the neighbor's fence." *New York Academy of Medicine*

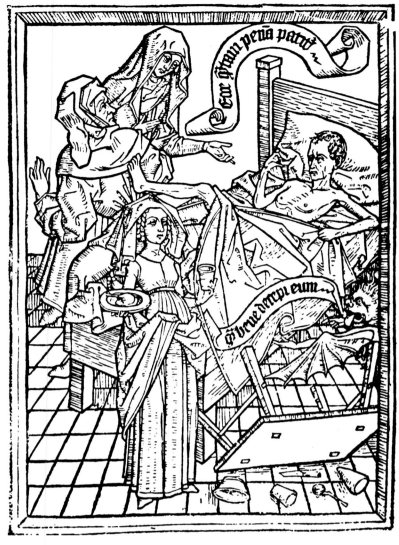

537

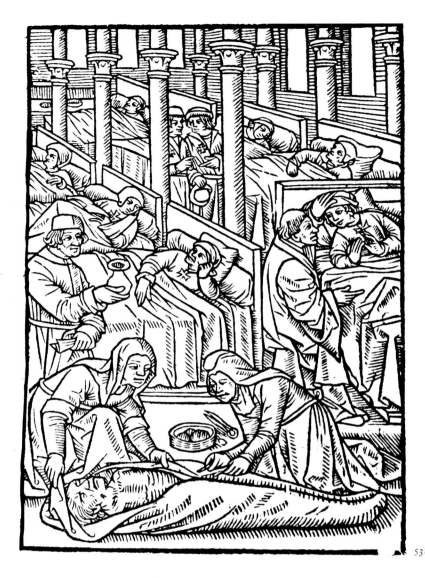

538

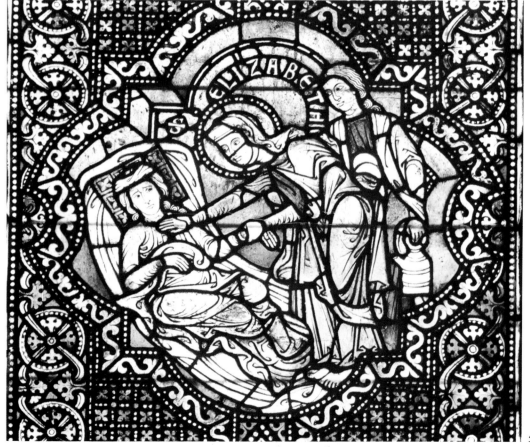

539

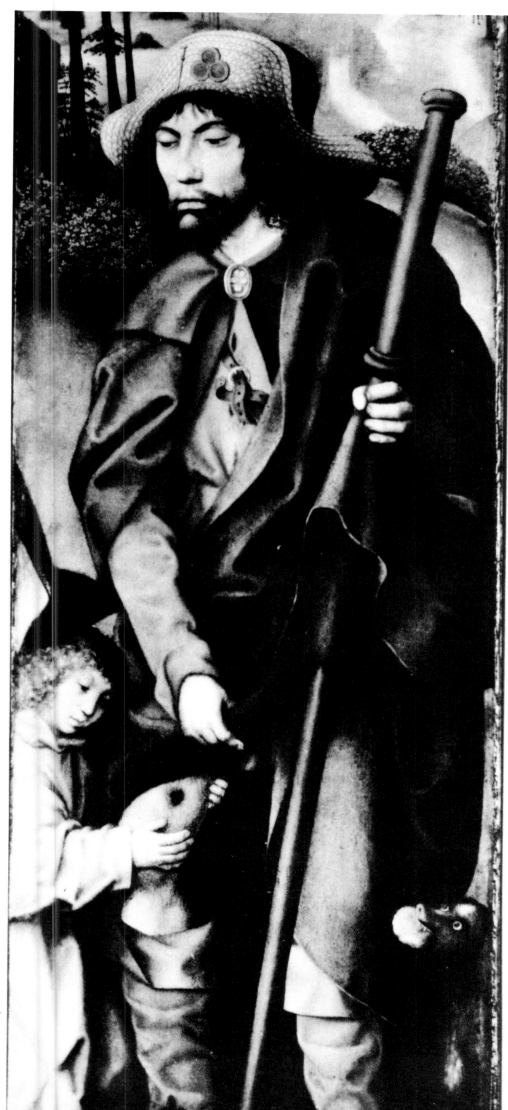

537 *Woodcut entitled* Impatience *from a Nether-landish* ars moriendi *(c. 1450), "the art of dying," in which a dying man tempted by the devil kicks doctor away from bedside, a typical leaf from such manuals of the Middle Ages. British Museum, London*

538 *Woodcut (c. 1500) from Jehan Petit's* Saint-Gelais, le Vergier d'Honneur, *showing everyday details of a medieval hospital: doctor examining urine, patient being comforted, and dead being sewn into shroud. Smith, Kline, and French Collection, Philadelphia Museum of Art*

539 *St. Elizabeth of Hungary seen tending a plague victim in a 13th-century stained glass window in the Choir Church of St. Elizabeth, Marburg*

540 *St. Roch (or Rocco) is shown in this painting (1460) by the Master of Frankfurt with the angel who guarded his recovery from plague and the dog that brought him food. Wallraf-Richartz-Museum, Cologne*

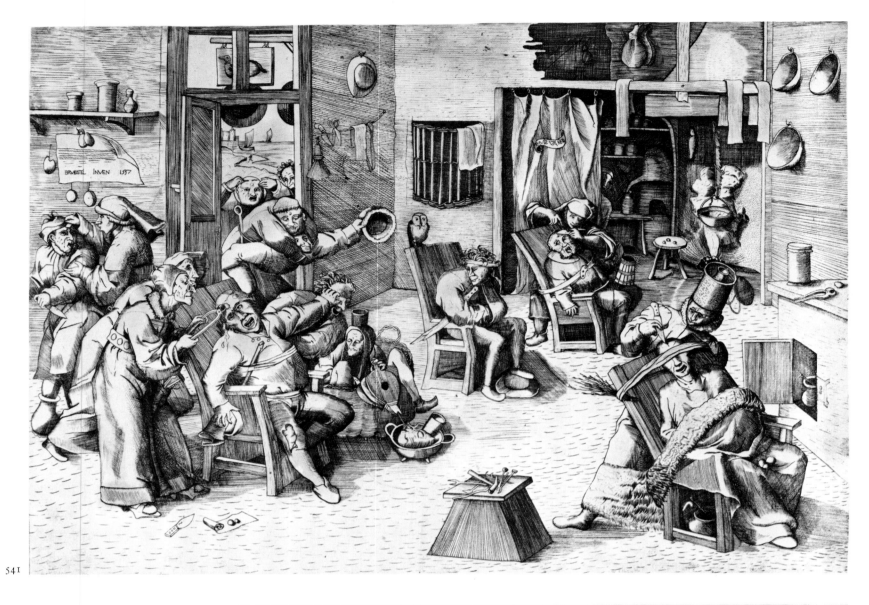

541

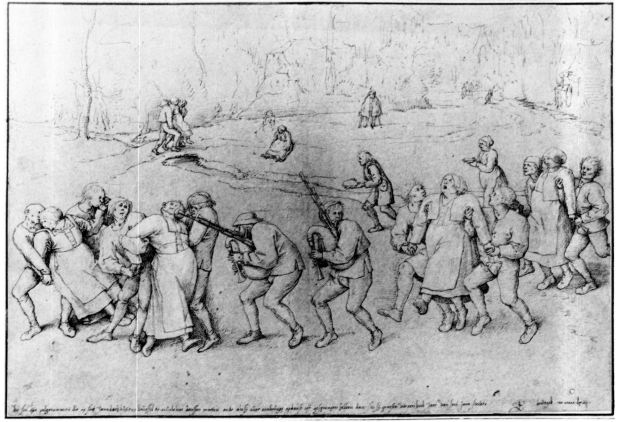

542

The major developments during the Middle Ages in medical disciplines were the regulation of physicians' training and organizations, the development of ideas of contagion and policies of public health, and the establishment of ongoing institutions to provide care, if not cure, for the hopelessly ill, aged, or unwanted.

The general populace had little contact with physicians. Thirteenth-century Paris had only a half dozen doctors in public employ, with little time to spend on individual patients. Even in northern Italy and the southern German countries, where physicians were more numerous, it was rare for a sick person to have a continuing therapeutic relationship with a doctor.

The distinction "doctor" in the Middle Ages was restricted to those with high rank and academic connections who spent more time thinking about disease in philosophical terms than in providing care. When supplied with the particulars of a difficult situation, the doctor would compose a *consilium*, generally at a high fee, but was rarely called upon to carry out his advice. In part, this derives from the later classical period when work with one's hands was considered distinctly inferior to that of the intellect.

Diet was thought extremely important in the treatment of illness, and prescriptions would cover the minutest of details for all sorts of conditions. Perhaps greatest general reliance was placed on broths, milk, and eggs; milk alone was given especial importance in the treatment of consumption. Drugs were used heavily throughout the Middle Ages, and virtually any source might be tapped at one time or another. Plant materials were most often used in the preparation of digestives, laxatives, emetics, diuretics, diaphoretics, styptics, and the like. The most frequently used medication was theriac, which was developed in the ancient world and utilized many ingredients (one of which was viper flesh, thought especially effective against poisons). Numerous imitations, like orvietan, were also used.

Mysticism became more prevalent during the Middle Ages, even as the sciences were more heavily utilized in the development of concepts and treatment of various disease states. Symbolic procedures were thought important not only when used alone (as in the saying of an appropriate chant in the presence of a diseased individual) but even in the preparation of drugs or during surgery. Astrology was also given great weight. Furthermore, with increasing frequency during the later Middle Ages possession by devils was thought to be causally related to specific illness, generally, though not always, with psychological manifestations. For this, only one remedy could possibly be beneficial: exorcism by a priest. Mysticism, however, was extended to many other aspects of medical care. Amulets were commonly used to ward off spirits, and animal parts, especially the genitals, were thought to possess great power. Even the person of the king was thought to be of therapeutic importance, especially in the use of the "royal touch" for the treatment of scrofula (tuberculosis of the neck glands).

Surgery ultimately derived from Greek and Byzantine traditions, at least as transmitted by the Arabists and the schools of Salerno and Montpellier. In general, surgery was limited to wounds, fractures, dislocations, amputations, and the opening of abscesses and fistulas, conditions not easily ignored—at least, not for long. The procedures themselves were generally the most simple and direct possible: cut it off or out. The Arab tradition of using cautery in preference to ligation persisted. Complicated procedures for the most part were eschewed if possible, and the repair of hernias and the removal of bladder stones were uncommon. Suturing (often with human hair for thread) was known but rare. Considerable advances, however, were made in the treatment of eye diseases, as both cataract operations and the use of spectacles became more prevalent.

Although medical treatment in the Middle Ages remains for us a bizarre combination of science and mysticism, this combination was not necessarily problematic to contemporary observers and derived ultimately from a redefinition

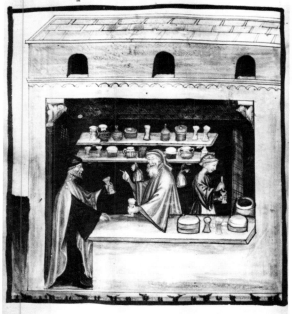

— 543

541 *Pieter Bruegel's engraving* The Extraction of the Stone of Madness (1556–57) *illustrates and satirizes medieval quackery. Bibliothèque Royale Albert 1er, Brussels*

542 *Belief in ritualistic cures is illustrated in Bruegel's drawing* The Pilgrimage of the Epileptics to the Church of St. John at Molenbeek (1569), *where victims of "falling sickness" are spared for a year from their affliction if they manage to cross a certain bridge. Graphische Sammlung Albertina, Vienna*

543 *Interior of a 13th-century pharmacy, from the* Tacuinum Sanitatis, *showing* triaca *(theriac) being dispensed. Series Nov. 2644, Österreichische Nationalbibliothek, Vienna*

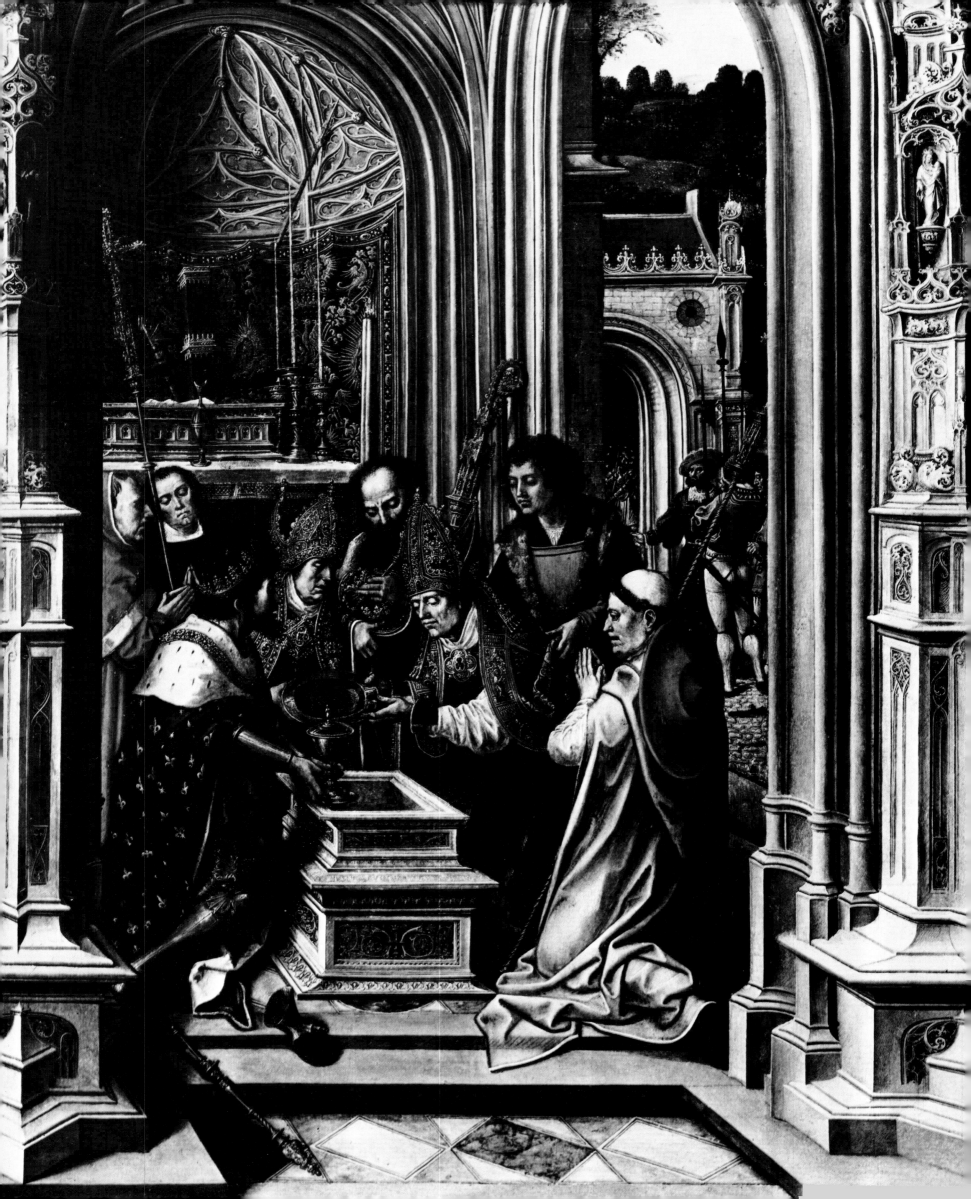

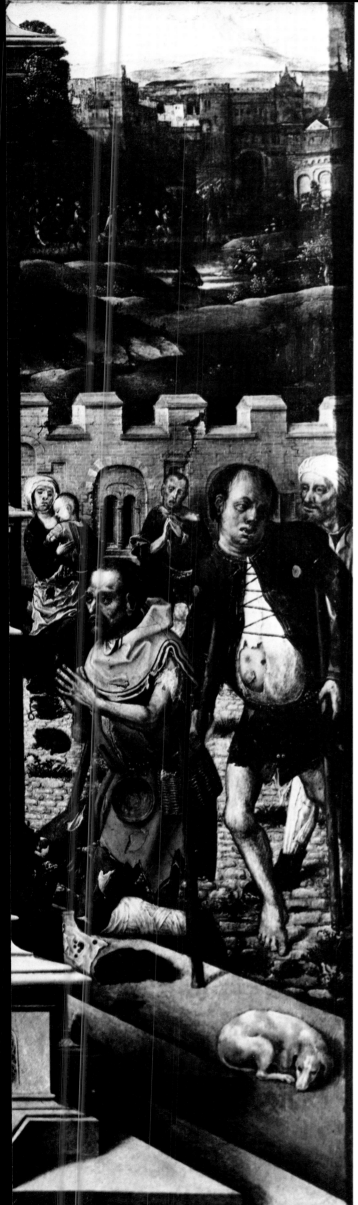

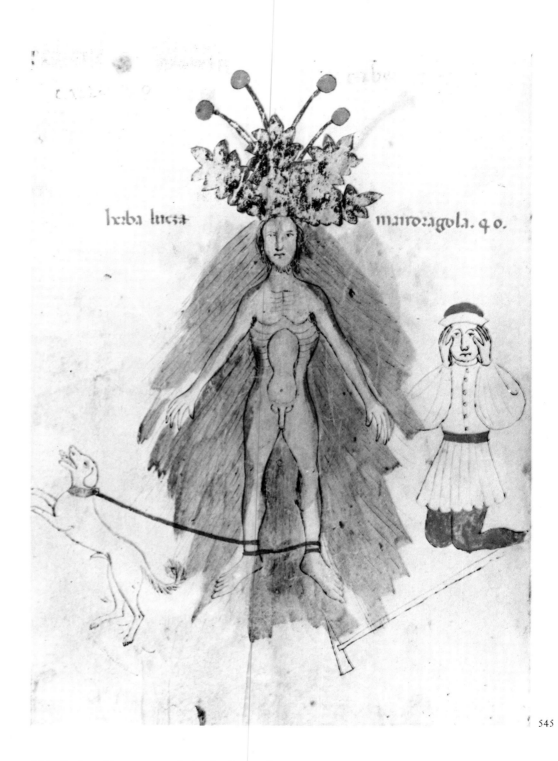

545

544 *Early–16th–century painting by Bernard van Orley showing a king taking part in a religious ceremony before applying the "king's touch" to heal scrofulous suppliants. Museo Civico di Torino*

545 *Fifteenth–century conception of the mandrake root, sometimes used as an anesthetic by Greek, Roman, and Arabic doctors. Believed to kill (through its screams) anyone pulling it from the ground, the mandrake was supposed to be uprooted by dogs. Ms. 130 E. 31, 211, fol. 20, Biblioteca Universitaria, Pavia*

544

357

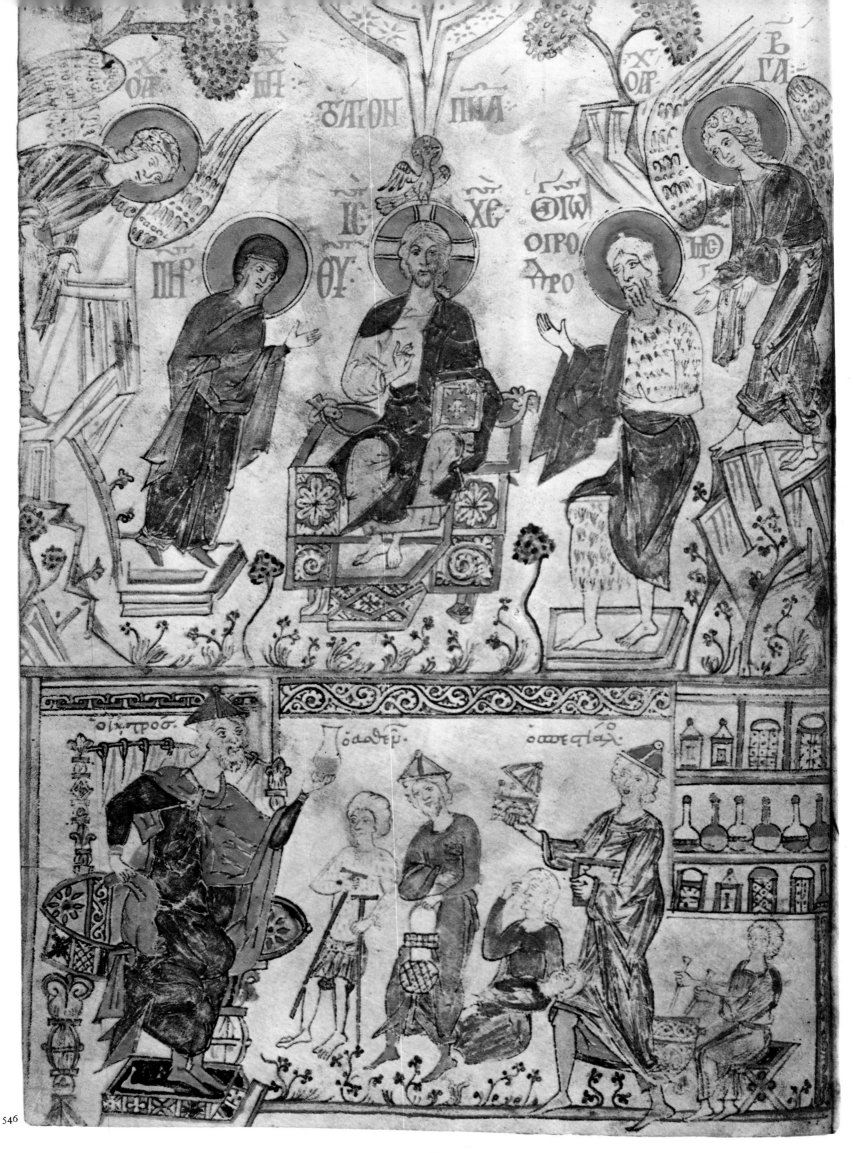

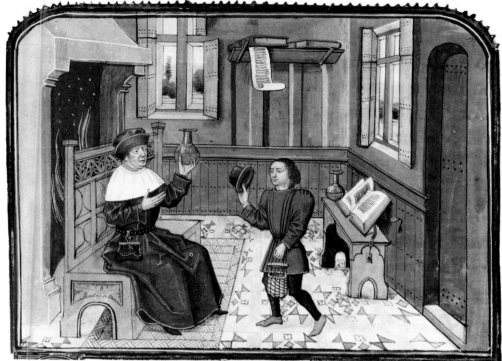

547

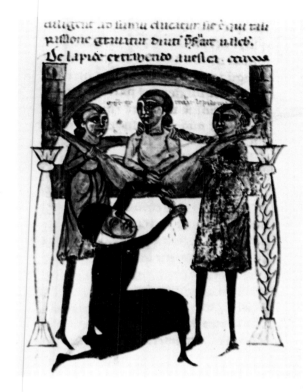

549

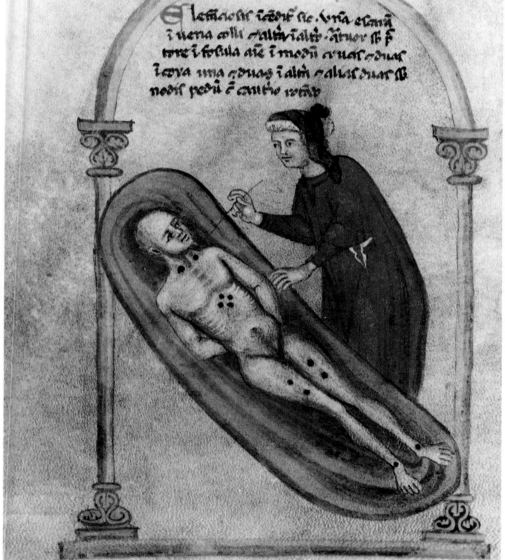

548

546 *Miniature from the 14th-century Greek manuscript* Antidotarium *of Nicholas Myrepsos, picturing a physician in a pharmacy examining urine while a cripple and a woman with a sick child wait their turns. Ms. grec 2243, fol. 10 v., Bibliothèque Nationale, Paris*

547 *Illustration from the 15th-century* Epistle of Othea *by Christine de Pisan, in which a physician examines a patient's urine brought by a messenger in a special carrying case, showing the reliance on uroscopy for diagnosis. Ms. 9392, fol. 42 v., Bibliothèque Royale Albert 1er, Brussels*

548 *Cauterization points indicated for the treatment of elephantiasis (marked swelling) as seen in this 14th-century manuscript illustration. Ms. anon. Rawl. c. 328, fol. 9 v., Bodleian Library, Oxford*

549 *Illustration in the 14th-century manuscript* Rolandus Parmensis Chirurgia, *showing an operation for removing bladder stones, a procedure with a low rate of success at the time. Ms. 1382, Biblioteca Casanatense, Rome*

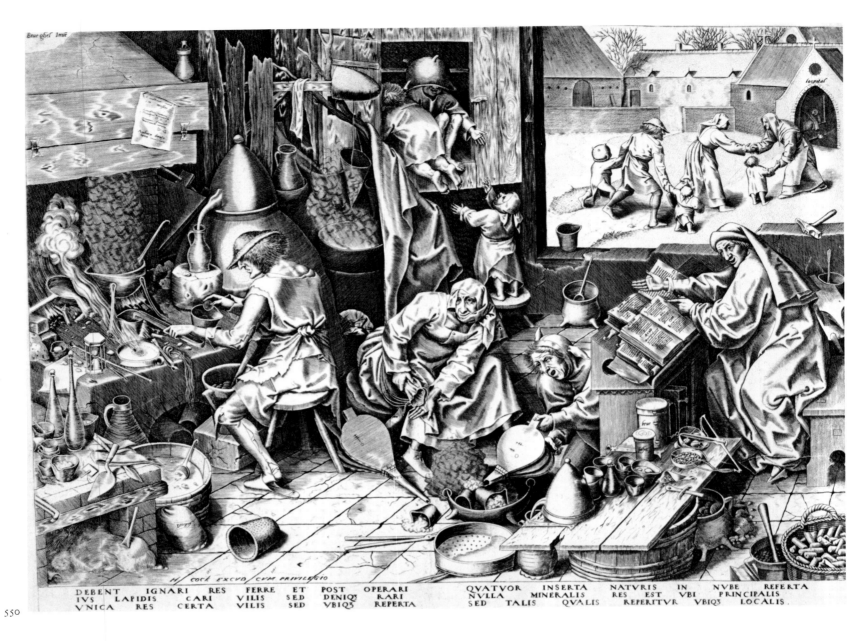

DEBENT IGNARI RES FERRE ET POST OPERARI QVATVOR INSERTA NATVRIS IN NVBE REFERTA
IVS LAPIDIS CARI VILIS SED DENIQ3 RARI NVLLA MINERALIS RES EST VBI PRINCIPALIS
VNICA RES CERTA VILIS SED VBIQ3 REPERTA SED TALIS QVALIS REPERITVR VBIQ3 LOCALIS.

550

550 *Engraving of an alchemist's shop done by Pieter Bruegel the Elder in 1558. The linking of alchemy, pharmacy, and astrology in the West was similar to the practices in Arabic countries. Bibliothèque Royale Albert 1ᵉʳ, Brussels*

551 *With rare access to formalized medical care, most people in the Middle Ages relied on folk-healers and, when necessary, devices such as the primitive crutches shown in the 12th-century* Topographia Hibernica *of Gerald of Wales. Ms. Roy. 13. B. VIII, fol. 30 v., British Museum, London*

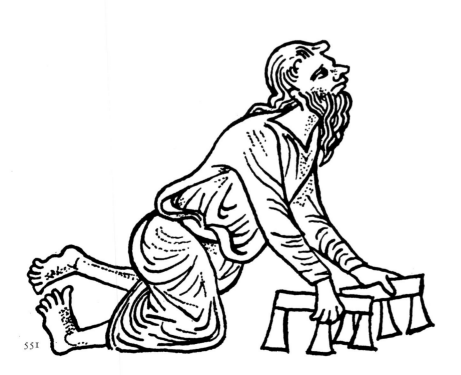

551

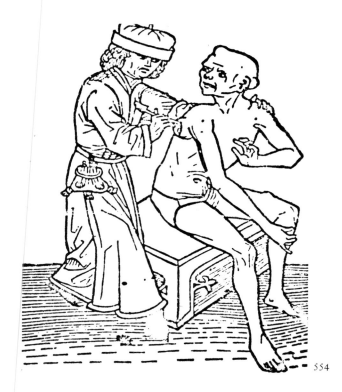

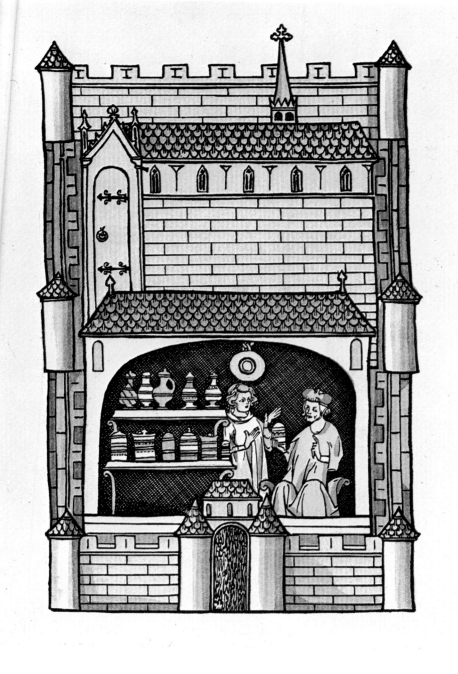

552 *Woodcut (c. 1490) showing a physician discussing the compounding of his prescriptions with a pharmacist in his pharmacy. National Library of Medicine, Bethesda*

553 *Astrologer shown, in German manuscript Henach Sagt . . . (1464), diagnosing and prognosticating by studying positions of the stars. Ms. CR 4.6, fol. 37, by permission of the Astronomer Royal of Scotland, Crawford Collection, Royal Observatory, Edinburgh*

554 *Fifteenth-century woodcut of surgeon lancing a plague-caused bubo, which probably only increased the likelihood of spreading the disease. World Health Organization, Geneva*

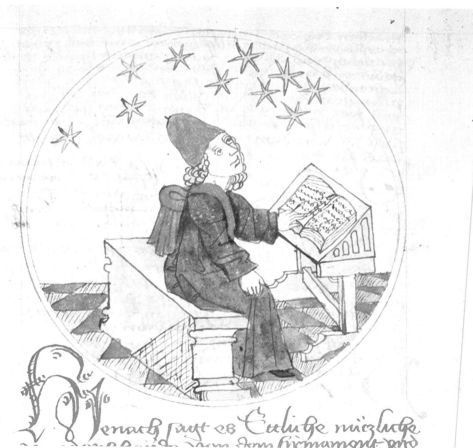

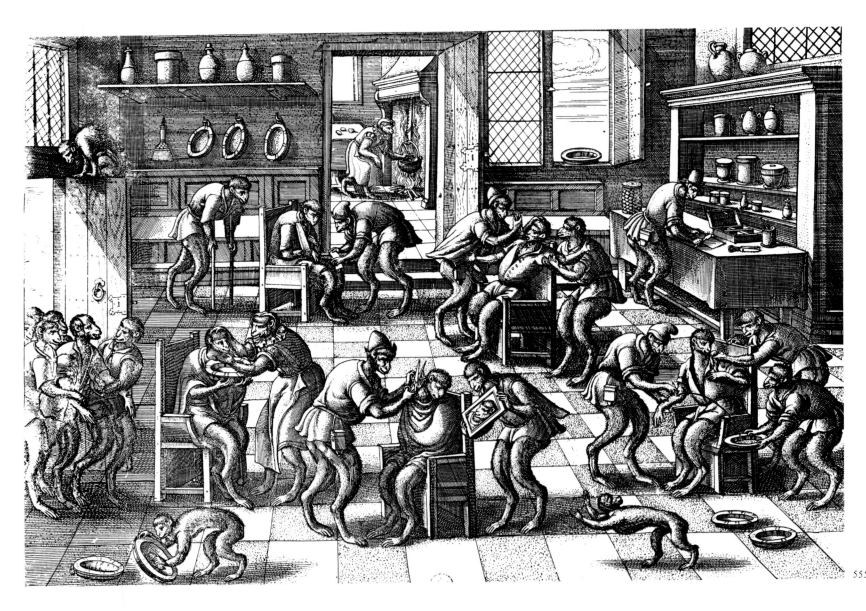

555

555 *Sixteenth-century engraving satirizing doctors and illustrating the wide variety of duties performed by barbers: bloodletting, tooth-pulling, hair-cutting, wound treatment, etc. Ms. RF 1 rés., fol. 66, Bibliothèque Nationale, Paris*

of the classical conception of humors. It didn't make much difference why there was an excess of a certain quality—or substance—in a portion of the body; it was more important to get rid of the imbalance. If an invocation or a purgative did the job, so much the better for not requiring anything more severe. But at times this would not be sufficient, and more drastic procedures were utilized. The most popular of these was bloodletting. Not unexpectedly, a physician might advise venesection but would rarely think of actually performing it. The surgeons who did this were thought unfit to receive any training beyond the obvious. Slowly, however, during the later medieval period, surgeons began to branch into two groups: those with greater education and those increasingly identified with the barbers. (It is difficult for us today to fathom the wide range of concerns allocated to barbers in the past—not just the care of locks and beard but also tooth-pulling, minor operations, the setting of bones and the like.) In France, the distinction between these two varieties of surgeons was given not only functional but legal definition.

If the pharmacy can be looked upon as the medieval workshop of the physician and of those whose vocations derived from the doctor, the public bath was the environment of the surgeon, although in the reliance of both upon diet a certain intermingling was obvious. There was much variety in the public baths. Many had tubs and vats, others often utilized steam therapeutically. Some baths were not restricted to one sex and gave bathing a notoriety which led to their being closed down. Often after a bath treatment, bloodletting would be performed, and the results were thought to be preferable to either being done separately.

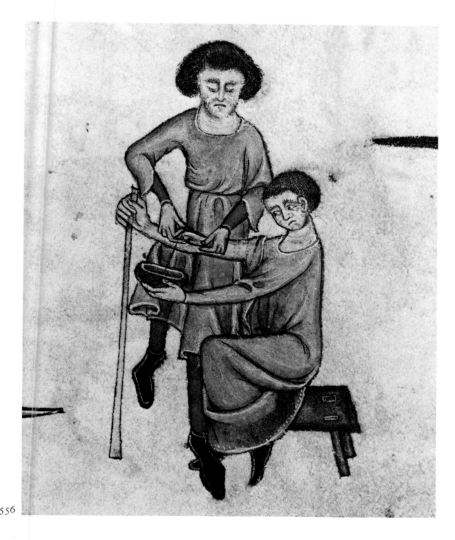

556

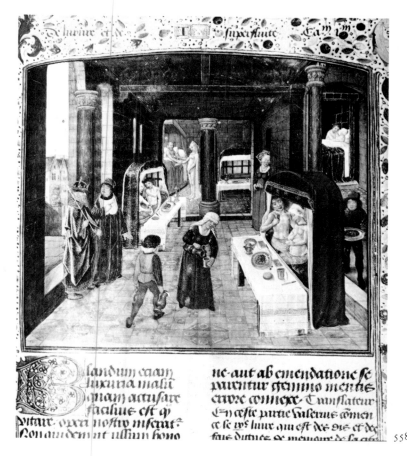

558

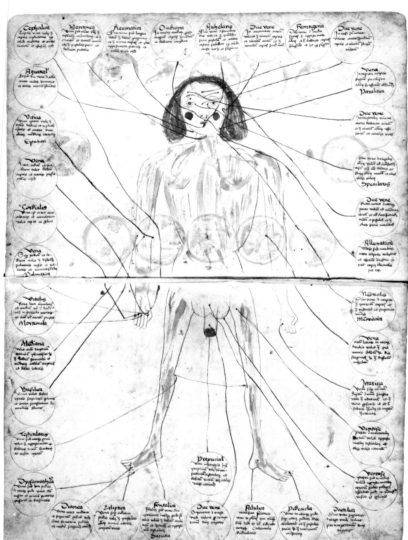

557

556 *Illustration from the* Luttrell Psalter (1340), *showing a barber-surgeon bleeding a patient who steadies his arm with a "barber pole."* Add. Ms. 42130, fol. 61, British Library, London

557 *Anatomically realistic chart in 15th-century manuscript showing points for bloodletting.* Ms. pal. lat. 1709, fols. 44 v. and 45 r., Biblioteca Apostolica Vaticana, Rome

558 *Illustration from the 15th-century* Deeds and Memorable Words of Valere Maxime, *showing mixed bathing in a public bathhouse, a practice leading to excesses and the eventual closing of such establishments.* Stadt- und Bezirksbibliothek, Leipzig

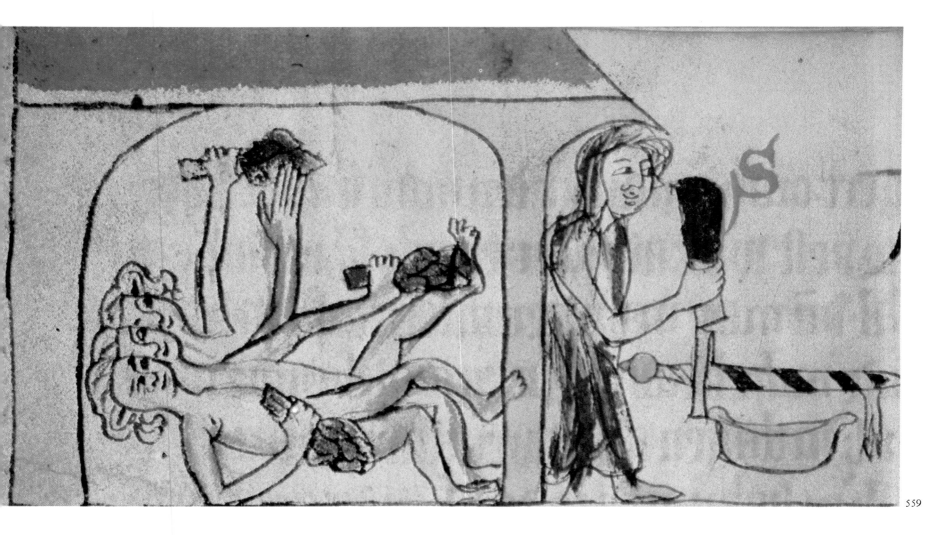

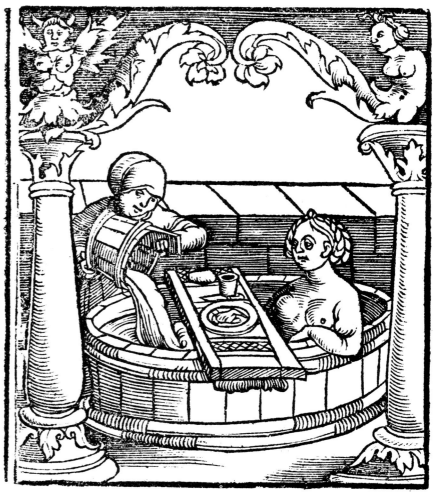

559 *Miniature from the 13th-century* Sachsenspiegel, *showing bathers massaging themselves with leaves and a barber, identified by his pole, ready to perform bloodletting, a service frequently combined with bathing. Universitätsbibliothek, Heidelberg*

560 *Woodcut from Brunschwig,* Buch zu Distillieren (1500), *in which a lady is seen dining in her thermal bath. Öffentliche Bibliothek der Universität Basel*

561 *Fourteenth-century miniature from Pietro da Eboli's* De Virtutis Balneorum Puteolanis, *showing banqueters and bathers and extolling the facilities at Pozzuoli. Ms. 1474, fol. 7, Biblioteca Angelica, Rome*

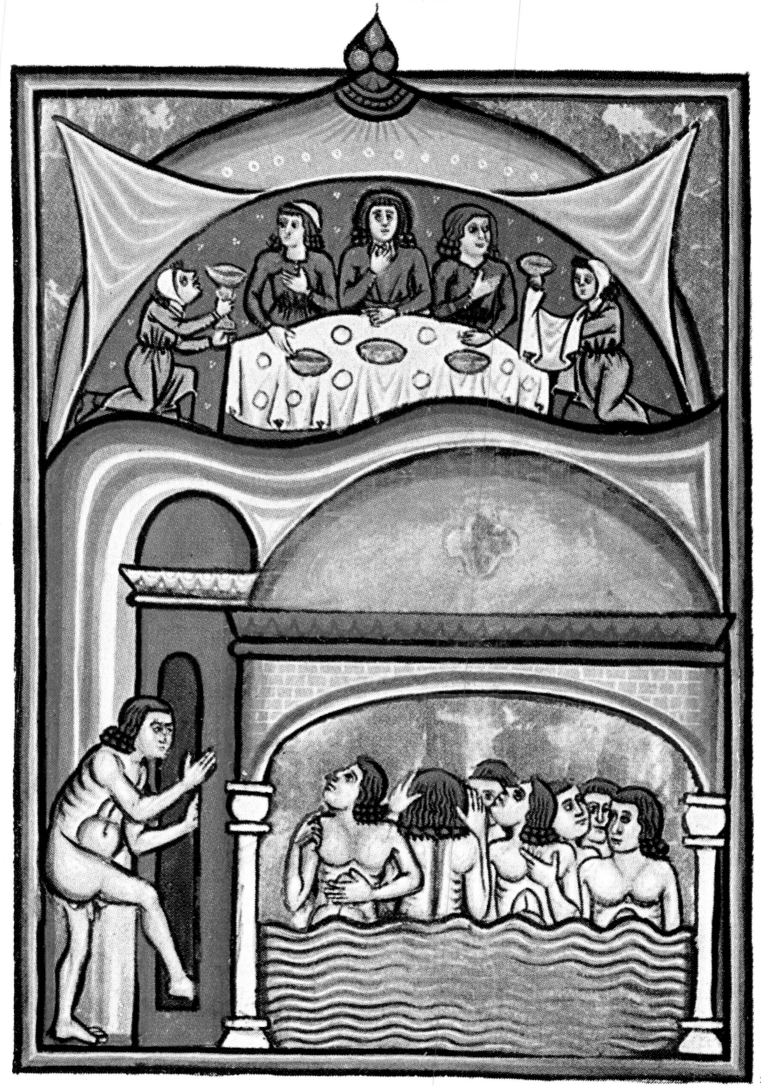

THE
FIFTEENTH
AND SIXTEENTH
CENTURIES

The Renaissance

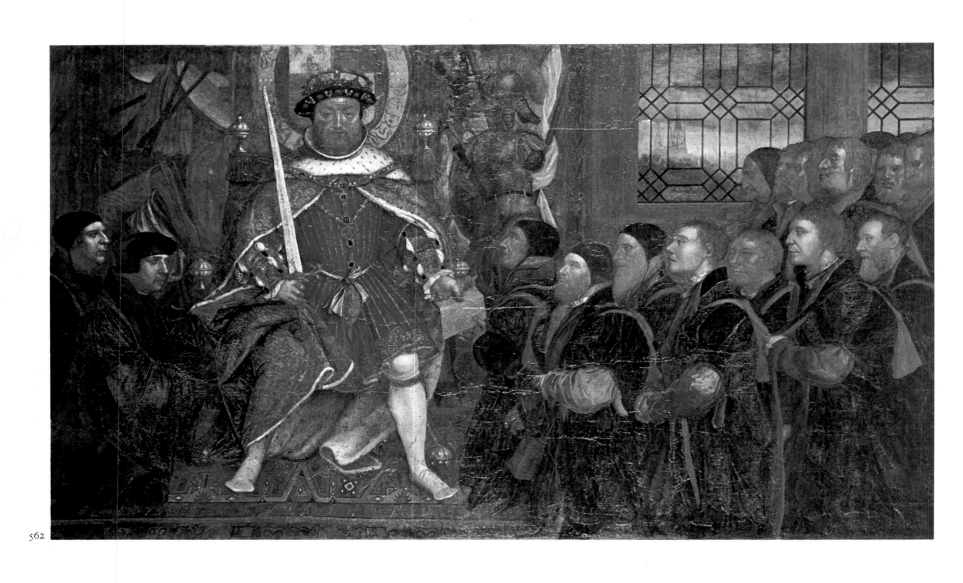

562

Even in the desperate depths of the Middle Ages, social, economic, and cultural events were underway which would burst forth in the mid-fifteenth century in that unparalleled phenomenon known as the Renaissance.

Giorgio Vasari (1511–74), Florentine artist, architect, and man of letters, dubbed the period a *rinàscita*, or rebirth, because of a common belief that the major force in its evolution was a return to the cultural priorities of ancient Rome and Greece. Although this was important, especially since the ancient civilizations were being looked at directly through their original writings, architecture, and works of art, other factors were also crucial. The invention of printing from movable metal type permitted the general dissemination of information at markedly reduced costs. The development of trade resulting from the Crusades and the establishment of local industry led to the creation of a money economy, and sophisticated speculative ventures were therefore possible in the private sector. The discovery of sea routes to India and the Americas suddenly opened up a vastly enlarged world with immense potential for exploration and exploitation.

Whereas these developments initially increased social and political tensions in most of Europe, in northern Italy conditions were ideal for their positive evolution. The political stalemate between the papacy and the Holy Roman emperors had permitted the development of several relatively independent city-states whose increasingly industrial and mercantile economies resulted in trading and banking empires which embraced the entire continent. The Turkish capture of Constantinople in 1453 led to an influx of Greek refugee scholars into Italy, greater than to any other country, and the universities of northern Italy, especially of Bologna, Padua, Ferrara, and Pavia, attracted students and scholars from all over Europe. Movable-type printing, invented just north of the Alps, was quickly introduced into Italy, and before long the publishing houses of Venice and Florence were among the best in all Europe. Thus, in the latter half of the fifteenth century, this constellation of social, economic, and political conditions in northern Italy encouraged a veritable burst of intellectual and creative activity which was further accentuated by the appearance of many individuals with excellent and even superlative talents.

The Medical Humanists

The earliest medical humanists tended to live in or, at least, to have studied at the universities of northern Italy, and the term "Renaissance man" has much historical justification. The first "modern" physicians were often also well-versed in physics and astronomy, like Copernicus (1473–1543), partly because of a continued interest in magic and astrology. Especially after the arrival of the Greek scholars from Constantinople, Italian philosophy took on a different, neoplatonic cast, and Aristotelian thought was in decline. Directly transferred to medicine, this meant that the study of Hippocrates and open-minded observation of natural phenomena were ascendant and Galenism and Scholasticism were increasingly out of favor. Until the controversy generated by the Reformation and Counter Reformation stamped out ease of intellectual discourse, the academic world of northern Italy was not only tolerant of new ideas but also extremely cosmopolitan. Nearly all the major courts and cities of Europe sent their finest to Italy for training and advanced education. This may have been just as important as printing to the victory of empiricism and (later) scientific experimentalism over Scholasticism.

Niccolò Leoniceno (1428–1524), one of the early medical humanists, taught medicine at the universities of Padua, Bologna, and Ferrara. "An elegant Latinist," he translated the *Aphorisms* of Hippocrates and worked on the writings of Galen. When he noted some five hundred botanical errors in Pliny's *Natural History*, Leoniceno refused to follow the humanist philological tradition of his day and he published them. The suggestion that this giant of ancient days might have erred

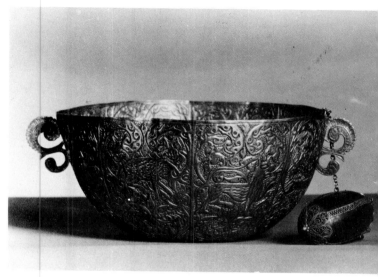

563

562 Henry VIII in 1540 Handing to Thomas Vicary the Act of Union between the Barbers and Surgeons of London, *by Hans Holbein the Younger. Convoked as the Masters and Governors of the Mystery and Commonalty of the Barbers and Surgeons of London, this group later became the Royal College of Surgeons of England. Royal College of Surgeons of England, London*

563 *Early-16th-century Portuguese gold basin with mounted bezoar stone, originally in the treasury of the Hapsburgs. This bezoar stone was prized for its magical properties and its ability to cure diseases. Kunsthistorisches Museum, Vienna*

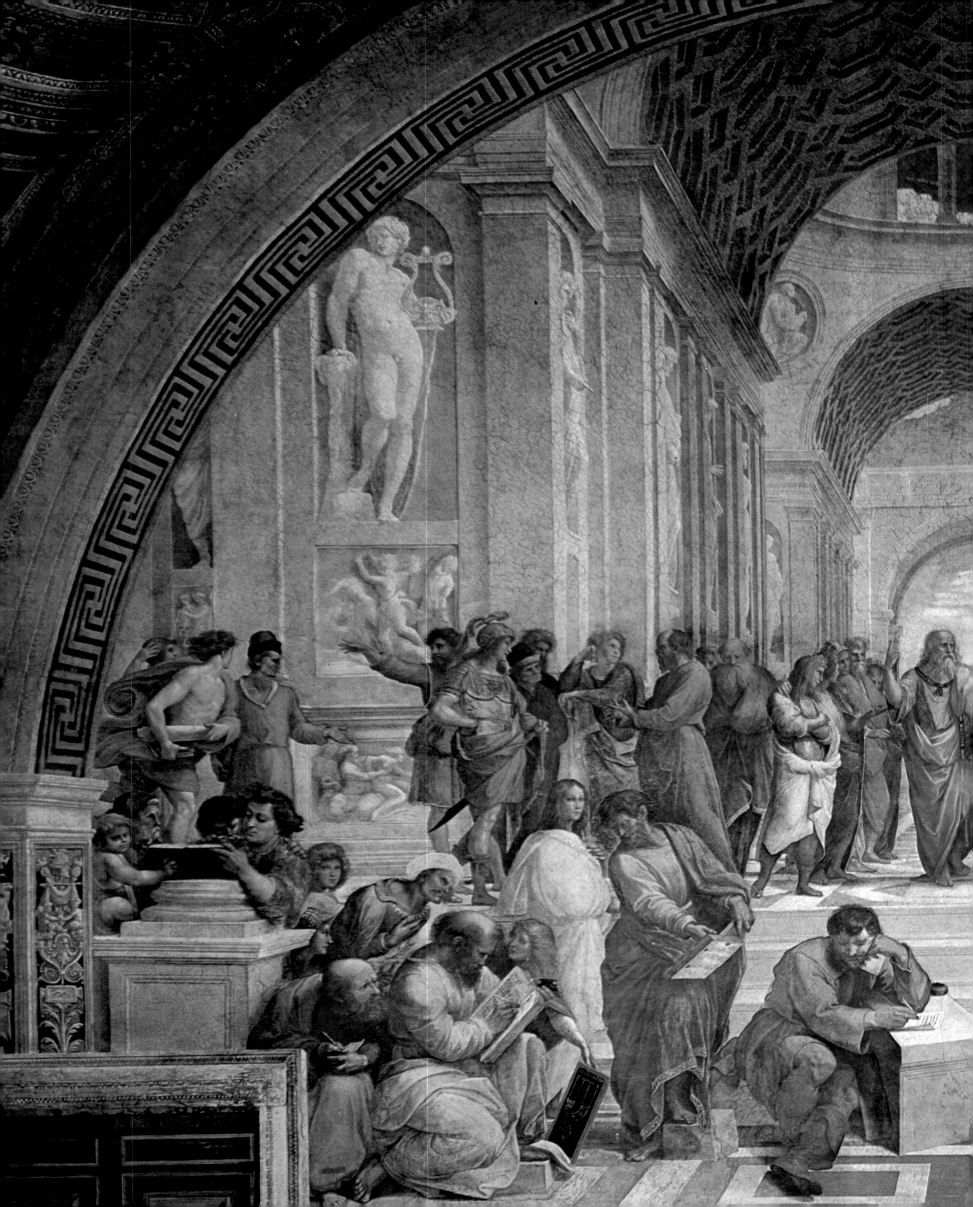

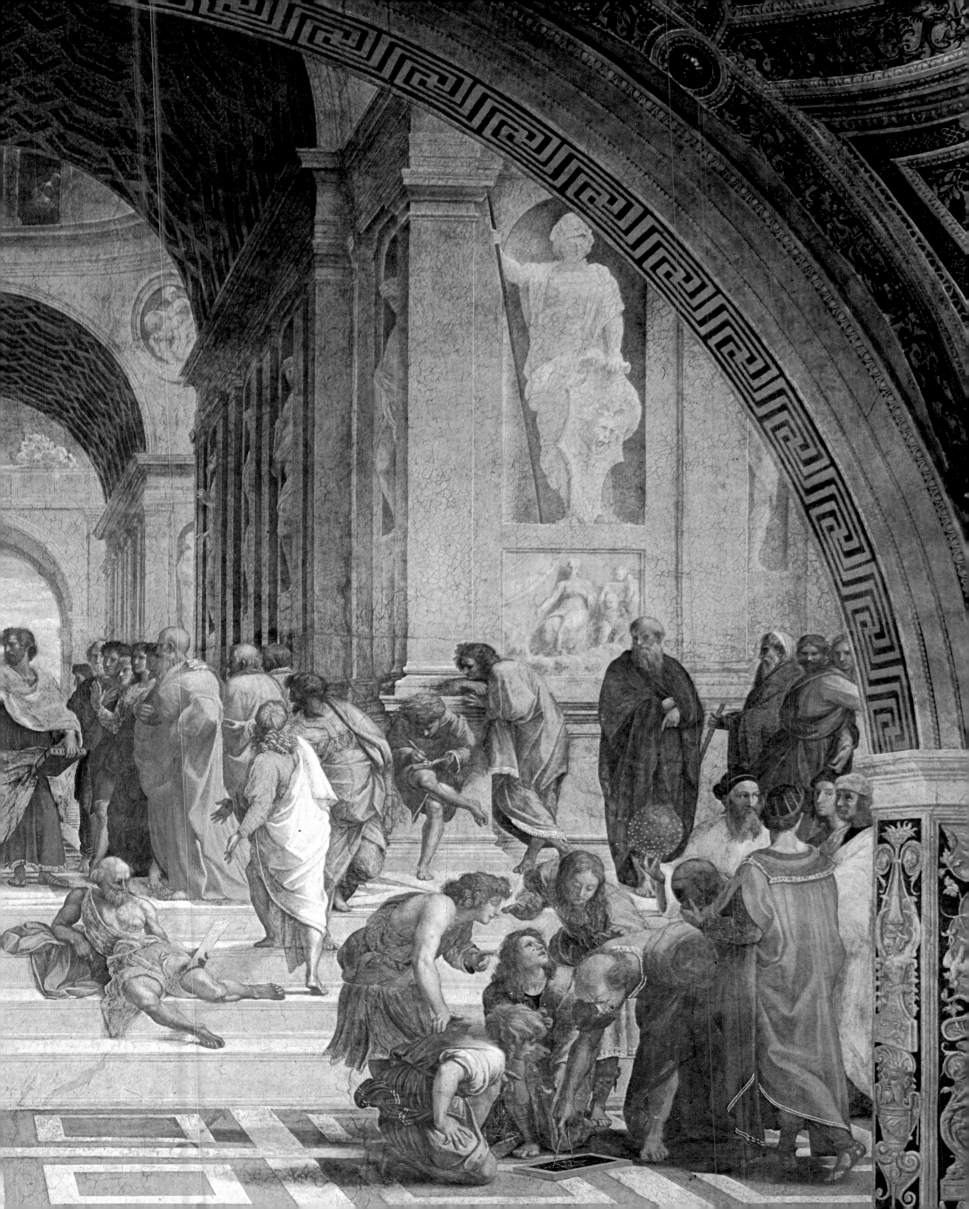

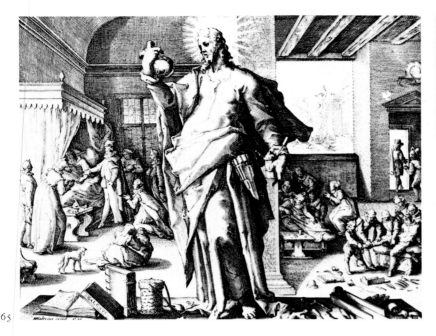

565

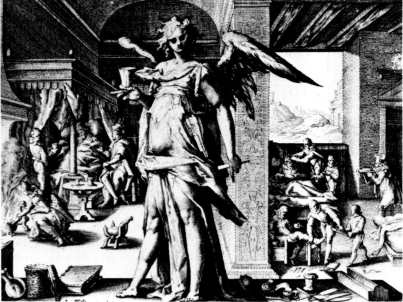

566

564 (*Preceding spread*) Raphael's *fresco* The School of Athens (*1510–11*) *was painted in response to the remarkable intellectual and artistic ferment in Renaissance Italy. This ideal group of philosophers and teachers included Socrates, Plato, Aristotle, Zoroaster, Ptolemy, Euclid, Anaxagoras, Heraclitus, and Epicurus. Stanza della Segnatura, Vatican Palace, Rome*

565–568 *Suite of engravings known as the* Allegory of the Medical Profession (*1587*) *by the School of Hendrik Goltzius. A god to the patient when he seeks help, the physician becomes, as the patient gets well, a devil who asks payment for his work. Smith, Kline, and French Collection, Philadelphia Museum of Art*

569 *Astrology was still closely tied in with medicine and the success of treatment in the Renaissance, as seen in this zodiac illustration from Johannes de Ketham's* Fasciculus Medicinae (*1522*). *Biblioteca Casanatense, Rome*

570 *From Biblical times onward, the physician was expected to be compassionate and helpful, as presented in this engraving by Crispin de Passe the Elder called* To Succor the Sick. *Smith, Kline, and French Collection, Philadelphia Museum of Art*

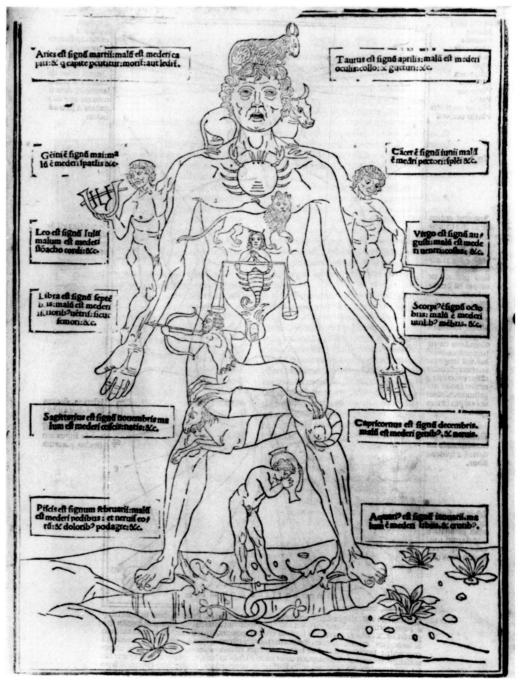

569

372

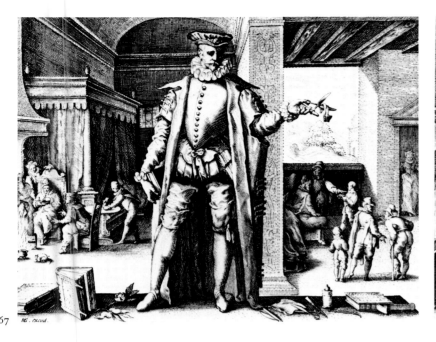

567

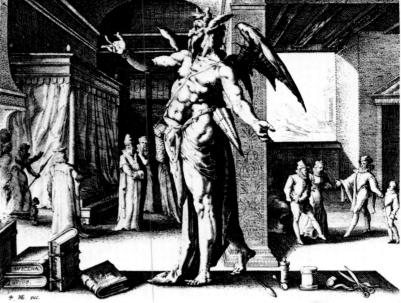

568

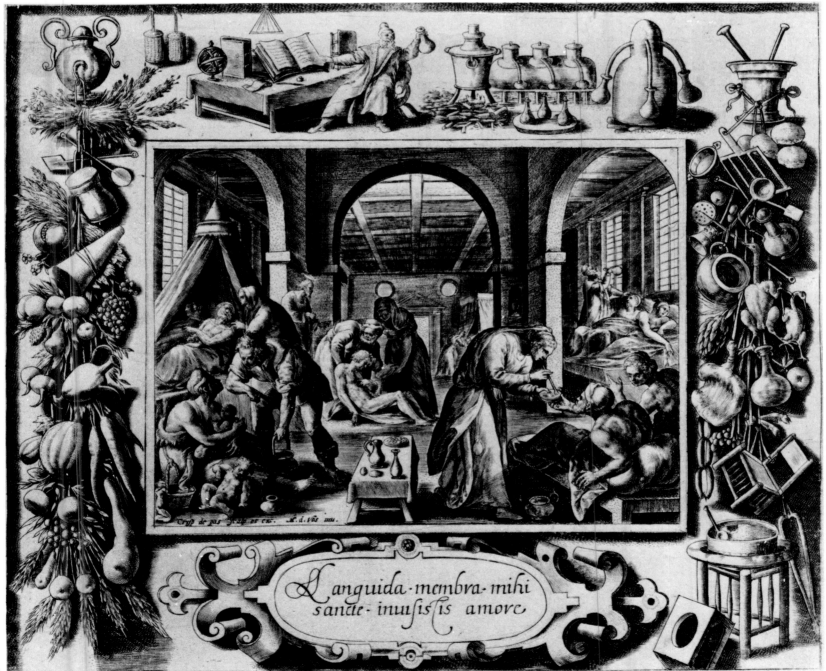

Languida membra mihi
sancte inuisistis amore

570

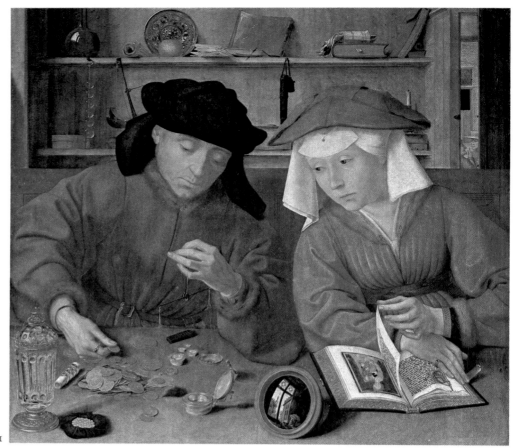

571

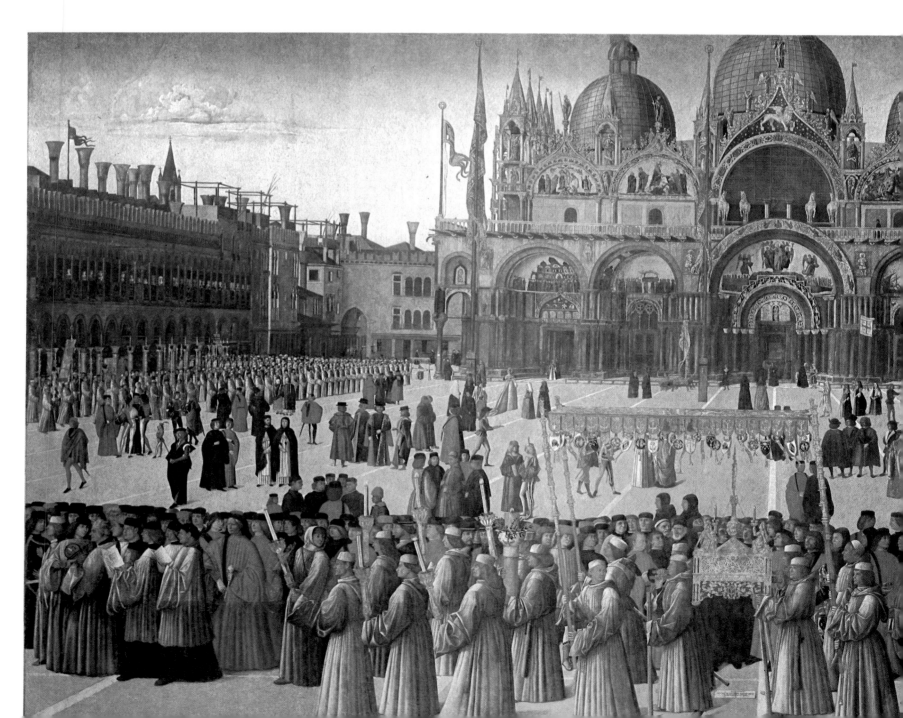

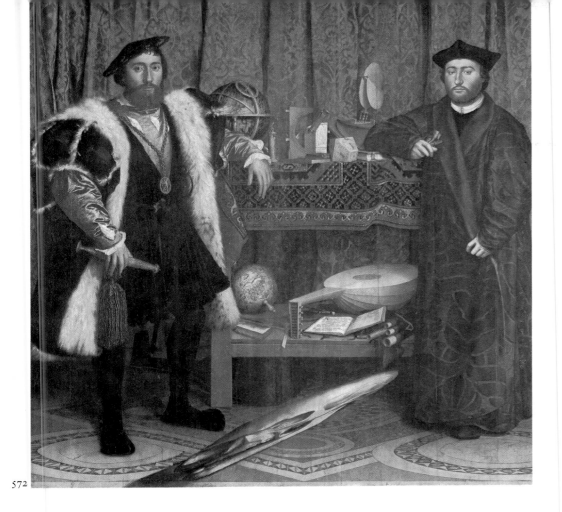

572

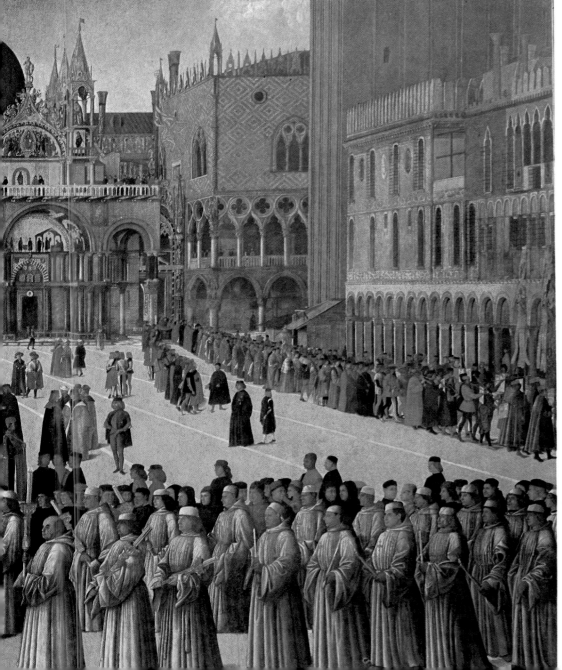

573

571 *Burgeoning commerce resulting from new trade routes and the discovery of America led to the creation of a money economy—evoked here in Quentin Metsys's* The Money Changer and His Wife *(1514)—and it enhanced the exchange of knowledge.* The Louvre, Paris

572 *With the invention of printing from movable type, the spread of scientific information quickened, and cultural exchanges became more frequent, as epitomized by Hans Holbein the Younger in* The Ambassadors *(1533).* National Gallery, London

573 *Venice, in the late 15th century, glittered with pomp, wealth, and intellectual ferment, as seen in this painting by Gentile Bellini of a procession in the Piazza San Marco.* Gallerie dell'Accademia, Venice

574 *Paracelsus, painted by Jan van Scorel, was a gigantic personality who introduced metals into pharmacology and taught reliance on one's own observations, not ancient authorities. He also subscribed to astrology and the occult sciences. The Louvre, Paris*

threatened the early humanists and showed how many attributes of medieval thinking outlived the Middle Ages.

Thomas Linacre (1460?–1524) also belonged to the early Renaissance period of philological study. Educated at Padua and Oxford, he was later physician to the English kings Henry VII and Henry VIII. Because of his Latin translations of Galen's treatises on hygiene, therapeutics, temperaments, natural faculties, the pulse, and semiology, he was responsible for the transmission back to England of an awareness of the importance of a critical and *accurate* reading of the authorities, earning him the title of "restorer of learning" in England.

Theophrastus Bombastus von Hohenheim, or Paracelsus (1493–1541), shirked neither challenging the ancients nor suggesting chemical therapeutics. Born near Zürich, he obtained his doctor's degree under Leoniceno at Ferrara. He also developed considerable interest in alchemy, astrology, and the occult sciences. With a reverence for Hippocrates, Paracelsus was a wandering spirit and, except for brief stays in Freiburg, Strassburg, and Basel where several remarkable cures gained him considerable fame, he journeyed about the German world quarreling with those in authority, especially for their blind and total acceptance of the classics. He sharply broke with tradition by teaching not in Latin but in the vernacular. More revolutionary was his growing tendency to subject the ancients (and their followers as well) to an unmitigatedly hostile criticism. To the same extent that he angered those in authority, he attracted the young and those in training. He took his considerable interest in alchemy to heart and, in applying this to the treatment of disease, earned for himself the title "father of pharmacology"—in spite of his limited pharmaceutical arsenal and his highly medieval pathophysiology wherein diseases were caused by influences of the stars and planets upon the "astral body" of man.

Jean Fernel (1497–1588) was trained at Paris and proved that not all medical progress during the Renaissance was directly dependent upon northern Italy. Though much of his time was somewhat reluctantly filled in treating the royal family, he did complete a masterly work entitled *A Universal Medicine*, in which he for the first time divided the study of medicine into the now standard disciplines of physiology (the normal functioning of the body), pathology (the abnormal functioning of the body), and therapeutics (those things which might resolve abnormalities). He also joined the debate as to whether syphilis and gonorrhea were different diseases or two forms of the same disease. Though most likely found in Europe at low incidence since primeval times, the first major epidemic of syphilis occurred among the sailors returning from Columbus's first voyage to the New World. The disease was then passed on to Spanish soldiers fighting for the king of Naples and finally reached the French troops of Charles VIII who had forced Naples to surrender after a three weeks' siege. As Charles's army returned north, the Italian peninsula was inundated with syphilis, which became known as the *morbo gallico*, or French disease. Girolamo Fracastoro of Verona (1483–1553), a poet, classicist, physicist, geologist, astronomer, and pathologist in addition to being a physician, gained fame through his *Syphilis sive Morbus Gallicus* (1530), a Latin poem drawing heavily on Ovid which not only gave the "French disease" its more general name but also suggested its venereal spread. His later treatise, *De Contagione* (1546), stated with marked clarity the modern theory of infection by invisible germs, which he called *seminaria*, except that he may not have viewed these contagious elements as living organisms. As the two venereal diseases syphilis and gonorrhea continued to overrun Europe, much interest was devoted to their nature and causation but also to their treatment. The ancients' lack of consideration of these diseases was bothersome, for it not only suggested that there were things of importance which had escaped the notice of classical authorities but which also required independent thinking. Fernel was the first to suggest that gonorrhea and syphilis were quite separate illnesses, sharing only a common mode of transmission.

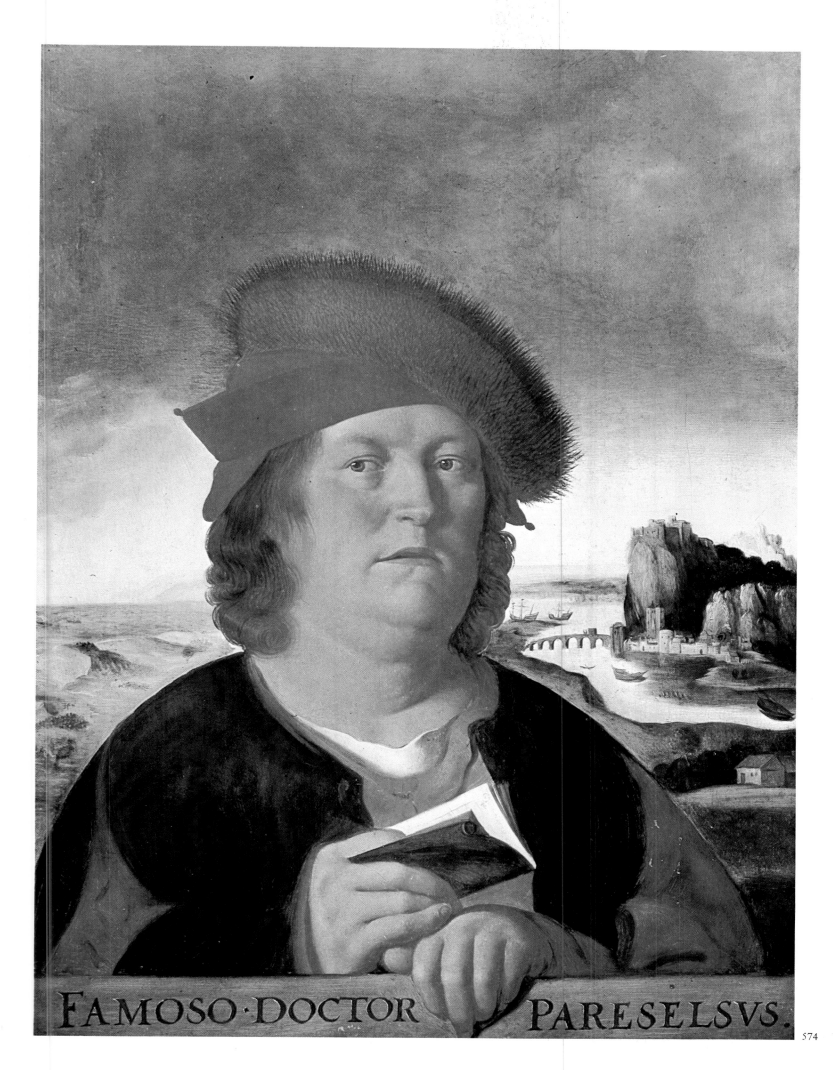

FAMOSO · DOCTOR   PARESELSVS.

574

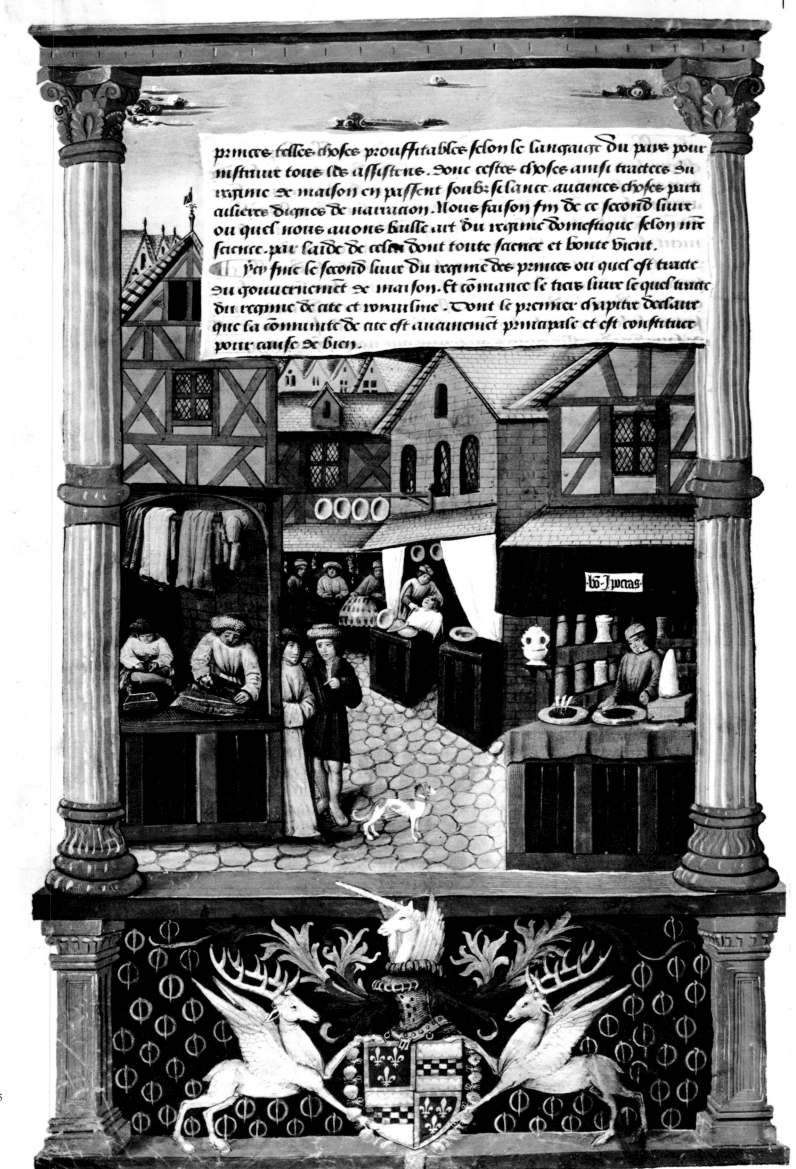

princes telles choses prouffitables selon le langaige du pais pour
instruire tous les assistens. Donc cestes choses ainsi tractees du
regime de maison en passent soubz silance. auances choses parti
ailleurs dignes de narracion. Nous faisons fin de ce second liure
ou quel nous auons baille art du regime domestique selon nre
science. par laide de celui dont toute science et bonte bient.

Cy fine le second liure du regime des princes ou quel est tracte
du gouuernement de maison. Et comance le tiers liure le quel tracte
du regime de cite et communisme. Dont le premier chapitre declaire
que la communite de cite est anciennement principale et est constituee
pour cause de bien.

575

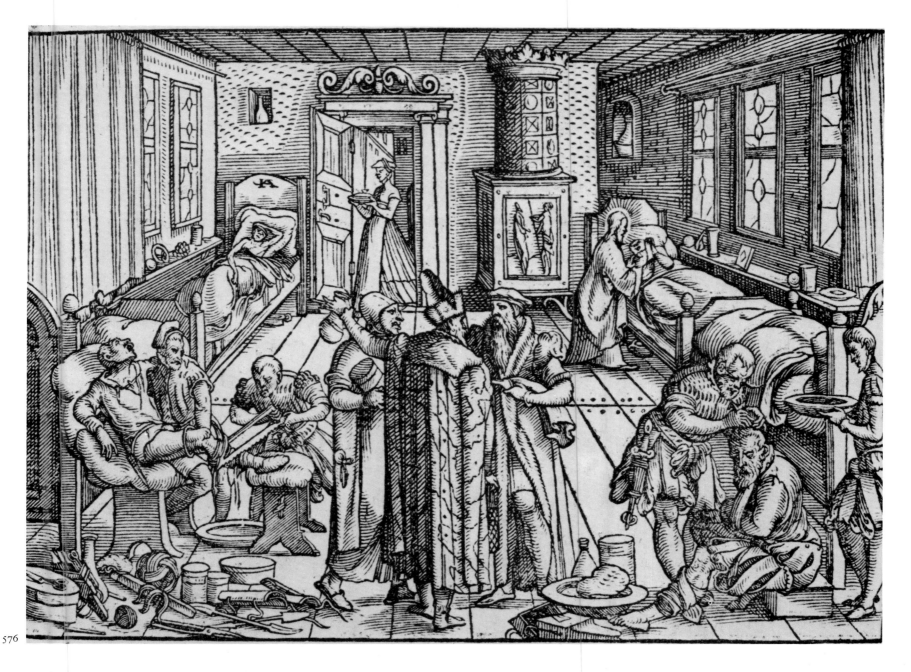

576

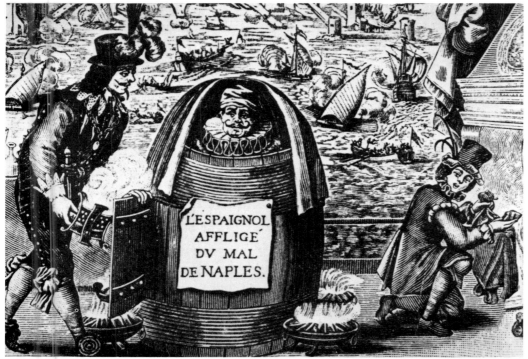

L'ESPAIGNOL
AFFLIGE
DV MAL
DE NAPLES.

577

575 *A street scene from the manuscript* Le Livre du Gouvernement des Princes, *showing an apothecary shop operating under the sign* Bon Ipocras ("*Good Hippocrates*"). *Ms. 5062, fol. 149 v., Bibliothèque Nationale, Paris*

576 *Woodcut from the title page of Paracelsus,* Opus Chirurgicum (1565), *showing the interior of a Renaissance hospital, where, increasingly, physicians received their training, rather than strictly in universities. National Library of Medicine, Bethesda*

577 *Spanish soldier shown being treated for syphilis (here called Naples disease, but later known as French disease), which first broke out in epidemic proportions among the sailors returning from Columbus's first voyage to the New World. World Health Organization, Geneva*

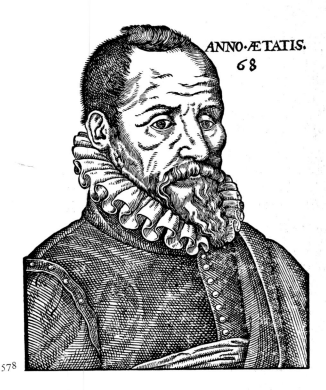

578

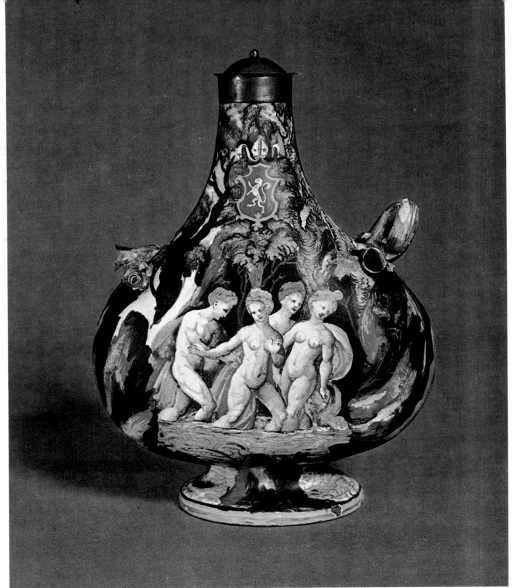

579

578 *Woodcut portrait of Ambroise Paré, at age 68, who, without academic training, revolutionized the treatment of battle wounds and wrote the innovative treatise* A Universal Surgery (1561). *New York Academy of Medicine*

579 *Pharmaceutical flask embellished with a mythological scene, from Urbino and dated 1535. Museo Civico, Forlì*

580 *Salts containers from Faenza, typical of the beautifully decorated receptacles for medicinal ingredients that were arrayed on the shelves of apothecary shops. Museo Internazionale delle Ceramiche, Faenza*

581 *Woodcut (c. 1560) showing Andreas Vesalius and Ambroise Paré in attendance at the deathbed of Henri II, who had named Paré a master surgeon on his merits despite a lack of academic credentials. National Library of Medicine, Bethesda*

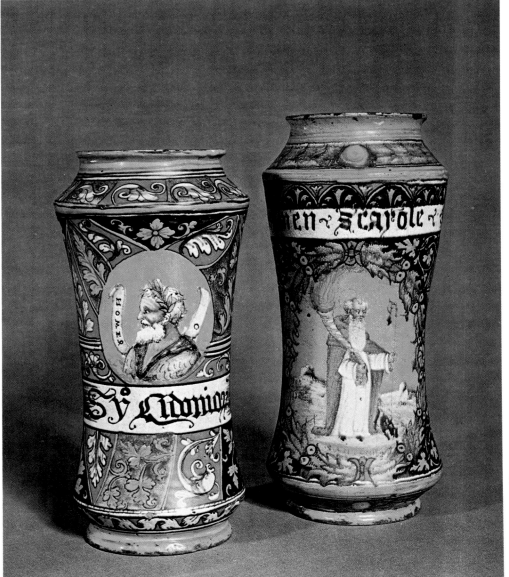

580

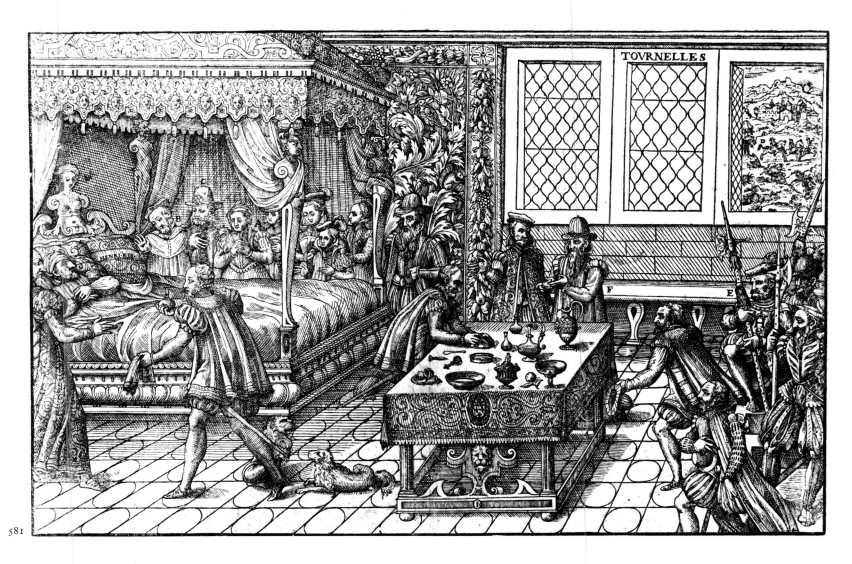

SURGERY

Clinical surgery during the Renaissance also owed much to France, though
almost entirely because of a single person. Ambroise Paré (1517?–90) came from
unusual circumstances for one who was to be so influential in the history of
medicine. From the countryside, he was first apprenticed to a barber and later
a wound-dresser at the Hôtel-Dieu in Paris. Snubbed by the Collège de St. Côme,
in 1537 he joined the army, where he was to achieve his fame. Giovanni da Vigo
(1460–1525) had written in his *Practica copiosa in arte chirurgica* (1514) that gunshot
wounds were poisonous, and from the pseudo-Hippocratic doctrine that "wounds
which are not curable by iron are curable by fire" Vigo and others concluded that
gunshot wounds should be first dressed with boiling oil. As Paré later related (in
French, for he knew no Latin) in *The Method of Treatment for Wounds Caused by
Firearms* (1545), one night after treating many gunshot wounds with boiling oil he
ran out of oil although many wounded remained uncared for. With trepidation, he
merely cleansed their wounds and dressed them. Arising before dawn the following
day, he dashed off to see how poorly those not treated with oil had done. To his
amazement, they were sleeping comfortably and their wounds were healing well.
In marked contrast, the soldiers treated with boiling oil were feverish and in much
pain, and their wounds were inflamed. As Paré's fame grew and this story was
made common knowledge, boiling oil was no longer used on the battlefield.

During later campaigns, Paré reintroduced the ancient method of stopping
hemorrhage by using ligatures and abandoned the cauterizing irons. In 1554 Henri
II made him a master surgeon (in spite of his poor education), and in 1561 he
published his magnificent treatise *A Universal Surgery*, wherein many novel
procedures and types of apparatus were presented.

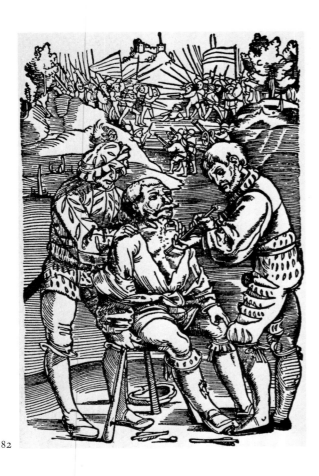

582

582 *Woodcut showing wound treatment on the battlefield, a practical training ground for Ambroise Paré, whose discoveries led to the abandonment of boiling oil as a treatment for gunshot wounds and a reduced reliance on the cautery. World Health Organization, Geneva*

583 *Sixteenth-century engraving illustrating a cataract operation, using instruments perfected if not conceived by Ambroise Paré. World Health Organization, Geneva*

584 *Cataract-removal instruments pictured in the Ten Books of Surgery (1564) by Ambroise Paré. New York Academy of Medicine*

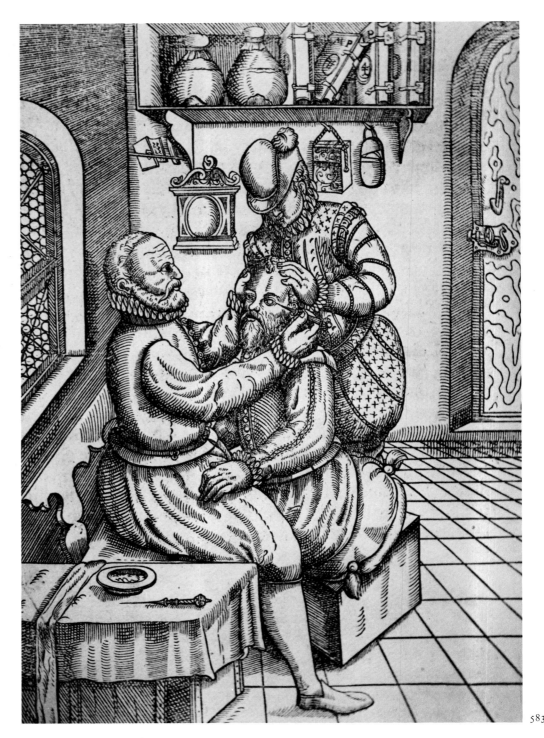

583

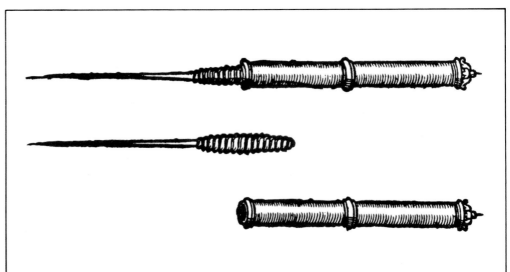

584

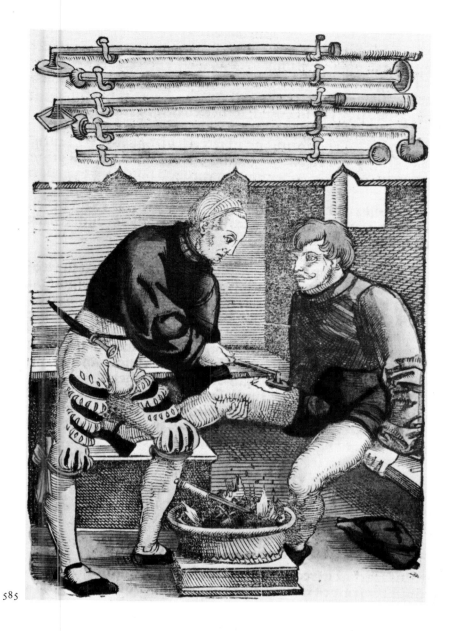

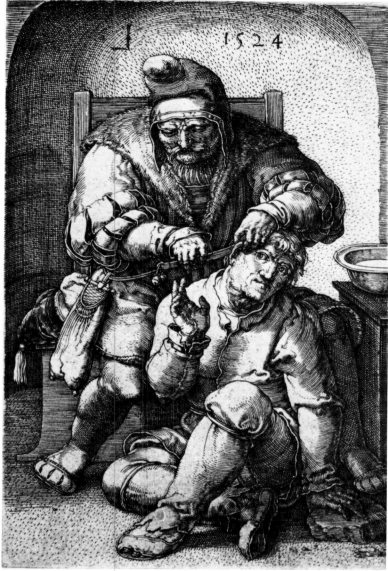

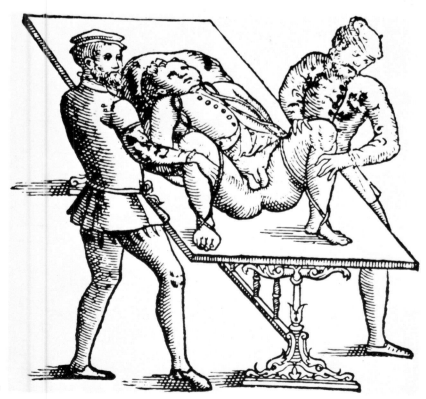

585 *Woodcut by Johannes Wechtlin from Hans von Gersdorff's* Feldtbuch der Wundartzney *(1540), showing a selection of cauterizing irons (at top) and a patient having his thigh cauterized after injury. Smith, Kline, and French Collection, Philadelphia Museum of Art*

586 *In his engraving* The Surgeon and the Peasant *(c. 1524), Lucas van Leyden shows a typical barber-surgeon plying his trade. Rijksmuseum, Amsterdam*

587 *Illustration of a patient properly positioned for an operation to remove a bladder stone, from the* Ten Books of Surgery *(1564) by Ambroise Paré. New York Academy of Medicine*

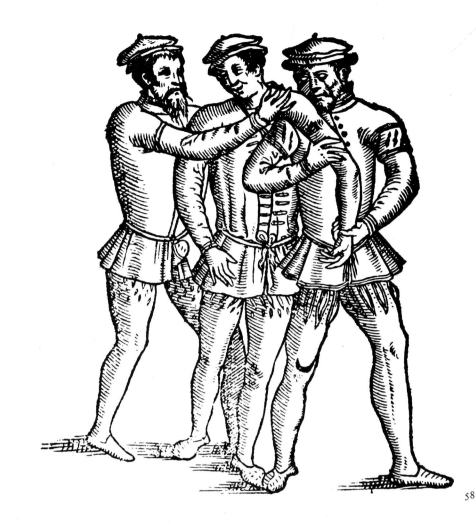

588

588 *The technique of reducing a complete dislocation of the left shoulder, as illustrated in* the Ten Books of Surgery *by Ambroise Paré. New York Academy of Medicine*

589 *Extension apparatus for a fractured arm, as shown in Hans von Gersdorff's* Feldtbuch der Wundartzney (1540) *in a woodcut by Johannes Wechtlin. Smith, Kline, and French Collection, Philadelphia Museum of Art*

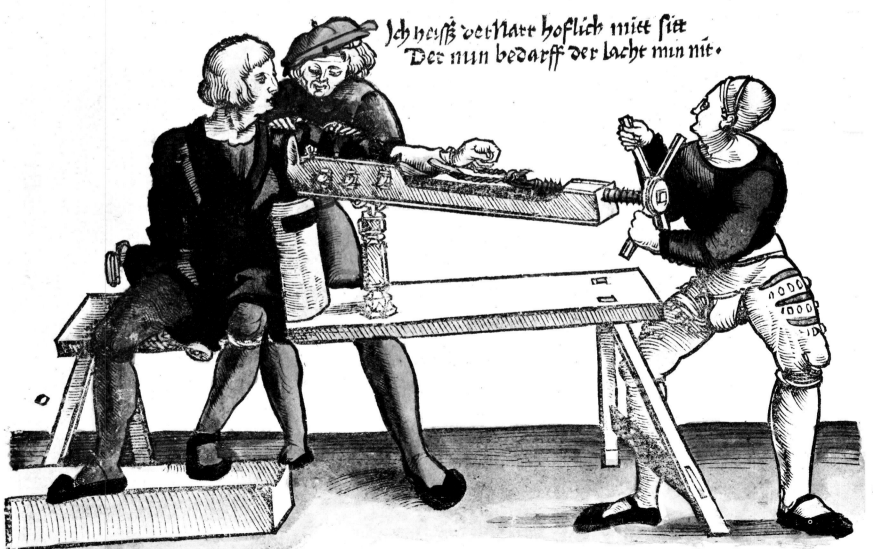

589

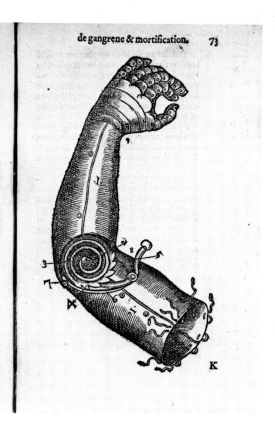

Traicté
Description du bras de fer
cy apres mis.

1 Le bracelet de fer pour la forme du bras.
2 L'arbre mis au dedans du grand resort
pour le tendre.
3 Le grãd resort qui est au coulde, lequel
doit estre d'acier trempé, & de trois piedz
de longueur ou plus.
4 Le rocquet.
5 La gaschette.
6 Le resort qui poise sur la gaschette, &
arreste les dentz du rocquet.
7 Le clouz à vis pour fermer ce resort.
8 Le tornant de la haulse de l'auant bras
qui est au dessus du coulde.
9 La trompe du gantelet faict à tornant
auec le canõ de l'auãt bras qui est à la main:
lesquelz seruent à faire la main prone & su-
pine:c'est à sçauoir prone vers la terre,& su
pine vers le ciel.

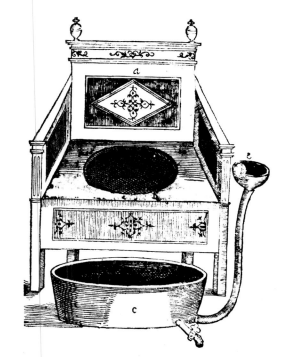

590

592

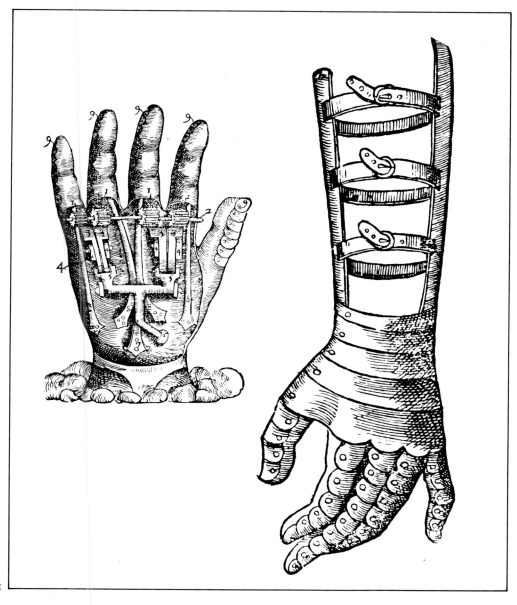

591

590 *Articulated artificial hand and arm, after Ambroise Paré. It is questionable how often these were actually used. Bibliothèque Nationale, Paris*

591 *Ingenious artificial hands, shown in Paré,* Ten Books of Surgery, *developed to replace the limbs lost to gangrene or battle injury. New York Academy of Medicine*

592 *Demi-bath chair developed by Ambroise Paré to alleviate the pains of bladder stones by sitting the patient over steam emanations. From the* Ten Books of Surgery. *New York Academy of Medicine*

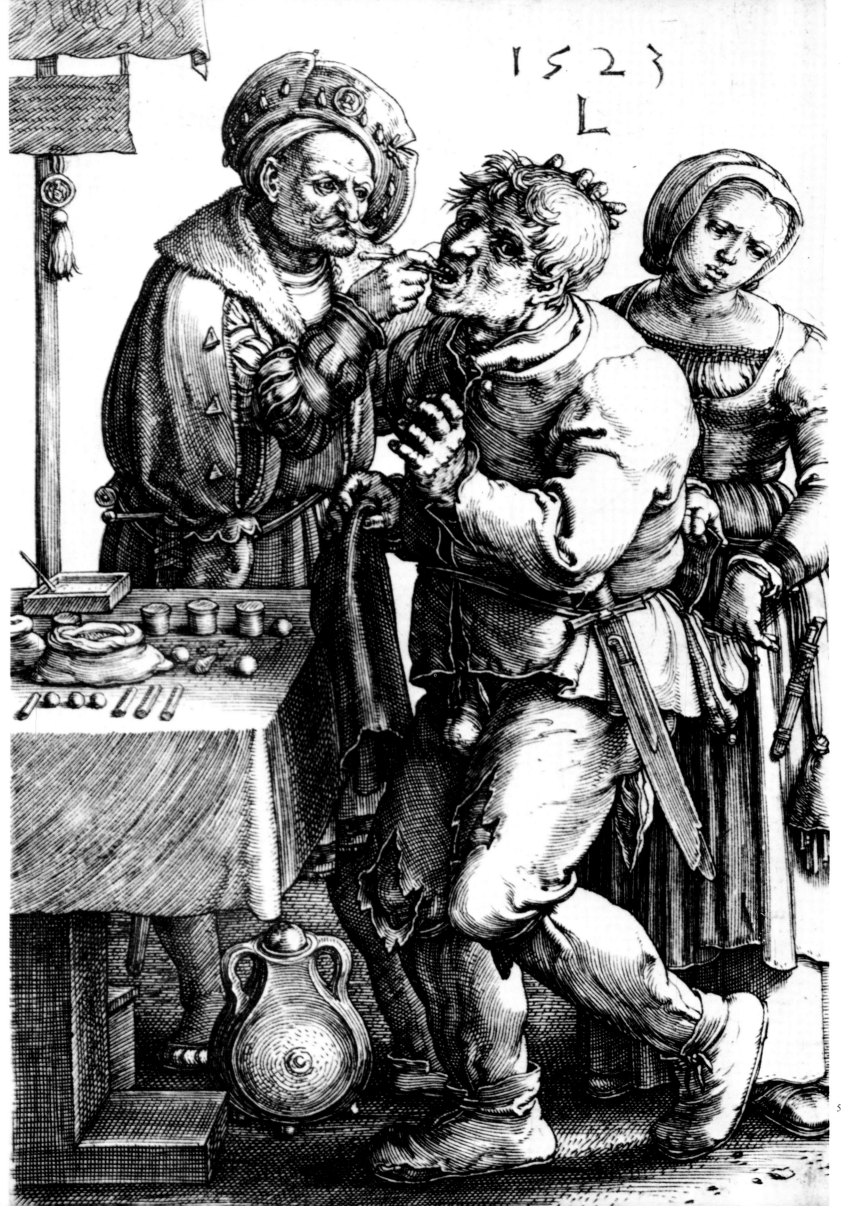

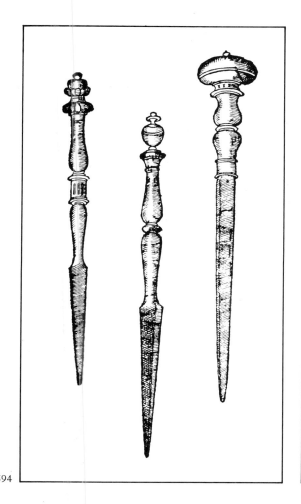

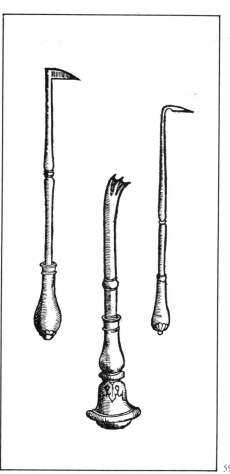

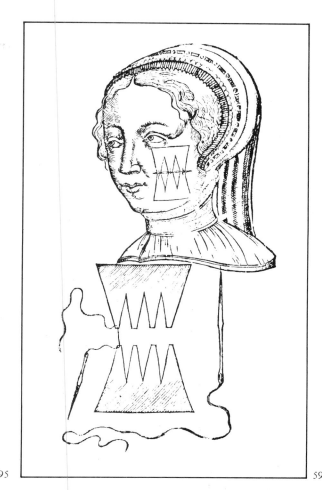

594

595

598

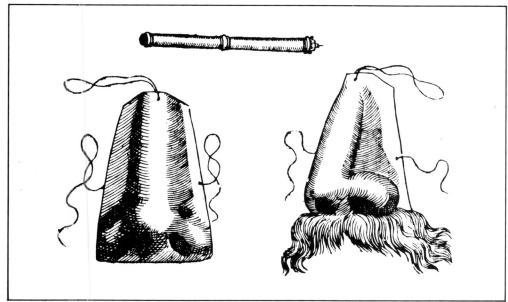

596

597

593 *Dentist shown treating patient in this engraving dated 1523 by Lucas van Leyden. Rijksmuseum, Amsterdam*

594–598 *Illustrations from the Ten Books of Surgery by Ambroise Paré, showing dental files, lancets, and thruster; artificial teeth; replacement noses; and the proper technique for suturing facial wounds. New York Academy of Medicine*

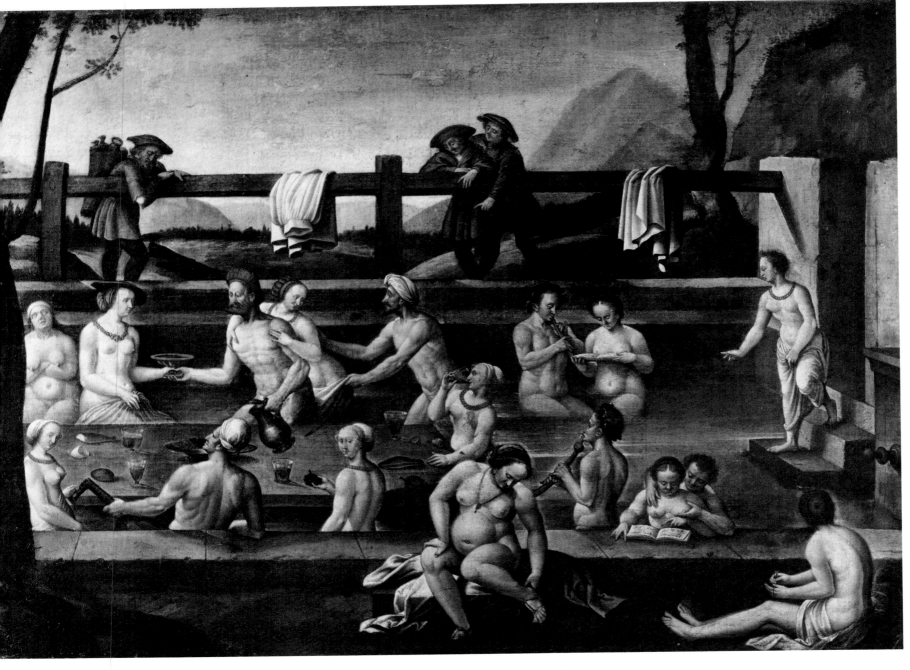

DISEASES

Epidemic diseases of the sixteenth century were quite different from those of the preceding century. The sweating sickness, leprosy, and epidemic chorea had almost ceased to exist. Syphilis, though less virulent, continued to be common, and the favored treatment was with mercury or guaiac. Gonorrhea became even more common. These two venereal diseases were directly responsible for the suppression of communal baths, which had been especially popular in the German countries (for both sexes, though usually segregated). In many areas this meant a loss of the only convenient means of personal hygiene, since adequate water was still generally unavailable to most of the population, at least in amounts sufficient for daily bathing or waste removal.

Other epidemic diseases became inexplicably more common in the sixteenth century, among them typhus, diphtheria, smallpox, and measles. In the north of Europe and among sailors, scurvy also increased in frequency, though neither cause nor cure was suggested.

Hospitals continued to be established and supported by municipalities. As leprosy became increasingly rare, most of the thousands of leprosaria closed. In

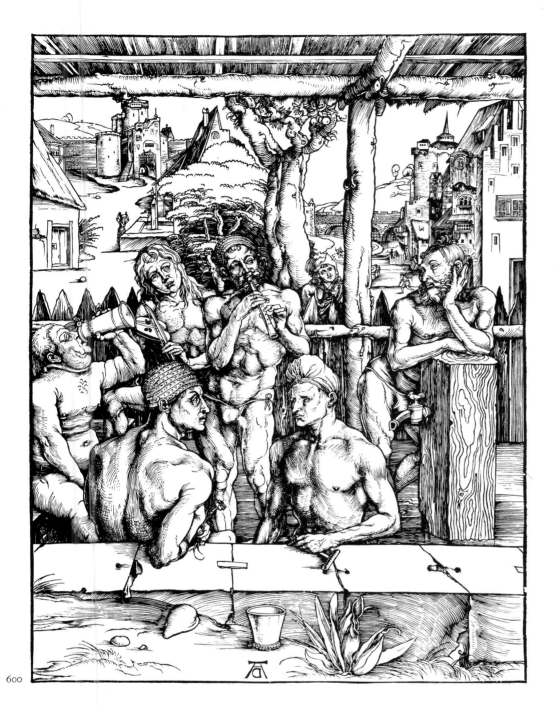

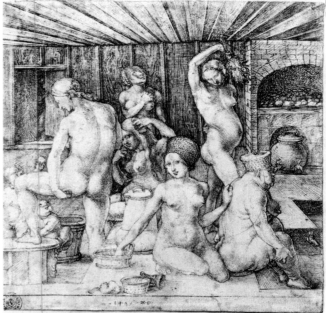

599 *Communal baths, such as those at Louèche painted by Hans Bock the Elder in the late 16th century, were eventually suppressed in part because of promiscuity and the spread of syphilis and gonorrhea. Öffentliche Kunstsammlung, Basel*

600 *Woodcut (1496) by Albrecht Dürer showing men relaxing at a public bathhouse, a convenient facility for personal hygiene at a time when most homes were not supplied with sufficient water for baths. Germanisches Nationalmuseum, Nuremberg*

601 Women's Bath, *as drawn by Albrecht Dürer in 1496, reflects the social as well as the hygienic benefits of a public bath during the Renaissance. Formerly Kunsthalle Bremen*

their place, however, institutions were increasingly built for the "lunatic" and the poor, who had been displaced from their feudal position without being made a part of the more urbanized society in which they lived. "Witch hunting" also grew by leaps and bounds. With the developing passions generated by the Reformation and Counter-Reformation, it was no longer necessary to blame misfortunes on Jews, for in the Catholic South a Protestant "heretic" would do quite nicely, as would a papist in the Protestant North.

It was to be some time before these attitudes would affect the universities. Many new ones were founded in the sixteenth century, especially in Germany and in central and eastern Europe. In the medical schools, the mainstays remained Avicenna's *Canon*, Galen's *Ars parva*, the *Aphorisms* of Hippocrates, and the works of Dioscorides. In 1543, Giambattista da Monte, or Montanus, (1498–1552) revived the Hippocratic form of bedside teaching at Padua. Though this was to lapse after 1551, it was later revived by his students Albertinon Bottoni and Marco degli Oddi. But this change was minor relative to the revolutions going on in the study of botany and anatomy, changes so important in the later development of the history of medicine that the next chapter will be devoted to them.

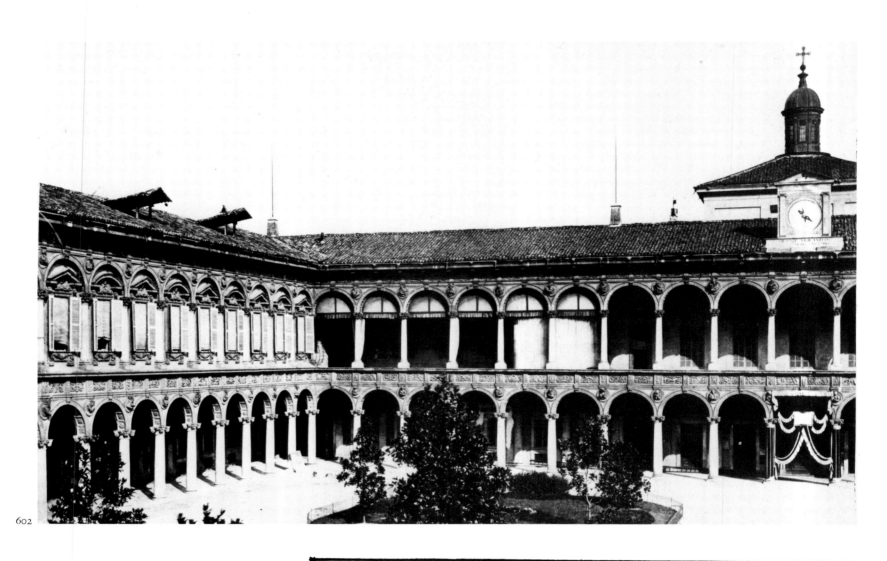

602

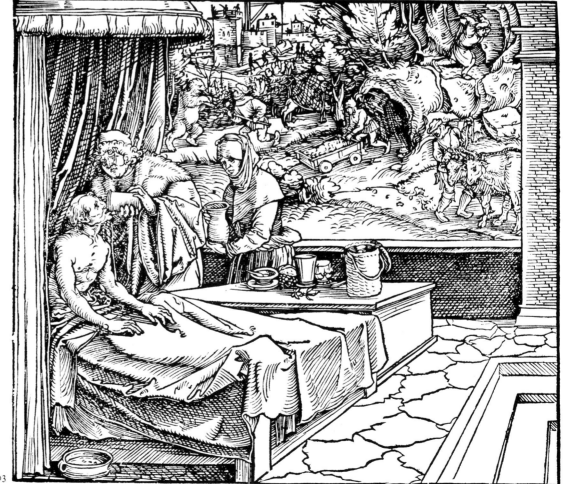

603

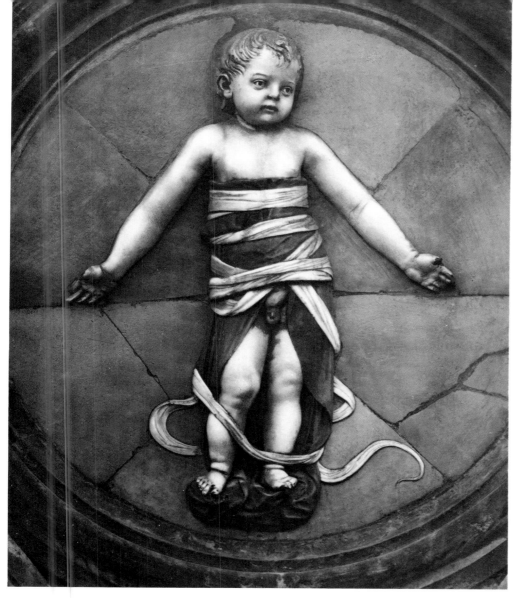

602 *Courtyard of the Ospedale Maggiore in Milan, a hospital founded in the 16th century. New York Academy of Medicine*

603 *Early-16th-century woodcut by Hans Weiditz, showing a physician caring for a patient at home. Only the poor and those with contagious diseases were cared for in hospitals. New York Academy of Medicine*

604, 605 *Glazed terra-cotta medallions of swaddled infants by Andrea della Robbia, on the facade of the Ospedale degli Innocenti in Florence, an early hospital for children, founded in 1419.*

604

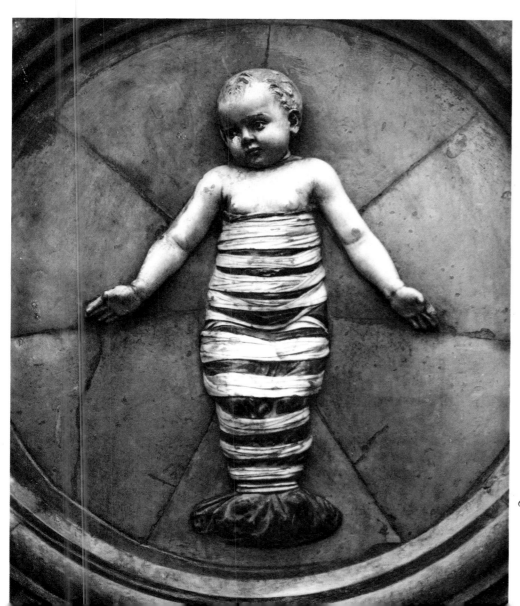

605

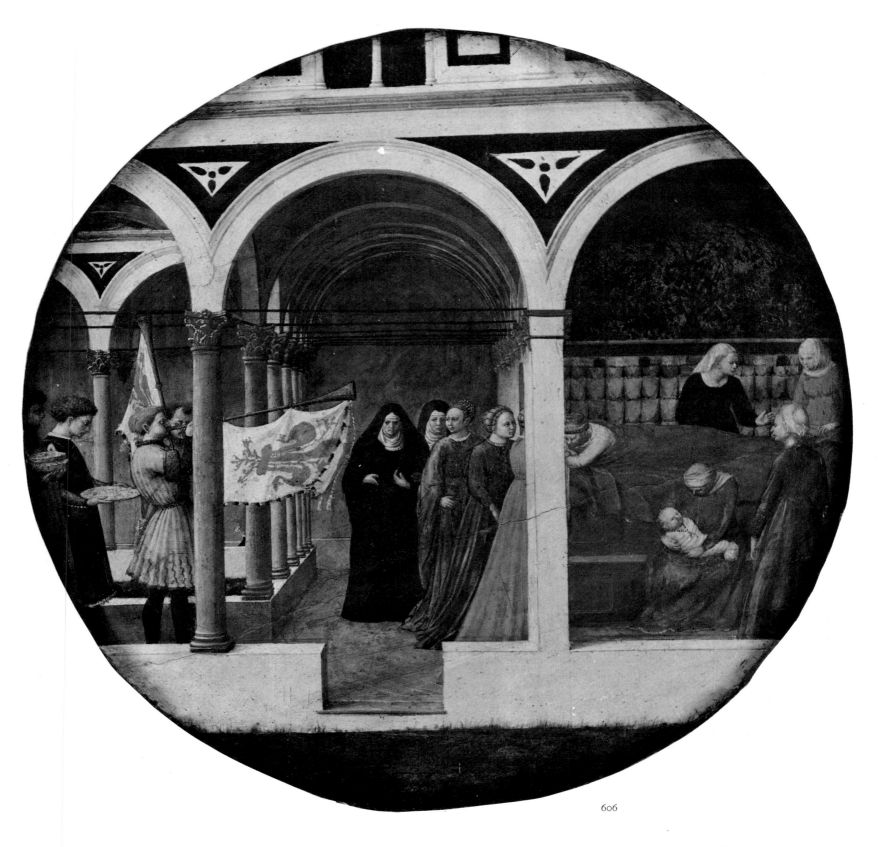

606

606 *Painting (c. 1426) by Masaccio showing visitors coming to wel-
come a newborn child and its mother. Staatliche Museen, Berlin*

607 *Illustration in Ambroise Paré,* Oeuvres *(1575), with the caption
"An admirable way for a woman to carry 20 infants in pregnancy."
National Library of Medicine, Bethesda*

608 *Childbirth scene in woodcut by Jost Amman, in Jakob Rueff's*
De Conceptu et Generatione Hominis *(1554), a famous and widely
used handbook for midwives. In the background, an astrologer casts
the child's horoscope. Smith, Kline, and French Collection, Philadelphia Museum of Art*

609 *A birthing chair illustrated in Rueff's* De Conceptu et Generatione Hominis *(1554). New York Academy of Medicine*

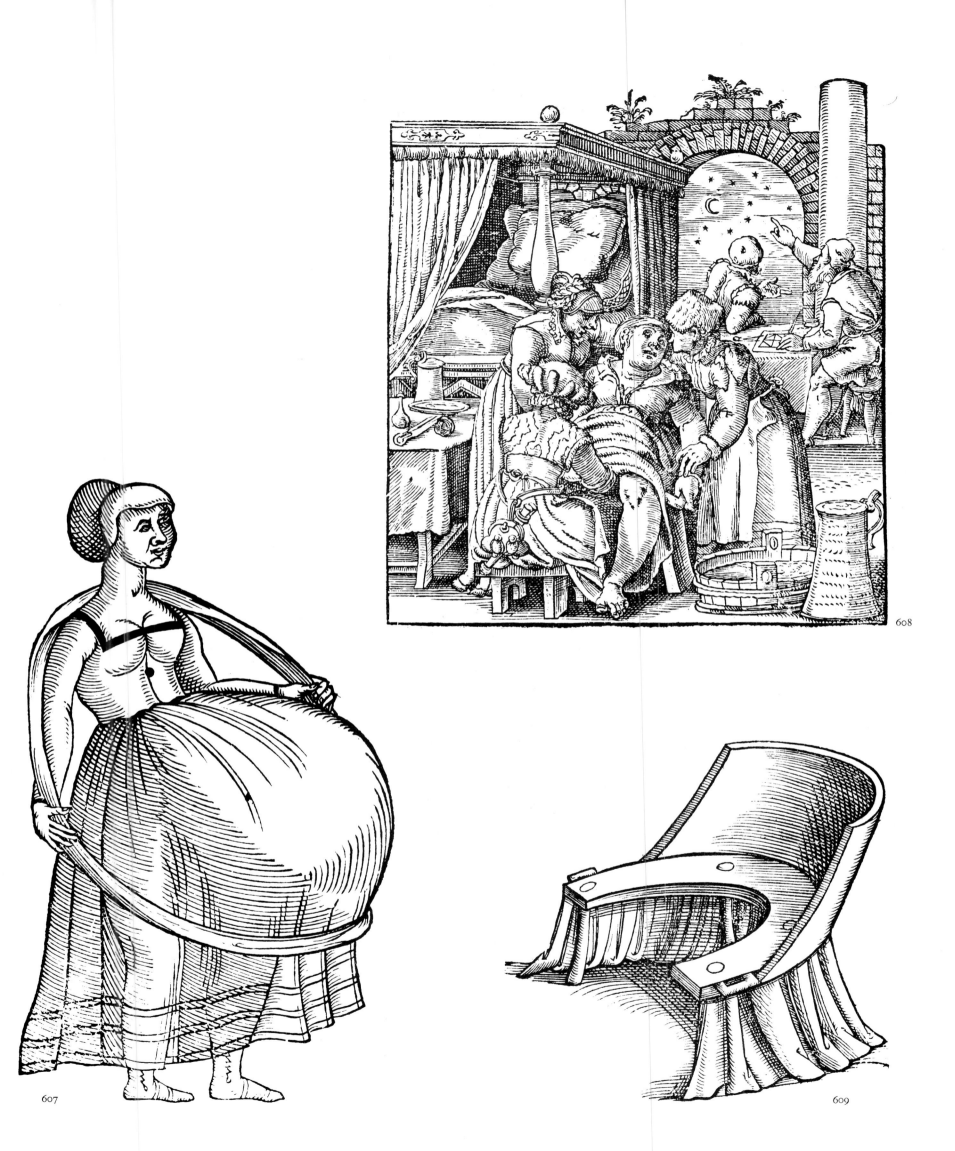

607

608

609

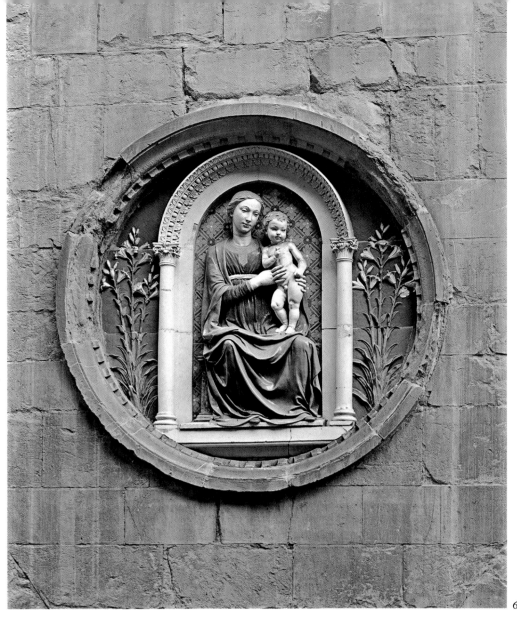

610

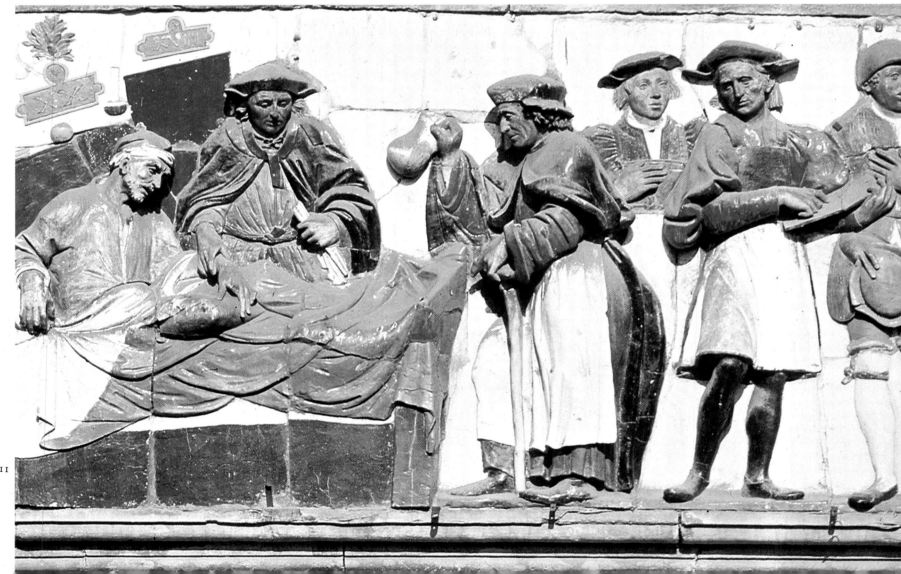

611

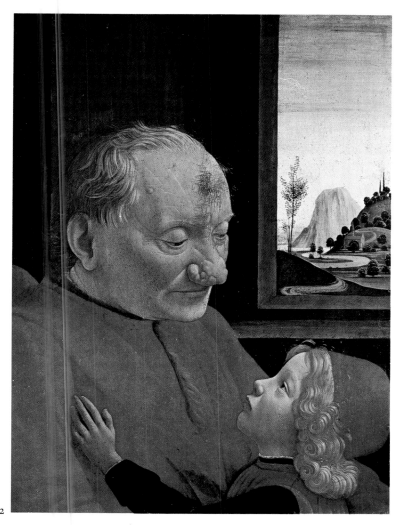

612

610 *Glazed terra-cotta medallion (1440–50), by Luca della Robbia, of the Madonna, Protectress of the Doctors Guild. Or San Michele, Florence*

611 Visiting the Sick *(1525), a glazed terra-cotta frieze by Giovanni della Robbia on the facade of the Ospedale del Ceppo in Pistoia. Hospitals increasingly were founded and supported by municipalities and combined the functions of hospice and infirmary.*

612 *Domenico Ghirlandaio's late–15th-century portrait of an old man and his grandson faithfully records the effects of the man's rhino-phyma (a nose condition sometimes present in the old), accentuating the contrast between youth and age. The Louvre, Paris*

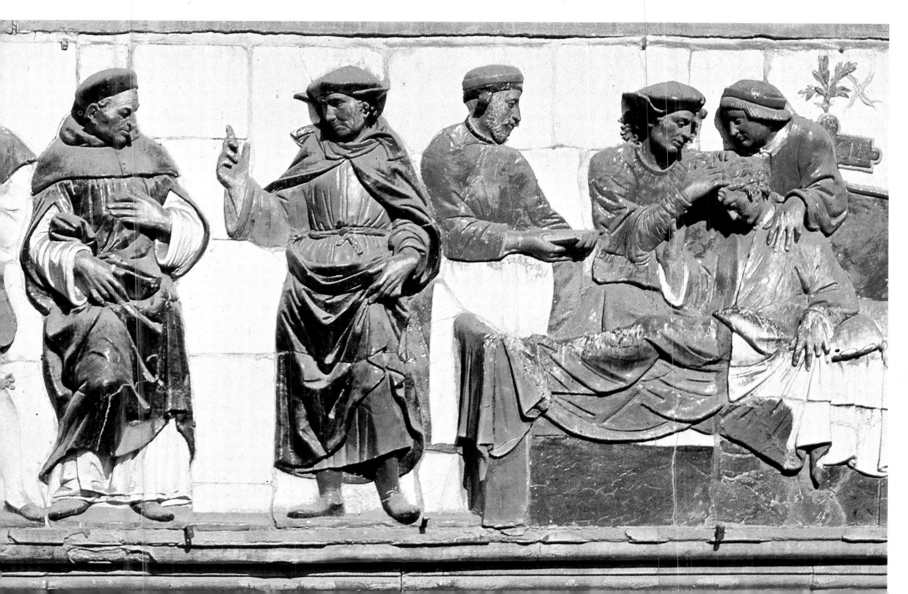

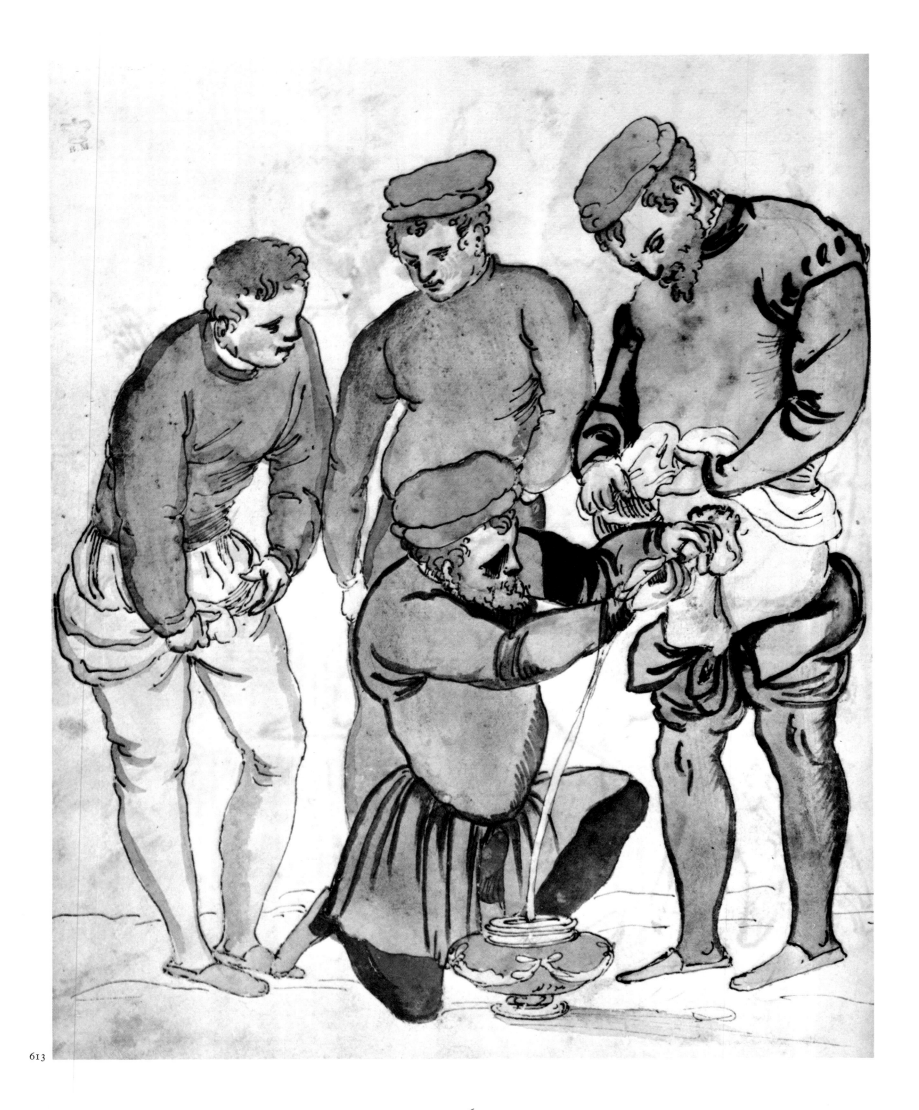

613

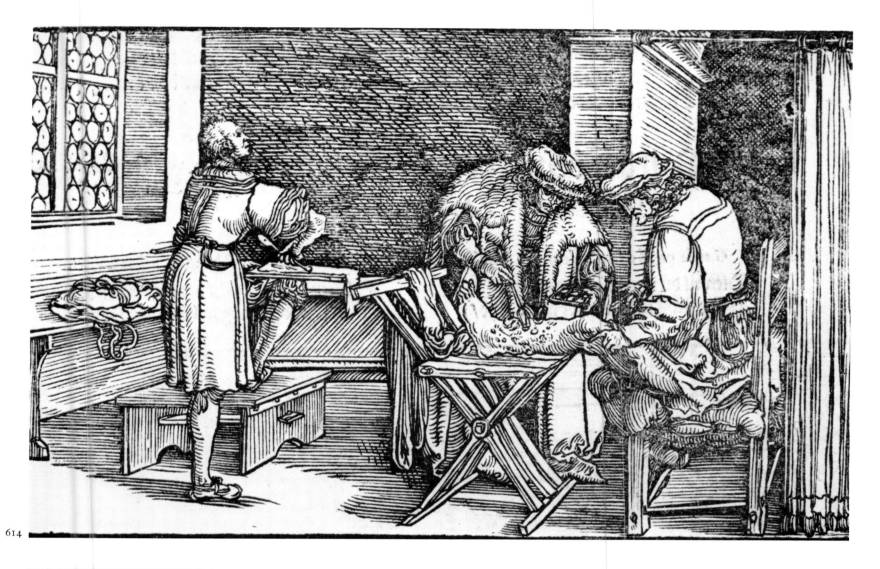

614

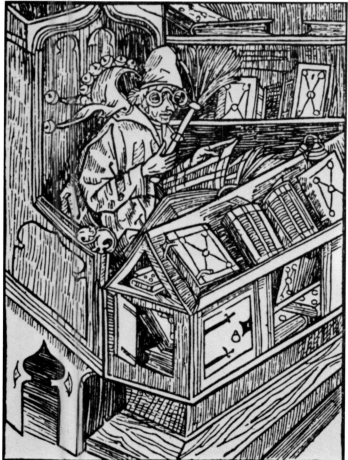

615

613 *Manuscript illustration showing an early cathe-*
terization for urinary stones. Ms. 197. d.2., fol.
19 v., British Museum, London

614 *Treatment for an ulcerated leg illustrated in*
Trost Spiegel in Glück und Unglück *(1572).*
National Library of Medicine, Bethesda

615 *A scholar wearing eyeglasses in a woodcut from*
Sebastian Brandt's Ship of Fools *(1494). Eyeglasses*
could free scholars from the limits imposed by poor
vision. New York Academy of Medicine

Art and Science

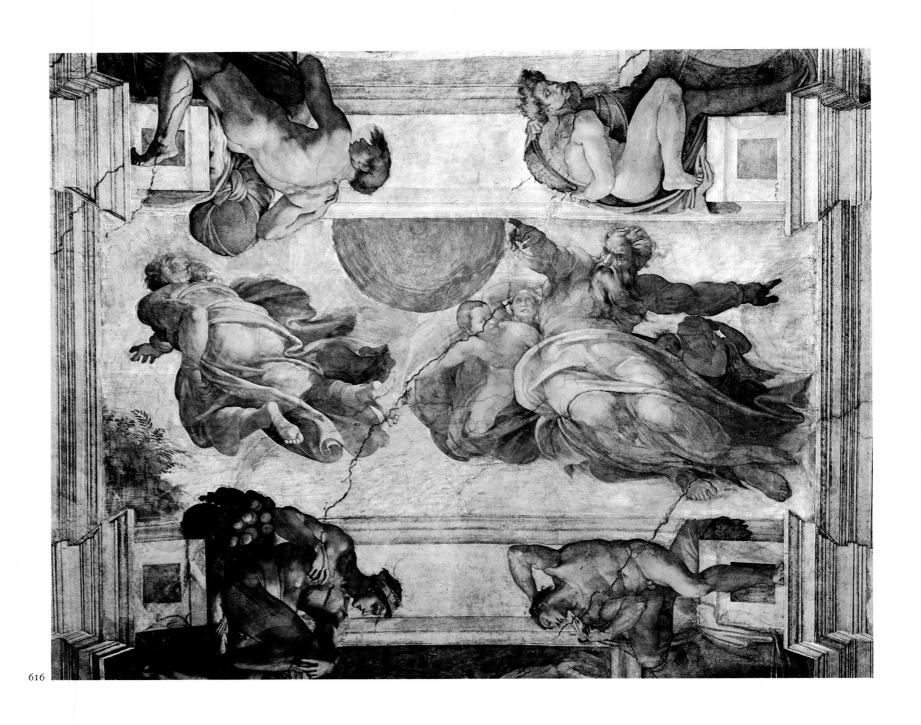

616

A RT and science were allied more closely in the Renaissance than during any other period in the history of man. Although this is commonly acknowledged for the study of human anatomy, it was equally true for many other fields including botany, zoology, engineering, the applied sciences, and even architecture.

During the earlier medieval period, supreme interest had been shown in a distant and at times vengeful God, whose goals and means of achieving them were often thought to be beyond the ken of man. Theology was therefore granted first rank within a heavily systematized hierarchy of scholarly endeavors, and belief and reason were thought to be mutually exclusive. Absolutes in all fields of human endeavor, from morality to economics, controlled the intellectual, social, and artistic life of man. Scholasticism was the natural result of this antiexperimental approach in which observed data were to be made consistent with previously assumed truths.

In contrast to this static view of reality in the Middle Ages, the quality most characteristic of the Renaissance was its dynamic versatility. The prospects of an otherworldly paradise beyond the grave—at best an uncertainty—paled before the new attractions of the natural world. Inevitably as absolutes lost favor particulars increasingly drew men away from a God in distant heaven toward themselves and the immediate environment.

During the Renaissance, the highest authority became the natural world itself, and even the writings of the ancient authorities were subject to independent verification; the experimental method had begun to take hold. When the early experimentalist-observer wanted to convey his findings to others, he found the older modalities of expression inadequate. Rather than utilizing observations to "prove" the validity of an assumed truth, he attempted through a close study of many independent events to determine generally applicable principles—a method we call empiricism. However, when the experimentalist acknowledged a lack of understanding of his observations, verbal description was often difficult and a pictorial account was the most expedient form of communication.

ANATOMICAL ILLUSTRATION

Five hundred years before Christ, human anatomy as a science was begun in southern Italy by Alcmaeon of Crotona, who performed dissections upon animals. Shortly thereafter a practical text from the Hippocratic School described the anatomy of the shoulder as if it had been learned through dissection. Aristotle alluded to anatomical illustration when he referred to *paradigmata*, which were most probably figures made following animal dissection. In the third century before Christ, the study of anatomy was advanced considerably at Alexandria, where many discoveries can be attributed to Herophilus and Erasistratus, who were the first to perform human dissections systematically. After 150 B.C., human dissection was again prohibited for religious and ethical reasons, a prohibition strongly enforced by Rome. The science of human anatomy, however, persisted in the Hellenistic world, although only animal dissections were acknowledged. In the second century A.D., Galen achieved the highest level of success in the utilization of animal dissection (mostly of Barbary apes and pigs) and its generally correct application to human anatomy; however, some errors were inevitable due to an inability to confirm findings on human cadavers. Galen also developed the doctrine of "final cause," a teleological system which required that all findings must be consistent with physiology as he understood it.

Although no specific examples of anatomic illustrations from the Classical period have survived, the medieval "five-figure series" of bones, veins, arteries, internal organs, and nerves were probably copies of earlier drawings. Invariably the figures were depicted in a froglike squatting position to demonstrate the various systems, and occasionally a sixth figure was added: either a pregnant woman or the male and/or female generative organs. In ancient bas-reliefs, cameos,

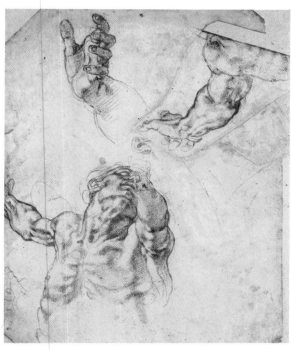

617

616 *In the 16th century, Michelangelo painted* The Creation of the Sun, Moon, and Planets *as the work of a supernatural force, but many Renaissance thinkers had already lost interest in this kind of force and were more concerned with discovering answers in the natural world. Sistine Chapel, Vatican, Rome*

617 *In these studies for Haman (1511) in the Sistine Ceiling, Michelangelo revealed his keen interest in anatomy. He spent years in careful human dissection. Ref. A 16 r., Teylers Museum, Haarlem*

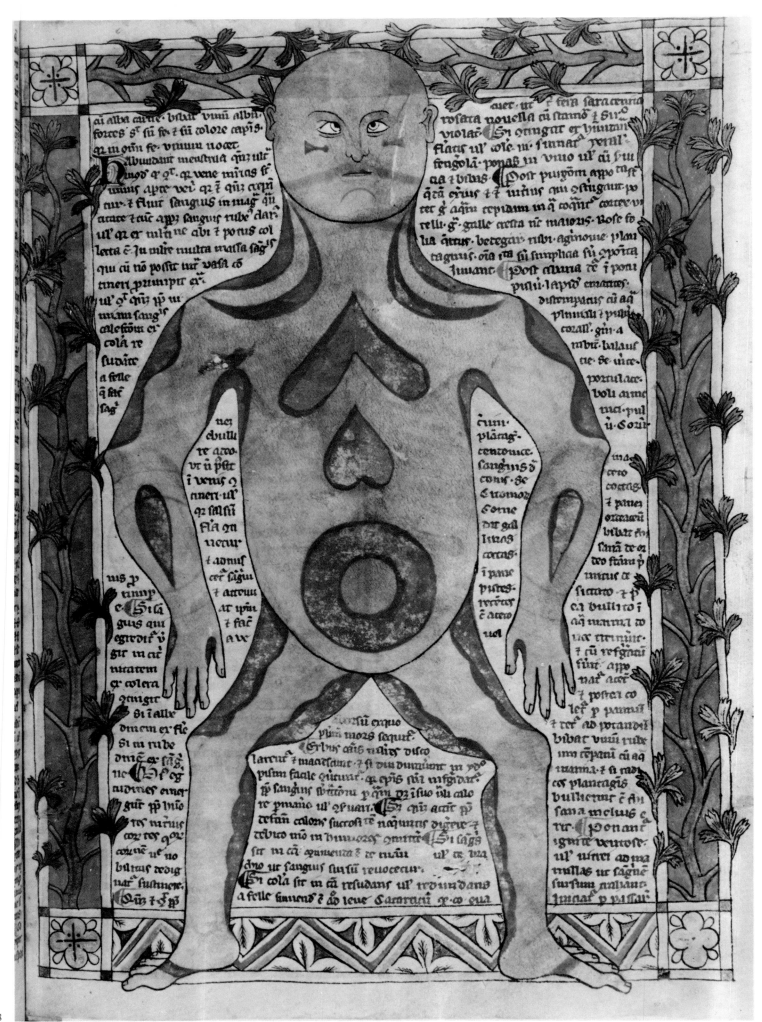

618

618, 619 *Pages from a 13th-century manuscript with anatomical figures in typical medieval postures, showing the limited knowledge*

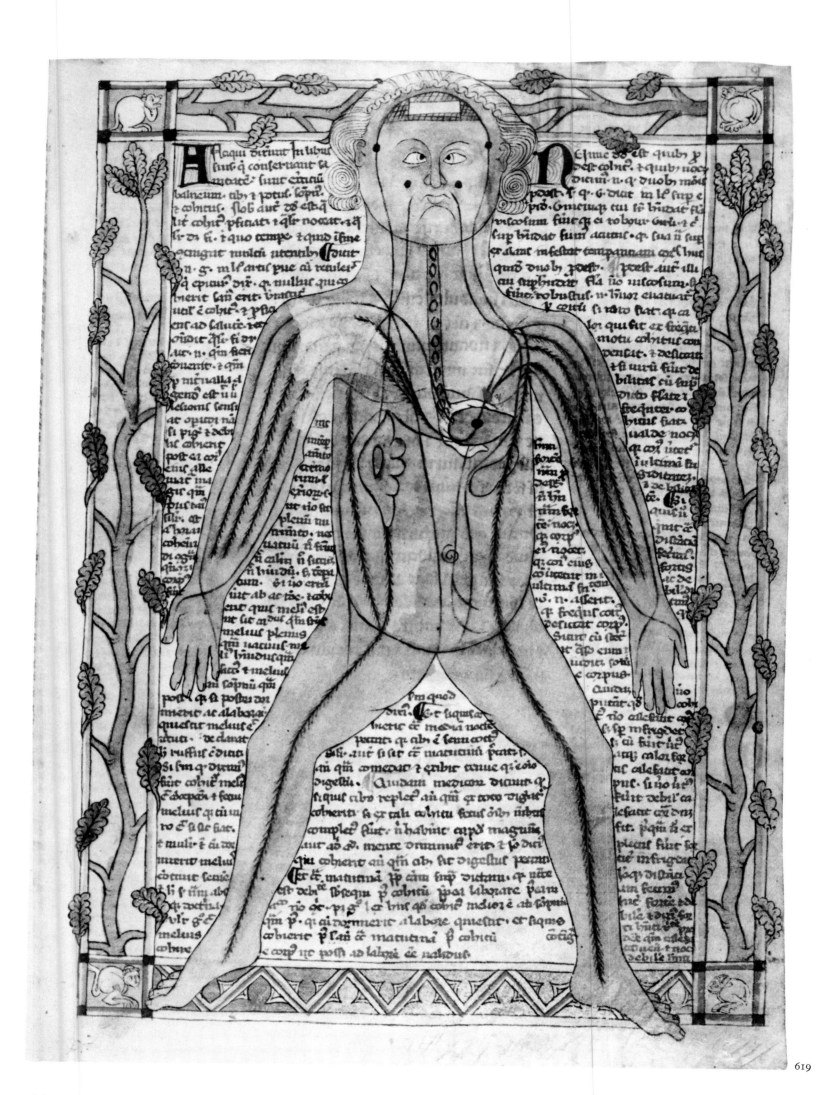

of the muscular system, left, and of the circulatory system, right. Ms. Ashmole 399, fols. 22, 19, Bodleian Library, Oxford

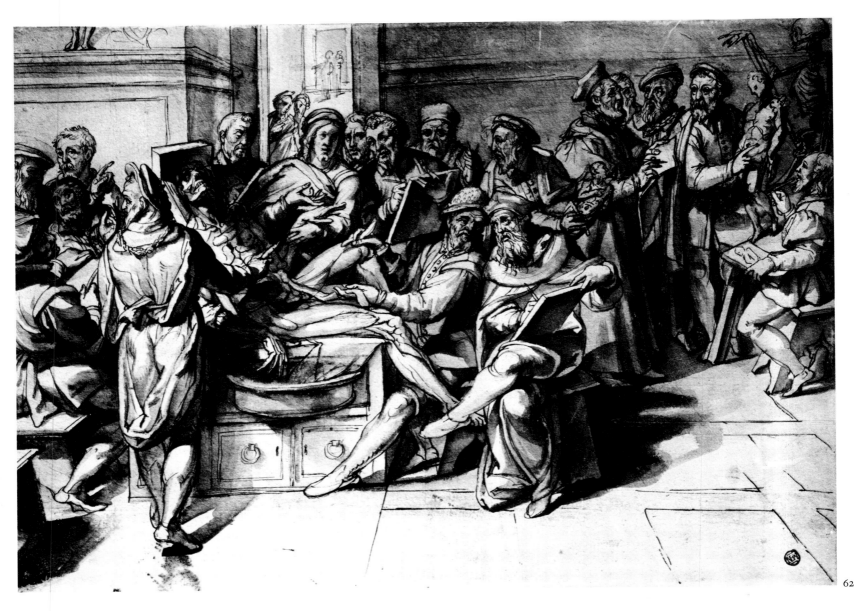

620

620 *This 16th-century aquatint by Bartolomeo Passarotti reflects the intense interest in studying the human form that developed in the Renaissance—not only among medical men but also among artists and scholars. The Louvre, Paris*

621 *The artist was likely to seize any opportunity for sketching the human form, as indicated by Antonio Pisanello's* Study of Hanged Men *(1433). British Museum, London*

622 *A rare, early-15th-century presentation of the range of female maladies. Ms. lat. 7138, fol. 239, Bibliothèque Nationale, Paris*

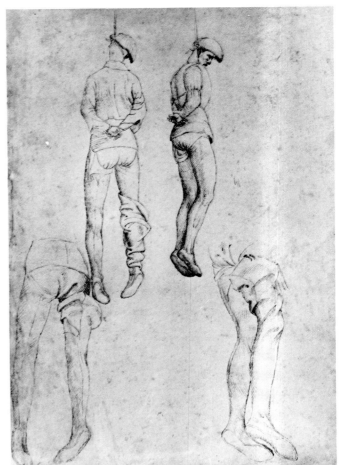

621

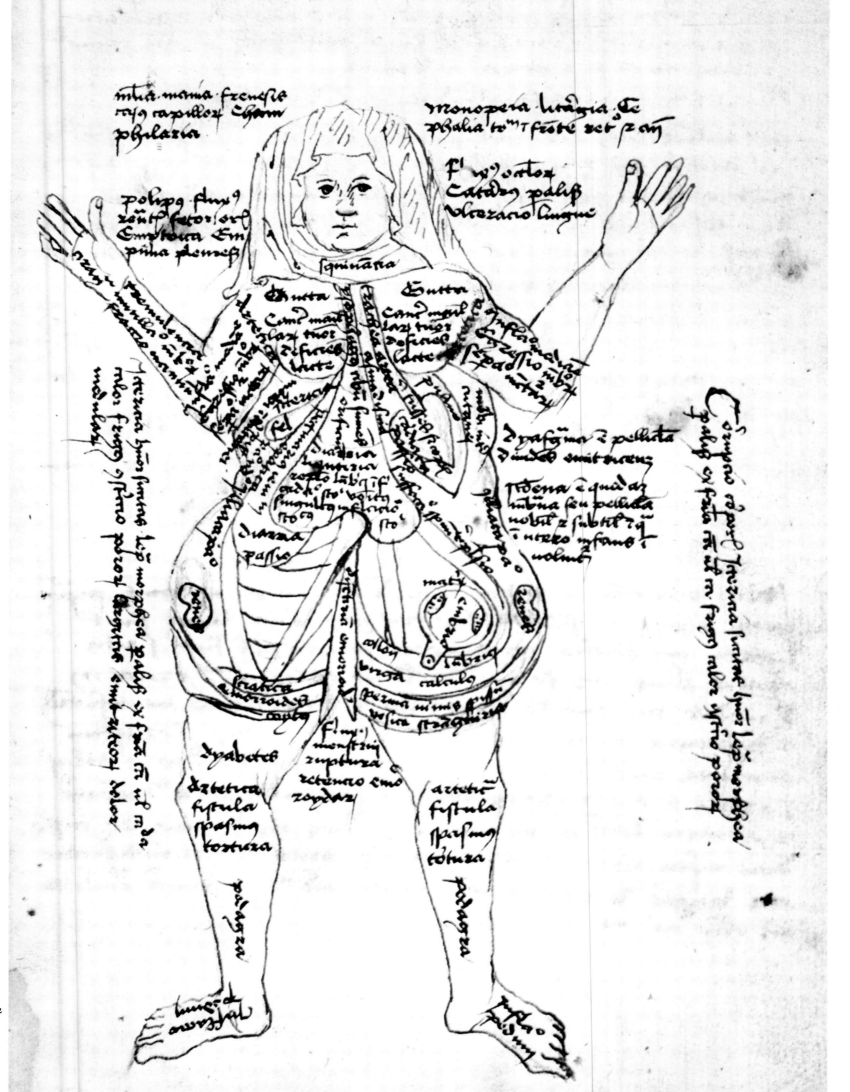

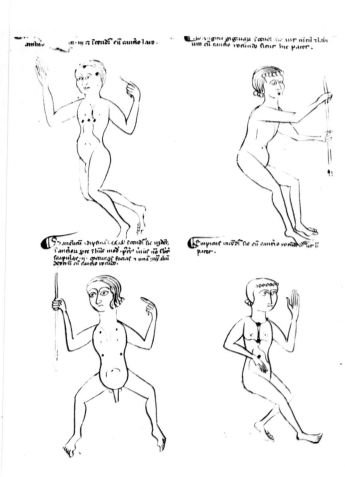

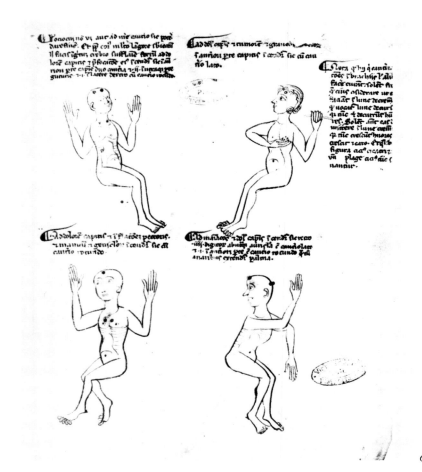

623

624

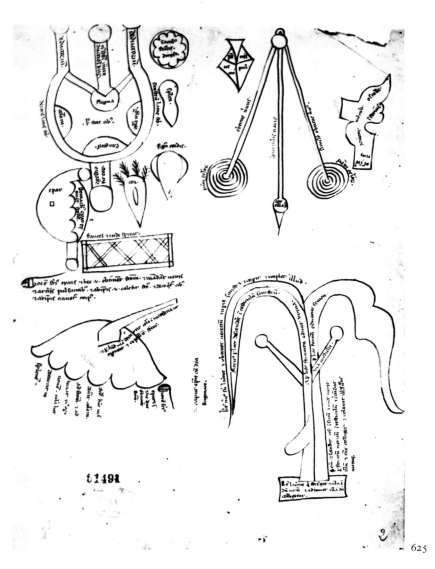

81491

625

and bronzes there often appeared figurations of skeletons and shriveled bodies covered with skin (called lemures), but these were emblematic rather than schematic and had no instructional purpose.

The study of human anatomy seems to have been recommenced more for practical than intellectual reasons. War was no longer strictly a local affair, and it was desirable to have the means of repatriating the bodies of those who had been slain. Embalming was sufficient for short journeys, but the greater distances common in the Crusades called for the custom of the "boiling of bones." The papal bull *De sepulturis* of Boniface VIII (1300), though often incorrectly thought to forbid human dissection, was intended solely to stop this practice. The greatest impetus to dissection of human cadavers was the desire to learn the cause of death for essentially medicolegal reasons, to ascertain what killed an important personage or to learn about the plague and other infectious diseases. The verb "anatomize" was also used to describe the increasingly frequent Caesarean section.

The manuscript tradition in the medieval period did not rely upon the natural world for reference. Rather, earlier illustrations were accepted and copied. In general, the ability of copyists was limited, and, not having examined the natural object, they often introduced errors of understanding as well as of technique. Things were often "seen" as they were thought to occur by the ancients, and realistic illustrations would have been considered an incorrect short-circuiting of the proper method of study. Anatomy was also not considered a separate discipline but, rather, an adjunct to surgery, which in that day was relatively crude and principally demanded a knowledge of the appropriate sites for bloodletting. So long as anatomy retained this antipractical quality, nonrealistic and schematic figures were sufficient.

The first book printed from type and illustrated with printed rather than painted pictures seems to have been Ulrich Boner's *Der Edelstein*, printed by Albrecht Pfister at Bamberg after 1460, but the illustrations were little more than coarse decorations. In 1475, Konrad Megenberg issued his *Buch der Natur*, which contained several woodcuts representing fish, birds, animals, and various plants. These figures, as well as many others from nature books and encyclopedias of that period, were well within the manuscript tradition and hardly recognizable.

Although many elements contributed to the development of technical illustration early in the sixteenth century, two factors seem to have been paramount. The first was the end of the manuscript tradition of copying earlier drawings and the institution of nature as the primary model. A conviction had developed that the most appropriate concern for man was the natural world and not the hereafter. The Scholasticism of St. Thomas Aquinas had inadvertently prepared for this development through its separation of natural and supernatural worlds, even though theology had remained supreme over natural science.

The second major factor influential in the development of scientific illustrations for teaching was the slow realization of the advantages inherent in the medium. Initially publishers had thought only in terms of quantity, that with the printing press large numbers of reproductions could be easily and cheaply produced. Only later did they recognize the significance of each illustration's being identical to the original. The ability to reproduce exactly similar pictorial representations of things observed became the hallmark of the various scientific disciplines as they discarded their former reliance upon tradition and accepted a descriptive and, later, an experimental methodology. Verification of empirical observation now became easier.

The first examples of printed anatomical illustrations remained in the medieval manuscript tradition. The *Fasciculus medicinae* was a collection of contemporary writings for practicing physicians that went through many editions. In the first edition (1491), the woodcut was first utilized for an anatomical figure. The illustrations contained large figures showing the location of appropriate bloodletting sites, and lines ran out to printed explanations at the margins. The

623, 624, 625 *Anatomical drawings from a manuscript dated 1220, showing,* top, *human figures in the typical medieval froglike posture, and,* bottom, *internal organs, which were probably copies from much earlier drawings. Ms. 735, Biblioteca Universitaria, Pisa*

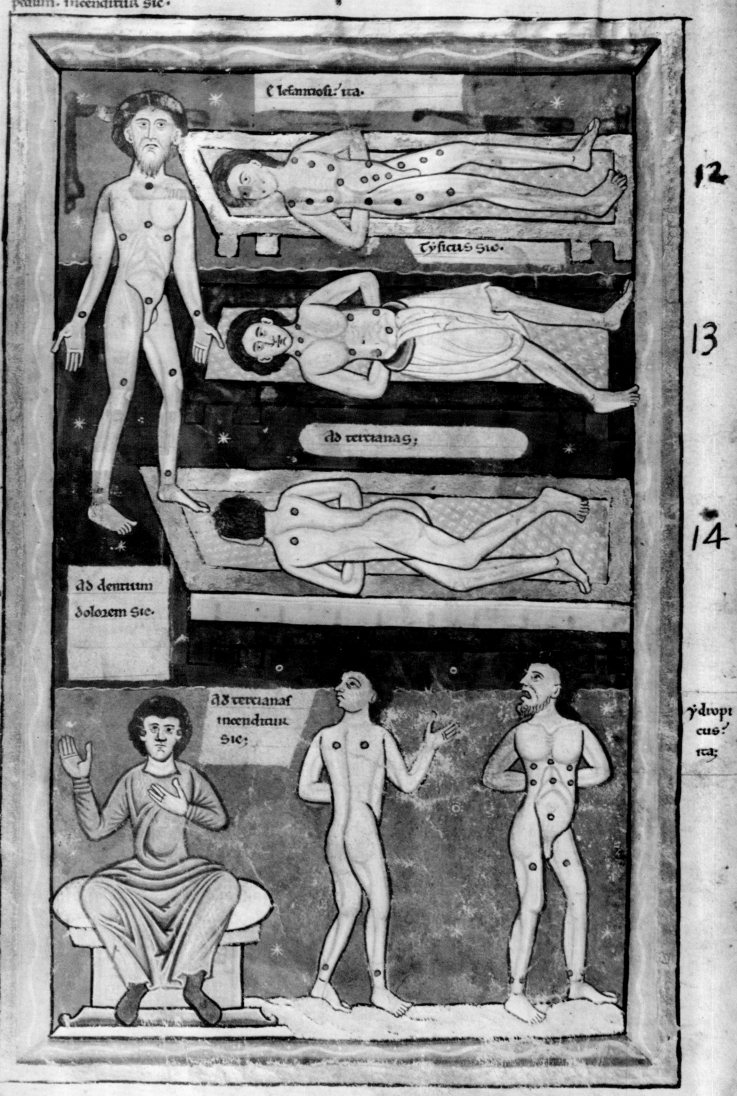

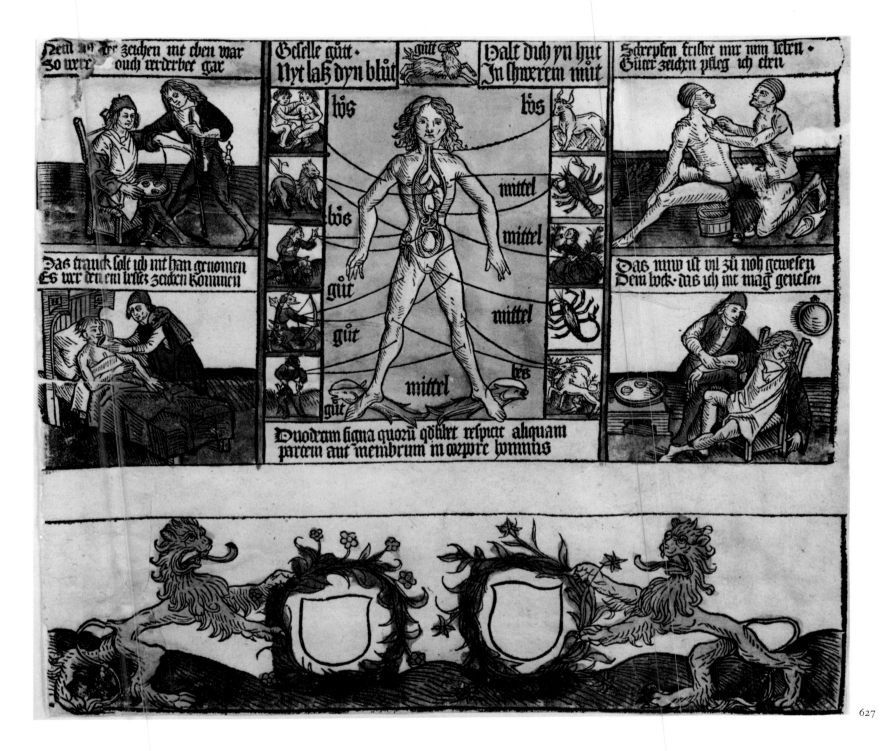

626 *Thirteenth-century chart showing points where hot cauteries could be applied to remedy certain maladies. Ms. Ashmole 1462, fol. 9 v., Bodleian Library, Oxford*

627 *Fifteenth-century woodcut displaying blood-letting points and their relation to the zodiac, with scenes of caring for the sick. Staatliche Graphische Sammlung, Munich*

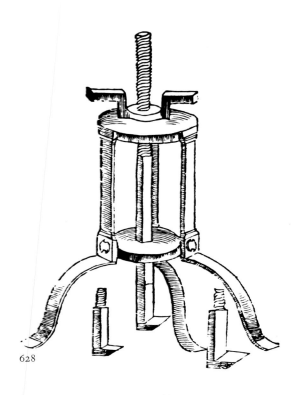

628

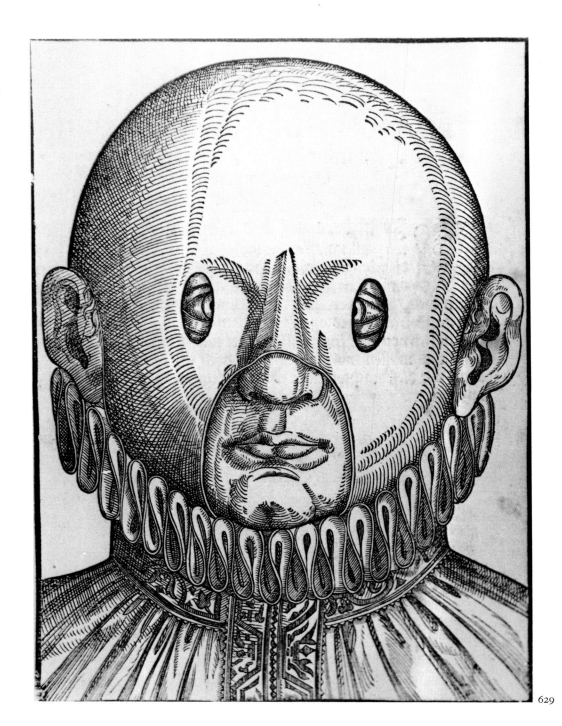

629

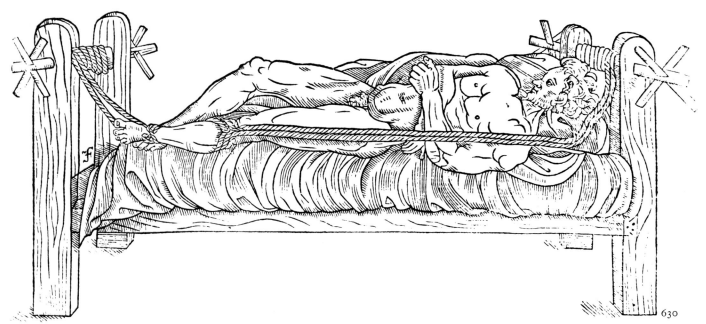

630

628 *Ambroise Paré used this device, illustrated in his* Ten Books of Surgery *(1564), for raising skull bones depressed by a blow. New York Academy of Medicine*

629 *A stratagem for correcting crossed eyes, as shown in a 16th-century woodcut. World Health Organization, Geneva*

630 *An apparatus for applying traction to dislocations was illustrated by Guido Guidi in his* Chirurgia e Graeco in Latinum conversa *(1544). New York Academy of Medicine*

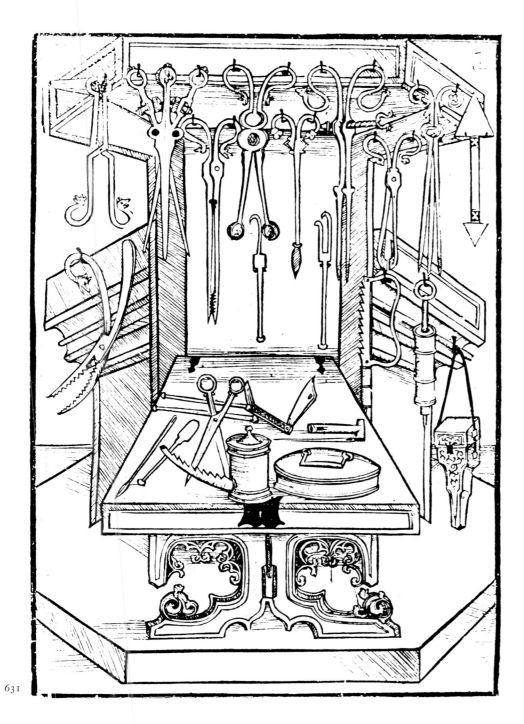

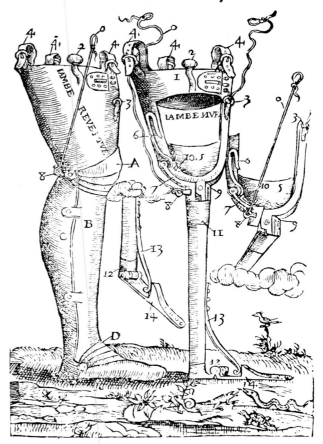

Pourtraict des iambes artificielles.

631 *A display of surgical instruments in Hieronymus Brunschwig,* Chirurgia (1497), *which detailed the variety used in medical practice at the time. New York Academy of Medicine*

632 *Ambroise Paré supplied careful drawings of his medical devices, as in this artificial leg from his* Oeuvres (1575), *so that others could duplicate them. National Library of Medicine, Bethesda*

633 *A method for immobilizing a limb with splints and bandages was presented by Guido Guidi in his* Chirurgia e Graeco in Latinum conversa (1544). *The value of careful, naturalistic illustration was increasingly appreciated in the Renaissance. National Library of Medicine, Bethesda*

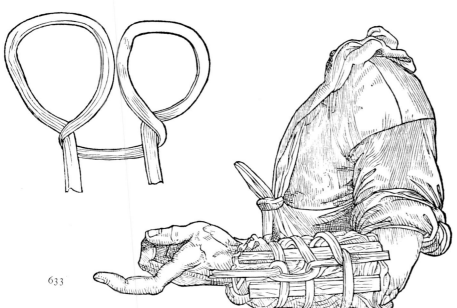

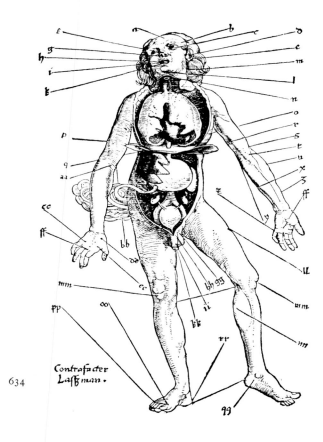

634 *Colored woodcut of bloodletting points by Johannes Wechtlin from* Treatise on Surgery *(1540). In the Renaissance, artists began to observe for themselves, and in anatomical drawings the size and placement of organs became more accurate. New York Academy of Medicine*

635 *An accurate knowledge of the human form gained from a dozen years of dissection is transformed into art in Michelangelo's drawing* The Resurrection *(1513–16). W.53, British Museum, London*

dissections were primitively and nonrealistically drawn. In the second edition (1493), the poses of the figures were more natural. In one scene a sick person was attended by his physician and several women. Another showed a dissection with the young, beardless professor sitting in the lecturer's chair while a barber surgeon dissected. The several texts of Hieronymus Brunschwig (c. 1450–1512) continued the use of narrative illustration. The final chapter of a work by Johannes Peyligk (1474–1522) was a brief anatomy of the entire body, but the eleven woodcuts included were little more than diagrammatic representations after the Arabists. In one, the intestines were cleverly but unrealistically represented as an interlaced love knot. In the *Margarita philosophica* by Gregor Reisch (1467–1525), an encyclopedia of all the sciences, several innovations were added to otherwise traditional woodcuts: the abdominal viscera were this time realistically represented.

In addition to those anatomical texts designed specifically for students and physicians, there were many separate printed sheets of anatomical figures captioned not in Latin (as were all works for physicians) but, rather, in the vernacular. There often was an intense interest in conception and the formation of the human fetus. The frequent use of the phrase "Know thyself" bespoke a philosophical and essentially nonmedical orientation. The Helain skeleton (Nuremberg, 1493) was the first example printed, and others quickly followed, but compared to renderings of many contemporary and even earlier artists it is inferior both anatomically and artistically. The "Dance of Death" had become an extremely popular subject, especially in the German-speaking countries after the Black Death, and, surprisingly, the artists' representations of skeletons and human anatomy were better than that of the anatomists.

The Renaissance artist of the fifteenth century became increasingly interested in the human form, and the study of human anatomy appropriately became a necessary part of the young artist's apprenticeship, especially in northern Italy. Leonardo da Vinci (1452–1519), however, was the first artist to consider anatomy for reasons beyond its practicality in depicting the human form. Leonardo himself made anatomical preparations from which he produced drawings, of which more than 750 are extant, representing the skeletal, muscular, nervous, and vascular systems. The illustrations were often supplemented with annotations of a physiological nature. Leonardo's scientific accuracy was greater than that of Vesalius, and his artistic beauty remains unchallenged. His correct assessment of the curvature of the spine went otherwise undiscovered for more than a hundred years. He depicted the true position of the *fetus in utero* and first noted certain anatomical structures. The sketches were seen by only a few contemporaries and were not published until the end of the last century.

Michelangelo Buonarroti (1475–1564) spent at least twelve years in serious pursuit of anatomical knowledge through personal dissection, especially at the Cloister of Santo Spirito in Florence. He later described his transition from an awareness of the usefulness to the artist of anatomy to an interest of and for itself, although this interest was always secondary to art.

Albrecht Dürer (1471–1528) wrote treatises on mathematics, chemistry, hydraulics, and anatomy. His treatise on human proportions was published after his death, but his concern for anatomy was entirely esthetic, deriving ultimately from an interest in classical canons by which beauty might be defined. With the important exception of Leonardo, whose drawings were almost certainly not available to the anatomists of the sixteenth century, the Renaissance artist was only secondarily an anatomist. Although important contributions to the realistic representation of the human form were made (such as the use of perspective and shading to suggest depth and three-dimensionality), true scientific advances awaited the collaboration of the professional anatomist and artist.

Once anatomists became aware of realistic representations of precise anatomical information, a period of intense experimentation began throughout Europe but especially in northern Italy and southern Germany. This is best represented in Jacopo

410

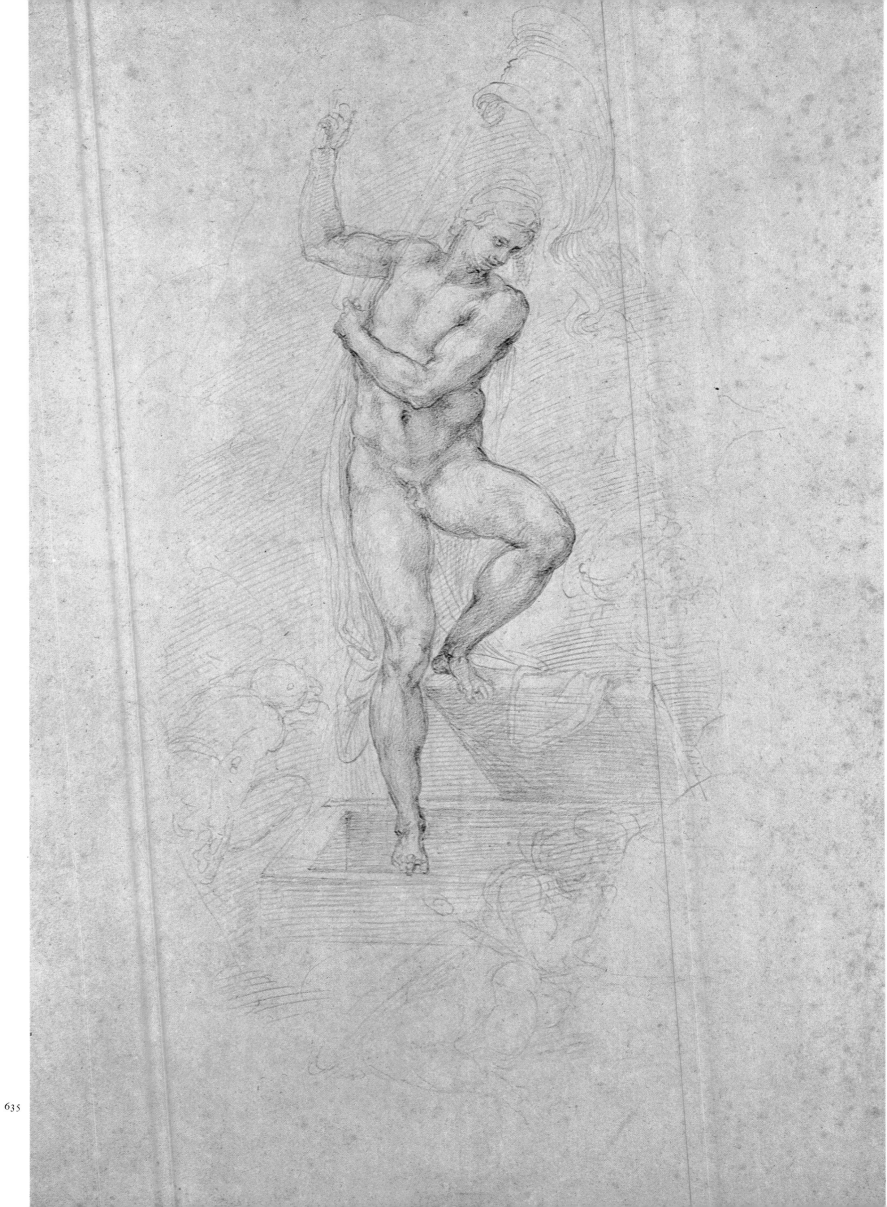

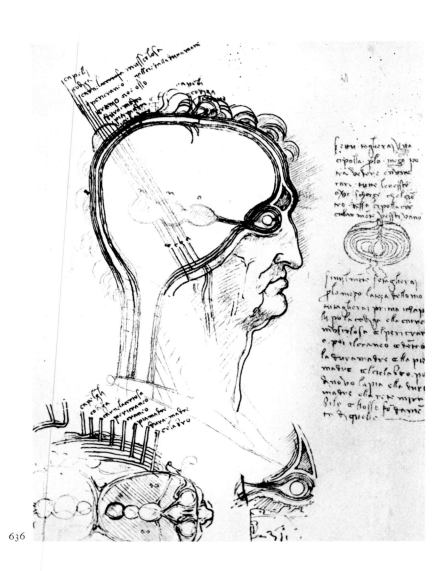

636

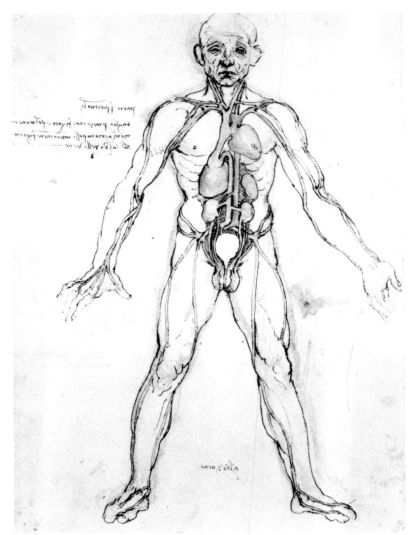

637

636–641 *Anatomical studies by Leonardo da Vinci, a selection from more than 750 extant drawings.* Above, courtesy World Health Organization, Geneva; *all others,* by permission of Her Majesty Queen Elizabeth II, Royal Art Collection, Windsor Castle

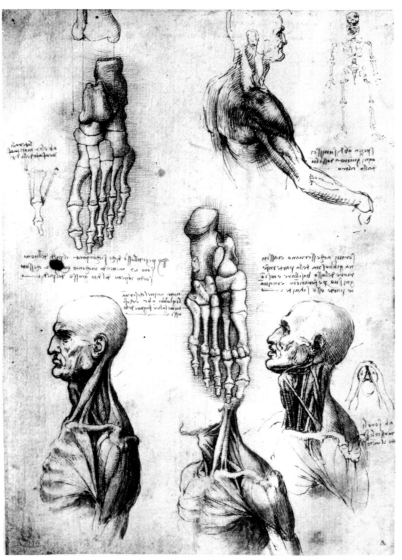

638

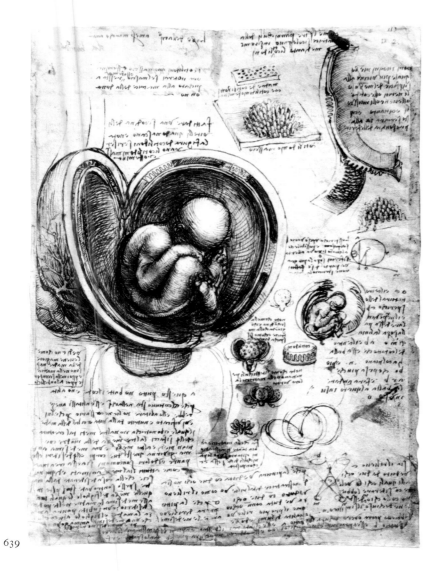

639

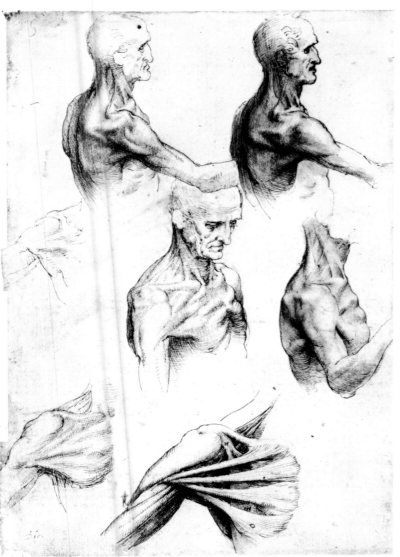

640

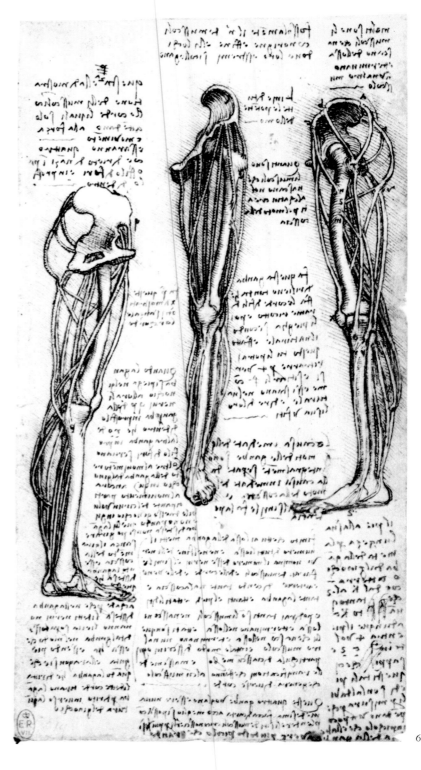

641

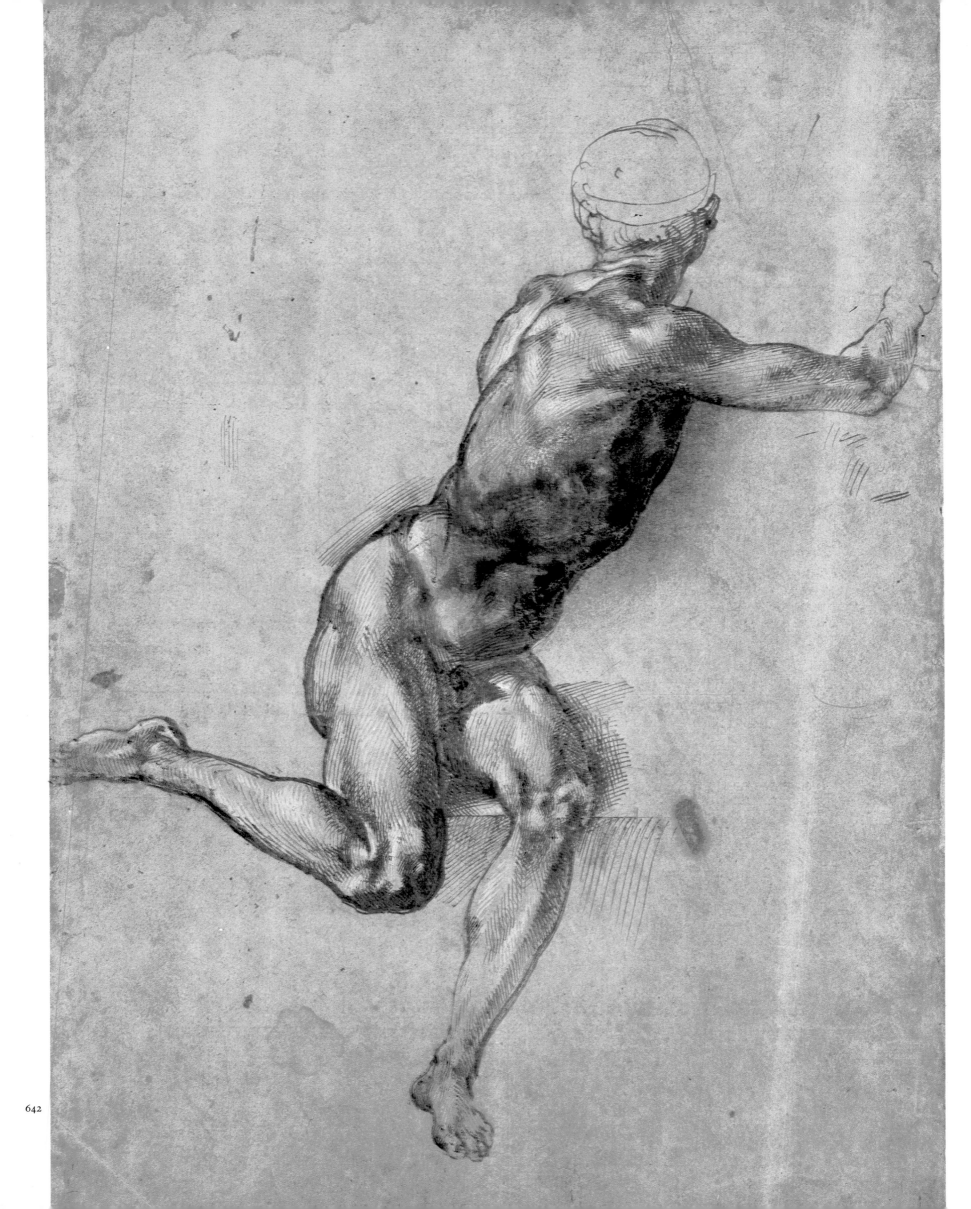

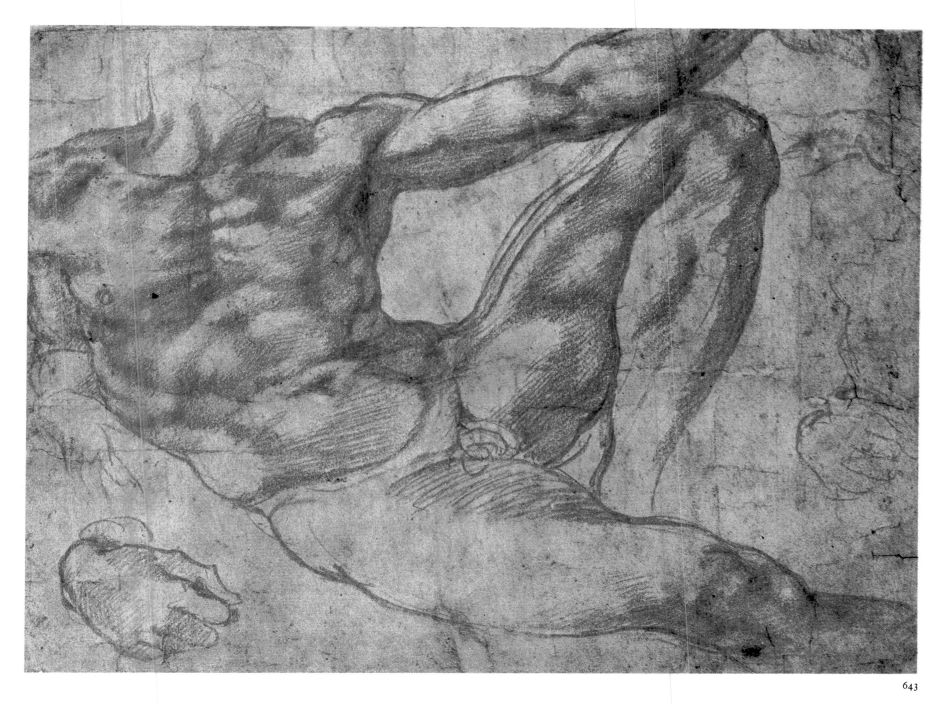

643

642 *Figure study by Michelangelo of a seated nude for* The Battle of Cascina (*1504*). *W.6 r., British Museum, London*

643 *Study by Michelangelo for Adam* (*1511*) *in the* Creation of Adam *for the Sistine Ceiling. W.11 r., British Museum, London*

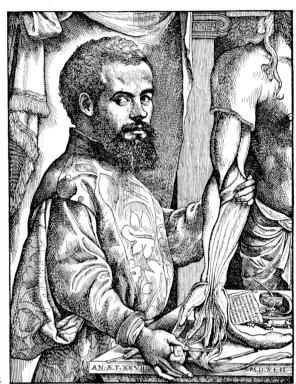

644

644 *Portrait of the great anatomist Andreas Vesalius at the age of 28, from his masterpiece* De humani corporis fabrica *(1543).* World Health Organization, Geneva

645, 646 *Plates from Vesalius's* De humani corporis fabrica, *showing the muscles and the entire vena cava (the principal vein of the body). The artist responsible for rendering the plates is unknown, but there is conjecture that it was Jan Stephen van Calcar, who was also credited with some earlier figures.* New York Academy of Medicine

647 *Figure study by Albrecht Dürer for Adam (c. 1506). Dürer was not only an artist but also a writer of treatises on mathematics, chemistry, hydraulics, and anatomy.* Graphische Sammlung Albertina, Vienna

648 *In this woodcut,* The Peddler *(1538), Hans Holbein the Younger, working in the* danse macabre *genre, reflects a more observant eye than many of the contemporary anatomists.* British Museum, London

Berengario da Carpi (d. 1530), author of *Commentaria super anatomica mundini* (1521), who presented the first anatomical illustrations made consistently from nature. In 1536, Cratander at Basel published an edition of the works of Galen which included figures, especially of osteology, rendered in a remarkably realistic fashion. As early as 1532 and through the next several years, Charles Estienne of Paris was preparing a work which stressed a complete pictorial account of the human body.

VESALIUS

One of the earliest and most successful solutions to reproducing exactly similar pictorial representations is to be found in the development of the illustrations published in the anatomical treatises of Andreas Vesalius (1514–64), culminating in his *De humani corporis fabrica* of 1543, one of the greatest books in the history of man. Vesalius had been born in 1514 in Brussels to a family with long-standing connections to the House of Burgundy and the Holy Roman emperor's court. His early medical training at the University of Paris (where his teachers included Jacques duBois and Guinter of Andernach) was interrupted by war between France and the Holy Roman Empire. Vesalius completed his studies at the renowned medical school of Padua in northern Italy. Immediately after graduation, he began teaching surgery and anatomy. After several preliminary works, in 1543, at the age of twenty-eight, he published his *opus magnum* which revolutionized not only anatomy but also scientific teaching in general. The *Fabrica*'s illustrations work precisely because of their close integration with the text. They were meant to fulfill needs which the text could handle only with difficulty, if at all. The scheme of organization used by Mondino, whereby those parts which decomposed most rapidly were discussed first, was abandoned, and each of the major systems (bones, muscles, blood vessels, nerves, and internal organs) was discussed and depicted separately. The various parts of each organ system were considered both together and isolated, and the relationships of all these structures were also considered. Vesalius recognized that all structures are not identical in all individuals.

Vesalius wrote of his surprise at finding numerous errors in the works of Galen, and much has been made of his refusal to accept something on faith solely because it was found in Galen. Though Vesalius could not confirm Galen's holes between the chambers of the heart, he nevertheless remained a genuine follower of Galenic physiology. Their differences in anatomical understanding have been magnified, not the least by Vesalius himself. Perhaps recognizing that a little controversy can go a long way toward gaining attention, Vesalius soon found himself in bitter controversy with his former teacher Jacques duBois (or Sylvius in the Latinized form). Sylvius was a complete Galenist whose only retort upon learning of the differences between certain structures as seen by Vesalius and as described by Galen was that mankind must have changed in the intervening twelve hundred years.

Although Vesalius attributed the artwork for three earlier figures to a fellow Fleming, in the *Fabrica* he gave no credit to any artist, and much controversy has arisen over the identity of the artist or artists. Much of this controversy has been accentuated by the question of who was more important, artist or anatomist. Even the brief discussion above should make it obvious that the illustrations were significant precisely because they were a combination of art and science, a collaboration between artist and anatomist. Too much anatomical information, especially of an innovative variety, was included for Vesalius not to have been involved in the preparation of the drawings. But it is equally obvious that the degree of artistic sophistication and the knowledge of techniques new even to artists in the Renaissance were too great for Vesalius to have been the sole person responsible. Whether Jan Stephan van Calcar (1499–1546/50), who had done the earlier figures and worked in the studio of Titian in nearby Venice, was the

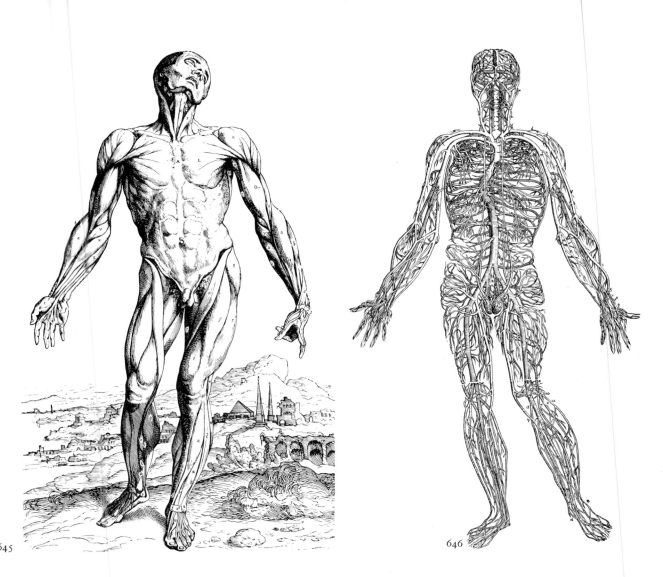

645

646

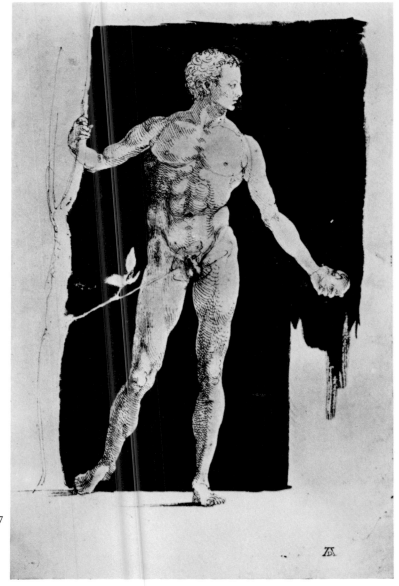

647

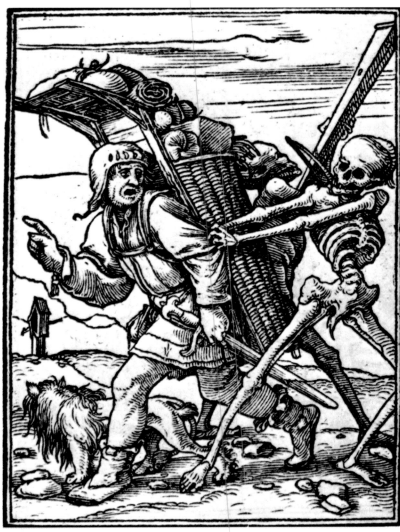

648

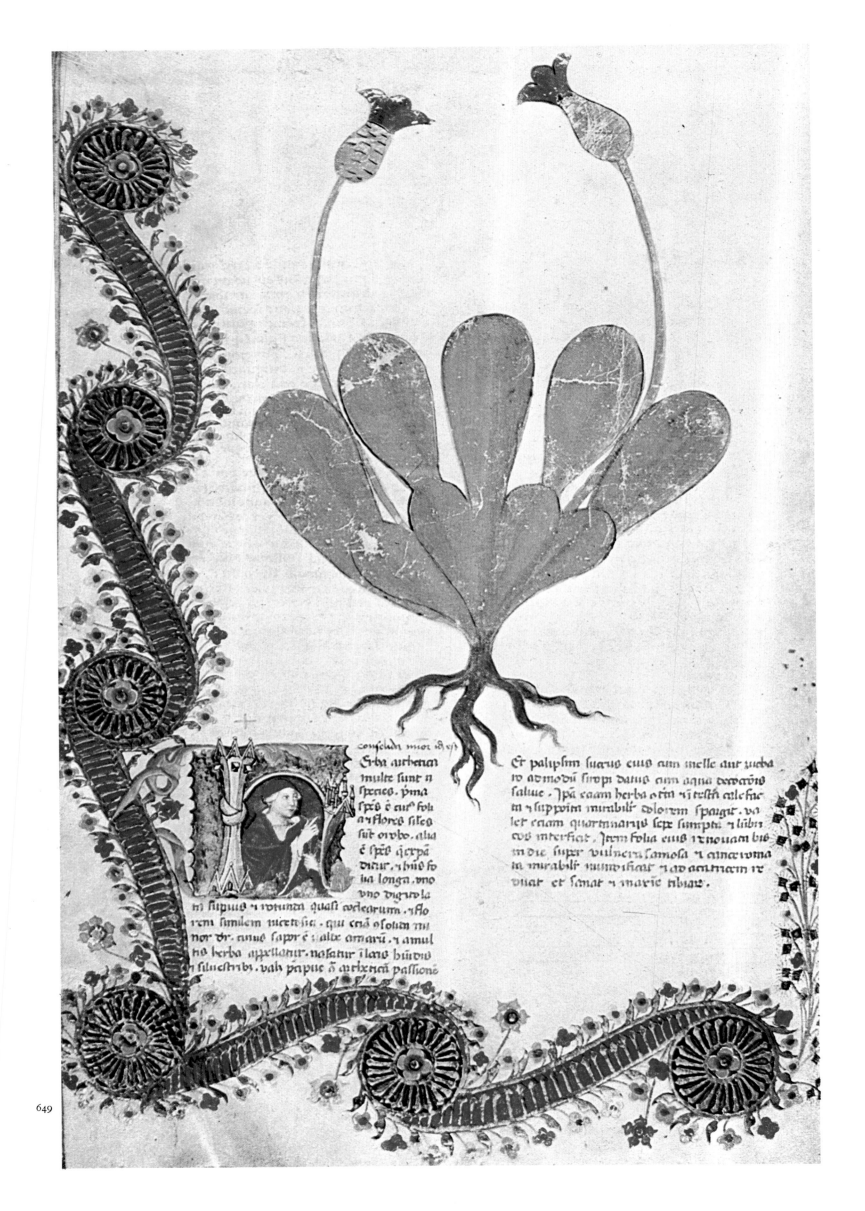

consolida mior id est

Erba autheuar
multe sunt n
species. pma
spes e eur soli
a flores siles
sut orbo. alia
e spes qerpa
ditur. i huis fo
lia longa. vno
vno diguola
n supius i rotuna quasi cocleaum. i flo
rem similem micteusta. qui eua osolan mi
nor dr. cuus sapor e : alte amaru. i amul
us herba appellatur. nosatur i laio biuons
n siluestribus. val papue d arthetica passioue

Et palipsim suauis eius aun melle aut ueba
ro admodu sirop datuis aun aqua devario
salue. Ipa eaam herba o in u testi cale hae
m i suppim murabili colorem spaigit. va
let eaam quartinarus sepe sumpta i lubn
cos mterficat. Item folia eius i rnouam bis
m die super vulnera samosa i auceroma
ta murabili numosicat i ab aurtricam re
uliat et sanat i marie tibiar.

artist, however, remains controversial and speculative. Nevertheless, a solution to the quest for the means of an adequate pictorial expression of natural phenomena had been found.

BOTANICAL ILLUSTRATIONS

Similar transitions from schematic medieval manuscript illustrations to realistic and easily reproduced renderings occurred in other disciplines of the natural and applied sciences. Of them only botany seems relevant to medicine in the Renaissance because of the heavy reliance of pharmacology on herbals and medications derived from plants. The medieval manuscript illustration of a plant, like that of an anatomical part, almost always had an earlier illustration as its model instead of the plant. Repeated copyings tended to simplify the drawing, and a kind of abstraction developed which was accentuated by the earlier tradition of using floral and animal motifs as manuscript decorations. Furthermore, the medieval propensity toward the exotic made it difficult to determine the truthfulness of an object pictured; for instance, in zoology the rich legends of the unicorn made it seem much more likely that it would be real than the giraffe or rhinoceros. The first published nature-books and encyclopedias contained illustrations quite similar to other drawings made at the same time: simplified, abstract, and having little resemblance to the natural object. The *Hortus Sanitatis* (1491) contained many colored woodcuts of real and fanciful plants and animals, but it was with Otto Brunfels (1488?–1534) of Mainz that we see the beginning of the transition from medieval to modern. His *Herbarum vivae eicones* (Strassburg, 1530–32) contained many illustrations of plants executed by Hans Weiditz although the textual description made no attempt at originality over Pliny and Dioscorides. Plant description really took its first start (after Theophrastus) with Hieronymus Bock, or Tragus, (1489?–1554) who wrote down numerous descriptions of plants in the vernacular in his *Kräutterbuch* (1539). Needless to say, a drawing by Leonardo da Vinci, or by many other artists, made decades earlier, possessed greater esthetic beauty and scientific accuracy than any of these primitive illustrations. Only with the publication in 1542 of the great *De historia stirpium* of the Bavarian Leonhard Fuchs (1501–66) do we find in botany a quality of rendering equivalent to that found in the *Fabrica*, and numerous reprints were to follow.

Once the works of Vesalius and Fuchs had been completed, much of the stimulus for development in the fields of anatomy and botany was lost, for so long as these disciplines were to remain descriptive, or empiric, there was little to do beyond adding detail. Thus, the works of Bartolommeo Eustachio (1524?–74), Matteo Realdo Colombo (1515?–59), Giovanni Battista Canano (1515–79), Gabriello Fallopio (1523–62), and Fabricius ab Aquapendente (1537–1619) in anatomy and Conrad Gesner (1516–65), Gaspard Bauhin (1550–1624), and Pierre Belon (1517–64) in botany seem inspired. Only when William Harvey (1578–1657) discerns the circulation of the blood from the discovery of the venous valves by his teacher Fabricius ab Aquapendente do we find an innovative use of empiricism, for which a long period of classifying was necessary before experimentation could proceed on strong footing.

649 *A typical medieval botanical illustration, from* Historia Plantarum (*14th century*), *based more on previous descriptions than actual plants. Ms. 459, fol. 125 v., Biblioteca Casanatense, Rome*

650 *Many plant illustrations in the Middle Ages were more reflective of mythology than botany, as exemplified in this fanciful woodcut of the mandrake root in a French edition (c. 1500) of* Hortus Sanitatus. *New York Academy of Medicine*

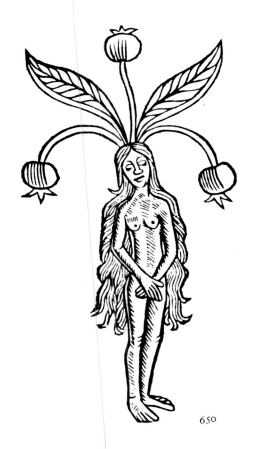

650

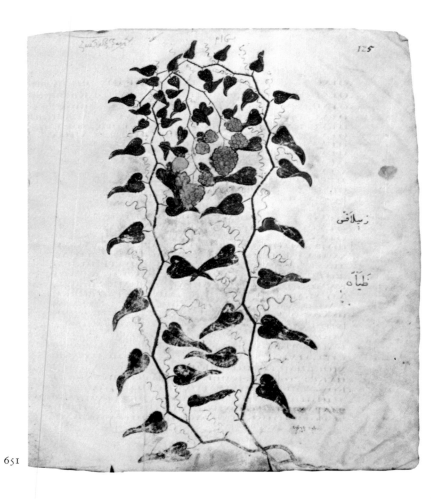

651

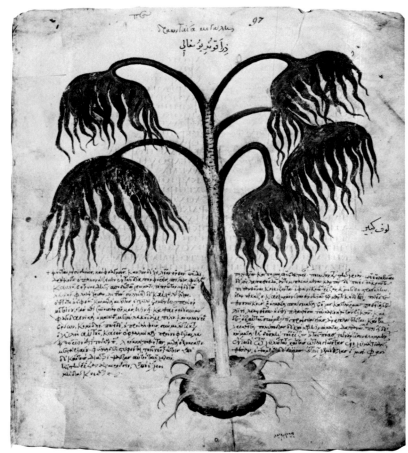

652

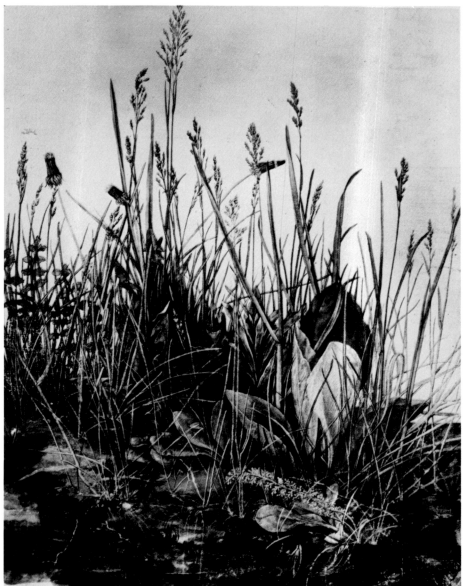

653

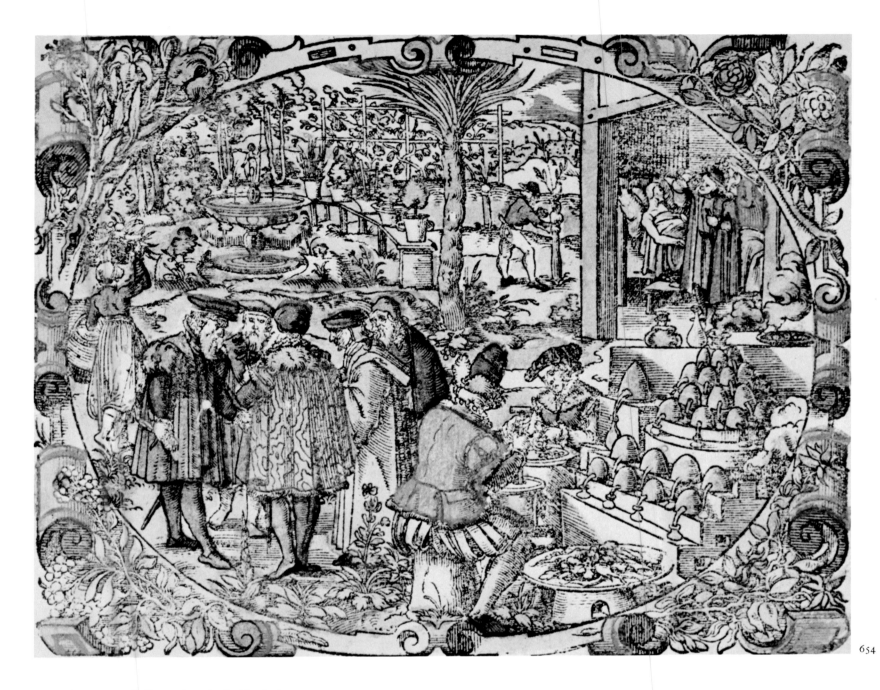

654

651, 652 *Botanical illustrations in the Dark Ages were often more decorative than informative, as evident in these two editions of Dioscorides,* De Materia Medica *(1st century). Left:* Codex Med. Graec 1 *(6th century); right:* Codex Constantinopolitanus *(485). Österreichische Nationalbibliothek, Vienna*

653 *In the Renaissance, artists began to rely more on direct observation than botanical precedent, with far more naturalistic results, as exemplified in Albrecht Dürer's* The Great Clump of Turf *(1503). Graphische Sammlung Albertina, Vienna*

654 *Vignette on the title page of Adam Lonizer,* Kreuterbuch *(1593), showing learned doctors in consultation while herbs are collected in background and distilled into concoctions, possibly for man in bed. National Library of Medicine, Bethesda*

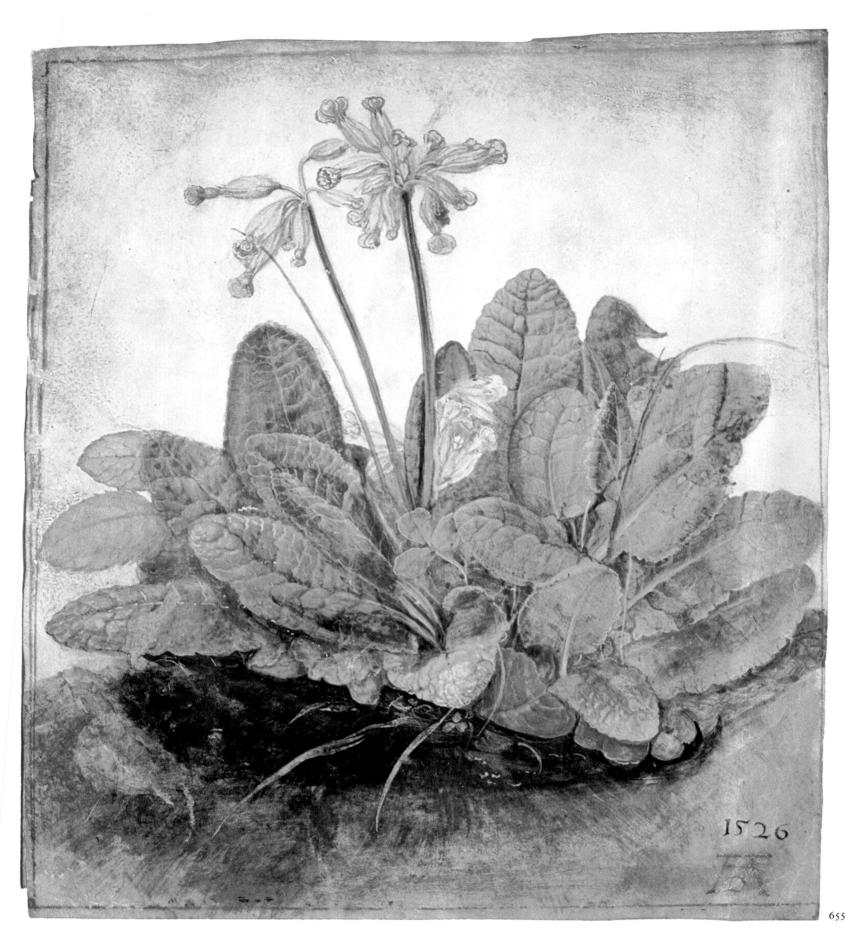

1526

655

655 *In this gouache on vellum,* Tuft of Cowslips *(1526), Albrecht Dürer presents a superb example of accurate rendering in scale and detail through close observation of nature. Collection Armand Hammer Foundation, Los Angeles*

656 *A page from the* Sketchbook *(1398) of Giovannino de' Grassi indicates that birds and animals were closely observed and accurately rendered much earlier than plants. Biblioteca Civica A. Mai, Bergamo*

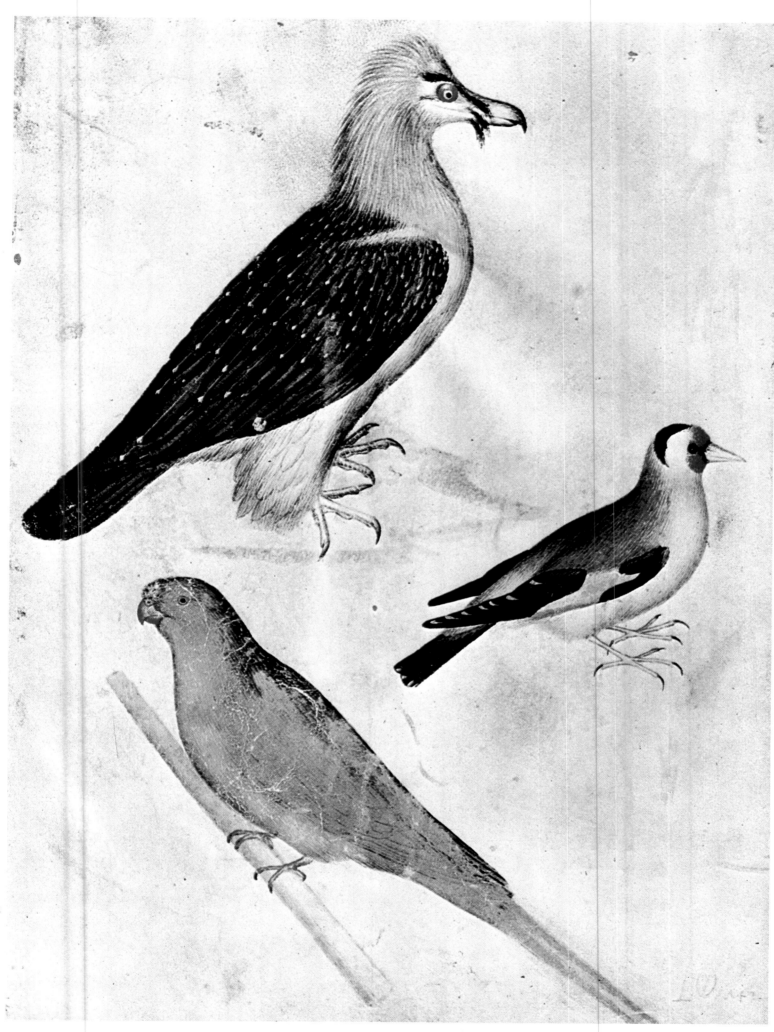

THE
SEVENTEENTH
CENTURY

The Seventeenth Century

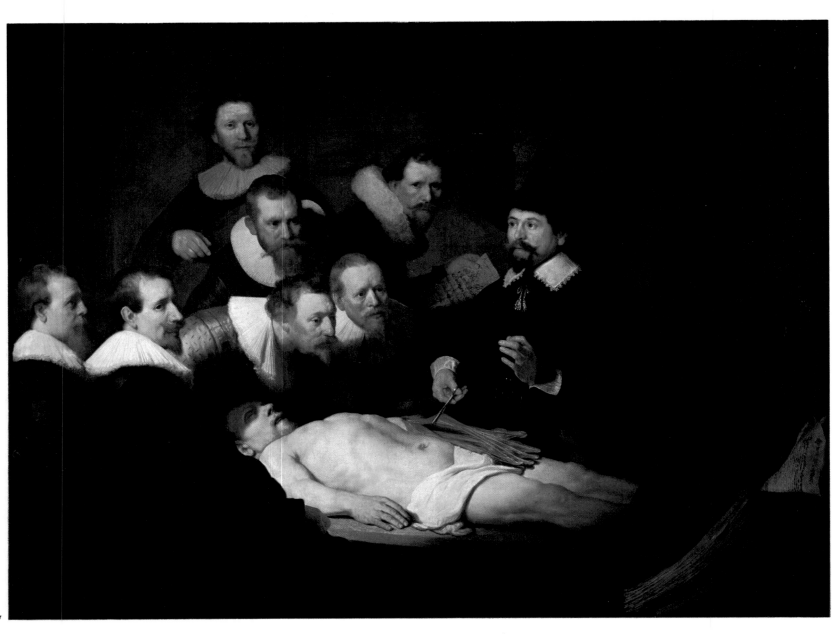

657

C ALLED the "Age of the Scientific Revolution," the seventeenth century represents a major turning point in the history of science. Instead of asking *why* things occur, scientists turned to *how* things happen—a shift in emphasis from speculation to experimentation. Interpretations became mechanistic, and the language of science became mathematical.

INFLUENCES FROM THE PAST

Three major influences from earlier centuries had to be reckoned with: Aristotelianism, Galenism, and Paracelsianism.

Aristotelianism in the seventeenth century was really a general view of nature, especially with respect to the physical sciences and biology. In the two thousand years following his death, Aristotle's original doctrines had gone through numerous changes by various cultures. Prior to the seventeenth century, the experimental method springing from Aristotle frequently consisted of no more than a single observation, often of a chance nature, and for the most part not quantified nor expressed in mathematical terms.

An influence on the seventeenth century reinforced by Aristotelianism was the intimate relationship between astrology and medicine. Aristotle's conception of a spherical earth in a spherical universe of finite size, moving according to mechanical plan, fitted well into the subsequent concepts of astrology. Chance was usually not a factor in the Aristotelian universe. However, the purpose of an occurrence was not necessarily obvious but rather an element of a plan that could be figured out. In astronomy there was a regularity and uniformity that was especially evident. This teleology, as seen in Galen's teachings, continued to be an important part of medicine until the seventeenth century, when Aristotelianism came under heavy attack.

Another influence on seventeenth-century medicine was Galenism, which, like Aristotelianism, embraced more than the concepts developed by Galen in the second century A.D. His works demonstrated a search for facts (although colored by preconceptions), a vigorous disrespect for authority (although he did worship Hippocrates), and a strong desire to see for himself. However, his numerous disciples tended to accept what Galen said he saw rather than follow his methods.

An additional important factor was Paracelsian thought inherited from the Renaissance. In opposing the long-term medieval reliance on the works of Galen and Avicenna, and in emphasizing observation and experience, Paracelsus was a revolutionary. He revived Hippocrates as the only physician of the past worth remembering, yet his own system was itself "un-Hippocratic." To him the physician was a magus who could direct the astral forces to heal. As the constellations changed so must diseases and their treatment; thus astrology became an important aspect of Paracelsian doctrine.

The most notable influence of Paracelsus was on chemistry in medicine. He concluded that the human body was a chemical machine, and whereas Galenic physicians had relied primarily on plant medicines Paracelsus popularized the use of minerals. This chemical medicine was to compete with the Galenic school for the next two hundred years and ultimately to find a place in the accepted pharmacopoeias.

PHILOSOPHIES OF THE CENTURY

René Descartes (1596–1650) represented ideas that were in some ways a transition between earlier systems of philosophy and the directions thought would take after the seventeenth century. Descartes's *Discourse on Method* in 1637 supported a generalization of the mathematical method and the development of a mechanistic picture of the world. Descartes began with general ideas arrived at intuitively from self-evident truths and from them deduced the phenomena of the world. To

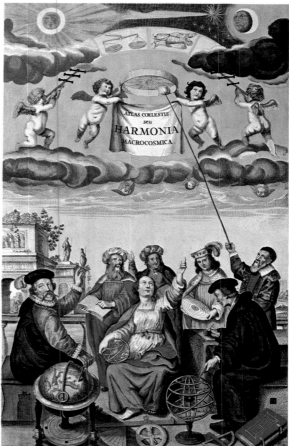

658

657 *Rembrandt's* The Anatomy Lesson of Dr. Tulp (*1632*) *indicates the importance of anatomy in the 17th century to medical teaching, an inheritance from the Renaissance. Mauritshuis, The Hague*

658 *The frontispiece of Andreas Cellarius,* Harmonia Macrocosmica (*1661*) *depicts the giants of the Age of Scientific Revolution, left to right, Tycho Brahe, Ptolemy, possibly St. Augustine, Copernicus, Galileo (with pointer), and (seated at right) the author himself. Library of Congress, Washington, D.C.*

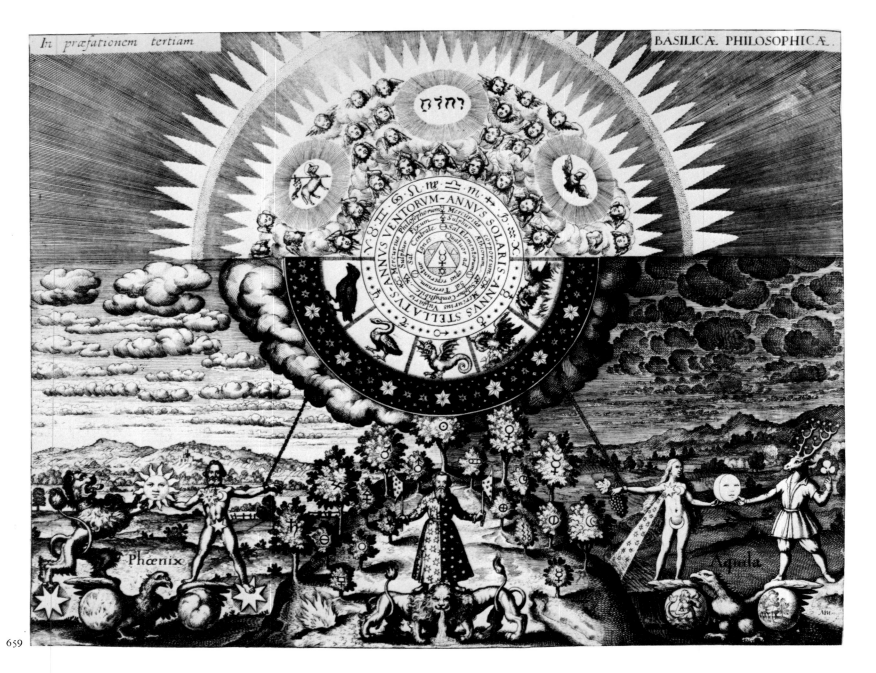

659

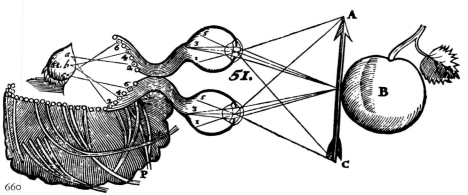

660

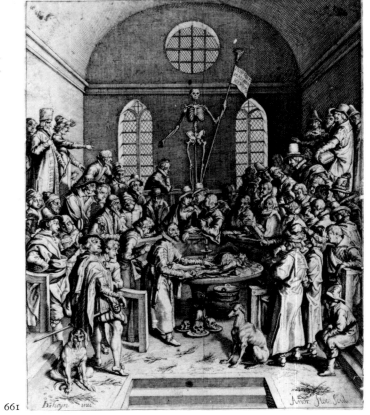

661

Descartes experiment was chiefly illustrative, but useful when deductive reasoning was inconclusive. Thus Descartes perpetuated the scholasticism and speculative tendencies of past tradition. On the other hand, he was generally opposed to an Aristotelian teleology, for to Descartes all natural objects were machines ruled by mechanistic principles.

Another philosopher of science was Francis Bacon (1561–1626). Apparently the inductive method he proposed did not have a marked effect on contemporary scientists, nor did he side with Copernicus (1473–1543), the advocate of a heliocentric world. Furthermore, some of his works were not well known until after his death. He was, nevertheless, an eloquent spokesman for experimentation and the inductive method, which was to collect particular facts with no hypothesis in mind and look for a general theory to emerge.

Bacon, like Descartes, viewed science as utilitarian. He saw humankind as ever moving ahead and accumulating the benefits of scientific endeavor, but the idea of Progress was something new to the seventeenth century. The Greeks had considered science primarily speculative and philosophical rather than the means of exerting power over nature. To most ancient people, time and the world were cyclical rather than progressive: civilizations rose and fell. Men generally felt that the present was in decline from a past Golden Age. Like Bacon, Descartes also subscribed to the idea of progress, but he believed that his own speculative thoughts could point the way ahead. Bacon on the other hand considered his method of reasoning from facts as merely a first attempt upon which others would improve.

NEW DIRECTIONS OF MEDICAL THOUGHT

Iatrochemistry, or medical chemistry, was the name given to the fusion of alchemy, medicine, and chemistry that was practiced by the followers of Paracelsus in the sixteenth and seventeenth centuries—an alternative to the new mechanistic philosophy which eventually dominated modern science.

Jan Baptista van Helmont (1577–1644) was the leading Paracelsian and iatrochemist of the seventeenth century. After taking a medical degree in 1599, Van Helmont became increasingly dissatisfied with the bookish Galenic medicine practiced in the schools and eventually took up a career of private research. His opposition to the established doctrines of medicine and to medical teachings of churchmen brought him into conflict with the Spanish Inquisition, which badgered him throughout much of his life.

Van Helmont advocated quantification and experiment, and his comparison of the weight of urine with that of water was the first measurement of its specific gravity. Another contribution was his recognition that air was composed of several gases. He actually coined the term "gas" (derived from the Greek and Latin "chaos").

Van Helmont believed that the basic substances of the world were not the four elements of Aristotle and Galen nor the three principles of Paracelsus. Instead he thought of all matter as reducible to water, which he said was supported by Scripture: on the second day God created the firmament to separate the waters above from the waters below, but nowhere in the Bible did it say that God created the water.

Like Paracelsus, Van Helmont was a founder of the concept of disease as a distinct entity existing parasitically in the body. This was in contradistinction to the Galenic concept that disease was part of the person and represented a derangement of the humors. Unlike Paracelsus, Van Helmont did not accept astrological principles as affecting disease, nor did he consider valid the Paracelsian analogy between microcosm and macrocosm.

By experiment he concluded that ferments (enzymes) were a fundamental part of all physiological mechanisms, which is not far from our contemporary views. Van Helmont's rejection of the Galenic conception of disease also caused him to

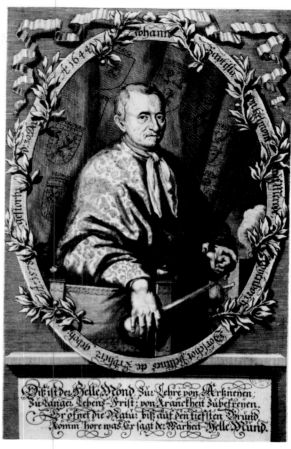

662

659 *The 17th century still looked upon the body as a microcosmic representation of the universe, as seen in this engraving,* Allegory of the Microcosm and Macrocosm, *by Matthäus Merian the Elder in* Opus Medico-Chymii Pars Altera *(1618–20) by Johann Daniel Mylius. National Library of Medicine, Bethesda*

660 *Philosopher-scientist René Descartes had great influence on mechanistic scientific thinking, but this drawing indicates that he was not aware of the crossing over of optic nerve fibers to the opposite side of the brain. World Health Organization, Geneva*

661 *Engraving by Andries Jacobsz Stock of a dissection taking place before a random group of onlookers, from Pieter Paaw,* Succentuiciatus Anatomicus *(1616). National Library of Medicine, Bethesda*

662 *Engraving by Johann Alexander Böner of the leading iatrochemist Jan Baptista van Helmont in the year of his death, 1644. He was an experimentalist who opposed the dogma of Galen, the astrology of Paracelsus, and many other established doctrines. Académie Nationale de Médecine, Paris*

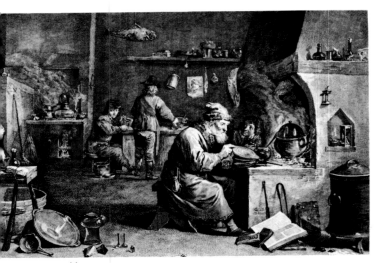

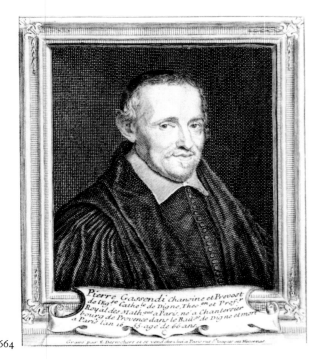

664

663 *The chemist, alchemist, and medical practitioner were often combined in the same person, as reflected in this engraving by David Teniers the Younger called* The Chemist. *Bibliothèque Nationale, Paris*

664 *Churchman, philosopher, scientist, and Epicurean, Pierre Gassend embraced the theory of atomism and taught that physical differences in objects were due to the arrangement and motion of their atoms. New York Academy of Medicine*

reject the therapeutics. Fever was not putrefaction of the humors but represented reaction to an invading, irritating agent. He declined to use bloodletting and purging, and rejected their supposed value in restoring the humoral balance. He used chemical medicines and improved on the use of mercury, which Paracelsus had so vigorously advocated.

Another important iatrochemist was Franz de le Boë, called Franciscus Sylvius (1614–72). His approach to medicine was empirical, making use of the newest discoveries in chemistry. His theory did not include the humors of Galen but was based on the concept of bodily acids, bases, and their neutralizations. In relying on direct observation and experience he was representative of the iatrochemists of the second half of the seventeenth century. Although his experiments, from which he made sweeping generalizations, were really little more than observations, he provided a foundation for a new system of medicine based on iatrochemical concepts. Furthermore, he made the laboratory an essential tool for the practice and teaching of medicine.

Sylvius's attitudes also helped to bring bedside teaching into its own again. For centuries there had been no systematic clinical teaching, for the universities awarded medical degrees on the basis of spoken disputations. Leiden, where Sylvius worked, was one of the first cities to institute clinical teaching (1636), and since Holland was a center of religious toleration students flocked into Leiden for instruction and study.

ATOMISM

The rise of atomism was of utmost importance to the development of science, and consequently of medicine. The concept had its origins in antiquity and was first fully developed by Democritus of Abdera and Leucippus of Miletus (c. fifth century B.C.). The differences in physical objects were due to the shape, arrangement, and motion of atoms, which were infinite in number and dispersed throughout an infinite void. Atomism had been revived in the third century B.C. by Epicurus, whose primary interests were in ethics rather than in natural science. However, the survival of atomism was due in no small part to the Roman poet Titus Lucretius Carus of the first century B.C., who put the doctrines of Epicurus in the form of an elegant poem, *De rerum natura*. Not popular in the Middle Ages because of its atheistic tone, the work was rediscovered during the Renaissance and given further currency in the seventeenth century through the efforts of Pierre Gassend (1592–1655).

Gassend was a Catholic priest with a wide scientific reputation and orthodox religious beliefs. To make atomism fully acceptable in religious thought he had to divest matter of its eternal nature. Since God had created the atoms, he should be able to destroy them. Moreover, their motions were not determined by chance or necessity but by God's constant intervention.

Robert Boyle (1627–91) was another important proponent of atomism. However, unlike most seventeenth-century physicists, he was not principally interested in mathematics. Boyle devised the air pump with which he demonstrated the necessity of air for life. He also formulated what has come to be called "Boyle's Law": the volume of a gas varies inversely with the pressure at a constant temperature. His writings covered a variety of subjects, including respiration, magnetism, blood chemistry, and even wine.

Although not a physician, Boyle did extensive work with medicinals, which brought him into contact with patients. Boyle's empiric use of "specifick medicine" was a more scientific approach than the employment of drugs according to their Galenic classification. The recognition that something worked, even if there was no explanation, was a step forward. On the other hand, his choice of medication sometimes betrayed his allegiance to an ancient idea of "like cures like" still prevalent in the seventeenth century: for instance, that jasper was of value in preventing hemorrhagic disease because of its red color. This principle of

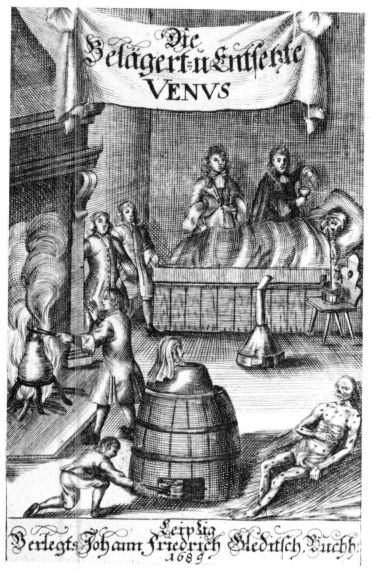

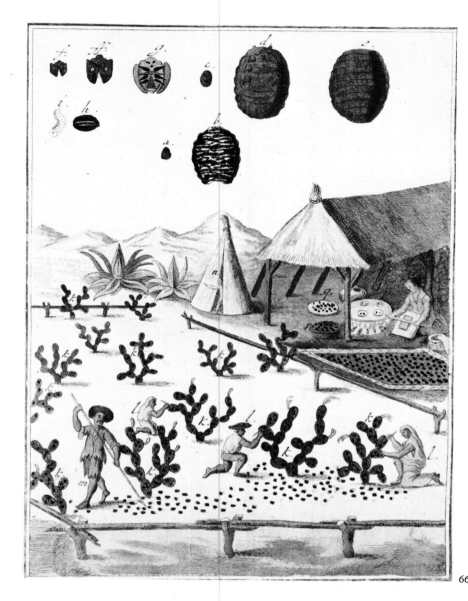

665

666

"sympathy," which was important to Paracelsus, was to continue into the nineteenth century and to find endorsement by Samuel Hahnemann (1755–1843) with his homeopathy.

 Another champion of modern science was Galileo Galilei (1564–1642). Some scholars believe that Galileo worked from experimental observations while others conclude that he worked from purely theoretical considerations, using experimentation to dress up his conclusions after the fact. Nevertheless his contributions were gigantic. Galileo formulated the laws of motion in a mathematical manner as they apply on the earth. It was the genius of Sir Isaac Newton (1642–1727) to extend these laws to the heavens by accurately describing the movements of the objects in our solar system under the influence of universal gravitation.

IATROPHYSICS

The explanation in medicine of phenomena as objects in motion resembling machines was iatromechanics, or iatrophysics. Giovanni Alfonso Borelli (1608–79) was the leading iatromechanist of the seventeenth century. Influenced by Galileo, he sought to apply his mechanical principles to medicine. Starting with a simple unit, the muscle, and then expanding his investigation to more complex systems in the body, he finally studied the whole organism.

 Giorgio Baglivi (1669–1707) represented the extreme use of iatromechanics, likening each organ to a specific machine. Another iatromechanic was Santorio

665 Mercury fumigation was used to treat syphilitic patients, whose various stages of illness were graphically depicted in this engraving from Steven Blankaart, Die Belägert und Entsetzte Venus (1689). National Library of Medicine, Bethesda

666 Engraving by Georg Peter Nusbiegel showing the collection and processing of cochineal lice into a drug and a dye. These cactus parasites were first obtained by the Spanish from the Aztecs. Senckenbergische Bibliothek, Frankfurt am Main

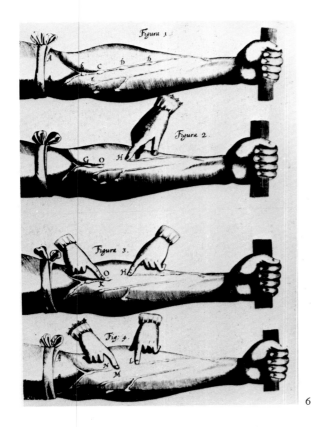

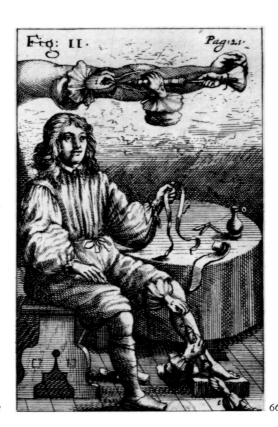

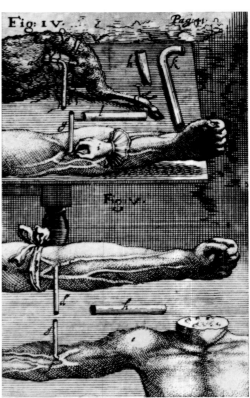

667

668

669

667 *Woodcuts used by William Harvey to demonstrate his proof of the circulation of the blood in* De Motu Cordis . . . (*1628*), *one of the most important books in medicine and biology. World Health Organization, Geneva*

668, 669 *Engravings in Johann Elshotz,* Clysmatica Nova (*1667*), *showing a man receiving an infusion in both an arm and a leg, and the techniques of transfusion from animal to man and man to man. Col. Brand., Bibliothèque Nationale, Paris*

Santorio (1561–1636), who constructed thermometers and is best remembered for his research into the physiology of metabolism. By means of a balance mechanism he measured the weight changes that result from eating, excreting, and perspiring.

EMBRYOLOGY

In 1677 Antony van Leeuwenhoek (1632–1723), a linen merchant of Delft, discovered the male spermatozoa with the aid of a microscope. Another Dutchman, Niklaas Hartsoeker (1656–1725), soon after Leeuwenhoek, published pictures showing tiny preformed men ("homunculi") in the spermatozoa he examined through a microscope. By the end of the seventeenth century there were two opposing views on how the embryo originated. Preformation, the dominant theory, saw a minuscule individual present in the sperm or egg, for which embryonic development was merely adding matter until the growing fetus reached newborn size. The other theory, epigenesis, taught that the organism began as a primitive substance that changed through a series of stages, gradually developing different structures and expanding others until the nature of the mature embryo was attained. In the seventeenth century preformation better fit the mechanistic attitude of science—the occurrence and maturation of the new organism was thereby explicable in secular, rational, and material terms. Epigenesis, on the other hand, seemed to require a spiritual, vitalistic theory to account for the seemingly occult change from formless matter into an organized creature.

William Harvey subscribed to the epigenetic explanation, and although some of his reports contained factual errors he made important contributions to embryology. It was his pioneer work on the circulation of the blood, however, which has gained him a prime position in the history of medicine.

CIRCULATION OF THE BLOOD

THE brilliant proof by William Harvey (1578–1657) of the continuous circulation of the blood within a contained system was the seventeenth century's most significant achievement in physiology and medicine.

Of course Harvey had had precursors. In Galenic physiology, blood was thought to be produced in the liver, where it received "natural spirit" and from which it flowed out to the periphery of the body due to a pulling or attractive force. Furthermore, blood obtained "vital spirits" in the heart and "animal spirits" in the brain. When Galen looked at the living heart in the second century A.D., he saw that it did not contract in a simple manner. First one side contracted and then the other, which did not seem to him the action of a pump. This movement was to Galen evidence of a displacement of blood from the right chamber of the heart into the left through tiny pores in the separating membrane.

The first person in the European tradition to propose a separate transit of the blood through the lungs was Michael Servetus (1511–53). Matteo Realdo Colombo (1516?–59) put forward a similar theory of the pulmonary transit solely on the basis of physiological reasoning. Since, contrary to Galen, the septum of the heart was solid, blood must follow another path from the right chamber to the left. The pulmonary artery coming from the right chamber seemed too large for the simple purpose of nourishing the lungs with blood, but blood in the pulmonary vein going into the heart's left chamber from the lungs was bright red whereas blood traveling to the lungs was dark red. He reasoned that it was the same liquid, but the change in color must be due to some action in the lungs.

Andrea Cesalpino (1519–1603) was perhaps the most important of Harvey's precursors. Not only did he use the expression "circulation" and think in terms of a closed circulatory system, but he had some straightforward ideas about the greater and lesser circulation (pulmonary transit). His astuteness was also shown in his proposal that fine vessels, or capillaries, connected the arterial and venous systems, so that there was no free, open effusion of blood into the tissues—as had been assumed for many centuries. On the other hand, Cesalpino believed that in addition to the capillaries there were major direct connections between the larger arteries and veins. Furthermore, Cesalpino believed that blood originated in the heart. He thought of circulation in terms of hot blood rising in the arteries and cold blood falling in the veins, but he had no clear conception of the veins as an exclusively centripetal system returning blood to the heart.

A much earlier predecessor was Ibn-Nafis (c. 1210–80), who also postulated the existence of the pulmonary circulation, but there is no evidence that Servetus knew of him. Although Alpago translated Ibn-an-Nafis in the Renaissance, he apparently failed to deal with the writings pertaining to pulmonary circulation.

Nevertheless, it was William Harvey who worked out most of the problems and is responsible for the present understanding of the blood's circulation. After being educated at Cambridge, he went to Padua, the apex of medical teaching at the time, where he found a direct link to Vesalius. Gabriello Fallopio (1523–62), after whom the Fallopian tubes are named, had been a pupil of Vesalius, and Fallopio was the teacher of Fabricius ab Aquapendente (1537–1619), one of the giants at Padua, who was in turn Harvey's teacher. The description by Fabricius of the valves in the veins was an important observation which Harvey used to support his circulation theory.

After returning to England from Padua in 1602 Harvey entered medical practice in London. There he rose quickly. Elected to the London College of Physicians, he gained a wide reputation and even became a court physician, first to King James I and later to King Charles I. During his many years as a practicing clinician in the monarchy, Harvey had managed also to engage in research. Although his lecture notes show that he believed in the circulation of the blood as early as 1615, he did not publish his findings until thirteen years later in *Exercitatio Anatomica de Motu Cordis et Sanguinis in Animalibus (On the Movement of the Heart and Blood in Animals)*, one of the most important works in medicine and biology.

How did Harvey reach his conclusions? For one thing, he concerned himself solely with the mechanical flow of blood, not with what happened in the heart,

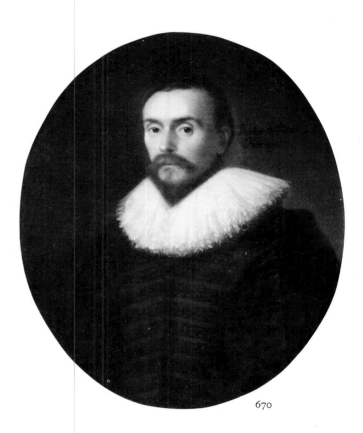

670

670 *William Harvey, whose experiments actually proved for the first time that the blood was pumped around the body in a closed system, is seen here in the Rolls Park portrait of 1627. National Portrait Gallery, London*

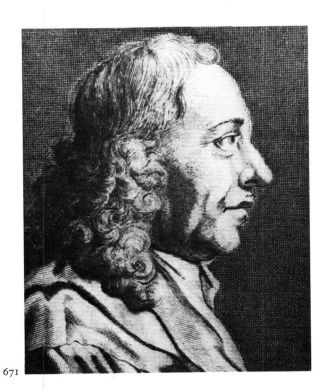

671

671 *Portrait of Marcello Malpighi, who discovered the capillary vessels postulated by Harvey and also described the finer structures of many tissues and organs. World Health Organization, Geneva*

672 *Painting by Robert Hannah in which William Harvey is shown demonstrating his experiments on deer to King Charles I and the boy prince. Royal College of Physicians, London*

liver, and brain. Nor was he involved with experiments on the role of the natural, vital, and animal spirits which were part of Galenic physiology. (Nevertheless, he continued to believe that the heart manufactured "vital spirit" which resided in the blood and was equivalent to the soul of man.) His arguments were based on morphological examples drawn from dissection and physiological experiments on animals. For instance, he showed that because of the valves in the heart and the veins, blood could flow in only one direction. In seeing that both ventricles of the heart contracted and expanded together, he concluded that there was no pressure difference between them which could drive blood through the thick septum. Moreover, the septum had its own system of arteries and veins, which would not be necessary if blood percolated through it. He also noted that after being removed from an animal, the heart continued to contract and expand like a muscle. Therefore, it was clearly a pump and not just an organ that sucked in blood. By experiment with a live serpent, Harvey demonstrated the direction of flow toward the heart in the great vein (vena cava) and away from the heart in the main artery (aorta).

In addition to anatomical dissections, physiological observations of humans, and direct experiments on animals, he also made use of quantitative data. If the human heart contained two ounces of blood (an observation from cadavers) and made about sixty-five beats per minute, then in one minute it pumped about eight pounds of blood. This amount multiplied by the minutes in a day gave a fantastic quantity of blood, far too much for the body to produce rapidly from food eaten. Harvey further supported these speculations with experiments on live sheep. Severing a sheep's main artery he collected and measured the blood expelled in a unit of time. It became obvious to him that blood circulated in a closed system. For the connection between arteries and veins to complete the circuit, Harvey assumed that there were capillaries even though he could not see them. The discovery of these microscopic structures was accomplished after Harvey's death by Marcello Malpighi (1628–94).

Although his contributions had enormous importance to anatomy and physiology, their impact on the practice of medicine was limited since the concepts and understandings of disease were little advanced by his demonstrations. However, after Harvey's proofs that a person's blood was continually recycling, the question of whether to bleed a patient from the same or opposite side of a disorder became irrelevant. Medicine adjusted to the circulation of the blood but still thought in terms of humors and of therapeutics relying on bleeding, purging, and vomiting.

Harvey's work was an important confirmation of the new mechanical science and the principles of experimental and quantitative analysis. His work formed a common front with that of Galileo, Kepler, Newton, Boyle, Borelli, Malpighi, and others. In his lecture notes Harvey compared the heart to a water bellows or a pump, which helped support the growing success of mechanistic philosophy.

How was Harvey's work received by his fellows? For twenty years after the publication of *On the Movement of the Heart and Blood in Animals* controversy raged over its conclusions. In this initial period many medical men ignored him, including those who had observed his demonstrations. For some of these men— surgeons concerned with achieving a respectable status denied them by the fraternity of physicians—adhering to Galenism made them more acceptable. His first major supporter was Robert Fludd (1574–1637), a mystic philosopher, physician, and friend who subscribed to the ancient concept of the human as a microcosmic analogy to the macrocosm. He concluded that the heart was the center of the body in the same way that the sun was the center of the universe. Another important champion of William Harvey was Jan de Waal (Walaeus) (1604–49), who performed new experiments that supported Harvey's findings.

James Primerose, an extreme adherent to Galenist doctrines, was the first to attack Harvey's ideas. He explained away the absence of pores in the septum of the heart by postmortem changes. Another critic was Caspar Hofmann (1572–1648).

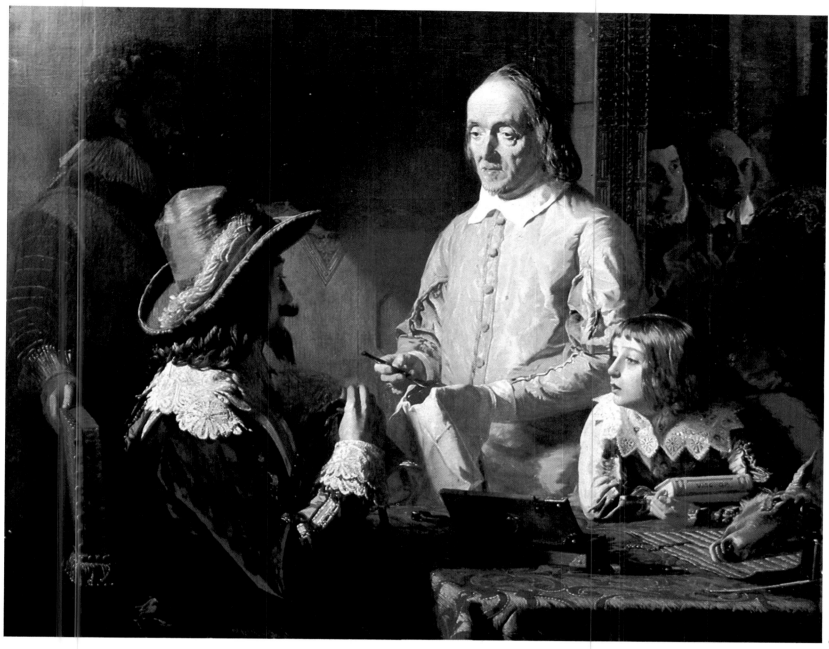

Although Hofmann was a supporter of Cesalpino and acknowledged the pulmonary transit (which he attributed to Realdo Colombo), he denied the muscular nature of the heart. He felt that Harvey had abandoned anatomy to the mathematical logic of calculation and quantitation. Hofmann also objected because Harvey's theories seemed to show that nature was acting superfluously by constantly circulating the blood. Harvey's response was simply that even if he did not know the reason for the circulation he saw that it happened.

Another critic of Harvey, Jean Riolan the Younger (1580–1657), an astute anatomist, tried to reconcile Harvey's teachings with Galen's. Using the same quantitative reasoning he arrived at a very different conclusion. By assuming that the heart pumped no more than a drop or two at each contraction, and by estimating how many drops were pumped each hour, he argued that no more than one or two circulations occurred per day. To account for Harvey's observations, Riolan explained that the heart, in the process of dying during vivisection, allowed blood to accumulate and so appeared to pump more blood. To him Harvey's results were therefore actually created by the experiments themselves.

Descartes also differed with Harvey. Earlier he had himself proposed a theory of the circulation of the blood, utilizing Aristotelian and Galenic notions. He

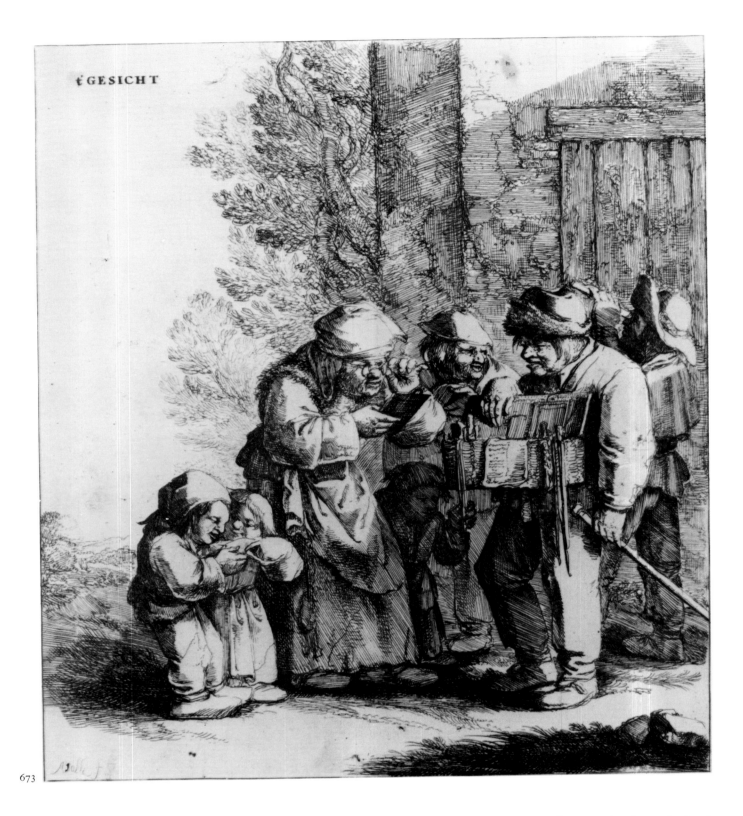

673

accepted the idea of a continuous circulation in a contained system but hypothesized that vaporization of blood in the heart forced it to dilate.

As a logical extension of the information obtained from Harvey's contributions, intravenous administration of drugs was introduced in the same century. Moreover, the first transfusions of blood into animals and then from animals into humans were also attempted with indifferent success and some outstanding failures.

The exact manner and careful experimentation of William Harvey has caused some historians to see him as a modern and to overlook the ancient prejudices he may have possessed. Others have seen Harvey as a representative of a strongly Aristotelian tradition and his quantitation as of only secondary importance. To them Harvey's idea of the circulation of the blood did not come from experimentation but from his belief in the Aristotelian principles that circular motion was the most perfect type of action and that the heart was the center of life. However Harvey is evaluated, his contribution is one of the most important in the history of medicine.

ANATOMICAL AND PHYSIOLOGICAL ADVANCES

THE story of the thermometer is an example of how clinical observation, physiological understanding, and technical development can intermingle in the achievement of a notable advance in medicine.

THE THERMOMETER

In the days of Hippocrates, the importance of body temperature was well recognized, but the physician had only his hand to evaluate the feel of a patient's skin. Later, in Alexandria, a patient's pulse became so important that body temperature was probably secondary. In the Middle Ages (because of the four humors and their qualities of hot, cold, dry, and moist), fever was considered a highly significant aspect of clinical observation even though scientific measurement of temperature was not attempted.

In 1592 Galileo constructed a thermometer (probably the first), but it gave only gross indications of temperature changes, had no scale of measurement, and was influenced by atmospheric pressure. Neither he nor his contemporaries appeared to see any medical application for the device. Santorio, however, showed a great interest in measuring body heat and devised ingenious but cumbersome thermometric instruments.

An essential step toward measurement was achieved in 1665 when Christiaan Huygens (1629–95) suggested a fixed scale in which the freezing point of water (designated as 0 degree) and the temperature of boiling water (100 degrees) were the parameters—the origin of the centigrade system. Gabriel Daniel Fahrenheit (1686–1736) in 1717 devised a scale which set the temperature of a mixture of ice and ammonium chloride as the lower fixed point and used smaller degree increments than in the centigrade scale. He found mercury more useful than water in his apparatus since its expansion and contraction are more rapid.

The first wide use of thermometry in clinical practice was by Hermann Boerhaave (1668–1738) in Holland and by his students Van Swieten and De Haen in Vienna. A voluminous study by De Haen reported the daily cyclical changes in the temperatures of healthy people, the rise in temperature produced by shivering, and the relationship of pulse to temperature. He emphasized the usefulness of temperature readings as a monitor of the course of illness, but most physicians of the day were not convinced. Not until about a century later did the thermometer become an integral part of medical practice.

The Swedish astronomer Anders Celsius (1701–44) in 1742 reintroduced the centigrade standard in clinical practice, and a series of improvements in the instrument and an increasing number of observations on the physiologic and pathologic significance of the temperature followed rapidly. Karl August Wunderlich (1815–77) by studying thousands of cases intensively was able to augment the realization that fever was a symptom, not a disease, and that the temperature of the patient was at least as important as the pulse. Yet many physicians still neglected to take temperatures, and some even scoffed.

Much of the resistance by practitioners was due to the complexities of measuring the temperature. The early thermometer was long and cumbersome and sometimes had to be maintained in contact with the patient for twenty-five minutes at a time. Aitkin in 1852 made the instrument more practical by narrowing the glass tubing above the bulb so that the column of mercury did not fall back again when the thermometer was removed from the patient. Finally, Thomas Clifford Allbutt in 1870 designed the size and shape employed today.

673 *One of a series (c. 1630) done by Andries Both on the five senses, this etching,* t'Gesicht, *or* Sight, *shows the trial and error method of choosing spectacles that prevailed until the late 19th century. National Library of Medicine, Bethesda*

674 *The first illustration of a mouth thermometer, one of several devised by Santorio Santorio, published in his* Commentaria in Primam Fen Priman Libri Canonis Avicenna *(1625). New York Academy of Medicine*

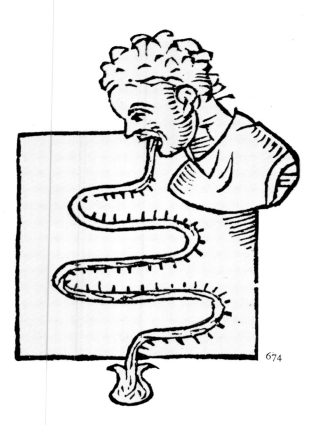
674

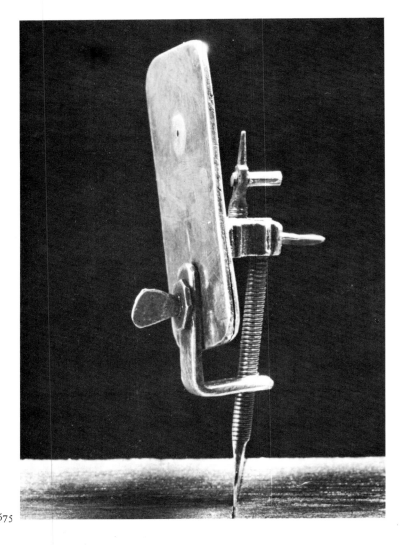

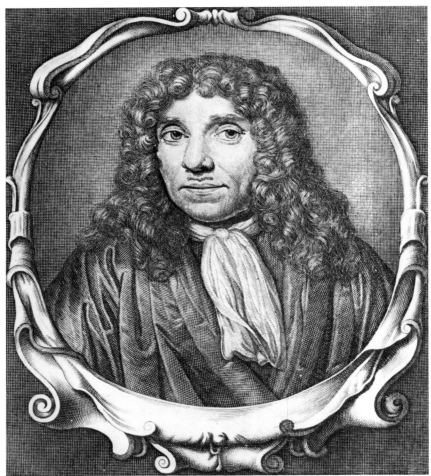

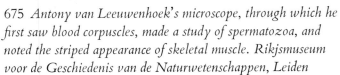

675 Antony van Leeuwenhoek's microscope, through which he first saw blood corpuscles, made a study of spermatozoa, and noted the striped appearance of skeletal muscle. Rikjsmuseum voor de Geschiedenis van de Naturwetenschappen, Leiden

676 Frontispiece portrait of Leeuwenhoek in his Epistolae ad Societatem Regiam Anglicam (1719). In his spare time, this linen draper developed microscope lenses so efficient that they were unsurpassed until the 19th century. Rijksmuseum van Oudheden, Leiden

677 This brass microscope, made by Negretti and Zambia of London in the late 19th century, comes close to modern types in achieving greater magnification by combining lenses. Semmelweis Medical Historical Museum, Budapest

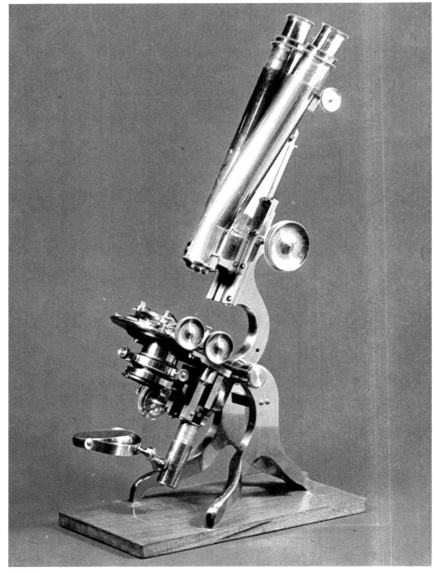
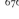

THE MICROSCOPE

One of the most important inventions in the development of medicine and general science was the microscope. The use of a ground lens as a magnifying glass was known in antiquity, and eyeglasses had been made in the Middle Ages. A Dutch spectacle-maker, Zacharias Janssen, and his son introduced the combination of more than one lens to increase power, but these earliest microscopes were crude and achieved a magnification of no more than ten times. The first scientific treatise making use of the microscope was done by Francisco Stelluti on the structure of the bee and was published in Rome in 1625. Pierre Borel may have made the first use of the microscope for medical inquiry. In 1655 he referred to wormlike creatures he saw in the blood of patients with fevers, but whether this was merely a fanciful elaboration of ancient views is not known. The two giants of seventeenth-century microscopy were Marcello Malpighi (1628–94) and Antony van Leeuwenhoek (1632–1723).

Leeuwenhoek was a cloth merchant in Delft, Holland, but he used his spare time to make lenses for microscopes so efficient that they were unsurpassed until the nineteenth century. Self-taught, and without Latin, he had difficulty keeping informed on scientific developments. Yet, eventually he was able to produce microscopes with a magnification power of 270 times. Before his death he had accumulated four hundred microscopes, some of which he bequeathed to the Royal Society in London, where he had sent the reports of his observations.

Leeuwenhoek looked through his microscope at everything imaginable, and his reports led the way to extraordinary advances. He was the first to recognize the blood corpuscles (which Malpighi had identified as "fat globules"). He also made a thorough study of spermatozoa and noted the striped appearance of skeletal muscle.

Malpighi, regarded as the founder of biological microscopy, also reported his findings in brief letters to the Royal Society in London. His contributions in both botany and biology affected the entire science of microscopy. By developing techniques for preparing tissues to be examined under the microscope, he and his successors were able to make observations otherwise impossible. Malpighi was the first to confirm by microscopic examination of the lungs the capillaries which Harvey postulated. He also corrected the previous view that the lungs were of a muscular consistency by showing that they consisted of many extremely thin-walled compartments connected to the smallest branchings of the windpipe. Indeed, hardly an organ escaped his discerning eye.

THE GLANDS

Many other advances were made in understanding the anatomy and physiology of the body. Francis Glisson (1597–1677) described in detail the liver, stomach, and intestines. Although his general biological views were basically Aristotelian, he also had modern ideas, as for instance that nerve impulses cause the evacuation of the gallbladder.

Thomas Wharton (1614–1673) in giving a comparative account of the glands took an important step by denying the old and persistent idea that the brain was a gland which secreted mucus. (However, he continued to believe that tears originated in the brain.) Wharton described the distinguishing characteristics of the digestive, lymphatic, and sexual glands, and the exit canal of the submaxillary salivary gland is now known as Wharton's duct. A highly significant contribution was his recognition that there were ductless glands (now called endocrine glands) whose secretions entered the blood, as distinguished from ductile glands whose secretions were discharged into cavities (exocrine glands). Niels Steensen in 1661 made clear the distinction between these glands and the lymph nodes (which are sometimes still called "glands" although not part of the glandular system). He also disproved the belief that tears came from the brain.

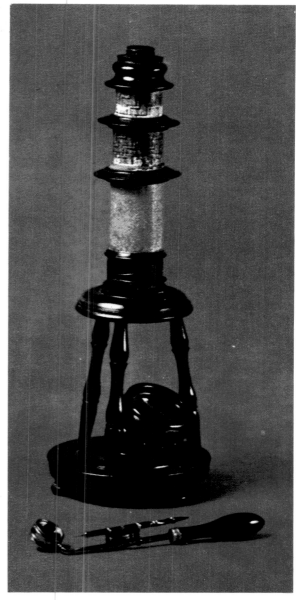

678

678 *Telescoping wooden-barreled microscope from Nuremberg (1750) and a brass-handled magnifying glass, both a few steps further along in ease of use than the Leeuwenhoek microscope. Semmelweis Medical Historical Museum, Budapest*

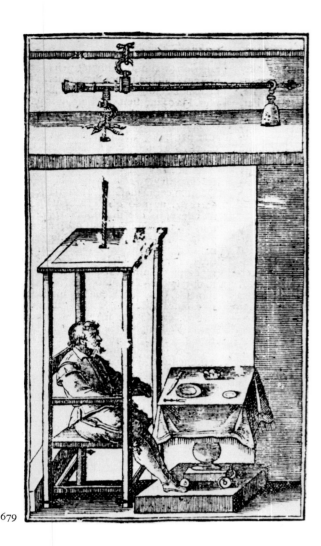

679 *Woodcut showing Santorio Santorio in his weighing chair. By attempting to weigh and compare the entire intake and output of a person, Santorio was one of the earliest savants to emphasize that the body operated on quantitative, mechanistic principles. National Library of Medicine, Bethesda*

The increased knowledge of the transport systems of the body attained through the work of a number of investigators helped to resolve the misconceptions of Galenic physiology concerning the production of blood. Gasparo Aselli (1581–1626) discovered that after a substantial meal the peritoneum (lining of the abdominal cavity) and the intestines of a dog became covered by white threads, from which a white fluid oozed when cut across. These vessels were the lacteals (the lymph channels of the intestines). Further details were clarified by Johann Vesling, Jean Pecquet, Thomas Bartholin, and Olof Rudbeck, who fought among themselves for recognition as pioneers.

RESPIRATION

Up to the time of Harvey, it was believed that respiration was meant to cool the heart for the production of vital spirits in the right ventricle. Though Harvey demonstrated that in the lungs blood was changed from venous to arterial, the basis for the change was unknown. The function of respiration took years for clarification, but there were notable increases in understanding during the seventeenth century. Boyle's experiments proved that both the combustion of a candle and the life of an animal were sustained by air. Robert Hooke (1635–1703) demonstrated that even without chest movement an animal could survive as long as air was pumped into the lungs. Richard Lower (1631–91), the first to transfuse blood directly, showed that the color difference between arterial and venous blood was due to contact with air in the lungs. John Mayow (1640–79) indicated that this reddening of venous blood happened because something was taken out of the air. He came close to a realization that respiration is an exchange of gases between the air and blood, believing that air gave up its "nitro-aerial spirits" and took away vapors yielded by the blood.

THE NERVOUS SYSTEM

In 1664, Thomas Willis (1621–75) published in *De Anatome Cerebri* (illustrated by Christopher Wren and Richard Lower) what was then probably the most thorough summary of the nervous system. His anatomical and physiological studies led to the use of his name in connection with the circle of arteries at the base of the brain, the eleventh cranial nerve, and also a type of deafness. However, in his zeal to localize mental processes anatomically, he drew unwarranted conclusions; among them, that the cerebrum controlled the motions of the heart, lungs, stomach, and intestines and that the corpus callosum (a tract connecting the brain hemispheres) was the site of the imagination.

MEDICAL PRACTICE

Few of the anatomical and physiological discoveries of the period were seen as useful to practical clinical medicine. Even the great Thomas Sydenham (1624–89), possibly the century's most famous clinical leader, placed little emphasis on the recent advances in science and medicine. Although he may have known of Harvey's blood circulation hypothesis, he would not have considered it medically useful, believing instead that observational skills and experience were far more valuable than scientific theories. He saw no practical value in microscopic anatomy, reserving his interest for visible anatomy readily correlated with the patient's state of health.

THE CLINICIANS

Sydenham has been called the "English Hippocrates." His detailed descriptions of gout, influenza, measles, scarlet fever, and other conditions were masterful, and

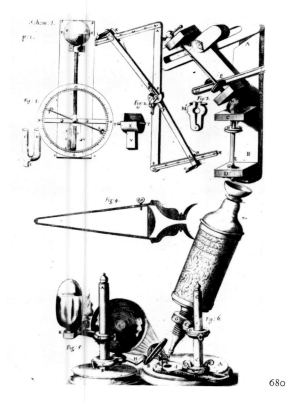

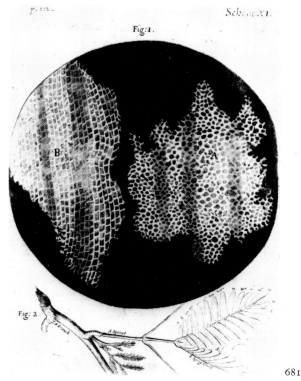

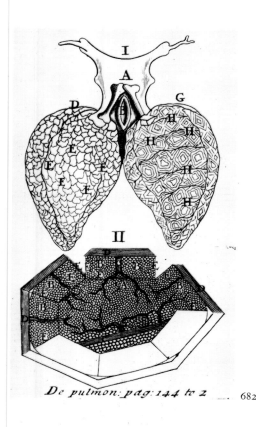

680

681

De pulmon: pag: 144 tv 2

682

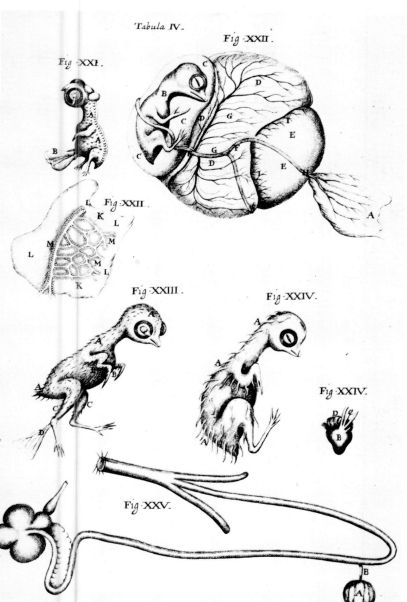

683

680 *Engraving from Robert Hooke's* Micrographia (1667) *depicting his microscope, which followed not too long after Leeuwenhoek's but seemed to show considerable development beyond the original idea. National Library of Medicine, Bethesda*

681 *Microscopic view of cork engraved in Robert Hooke's* Micrographia (1667). *His observation that cork was composed of compartments, which he called "cells," was to be used for the 19th-century theory that a cell was the basic unit of all living organisms. National Library of Medicine, Bethesda*

682 *Engraving of the cardiovascular system of a frog, from Marcello Malpighi,* Opera Omnia (1687). *At bottom, a microscopic view of the lungs showing capillaries—the minute vascular structures postulated by Harvey to connect the smallest arteries to the smallest veins—which Malpighi demonstrated under the microscope. National Library of Medicine, Bethesda*

683 *Illustration from Malpighi's* Dissertatio Epistolica de Formatione Pulli in Ovo (1673), *indicating that Malpighi followed the theory of epigenesis, which held that organisms begin as primitive substance and develop into mature embryos through a series of stages. New York Academy of Medicine*

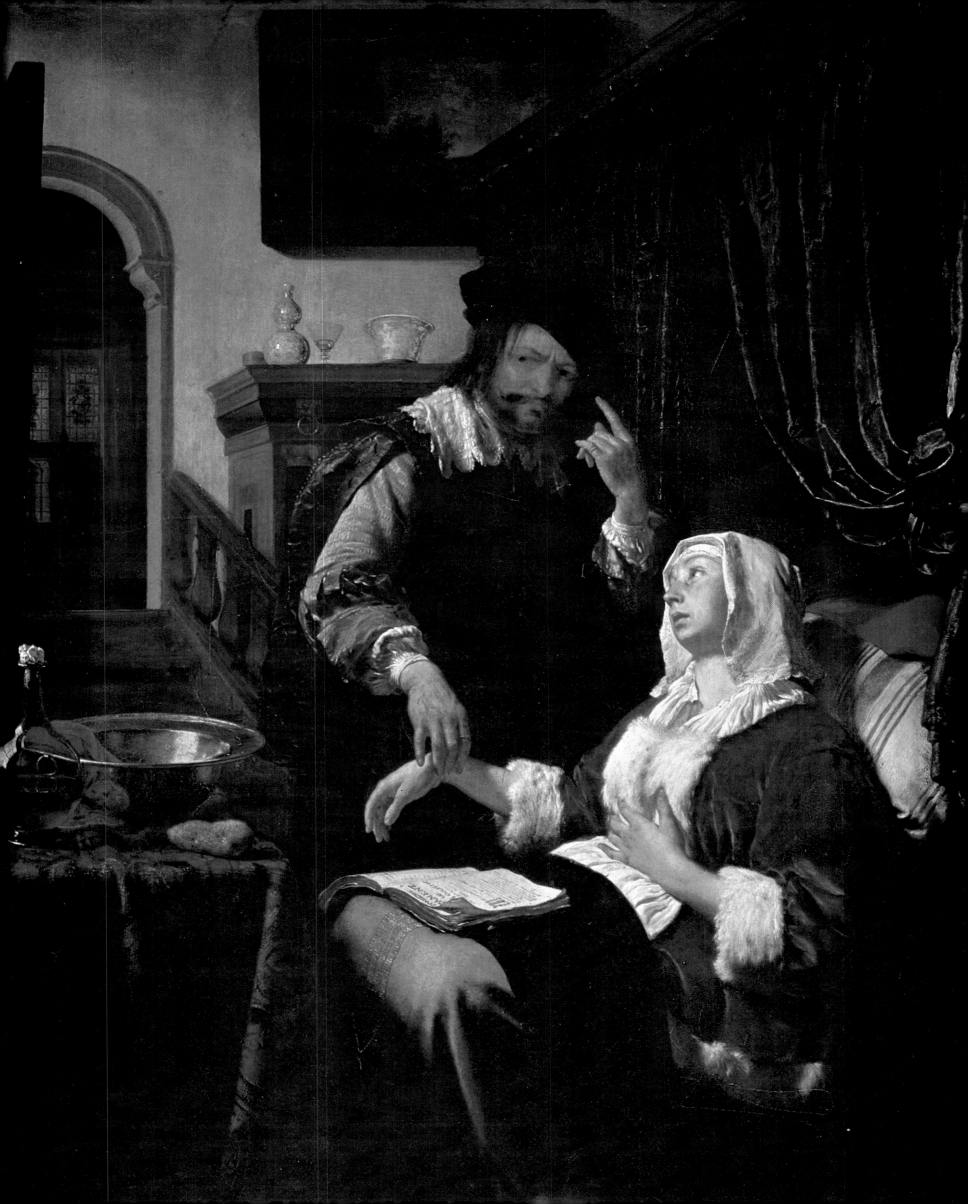

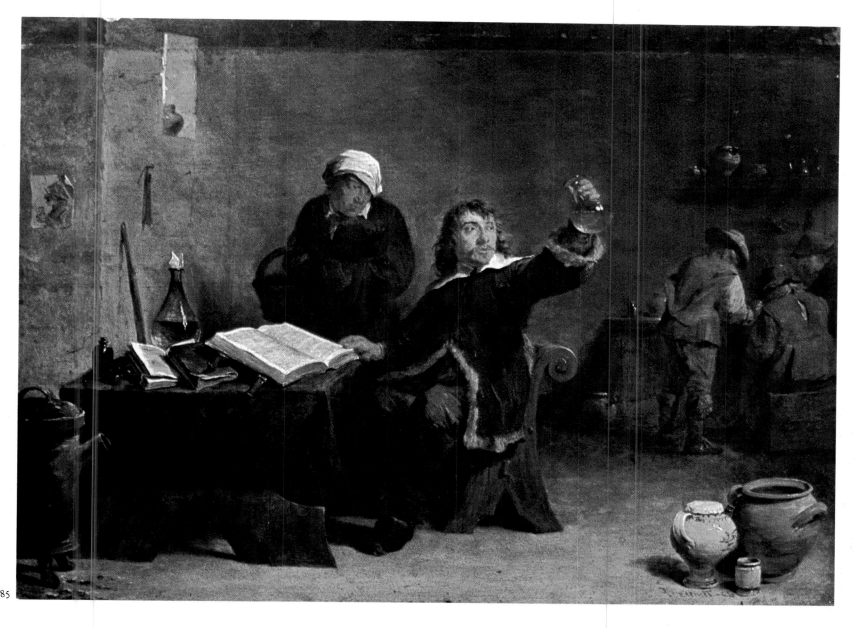

685

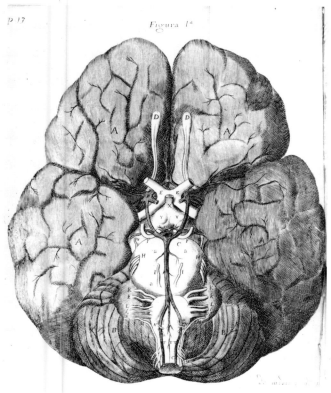

Figura 1ª

686

684 *Doctor checking the pulse of a patient, as painted by Frans van Mieris the Elder in* The Doctor's Visit. *Although emphasized since Galen, it was not until the advent of watches with minute hands, around 1700, that the rate of the pulse could be accurately counted. Kunsthistorisches, Vienna*

685 *The ancient art of uroscopy was still practiced by men of medicine in the 17th century, as evidenced in* The Village Doctor *by David Teniers the Younger. Musées Royaux des Beaux-Arts de Belgique, Brussels*

686 *This drawing of the circle of arteries named for Thomas Willis at the base of the brain was done by Christopher Wren, architect of St. Paul's in London. Ms. Lister B.66 Alt.BTW.12-13, Bodleian Library, Oxford*

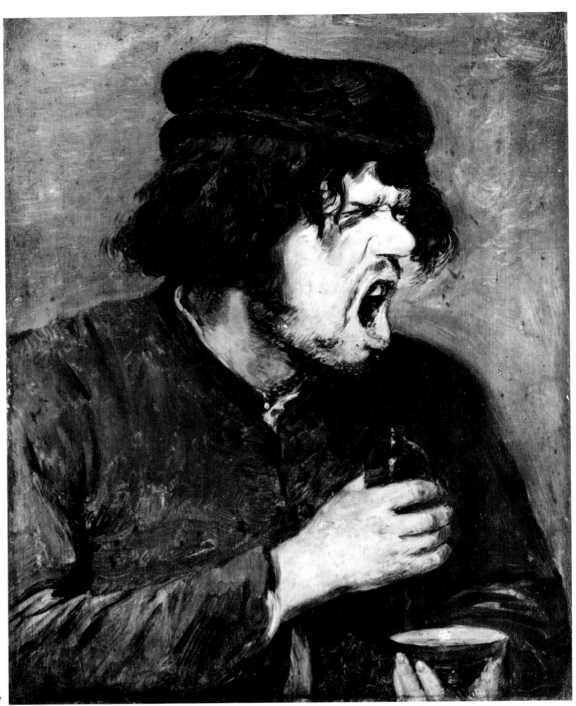

687

his attention to bedside medicine rather than to books was in the Hippocratic tradition. He taught that each patient was a unique dynamic entity in whom a disease could vary from person to person, but, unlike Hippocrates, he did concern himself with classifying diseases. Classification, however, became far more characteristic of the next century, when Linnaeus and others developed detailed categorizations of plants and animals.

As a follower of Francis Bacon, Sydenham also collected random scientific observations until he could induce a generalization. Nevertheless, while he supported the idea of experimentation, he preferred to reason out the causes of disease, using his senses to gather clues. Ultimately, to him, health or illness depended on the adequacy or foulness of the air, the sufficiency and character of food, the amount of exercise, rest, sleep, and alertness, the retention or evacuation of body fluids, and the calmness or perturbations of the mind. Sydenham's reputation was enormous, as was his influence on practice.

Another great clinician, Thomas Willis, was more in tune with the new methods of science, since his views were for the most part arrived at by experiment.

For instance, to understand nerve function he tied off the vagus nerve in a live dog and observed the effects on its heart and lungs. To match clinical symptoms with anatomical abnormalities (pathology), he performed many autopsies. He was also one of the first to emphasize the sweetness of urine in diabetes, thus differentiating it from another unrelated condition formerly called diabetes insipidus.

THE PROFESSION

The seventeenth century was not an innovative period in medical education. Anatomy was inadequately presented, and most teachings were dependent on works of antiquity or the writings of Muslim authors such as Avicenna. Standards and requirements for medical students varied greatly from country to country and even within a country. Degrees from Leiden which could be bought after a brief visit of a few weeks were nevertheless honored at Cambridge. Students were frequently disrespectful and rowdy, and it was during this century that much of the influence of students in shaping the curriculum and controlling the operation of universities began to wane.

In France three kinds of medical degrees were given: the baccalaureate, the license, and the doctorate—with different privileges attending each degree. The pattern was similar in other European countries and England. Sometimes a Bachelor of Arts degree (or equivalent) was a prerequisite to entering medical training, and so it might take thirteen years to complete a doctorate. Most medical students came from the middle class, and, while entrance into medical training was relatively easy for sons of physicians, prohibitions were stiffened against nonconverted Jews, bastards, and sons of hangmen. Among the upper classes, generally it was the petty nobility rather than the highly placed who entered the profession. They were well-paid and socially recognized as part of the intellectual elite, but the passing of medical examinations was often mainly a demonstration of competence in Latin.

In France, of the twenty-four medical schools four were dominant: Montpellier, Paris, Toulouse, and Strasbourg. Montpellier, one of the oldest, imparted the most classical education, but it was also more intellectually free and independent of the church than the Paris school. Some countries of Europe had many medical schools, while others such as the Netherlands (which from 1580 to 1625 graduated approximately three students per year) had few. In Russia, for many centuries the only physicians available had been trained abroad and usually ministered only to the nobility and the court. The majority of the population was treated by monks, women who knew the medicinal value of plants, and lay surgeons who treated wounds. At the beginning of the seventeenth century there were approximately twenty physicians in all of Russia trained in Western methods. However, responding to the need for more physicians to treat the wounded and sick of the Russo-Polish war, Czar Alexei Mikhailovich (1645–76) finally created a medical school. In the British Isles, Italy, Germany, and Spain, there had been universities since the Middle Ages.

Scientific progress in the seventeenth century came less from the universities than from new public and private scholarly societies. Whereas the universities were Aristotelian in outlook, that is, deductive and backward-looking, the scientific societies were experimental, inductive, and empirical. The *Accademia dei Lincei* (Academy of the Lynx) evolved in Rome in the early part of the century as a discussion group, which included Galileo among its members. The first truly empirical society was the *Accademia del Cimento* (Academy of Experiment) in Florence, in which the members worked together on questions of an experimental nature. They published their first work in 1667. Informal scholarly groups in other parts of Europe gradually arose. Initially scientific discoveries had been propagated through correspondence, but eventually a few journals, such as the very important *Philosophical Transactions* of the Royal Society in England, were created to disseminate this information.

687 *Adriaen Brouwer in* The Bitter Medicine (1635) *illustrates the universal precept that to be good for you medicine must taste bad. Städelsches Kunstinstitut, Frankfurt am Main*

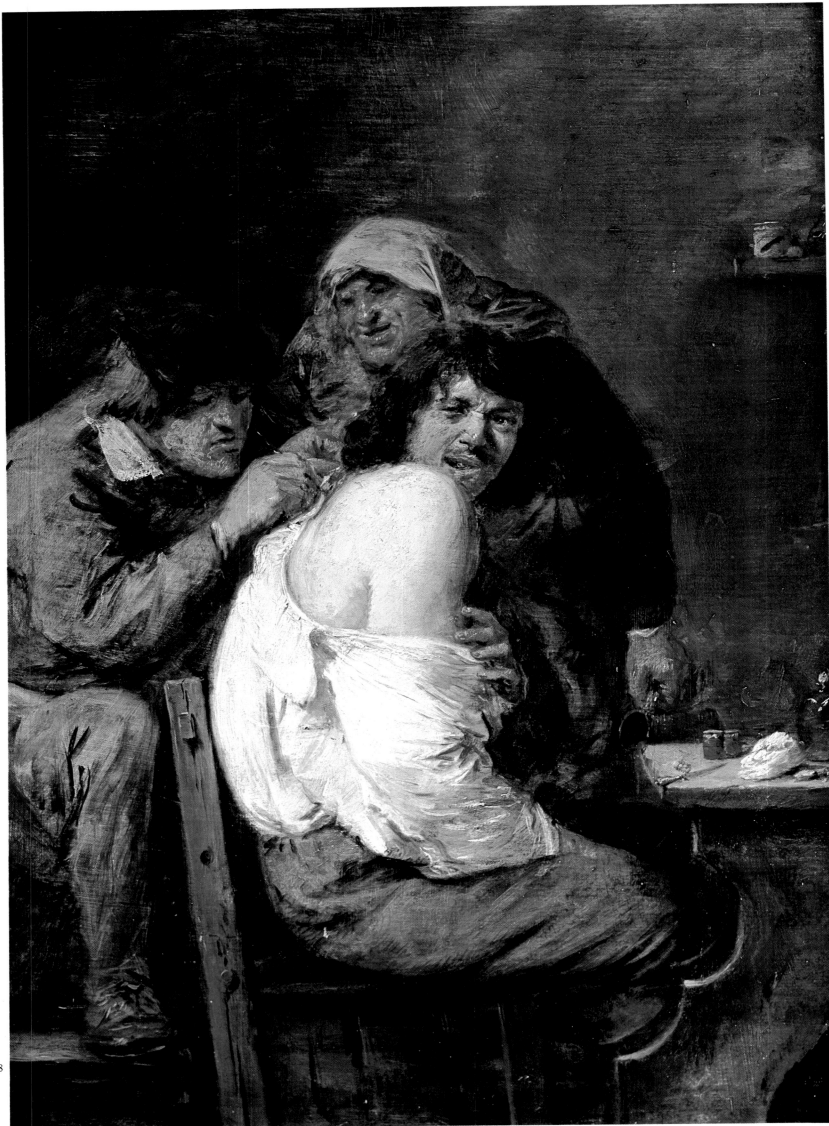

688

England and France took different approaches to scientific societies. In France, the *Académie des Sciences*, which had only a small membership, was founded to bring together the leading scientists of France and the world. The French government appointed the members and paid their salaries. They were the best-equipped scientists in Europe, but their arrangement had a price, for the government had a controlling influence. In England, the Royal Society was organized as a public group with little but moral support from Charles II, its doors open to anyone who showed an interest in scientific endeavors. However, amateurism among the membership in the 1670s almost caused the society's collapse, but it survived and today may be the oldest scientific society still in existence.

Besides the Royal Society, of which physicians made up the largest group, there was an entirely separate College of Physicians, whose functions included policing the profession, controlling quackery, regulating competition from other medical groups such as the apothecaries, overseeing fees, and limiting personal feuds between physicians. Whereas the College of Physicians was parochial, the Royal Society had numerous foreign members including Leeuwenhoek and Malpighi. There was an extraordinary openness with respect to research and medical information in the society, and its *Philosophical Transactions* was circulating at a time when special remedies and medical techniques were often kept secret.

An interesting overview of the medical profession in the seventeenth century may be obtained by noting the conflicts between apothecaries and physicians in London. By 1617, apothecaries had dissociated themselves from grocers and formed their own society. Originally apothecaries were restricted to filling prescriptions exactly as physicians ordered, but they could perform bleeding. While physicians wished to maintain the status quo, the apothecaries sought to liberalize the restrictions. By the end of the seventeenth century the apothecaries had overcome the opposition and were permitted to practice medicine—without a physician's license. But the battle was bitter and stormy.

Because of the relative paucity of educated, licensed doctors, apothecaries filled a void, often performing the treatments physicians had advised after examining the patient. However, to prevent a patient from relying too much on an apothecary, the practitioner sometimes wrote a prescription without directions for its use, giving these only to the patient. Apothecaries retaliated by favoring with referrals only those doctors who would prescribe large numbers of drugs, since apothecaries were not permitted to charge a fee for direct advice. The culmination of the antagonism occurred in 1704 when an apothecary who had brought charges against a butcher for nonpayment for medical services won his case, after a turbulent legal battle and an appeal. Apothecaries thereby emerged as sanctioned general practitioners.

Dentistry was practiced by any who could acquire the skills. Although there were legitimate doctors, barber-surgeons, and apothecaries who could take care of teeth, many quacks also posed as tooth-drawers and often displayed their techniques in the street before audiences of passersby. In 1699 an edict of Louis XIV established the professional status of dentists in France. Two years of study were required, followed by an examination before the College of Surgeons on theory and practice. In addition a special category was created for surgeon-dentists, that is, surgeons who had specialized in dentistry.

Although doctors were generally held in high regard, the limitations of medicine and the arrogance of some of its practitioners did not escape the biting satire of cartoonists and writers. Molière, for example, exposed the petty frailties of physicians in his plays. Ironically, in Molière's last performance as an actor, in *The Imaginary Invalid*, his uncontrollable coughing—associated with tuberculosis— was applauded by the audience as brilliant acting. Shortly after, the great playwright-actor expired. The helplessness of the medical profession in treating Molière's illness may have contributed to his scornful attitudes.

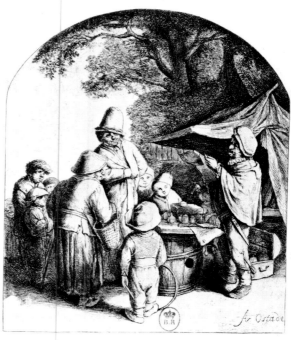

689

688 The Village Quack (*1636/37*) *by Adriaen Brouwer. Often the untutored barber-surgeon was the principal available healer. While some indeed may have been quacks, others were effective therapists. Städelsches Kunstinstitut, Frankfurt am Main*

689 *The peddling of nostrums was a common sight in the 17th century, as depicted in this engraving,* The Street Healer, *by Adriaen van Ostade. Cb 22, Bibliothèque Nationale, Paris*

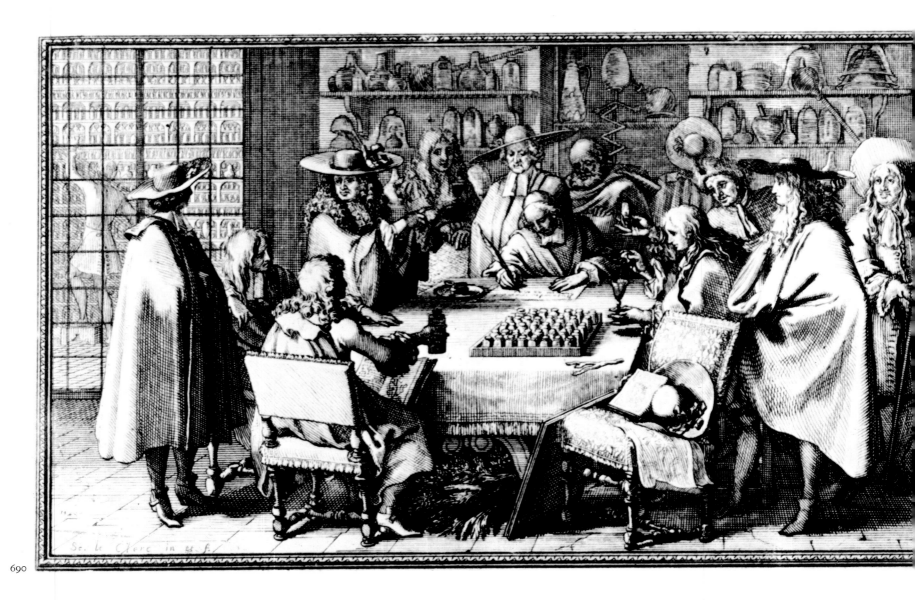

690

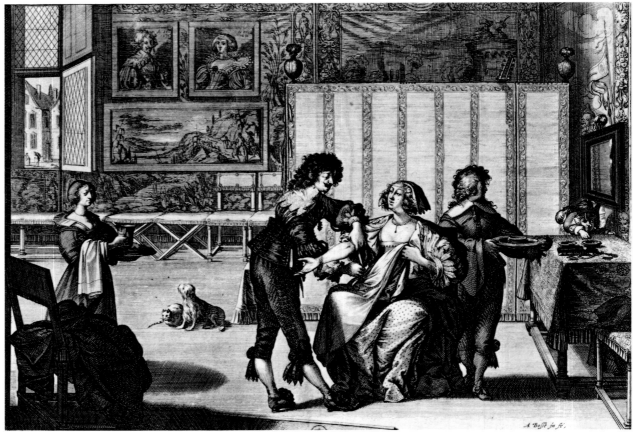

691

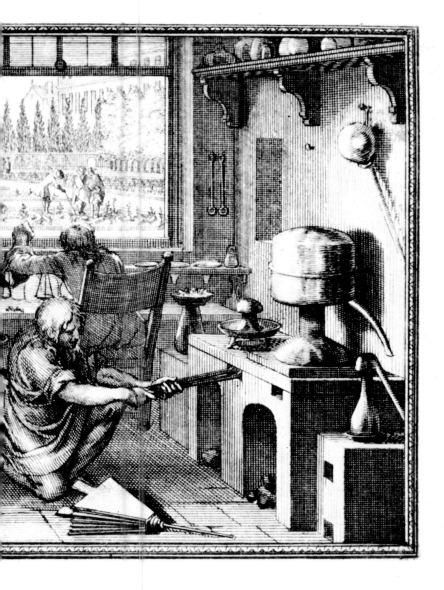

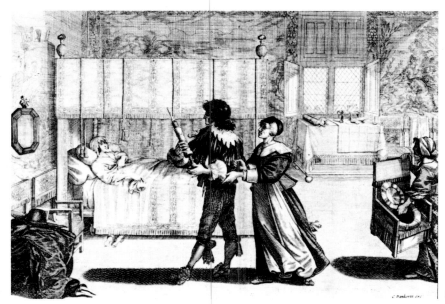

690 *Woodcut by Sebastien Leclerc showing a group of doctors in an apothecary laboratory. Physicians were often assigned to inspect and oversee the work of apothecaries. Kunstsammlungen, Veste Coburg*

691 *Abraham Bosse depicts a scene of blood-letting by venesection amidst luxurious surroundings in this etching of 1635. Ed 30 rés. fol., Bibliothèque Nationale, Paris*

692

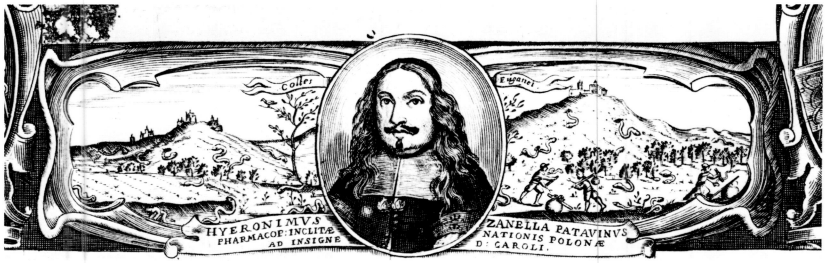

693

692 *In an engraving by Cornelius Danckerts after Abraham Bosse, an apothecary approaches his patient with a clyster. Enemas were a popular method of therapy since ancient times. National Library of Medicine, Bethesda*

693 *Cartouche from a batch certification of troches of viper signed May 25, 1676. The ancient panacea theriac, of which viper flesh was an important ingredient, was still produced in the 17th century. Germanisches Nationalmuseum, Nuremberg*

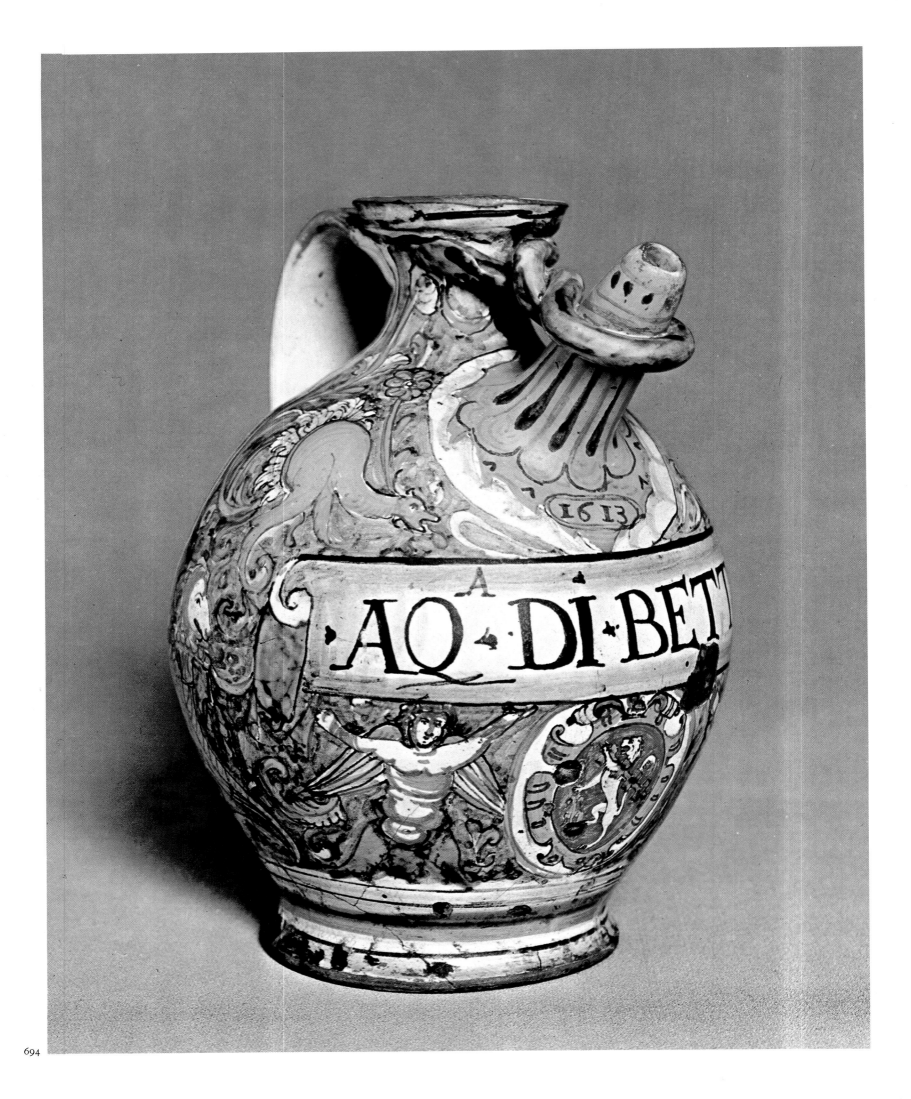

694

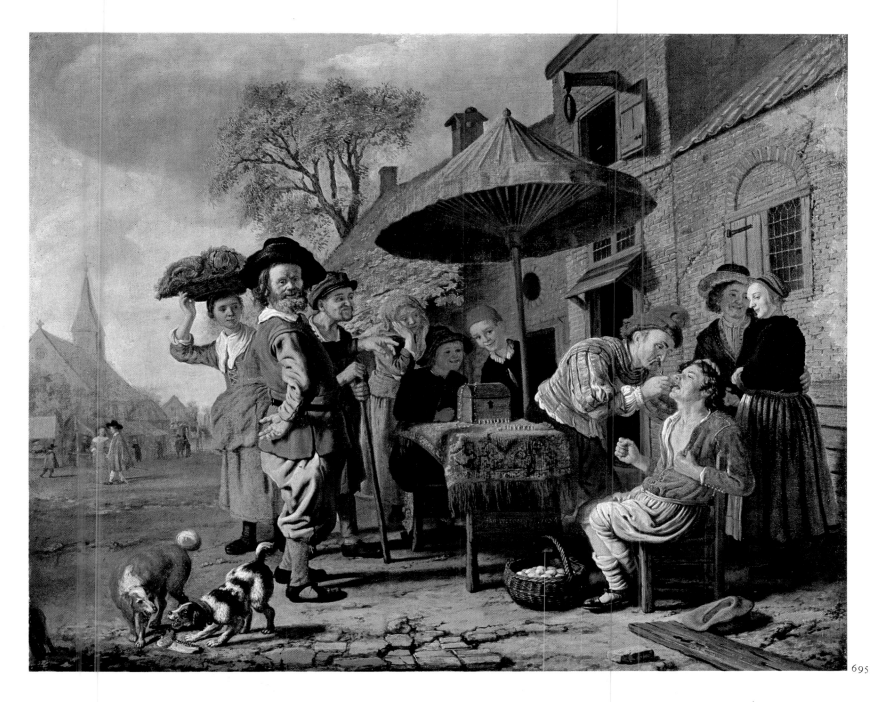

695

694 *Pharmaceutical jug, decorated with escutcheon,*
putti, and dragons, was made in Faenza and dated
1613. Civica Raccolta dell'Arte Applicata, Milan

695 The Country Dentist (*1654*) *by Jan Victors.*
Dentistry was the province of anyone who decided
to do it: regular medical practitioners, barber-surgeons,
apothecaries, and self-ordained tooth-pullers.
Rijksmuseum, Amsterdam

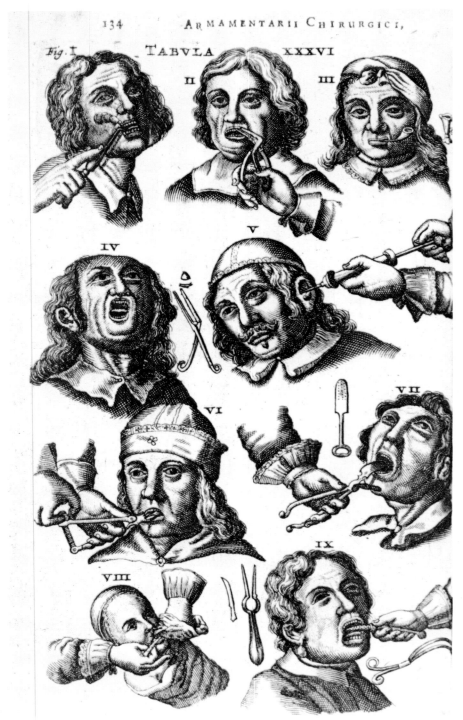

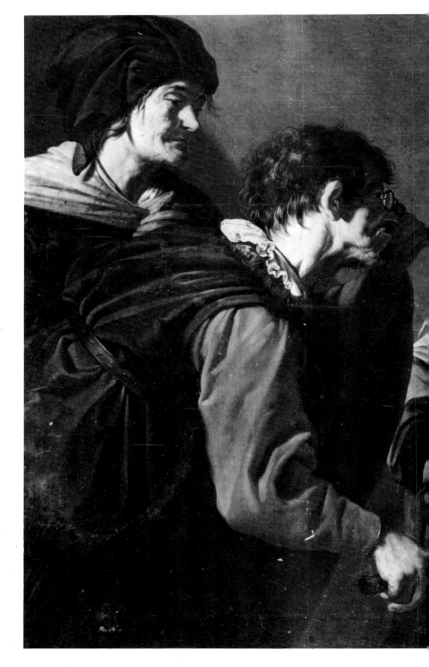

696 *Engraving of various dental operations from* Armamen-tarium Chirurgicum *(1665) by Johannes Scultetus, an advanced authority on surgery during the 17th century. Although anesthetics had not been invented, alcohol and other drugs were doubtless used to lessen pain. National Library of Medicine, Bethesda*

697 *Itinerant tooth-pullers, such as this one painted by Theodor Rombouts, were numerous until the professionaliza-tion of dentists. The pile of teeth on the table attests to the willingness of patients to make use of this service. The Prado, Madrid*

698 *Various treatments for eye diseases were recommended in 17th-century treatises, including wicks soaked in honey, vinegar, and verdigris threaded through the eyelids, as well as piercing the nape of the neck. World Health Organization, Geneva*

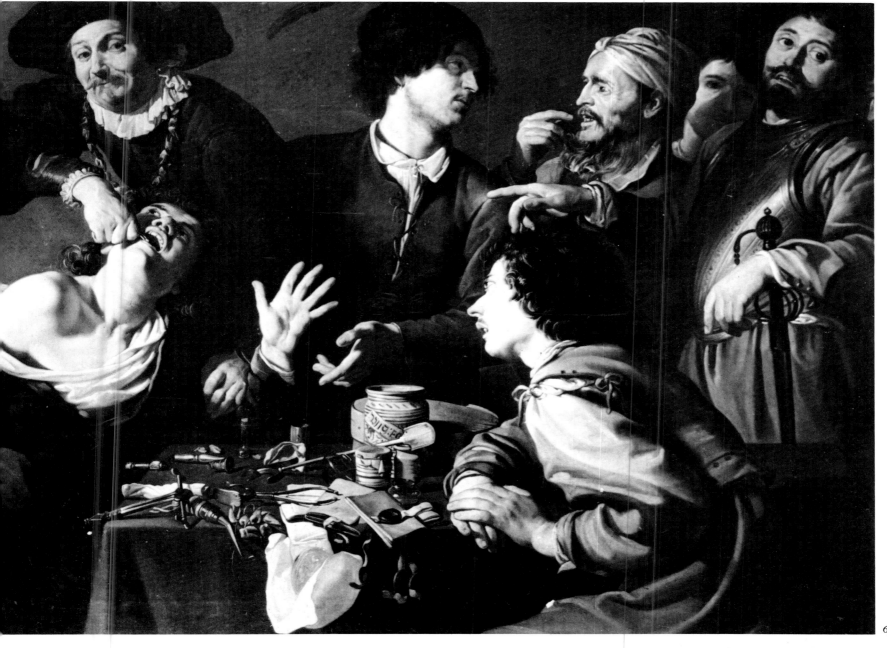

697

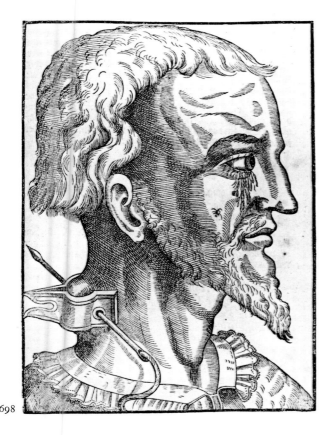

698

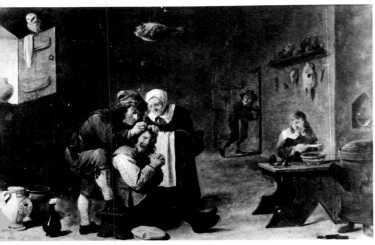

699

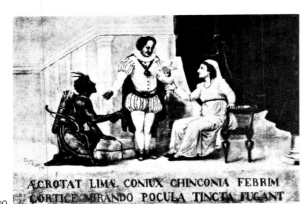

ÆCROTAT LIMA. CONIUX CHINCONIA FEBRIM
CORTICE MIRANDO POCULA TINCTA FUGANT

700

699 *Surgical procedures, such as the one depicted by David Teniers the Younger, were done mainly on external parts of the body. Amputations also were sometimes performed in the home. The Prado, Madrid*

700 *Fresco picturing the fanciful legend of the introduction to Europe of quinine as a medication for malaria by the Countess of Chinchòn, vicereine of Peru. Ospedale di Santo Spirito, Rome*

TREATMENT

THERAPY in the seventeenth century was mainly a continuation of the past in terms of bleeding, purging, dietary restriction, exercise, and the use of nonspecific plant, mineral, and animal drugs. One new medication, however, was a striking departure in effectiveness and in general influence on the principles of therapy: quinine—as a treatment for malaria.

MALARIA

Malaria affected much of Europe and had been a disease of considerable impact in all centuries. In the seventeenth century, it was still called "ague," and not until the eighteenth century did its present name (from *mal aria*, "bad air") become common because of the disease's association with swamps. The first effective remedy for it, a plant derivative from Peru, was called cinchona by Europeans because of a fanciful story that the Spanish countess of Cinchón had introduced the plant into Spain from Lima, where her husband the viceroy was supposed to have been cured by the "fever bark." Apparently cinchona was introduced into Europe about 1633 after having been cited by Antonio de la Calancha as a substance that "produced miraculous results in Lima." Word of the medicinal bark spread rapidly, as did demand for it. Because Jesuit priests held a virtual monopoly on its importation into Spain and Italy, it was also called "Jesuit's Bark."

The introduction of cinchona had an enormous influence on venerable concepts of illness. At the time malaria had been a chronic disease that took many months to alleviate, but since cinchona cured quickly and acted specifically on only a certain kind of fever, the belief in fever as a general manifestation of unbalanced humors received a severe blow. It was then felt that each fever could be a different disease. In modern times, we have returned to the idea of fever as a general manifestation of various different specific illnesses.

Quinine was isolated from cinchona in the first quarter of the nineteenth century and received its present name from the quina-quina plant, which, although it had no antimalarial properties, had been mistaken for cinchona. Quinine remained the only effective antimalarial until well into modern times. However, many knowledgeable physicians continued to use the ancient arsenical preparations because they were thought to produce a more permanent cure and also because cinchona cost so much. Indeed, arsenic salts were to continue for centuries as mainstays in therapeutics. Even those who appreciated the dangers still used arsenic confidently, though cautiously, for a multitude of external and internal conditions. Well into the nineteenth century, an arsenic compound called Fowler's solution became so popular that it was mocked in cartoons.

SURGERY

Surgery in the seventeenth century did not keep pace with the progress in anatomy and physiology. The means for making surgery safe—anesthesia and control of infection—had not yet arrived. Nor did surgeons reach the social and academic level of physicians. One exception was Charles-François Félix, who operated successfully on an anal fistula of Louis XIV and gained for surgery the support of the crown. Nevertheless, French surgeons alternately competed with barbers and then joined with them against the physicians, as English surgeons had done in the previous century.

There were two kinds of surgeons and various grades within the subdivisions. "True" surgeons concerned themselves with the major operations: suture of holes in the intestines, removal of tumors, plastic operations on the lips and nose, repair of rectal fistulas. The barber-surgeons were wound doctors who also performed

454

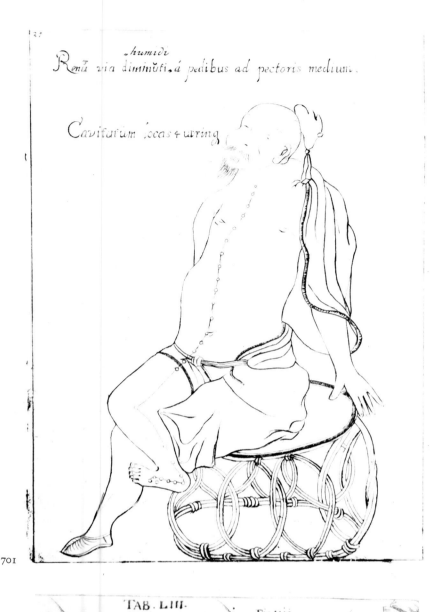

humidi

Renū via diminūti. á pedibus ad pectoris medium.

Cavitatum siccas + utring

701

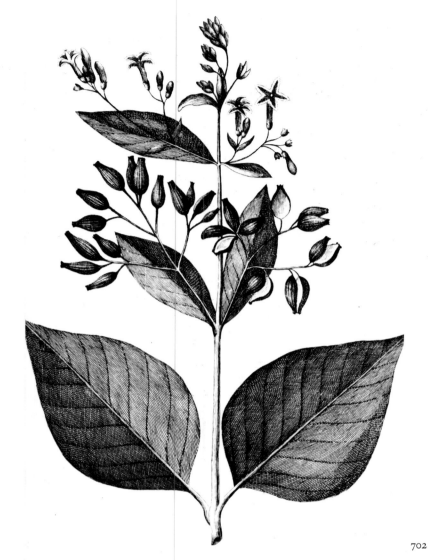

702

TAB. LIII.

Fig. i.

Fig. vij.

Fig. ii.

Fig. viii

Fig. iij.

Fig. iv.

Fig. ix.

Fig. v.

Fig. x.

Fig. vj.

Fig. x j

703

701 *Engraving in Andreas Cleyer,* Specimen Medicinae Sinicae *(1682) indicating that acupuncture was known in the West during the 17th century. The points marked are for kidney treatment. National Library of Medicine, Bethesda*

702 *Seventeenth-century engraving of the cinchona plant, the bark of which was used in the treatment of malaria. Later, this was found to contain quinine. World Health Organization, Geneva*

703 *Engraving from J. Scultetus,* Armamentarium Chirurgicum *(1665) showing the procedure, instruments, and method of bandaging for amputation. National Library of Medicine, Bethesda*

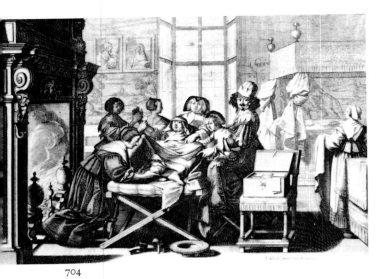

704

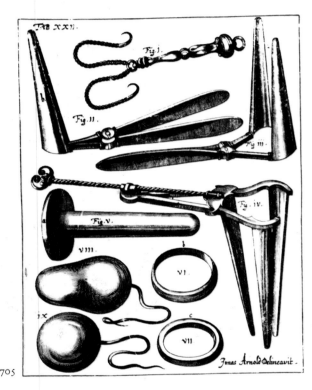

705

bloodletting, cupping, the extraction of teeth, and the management of fractures, dislocations, and external ulcers. In addition, there were untutored, itinerant wound-doctors who operated for cataracts, bladder stones, and hernias—apparently with results so bad that reputable surgeons avoided association with them.

The names of a few surgeons should be mentioned. In Italy, Cesare Magati (1579–1647) followed Paré's teachings that gunshot wounds should be treated by plain water and mild applications rather than with the cautery or boiling oil. Pietro de Marchette reported many complex case histories, and Giuseppe Zambeccari was a pioneer in experimental surgery. Peter Uffenbach compiled a noteworthy surgical anthology which relied exclusively on the practices of sixteenth-century surgeons. Johann Schultes (1595–1645) was a great illustrator of surgical treatises. Matthaeus Gottfried Purmann (1649–1711) emphasized the anatomical basis of surgery.

Wilhelm Fabry of Hilden (1560–1634), considered the "Father of German Surgery," was an innovator and one of the first to emphasize amputation through healthy tissue rather than the gangrenous part. Yet he continued to utilize the cautery and to rely on "weapon salve," an accepted method of the time whereby the medicament was applied to the weapon rather than the injured part. This idea seemed to fit the new atomism, which saw the weapon, especially gunpowder, as giving off atoms of the same material it had deposited in the wound. In a manner of "like attracting like," the atoms of the weapon together with the medication would be brought to the wound. This method, fanciful as it was, nevertheless may have been beneficial to the patient since the wound was spared frequent applications of ointments and injurious substances.

OBSTETRICS

Male attendants had rarely been present at the birth of a child, but by the end of the seventeenth century male midwifery had become the fashion in certain parts of Europe. In 1628 Peter Chamberlen attended Queen Henrietta Maria in a miscarriage, and in 1692 another Chamberlen was responsible for delivering a child to the future Queen Anne. The Chamberlen family had a secret obstetrical forceps which was guarded carefully and was thought to be the reason behind their successful results. More and more, men began to assist in delivery and to take an active part in the medical supervision and examination of women.

MENTAL ILLNESS

The attitude of the period toward mental illness continued to be ambivalent. Felix Platter (1536–1614) categorized insanity as follows: imbecilitas, consternatio (febrile delirium and catatonic states), alienato (dementia, alcoholism, love and jealousy, melancholia and hypochondriasis, possession by the devil, raving mania, St. Vitus's dance, and "phrenitis"), and defatigatio (insomnia which was supernaturally caused by God or the devil).

Belief in witches continued to decline, but it was not until 1680 in France that the death penalty for being a witch was abolished. As supernatural causes were gradually abandoned, the mentally ill came to be considered merely "asocial." However, one bad effect of this notion was their incarceration along with criminals and paupers.

The new technique of transfusing blood was extended by Jean-Baptiste Denis (1620–1704) to the treatment of mental patients. When arterial blood of lambs was injected into the venous system, the patients seemed to recover. However, when one patient died, the method was discontinued.

The quackery of the time, which seemed to become ever more common, was in part due to the bitter controversies between the Paracelsians and Galenists, who reviled each others as "quacks," and to the obvious failure of even reputable physicians to stem the course of the epidemics which recurred frequently.

704 *Etching by Abraham Bosse, entitled* L'Accouchement *(1633), depicting a lying-in scene, with no other male but the husband present. Smith, Kline, and French Collection, Philadelphia Museum of Art*

705 *Instruments for use in gynecology and obstetrics pictured in J. Scultetus,* Armamentarium Chirurgicum *(1665). By the end of the 17th century, male midwifery was the fashion in many cities. National Library of Medicine, Bethesda*

706 *Etching by Jacques Callot, entitled* Gypsy Encampment *(1621). There is no evidence that childbirth under these circumstances was any more hazardous than in a hospital of the time. Philadelphia Museum of Art*

707 *Francisco Goya,* The Madhouse *(c. 1812–19). Although belief in supernatural causes for insanity was abandoned by the 17th century, the insane were often kept under frightful conditions. Real Academia de Bellas Artes de San Fernando, Madrid*

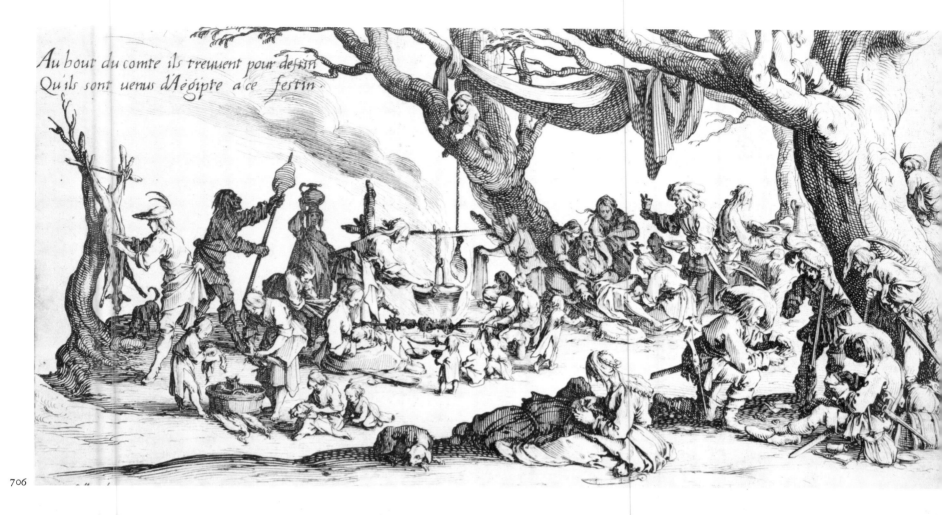

Au bout du comte ils treuuent pour deftin
Qu'ils sont uenus d'Aegipte a ce festin

706

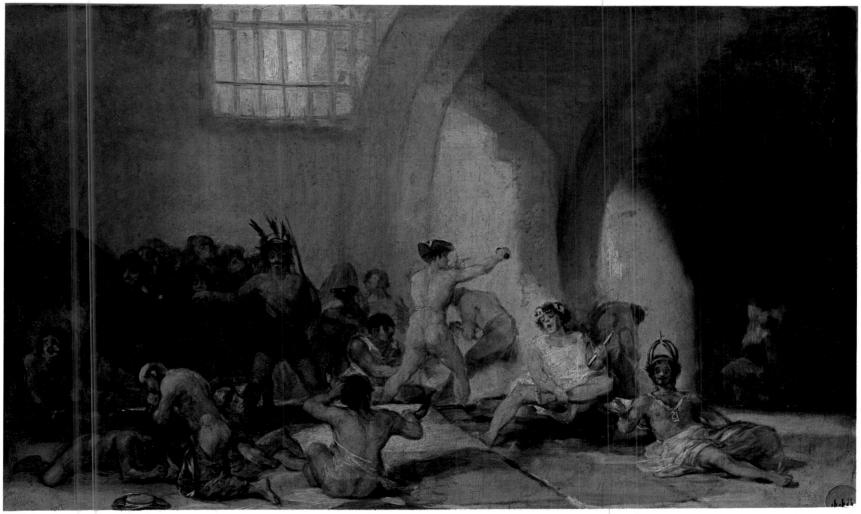

707

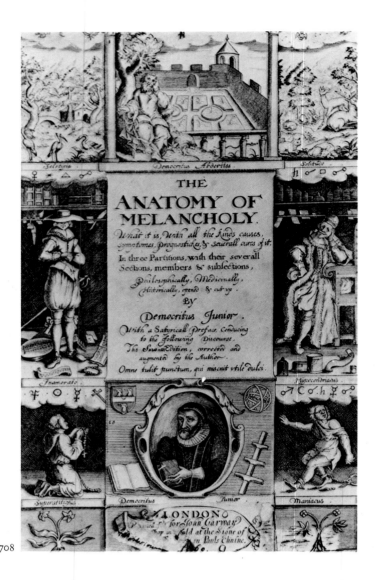

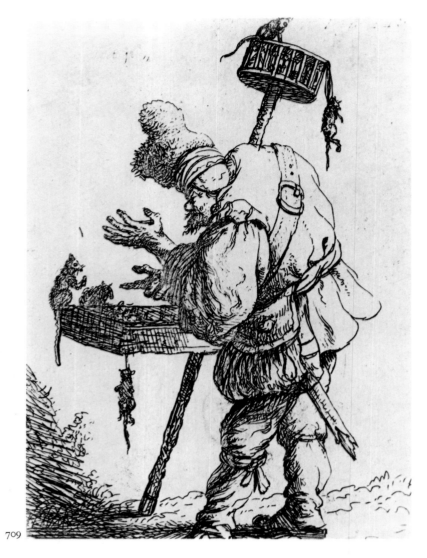

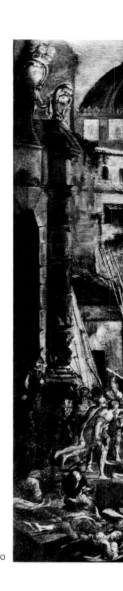

708 *Title page of* The Anatomy of Melancholy
*(1660), an excellent account by Robert Burton of
depression, which included repetitions of old myths
but also some perceptive insights, such as the benefits
of confessing grief to a friend. National Library of
Medicine, Bethesda*

709 *Etching entitled* The Rat Killer *by Jan Georg
van Vliet. The association of rats with bubonic
plague had been known since Biblical times, and so
this man performed a public health service. Gift of
Associated American Artists, 1969, National Library
of Medicine, Bethesda*

PUBLIC HEALTH

The state of concern for public health in seventeenth-century England may
be amply illustrated in the care of children. Many unwanted sons and
daughters were simply abandoned, and they roamed the streets in bands.
Youngsters of four or five were frequently put into workhouses, and older orphans
might be shipped to America. It seems that children of the poor had little or no
access to medical attention. Of the many texts available on treatment and rearing
of children, one of the most popular was actually written in Roman times—the
work of Soranus.

Epidemics of plague, measles, smallpox, scarlet fever (carefully defined by
Sennert but nevertheless confused with measles), chicken pox ("swine pox" on the
bills of mortality), diphtheria (under various names), and other acute febrile illnesses
took an especially heavy toll of the young. Congenital syphilis first appeared in a
pediatric text during this time, to join gonorrhea, scurvy, lumbago, and rickets as
diseases believed to be transmitted by inheritance. Infants with syphilis were often
abandoned by everyone (including their mothers) because of the fear of transmission
—especially to wet nurses, who frequently passed from infant to infant. Among the
well-to-do, wet nurses were carefully chosen since it was believed that breast milk
could influence the health and behavior of the young.

Tongue-tie was treated by midwives, who grew the right thumbnail long to
cut the frenulum. Ear infection (otitis), since it occurred so frequently, was considered
virtually a normal condition, as were discharges from the nose and ears which were
presumed to issue from the brain. Dental diseases sometimes caused death, and
"worms" were implicated when another diagnosis was not apparent— an idea with

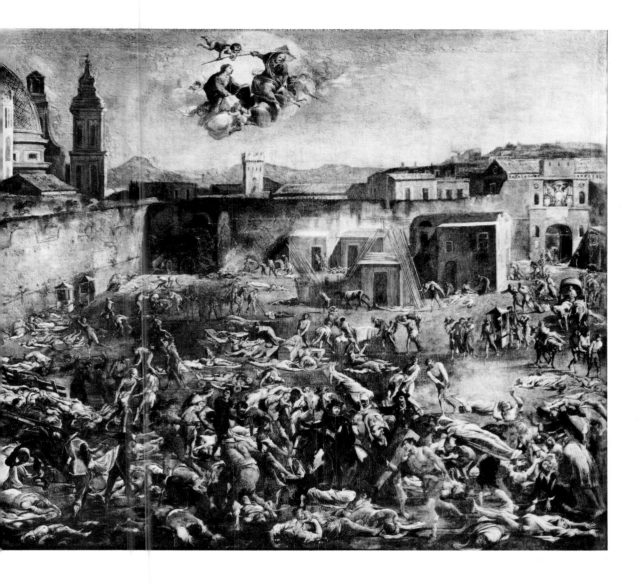

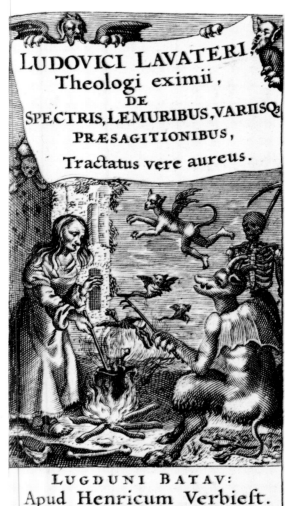

an ancient history. In addition, congenital and acquired blindness were common.

Nor were health conditions much better for adults. In some places, epidemics of the plague killed over half the population: 80,000 in Milan and 500,000 in Venice. Furthermore, the Thirty Years War was devastating to life and hygienic conditions, especially in Germany. Organization and administration of public health controls remained virtually the same as in medieval times. Whatever organization there was centered around the towns, for the leaders had begun to recognize that a healthy population was beneficial to the state.

STATISTICS

There was a start at gathering some health and vital statistics in the sixteenth century, but significant attention to the statistical analysis of medically related phenomena only developed in the latter half of the seventeenth century. In England, at the beginning of the century, christenings, marriages, and burials were recorded by local parishes, and this information was passed to the king on a weekly or annual basis. In 1629 these "bills of mortality" were expanded to include fatal diseases other than the plague.

Generally the medical profession had little interest in statistics. The collection and analysis of everyday numbers did not at first seem to them valuable in the treatment of patients. Indeed the first person to utilize medical statistics was a tradesman, John Graunt (1620–74), who was also a ward politician. The spirit of quantitation which began to pervade scientific thinking, however, finally influenced many medical leaders to see the importance of the numbers. Graunt's book, *Natural and Political Observations . . . made upon the Bills of Mortality* (1661),

710 *Epidemics continued to take their toll, as demonstrated in this depiction of* The Plague of Naples *(1656) by Domenico Gargiulio. Museo Nazionale di San Martino, Naples*

711 *Engraved title page of Ludwig Lavater, De Spectris, Lemuribus et Magnis . . . (1659) showing a witch stirring a cauldron. Although the death penalty for being a witch was abolished in France in 1680, belief in witches persisted into the 18th century. National Library of Medicine, Bethesda*

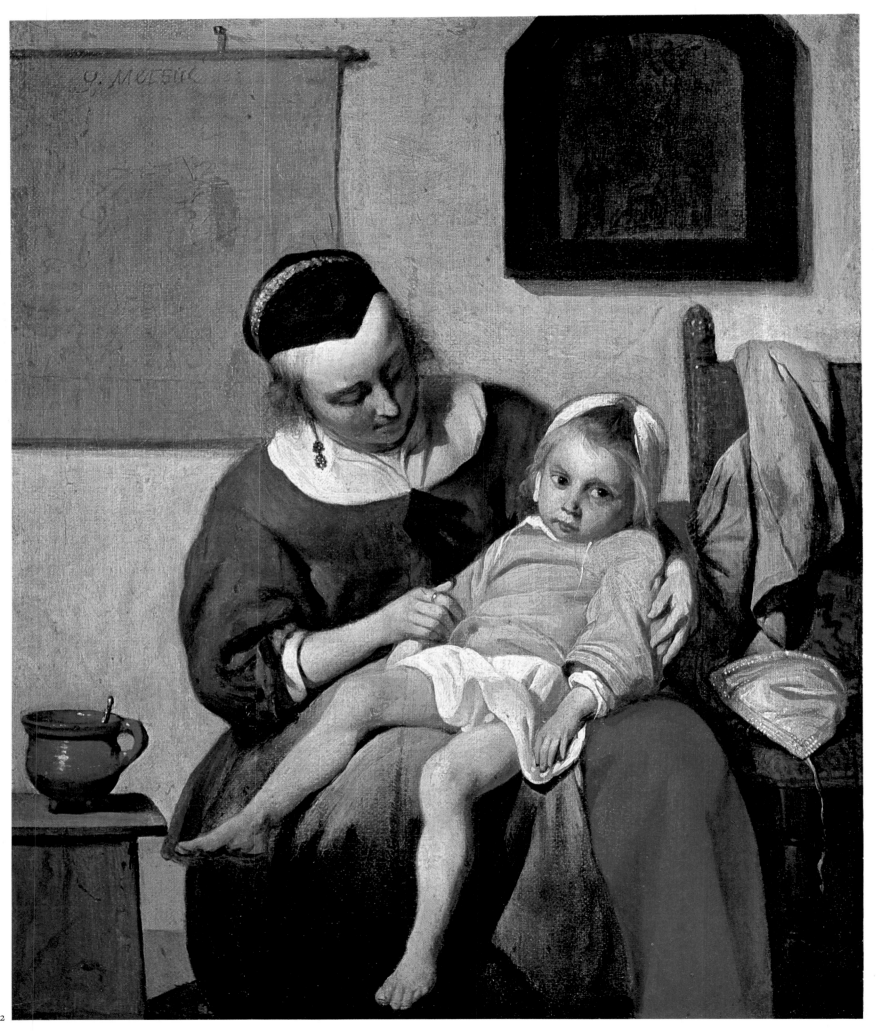

712

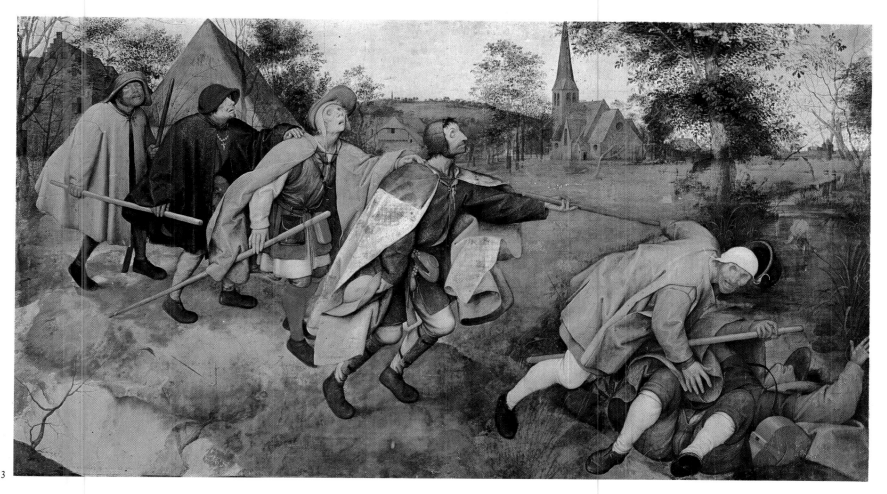

713

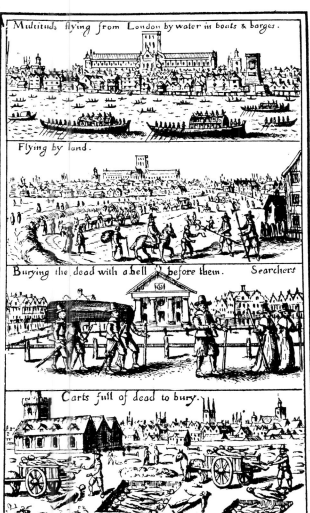

714

712 The Sick Child (*c. 1660*) *by Gabriel Metsu. This child is sympathetically cared for, but the children of the poor had little chance for medical attention in the 17th century. Rijksmuseum, Amsterdam*

713 *That congenital and acquired blindness were common afflictions in Europe is recalled in Pieter Bruegel the Elder's* The Blind Leading the Blind (*1568*). *Museo e Gallerie Nazionali di Capodimonte, Naples*

714 *Print showing scenes in London during the Great Plague of 1664. Pepysian Collection, Clarendon Press, Oxford*

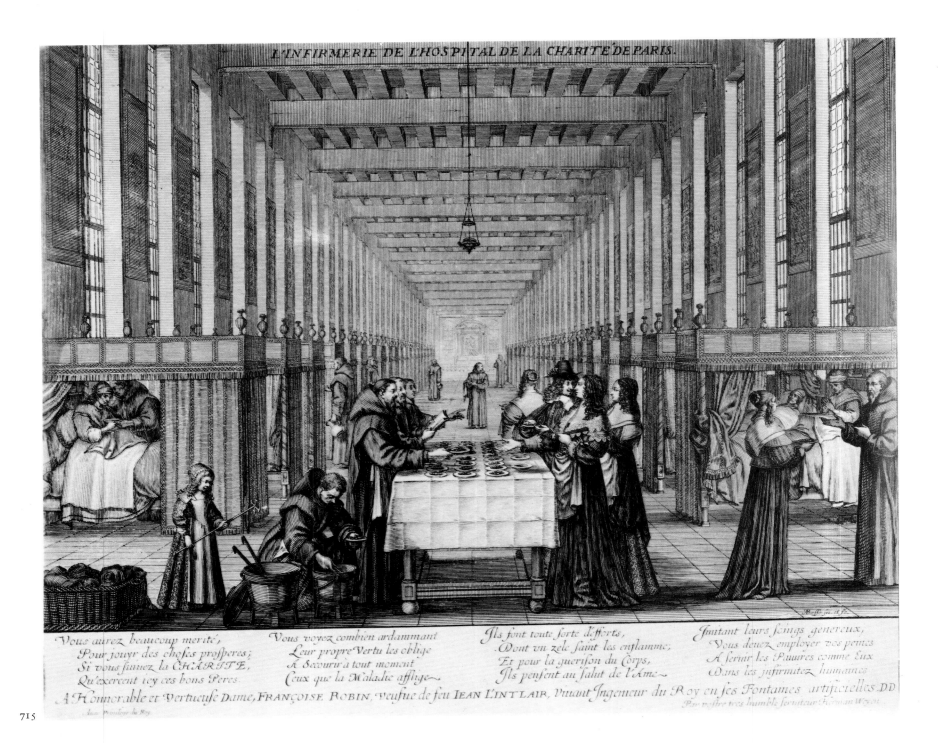

L'INFIRMERIE DE L'HOSPITAL DE LA CHARITE DE PARIS.

Vous aurez beaucoup merité,
Pour jouyr des choses prosperes;
Si vous suiuez la CHARITE,
Qu'exercent icy ces bons Peres.

Vous voyez combien ardammant
Leur propre Vertu les oblige
A Secourir a tout moment
Ceux que la Maladie afflige~

Ils font toute sorte d'efforts,
Dont vn zele saint les enflamme;
Et pour la guerison du Corps,
Ils pensent au salut de l'Ame~

Imitant leurs soings genereux,
Vous deuez employer vos peines
A seruir les Pauures comme Eux
Dans les infirmitez humaines

A l'Honnorable et Vertueuse Dame, FRANÇOISE ROBIN, Veufue de feu IEAN L'INTLAIR, Viuant Ingenieur du Roy en ses Fontaines artificielles DD

Par nostre tres humble seruiteur Herman Weyen

715

715 *Etching (c. 1635) by Abraham Bosse showing the infirmary of the Charity Hospital in Paris. Until the 18th and 19th centuries, hospitals did not focus on caring for the acutely ill but on the poor, crippled, and chronically ill. Smith, Kline, and French Collection, Philadelphia Museum of Art*

716 *Etched portrait of Bernardo Ramazzini, who wrote the first comprehensive treatise on occupational health problems. New York Academy of Medicine*

analyzing and evaluating the bills over a sixty-year period, so impressed the medical fraternity that Graunt was admitted to membership in the august Royal Society, a particularly signal honor for a layman.

One of Graunt's supporters was Sir William Petty (1623–87), who had helped him with his book. Since Petty believed that a large population was an asset to a country, he favored all measures which preserved and restored health. He saw that hospitals should be the focal point not only for treating the sick but also for training physicians and developing research. He offered many brilliant, far-reaching proposals, such as separate hospitals for plague victims, specialized maternity institutions, governmental concern for the health of occupational groups, and the establishment of a central health council to organize public health. However, these measures were too far in advance of the times, and very few of Petty's suggestions were then carried out.

Graunt's ideas, however, did have important influences. In 1669 Christiaan Huygens and in 1693 Edmund Halley (1656–1742) used their mathematical talents to arrive at tables of life expectancy, which later would be of use in life insurance. Of course statistics worked into medical thought from other sources besides Graunt: the collection of meteorological information, the popular accent on mathematics, the interest in precision instruments, and the beginnings of experimental data on physiological phenomena.

The growing concern of the state for its citizens was especially exhibited by the German principalities, where the concept developed that government through its agents was responsible for the care and supervision of its citizens in regard to disease.

In several areas of Europe, public health remained primarily the responsibility of the inhabitants (for example, street cleaning and drainage), but laws were created and inspectors were assigned for enforcement. "Scavengers" were appointed to collect the garbage, and space outside of town was assigned for the dumping.

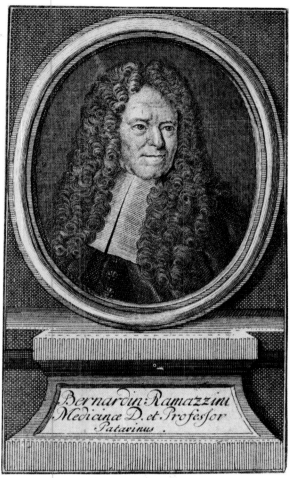

Town water resources initially were springs and wells, and later the rivers. When technical innovations such as pumps gradually came into public service, water was usually conveyed to a central cistern and from there to local cisterns; however, most of it was polluted by the time it reached the consumer.

Hospitals for the crippled were a local responsibility and usually were intended for the care of the poor, the aged, and the sick. The adaptation of hospitals for their separate task of treating the acutely ill did not occur until the eighteenth and nineteenth centuries, but in the seventeenth century hospitals began to be used for medical research and teaching.

Among the outstanding contributors of the time to public health were Lancisi, Kircher, and Ramazzini. Giovanni Maria Lancisi (1654–1720) came close to understanding that an insect transmitted malaria, believing that swamps emitted animate creatures (later found to be mosquitoes) and also inanimate particles that produced disease.

Athanasius Kircher (1601–80) was among the first to point explicitly to microorganisms as the cause of infectious disease. However, it is likely that the "worms" he saw in the blood with his low-power microscope were actually red cells and not bacteria. His work attracted attention throughout Europe, but because of technical and theoretical difficulties some followers fancifully reported seeing more than actually existed—which caused a reaction that led to a general condemnation of claims that disease was due to microscopic creatures.

Bernardino Ramazzini (1633–1717) wrote the first full-scale treatise on occupational health, which examined the potential sources of illness in more than forty-two different occupations, including those of miner, gilder, midwife, apothecary, singer, painter, soldier, and baker. Ramazzini's work was an important synthesis of all the knowledge then available on occupational disease and served as a source for further investigation by students of public health until the nineteenth century.

THE
EIGHTEENTH
CENTURY

The Eighteenth Century

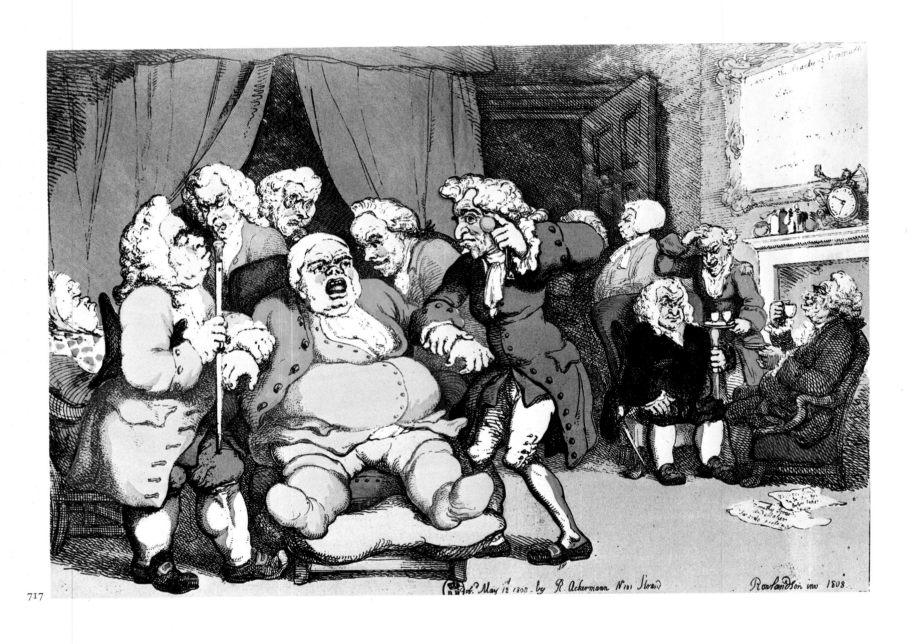

I T is often thought that the eighteenth century—with its insistence on a rational and scientific approach to all the historic issues confronting mankind—succeeded in sweeping away forever the tyranny of medieval dogma. Undoubtedly the vistas unfolded in the previous century by the genius of Newton, Descartes, Boyle, and Bacon led men away from a blind belief in authority to a new faith in progress and the inexorable triumph of the human spirit. Nevertheless, the physician, always noted for his conservatism, has seldom been able to keep pace with contemporary scientific advances, especially in other fields, or to put such advances to immediate practical use. The men of medicine could hardly disregard the rapid succession of startling advances in physics and chemistry, but the resultant revival of interest in the systems of the iatrophysicists and iatrochemists did nothing to advance the practice of medicine, and it may have contributed to a period of stasis or decline.

Of special interest to eighteenth-century medical theorists was the celebrated philosopher Gottfried Wilhelm Leibnitz (1646–1716). His basic tenets of logic, natural law, and a vital force governing the body were to find their way into many of the medical systems which came into vogue during the early years of the century. Of these, one of the most influential was that of Georg Ernst Stahl (1660–1734), who rejected the view of Descartes that the body was simply a machine. Instead, Stahl's theory of vitalism postulated the existence of an "anima" or sensitive soul which regulates the body health in a manner not unlike that of the "physis" of Hippocrates or the "psyche" of Aristotle. Disdainful of anatomy and physiology, Stahl was a strong advocate of bloodletting and other methods aimed at reducing "plethora." His support of the phlogiston theory of combustion may have delayed the discovery of oxygen by several decades.

A colleague of Stahl's at the University of Halle (destined to become his bitter rival) was Friedrich Hoffmann (1660–1742). Unlike Stahl, Hoffmann was a warm, inspiring teacher, who attracted to his lectures a host of students. His openly mechanistic system taught that the fibers of which the entire body was composed could dilate or contract in response to a property known as "tonus." This in turn was controlled by a "nervous ether" emanating from the brain. Health depended on the proper regulating of tonus, and Hoffmann's relatively simple therapy consisted of administering relaxing sedatives or irritating stimulants—a system reminiscent of the theory of the "pores" which Asclepiades championed in Roman times. In France, Hoffmann's mechanistic views reached a wide audience through the writings of the medical philosopher Julien de La Mettrie (1709–51) whose *L'Homme machine* (1748) was greatly admired.

Hoffmann's system also had great influence on the English-speaking world, having been adopted with some modification by William Cullen (1710–90), professor at Glasgow and Edinburgh, whose *First Lines of Physic* (1776) was to become the vade mecum of generations of students and practitioners. Cullen's theory of "nervous energy" as the determinant of the normal state of the body was further simplified, or debased, by a former pupil, the drug- and alcohol-addicted John Brown (1735–88), who considered "excitability" to be the basis of bodily health and who therefore recommended the use of stimulants or sedatives to bring about the desired harmonious balance of "stimuli." Brown's classification of all diseases as "sthenic" or "asthenic" had great appeal to the hard-working physician on the American and Canadian frontiers, having received the blessing of no less an authority than the eminent American medical leader Benjamin Rush (1745?–1813).

Still another theory, also highly speculative, had considerable influence in France. Adopting Stahl's doctrine of a "vital force," Theophile de Bordeu (1722–76) proposed his own version of vitalism in which he maintained that the three important organs of the body—the stomach, heart, and brain—elaborated a secretion whose proper concentration in the bloodstream helped to maintain health. Bordeu has thus become known as a pioneer in endocrinology. His insistence that every disease ended in a crisis restored interest in this ancient doctrine of

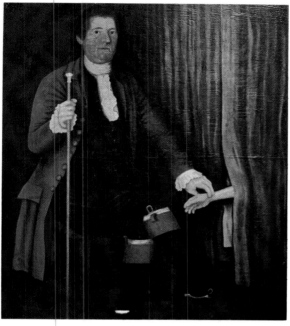

718

717 *The helplessness of physicians in the face of severe illness is caricatured by Thomas Rowlandson in* The Consultation *(1808): "The last hope, when the masters shake their heads, and bid their Patient think on Heaven—All's over, good Night." National Library of Medicine, Bethesda*

718 *Winthrop Chandler's painting of about 1780 shows Dr. William Clysson discreetly taking the pulse of a female patient, one of several ways of arriving at a diagnosis. Ohio Historical Society, Campus Martius Museum, Marietta, Ohio, on loan to the Art Institute of Chicago*

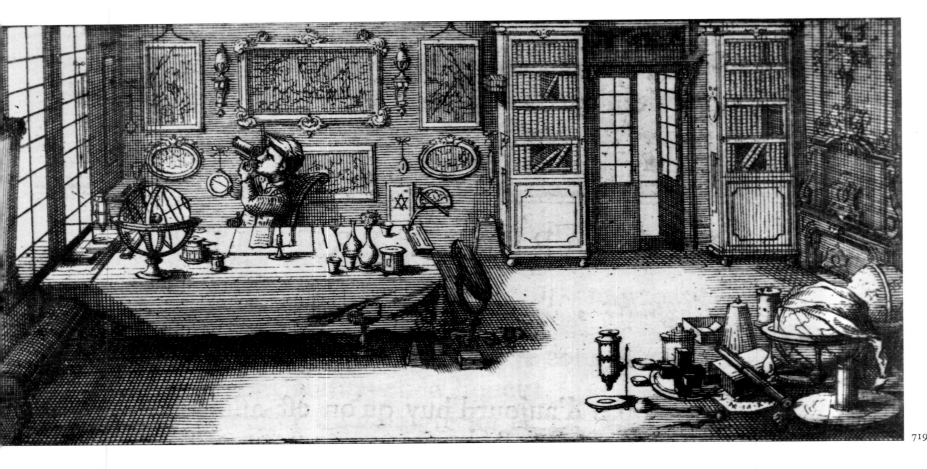

719 *Engraving from Louis Joblot*, Descriptions et Usages de Plusieurs Nouveaux Microscopes (1718). *Startling advances in physics and chemistry led to a revival of interest in the works of the iatrophysicists and iatrochemists. National Library of Medicine, Bethesda*

720 *Portrait of Dr. Georg Ernst Stahl, who taught that a life force, anima, controlled health, that fever was an agent of anima to combat disease, and that bleeding and purging were beneficial. New York Academy of Medicine*

721 *Engraving (1800) by Edward Savage of the likeness of Benjamin Rush, the outstanding American physician of his time. Mabel Brady Garvan Collection, Yale University Art Gallery*

722 *Benjamin Rush's medicine chest. Mutter Museum, College of Physicians of Philadelphia*

723 *Engraving by Jean-Baptiste Hilaire of the Jardin des Plantes, where, under government auspices, scientific studies were pursued to provide botanists and zoologists with detailed information. No. 737, Ve 53f, rés. fol. 103, Bibliothèque Nationale, Paris*

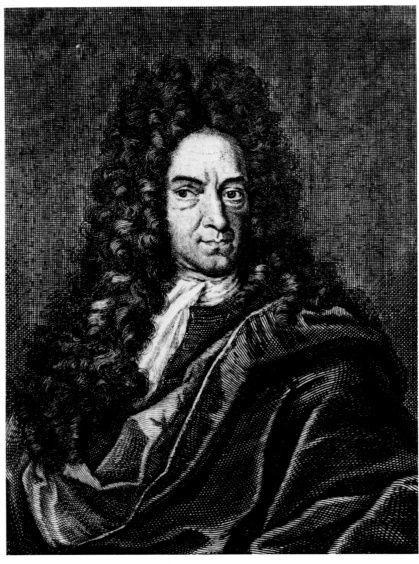

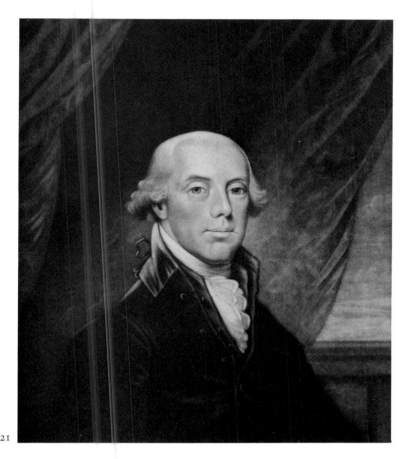

721

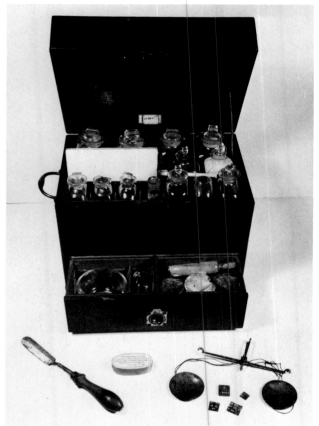

722

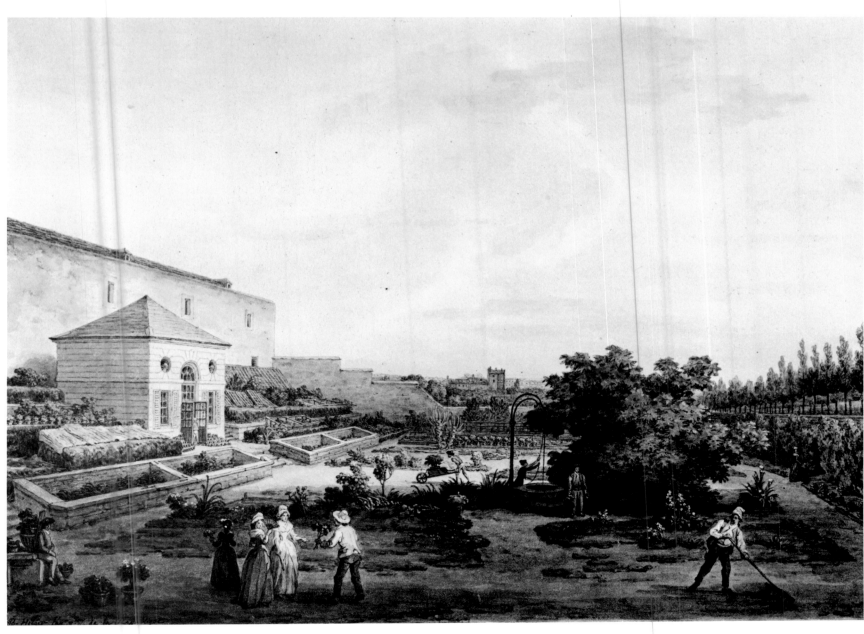

723

724 *Eighteenth-century lifesize anatomical figure made of wax, similar to many used as teaching tools in the universities. Semmelweis Medical Historical Museum, Budapest*

725 *Bleeding knife with three blades and a lancing pin (c. 1790). Bloodletting was still a respected method of treatment in the 18th century, along with cupping and purging. Private collection*

726 *Dove-shaped sucking bottle used in feeding patients flat on their backs. Semmelweis Medical Historical Museum, Budapest*

727 *One of many caricatures of the medical profession done by Thomas Rowlandson. National Library of Medicine, Bethesda*

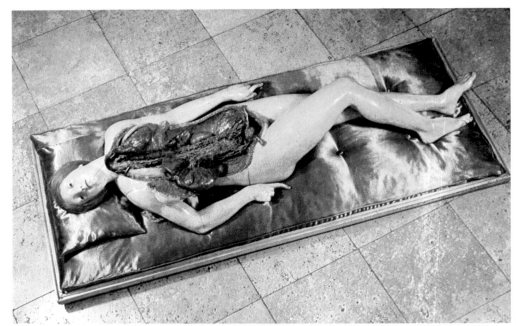

724

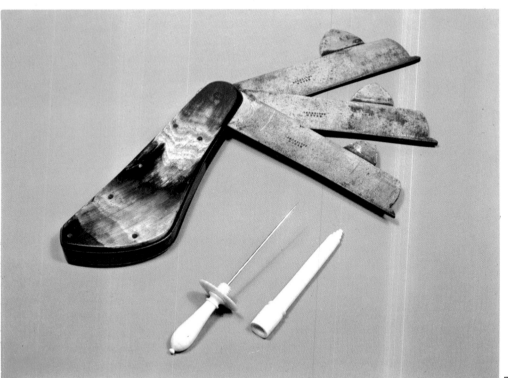

725

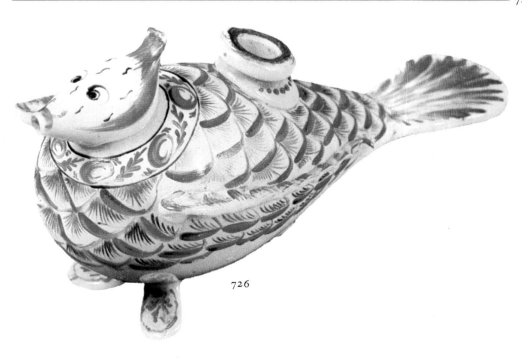

726

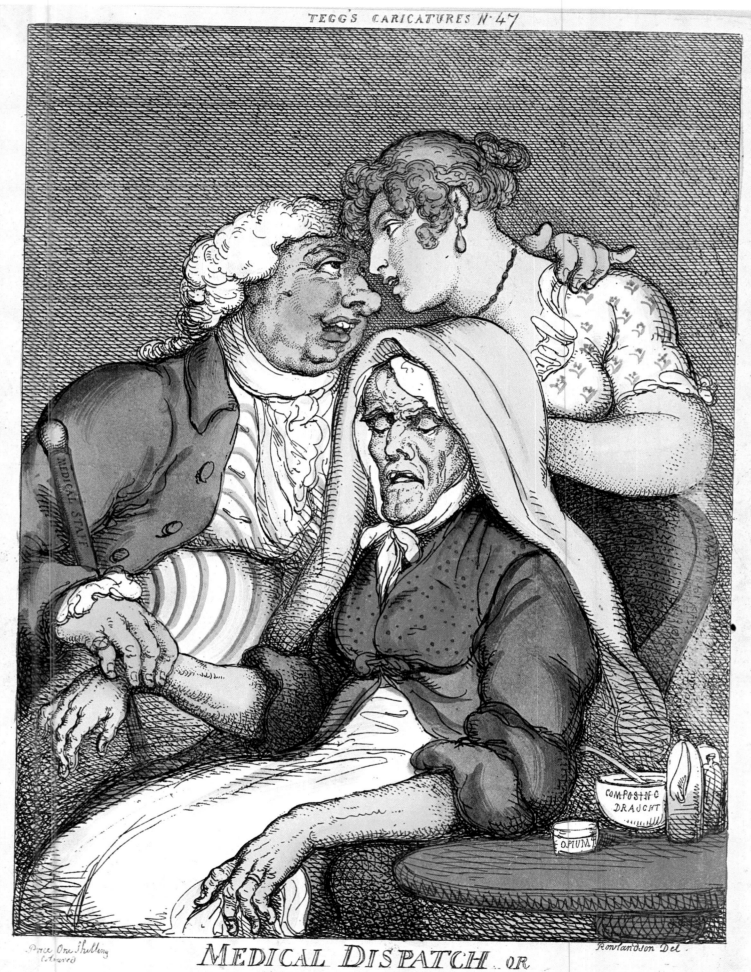

MEDICAL DISPATCH..OR

DOCTOR DOUBLEDOSE KILLING TWO BIRDS WITH ONE STONE.

471

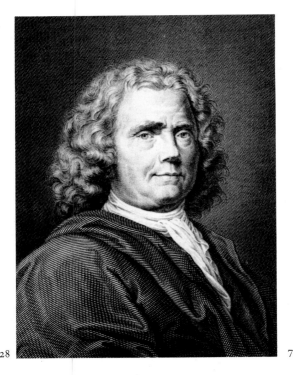

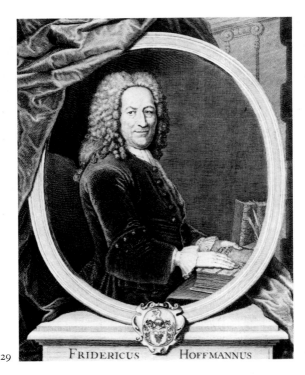

FRIDERICUS HOFFMANNUS

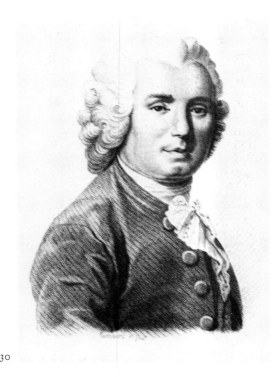

728   729   730

728 *Hermann Boerhaave, great teacher and clinician, was the central figure at Leiden, where students of medicine flocked. New York Academy of Medicine*

729 *The influential medical philosopher Friedrich Hoffmann believed that scientists should investigate nature by using mechanics, chemistry, and anatomy. New York Academy of Medicine*

730 *Engraved portrait of Theophile de Bordeu, a pioneer in endocrinology. New York Academy of Medicine*

731 *Anatomical drawing (1756) by the American artist John Singleton Copley. British Museum, London*

732 *Engraving by Claude Perrault that commemorates a visit by Louis XIV to a mathematics class at the Academy of Sciences at the Jardin des Plantes. State patronage of the sciences gave impetus to steady development. Va 257 fol., Bibliothèque Nationale, Paris*

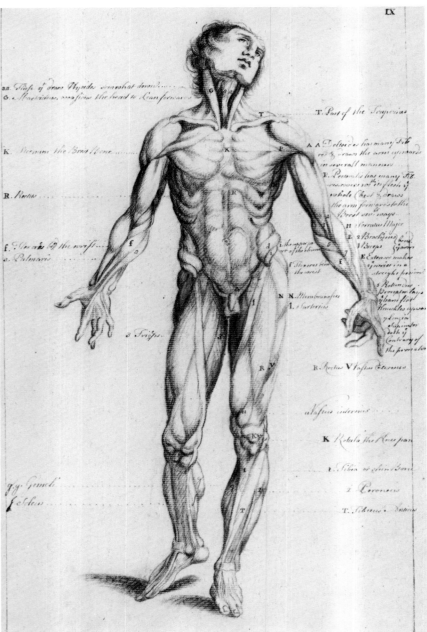

731

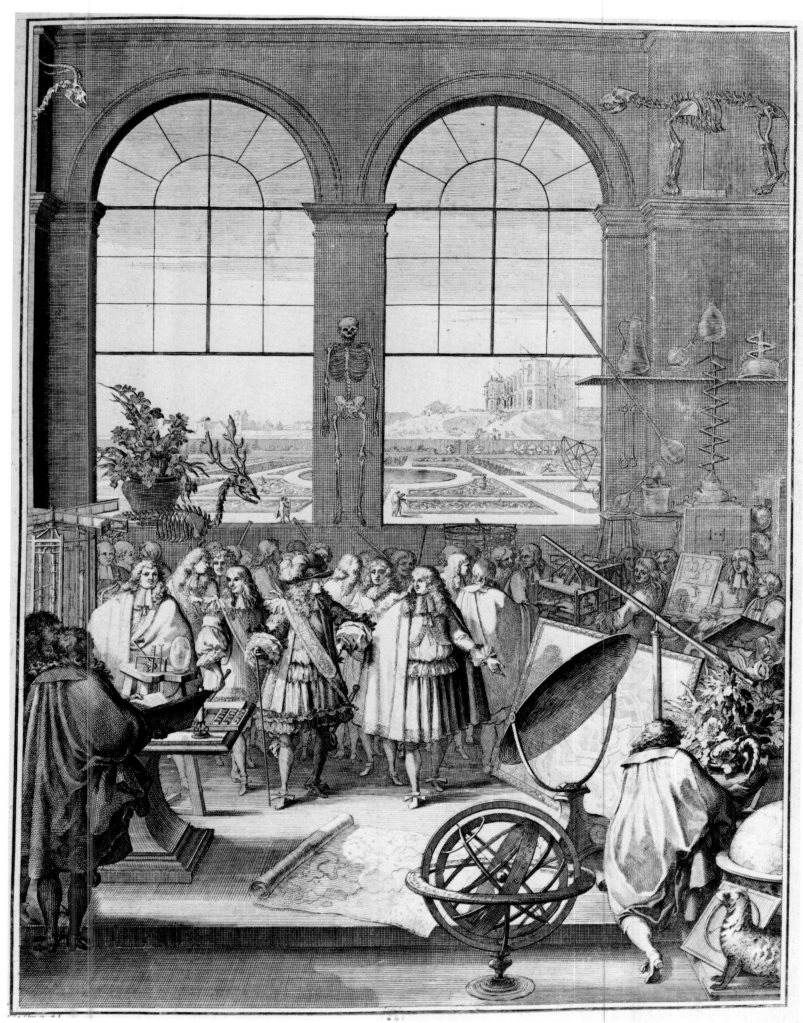

732

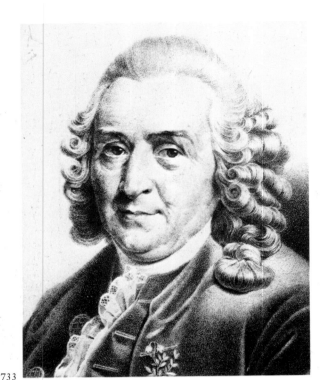

733

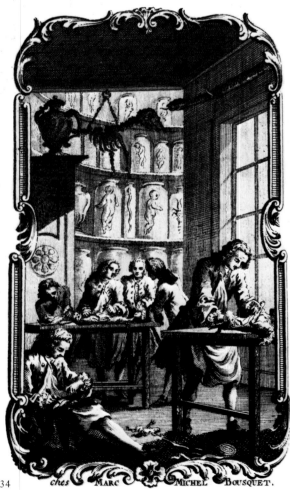

734

Hippocrates. Vitalism continued to exert great influence throughout the century, reaching new heights of popularity through the efforts of a Montpellier professor, Paul Joseph Barthez (1734–1806).

Attempts to classify all diseases were sparked by the success of Carl von Linné or Linnaeus (1707–78), the Swedish botanist-physician, originator of the binomial nomenclature still used to this day in botanical and zoological classifications. Nevertheless the medical classifications of Linnaeus, and later those of Philippe Pinel (1745–1826) and others, proved to be worthless. Only the systematic listings of Boissier des Sauvage were of sufficient validity to entitle him to lasting fame as the founder of medical classification.

EDUCATION AND THE TEACHERS

BY the beginning of the eighteenth century the older medical centers of northern Italy had lost their preeminence, and many new schools founded north of the Alps were vying actively for students. It happens not infrequently that a medical school will benefit greatly from the magnetic presence of a single great teacher. We have already noted the success of Hoffmann at Halle, but this was easily surpassed by the throngs which made their way to the University of Leiden to hear the great Hermann Boerhaave (1668–1738). This charismatic individual succeeded in making Leiden the temporary medical center of all Europe. A true humanist in the Renaissance mold, Boerhaave's interests wandered far beyond medicine to encompass all the arts, including music as well as literature. An eclectic by choice, he was not an outstanding original thinker nor a noted contributor to therapy, but as an observer and instructor he was unsurpassed. Like Sydenham, whom he ardently admired, Boerhaave placed the greatest emphasis on bedside instruction, thus reviving this important aspect of the Hippocratic method. He also insisted that the student follow a patient's corpse to the autopsy table to fix clearly in mind the correlation between lesions (abnormal changes) and symptoms. Fortunately students at Leiden had the advantage of instruction in dissection from Bernhard Siegfried Albinus (1697–1770), one of the most famous anatomists of the day.

Among the many pupils of Boerhaave who spread the teachings of the master to all parts of Europe was the Dutchman Gerhard van Swieten (1700–72), author of a famous commentary on the *Aphorisms* (1709) of his teacher. Called by Empress Maria Theresa to Vienna to serve as her personal physician, Van Swieten was also granted a free hand in reorganizing the teaching of medicine at the ancient university after the pattern of Leiden. To assist him in this undertaking Van Swieten called on a fellow-alumnus, Anton de Haen (1704–76). An excellent clinician and hygienist, De Haen did much to popularize the use of the thermometer in medicine and the use of a methodology in solving puzzling cases.

This so-called old Vienna school reached an acme of popularity just after mid-century, drawing flocks of students from all over Europe. Possibly its most illustrious alumnus was Leopold Auenbrugger (1722–1809), whose *Inventum Novum* (1761) clearly outlined the procedure of percussing the chest (tapping with the fingers) to diagnose abnormalities of the thorax. Although this technique was ridiculed by contemporaries of Auenbrugger, fifty years later his book was rediscovered and translated into French by Jean-Nicolas Corvisart (1755–1821), reintroducing one of the lasting diagnostic tools of the profession. In the construction of the famous Allgemeines Krankenhaus (1784), Vienna set a model for all Europe of a hospital devoted not only to teaching but also to care of the underprivileged.

Earlier in the century, while Boerhaave was still teaching, another of his pupils, Alexander Monro (1697–1767), returned to his native Scotland to add vigor to the ancient University of Edinburgh. A master anatomist, Alexander was succeeded by a son and grandson of the same name, thus providing a dynasty which

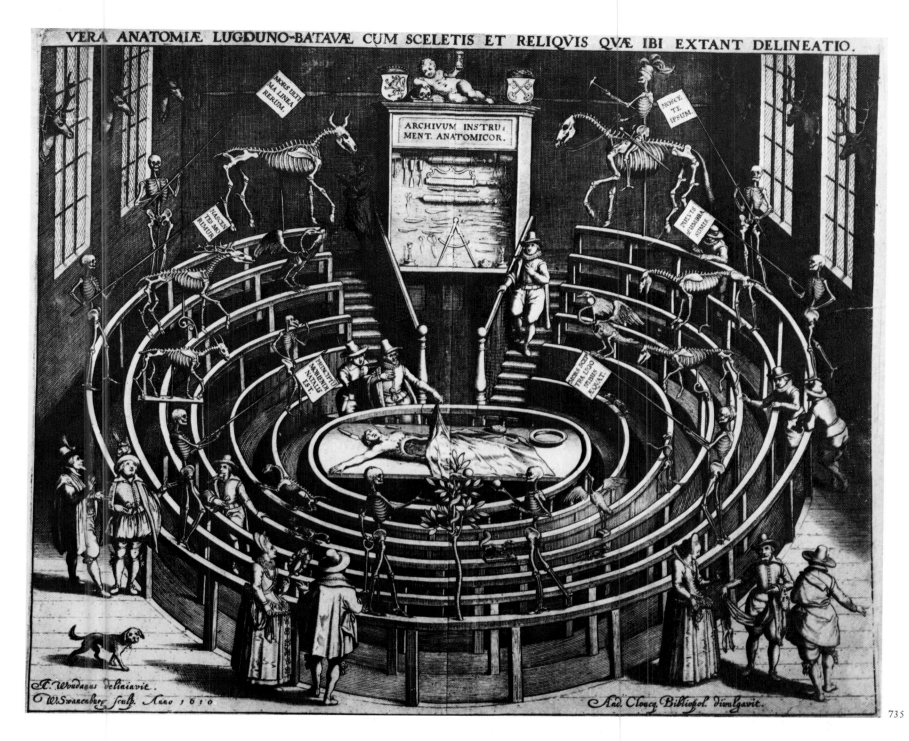

735

733 *Portrait of the Swedish botanist-physician Linnaeus, whose success in developing a system of botanical and zoological classifications led to similar attempts to classify diseases. New York Academy of Medicine*

734 *Illustration from Albrecht von Haller,* Memoires sur la Nature Sensible et Irritable des Parties des Corps Animals (*1756*). *A towering figure, Haller illuminated the physiology of the nervous system, establishing the function of the nerve fibers and their relationship to the brain. National Library of Medicine, Bethesda*

735 *Bernhard Siegfried Albinus taught anatomy at Leiden and was so famous that fashionable folk often dropped in on his lessons, creating a scene similar to the one portrayed in this engraving. Rijksuniversiteit, Leiden*

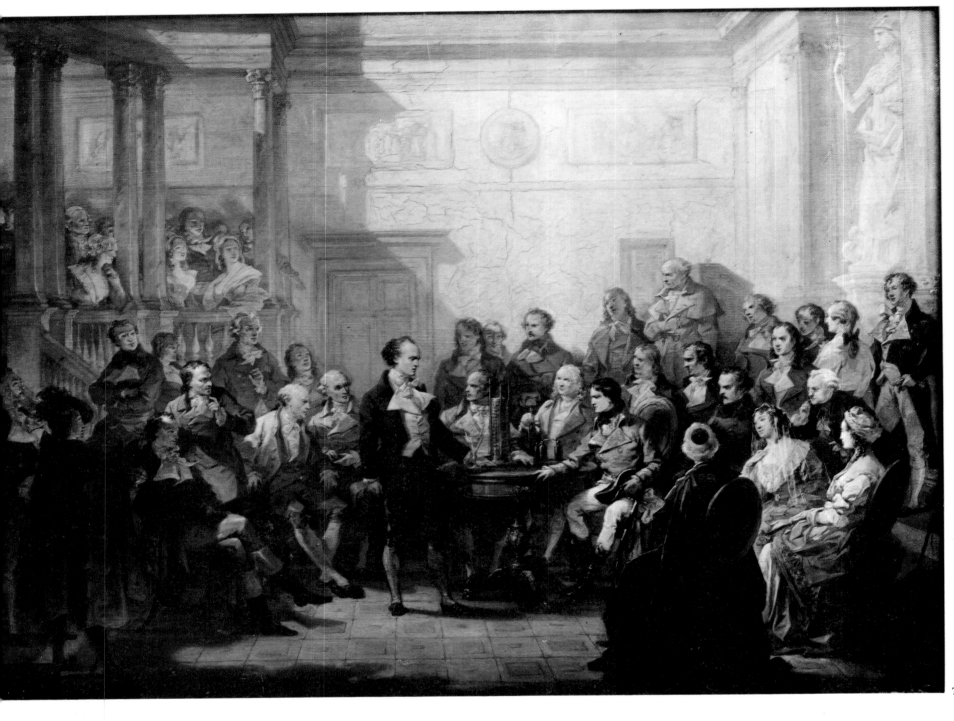

736

736 *Italian physicist Alessandro Volta is shown here, by Alexandre-Evariste Fragonard, explaining to Napoleon the workings of his pioneer battery. Collection Wildenstein, Paris*

737 *Antoine-Laurent Lavoisier and his wife, as painted by Jacques-Louis David in 1788, working together, revolutionized the science of chemistry and established the importance to living cells of oxygen, which Lavoisier named. Metropolitan Museum of Art, New York*

was to endure for well over a century. Edinburgh rapidly became the principal center of medical instruction for the English-speaking world.

The most notable of all Boerhaave's disciples, and one of the towering figures of the century, was the Swiss Albrecht von Haller (1708–77), a man of unlimited energy and imagination. He emulated and easily surpassed his own master in humanistic interests. Poet, novelist, writer of thousands of letters, and master bibliographer, Haller has often been described by his admirers as a universal genius. At the University of Göttingen, which he helped to create, he gave courses in a variety of subjects. His botanical garden attracted savants from all over the world, and even in this special field Haller could compete on equal terms with the great Linnaeus.

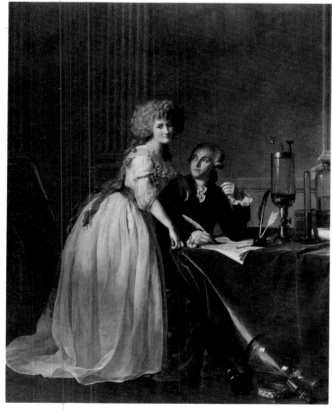

737

In the performance of physiological experiments Haller confined himself almost exclusively to the nervous system, refusing to accept the age-old concept of a fluid traversing the nerves as the cause of nerve action. He focused his observations on the nerve fiber itself, demonstrating clearly that while "irritability" was a property of muscle fiber, another factor, "sensibility," was characteristic of the nerve fiber. He outlined our current theory of the relationship of the brain cortex to the peripheral nerves, and although he still regarded the central area of the brain as the seat of the principle of life, or soul, he decried all mystical systems, and may be regarded as the founder of modern physiological thought.

Other experimenters in physiology whose studies were applicable to medicine were: René de Réaumur (1683–1757), inventor of a thermometer and a scale which bear his name and a pioneer in the study of gastric digestion; Lazzaro Spallanzani (1729–99), who helped put to rest the ancient concept of spontaneous generation and who was a pioneer in experimental fertilization; Stephen Hales (1677–1761), who demonstrated the dynamics of blood circulation, stressing the importance of the capillary system and recording blood pressure with a manometer, a forerunner of today's apparatus.

As the century drew to a close, Luigi Galvani (1737–98) launched the new science of electrophysiology with his observation that nervous action in muscle could be induced by an electrical charge. The erroneous theories and quackeries of "animal electricity" which resulted were disproved by the studies of Alessandro Volta (1745–1827), who not only demonstrated that the galvanic effect did not require the contact of an animal but also pioneered in the development of a battery.

The physiology of respiration received additional impetus in this period, stimulated by exciting advances in knowledge of the composition of air. The isolation of oxygen by Karl Wilhelm Scheele (1742–86) and Joseph Priestley (1733–1804) led to the disappearance of the phlogiston theory which had postulated the presence of a special substance in combustible materials yielded to the air on burning. Antoine-Laurent Lavoisier (1743–94) repeated many of Priestley's experiments but understood the significance of the results more clearly. Whereas Priestley still steadfastly supported the phlogiston hypothesis, Lavoisier proved its fallaciousness, gave the name "oxygen" to the substance in air responsible for combustion, and even perceived that respiration was necessary to the process we call oxidation in living tissue. Ironically, the pioneer who had advocated adequate housing space so that people could obtain sufficient oxygen was guillotined in the aftermath of the French Revolution by those whose benefit he sought. Eventually his demonstration of the role of oxygen in combustion revolutionized the entire science of chemistry.

The study of anatomy continued an orderly advance during this period, but more interest was directed to the newer subsciences of pathologic anatomy, comparative anatomy, and embryology. One of the greatest names of the century was that of Giovanni Battista Morgagni (1682–1771), whose five decades as professor at Padua were crowned by the publication of one of the acknowledged masterpieces of medical literature. In contrast to the earlier, poorly organized

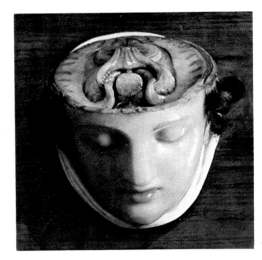

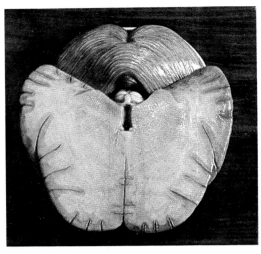

738

739

738, 739 *Two views of a wax anatomical model (c. 1800) designed for use as a teaching aid in the study of the skull and brain. Semmelweis Medical Historical Museum, Budapest*

740 *Another caricature of the medical profession by Thomas Rowlandson. National Library of Medicine, Bethesda*

741 *Used to power a defibrillator (as well as for other purposes), this "Ramsden"-type plate electrostatic generator (c. 1790) was one of the instruments that grew out of Luigi Galvani's experiments associating electricity and muscles. Museum of Electricity in Life at Medtronic, Minneapolis*

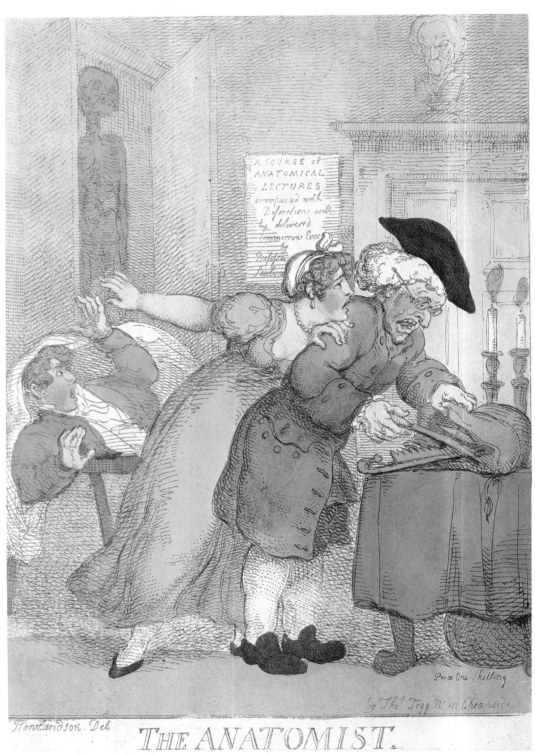

THE ANATOMIST.

740

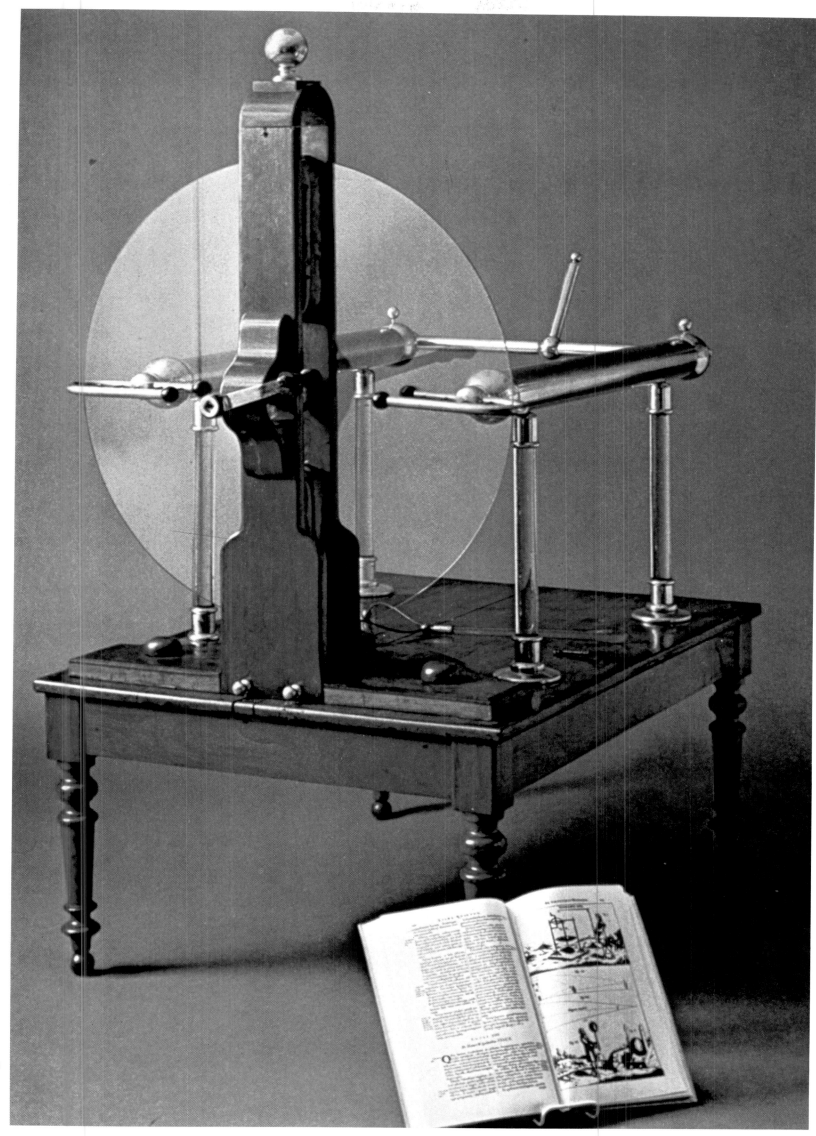

742 *One of the greatest medical men of the 18th century, Giovanni Battista Morgagni demolished the ancient humoral theory of disease through the publication of his* On the Sites and Causes of Diseases (1761) *which proved that pathologic anatomical changes in the internal organs were responsible for the symptoms of diseases.* New York Academy of Medicine

743, 744 *Two engravings by Martin Engelbrecht, entitled* A Surgeon or Barber *and* The Barber's Wife, *showing some of the surgeon's varied equipment, ranging from scissors and comb to saw and trepan.* Bibliothèque des Arts Décoratifs, The Louvre, Paris

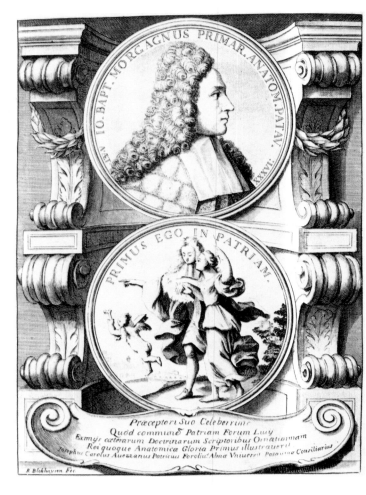

742

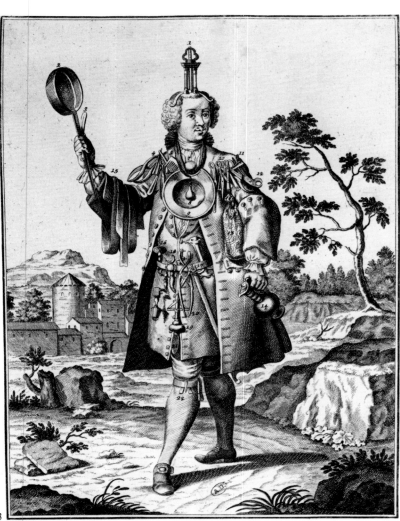

743

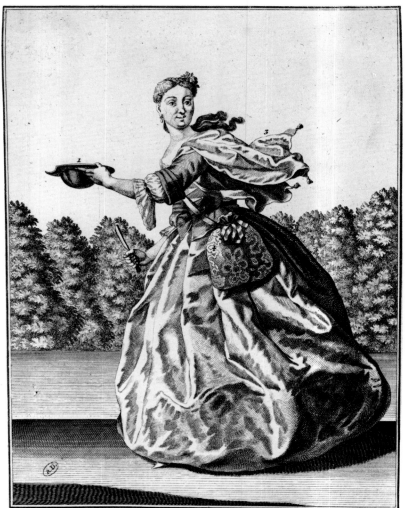

744

Sepulchretum of Theophile Bonet (1629–89), to which Morgagni paid due respect, his own *De Sedibus et Causis Morborum* (*On the Sites and Causes of Diseases*) (1761) contained beautifully arranged descriptions of the five hundred cases which he saw at autopsy, including in each instance a strict correlation of clinical symptoms with postmortem findings. Morgagni's work disposed of the ancient humoral theory of a single morbid cause for all disease and established the concepts and methods of study which provide to this day the basis of medical investigation and teaching. Among individual entities first clearly identified by Morgagni were hepatic cirrhosis, renal tuberculosis, syphilitic lesions of the brain, and pneumonic solidification of the lung. One of the followers of Morgagni was the brilliant Frenchman Xavier Bichat (1771–1802), who in his short lifetime studied over six hundred cadavers before dying of an infection contracted in the dissecting room. Without the use of a microscope Bichat succeeded in identifying twenty-one different tissues. His insistence that tissue was the prime element in the study of pathology facilitated the transition from Morgagni's theory of organs as principal components of the body to the doctrine of Rudolf Virchow that the cell was the basic unit.

The first systematic illustrated textbook of pathology, the work of Matthew Baillie (1761–1823), had been anticipated in part by the Irish anatomist Samuel Clossy (1724–88) whose *Observations* had appeared as early as 1763. What are now the modern concepts of embryology were given considerable impetus by the work of Caspar Friedrich Wolff (1733–94), who dared to oppose the great Haller's teachings on the development of the embryo. In opposition to the ancient accepted theory of embryonic preformation in miniature, Wolff reintroduced the doctrine of epigenesis, that is, the elaboration of the embryo by division from a single undeveloped form.

The dominating figures in the study of anatomy in England during the latter half of the century were the Hunter brothers. William (1718–83), a pupil of Cullen, founded the famous Great Windmill Street School of Anatomy, the first medical school in London. He also published works of fundamental importance on the human teeth and the pregnant uterus, having succeeded his master William Smellie (1697–1763) as the most fashionable "man-midwife" in the English metropolis. The introduction of the hitherto secret Chamberlen obstetrical forceps into general use (1727) and the delivery of members of the royal family by William Hunter were factors which helped to raise the science of obstetrics from medieval obscurity. Of equal importance in reducing maternal mortality was the establishment of the famous Rotunda in Dublin. This obstetrical hospital under the supervision of Sir Fielding Oulds was to set a standard of cleanliness and efficiency for all the continent to follow. William Hunter epitomized the courtly, humanistic physician of the early Georgian period. Following in the footsteps of Sir Hans Sloane (1660–1753), whose great collections helped form the nucleus of the British Museum, and of Richard Mead (1673–1754), one of the great bibliophiles of all time, Hunter himself became one of the most famous collectors of the period. Fortunately all his books, manuscripts, works of art, and unrivaled Greek and Roman coins can be studied today at the University of Glasgow.

But it was William's younger brother John (1728–93), brilliant surgeon and experimentalist, who has left a greater impress on the history of medical science. Having become an expert anatomist at his brother's school, John proceeded to study surgery under the two men who dominated the field in England during most of the century, namely William Cheselden (1688–1752) and Percivall Pott (1714–88). An expert in the practice of lithotomy (removal of bladder stones) when speed in any surgical procedure was of the essence, Cheselden was reputed to have performed this operation in less than one minute. The equally brilliant Pott is the eponym for several medical conditions, including Pott's fracture of the ankle and Pott's curvature of the spine. It was this keen observer who first traced the relationship of scrotal cancer in chimney sweeps to their constant exposure to soot.

Following in the footsteps of these famous masters and basing his own work

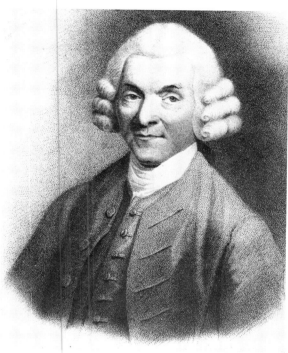

745

745 *Portrait of William Hunter, who, together with brother John Hunter, founded the first school of anatomy in London. His published works included studies on human teeth and the pregnant uterus. New York Academy of Medicine*

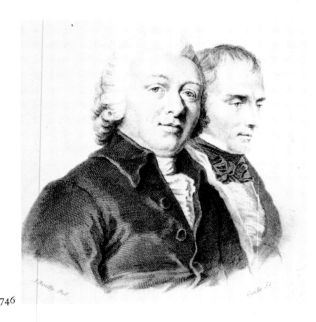

746

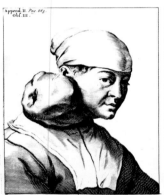 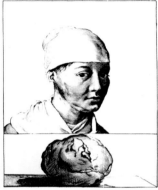

747

746 *Double portrait of Pierre-Joseph Desault, influential surgeon and teacher whose bandage for fractured clavicle is still used, and Marie-François-Xavier Bichat, whose extensive dissections showed that the fundamental sites of disease were in the tissue structure of organs. New York Academy of Medicine*

747 *Illustrations from a 1741 edition of Johannes Scultetus,* Armamentarium Chirurgicum *(1665) showing a neck tumor before and after removal. New York Academy of Medicine*

on a firm knowledge of anatomy and physiology, John Hunter was well prepared to raise surgery from a technique to a science. In operative surgery, possibly his single greatest contribution was a new method of closing off an aneurysm (outpouching of an artery), thus preserving the limbs of thousands of soldiers and civilians from unnecessary amputation. A man of the utmost precision in his work, he has been called the founder of experimental surgery and pathology and a pioneer in comparative anatomy. The hundreds of specimens he collected formed the basis of the Hunterian Museum now housed in the College of Surgeons of London. Only once did a Hunter experiment prove fallacious: in an attempt to prove that the two great venereal diseases had a common origin John had himself inoculated with matter from a case of gonorrhea. Unfortunately the donor was suffering from both diseases, and the development of syphilitic signs naturally convinced Hunter of his original hypothesis, which others had also held before him. It was not until a half century had elapsed that Philippe Ricord finally cleared up the confusion. The host of pupils left behind at John Hunter's death constitute a roster of distinguished names. Of these one may mention the surgeons Astley Cooper (1768–1841) and John Abernethy (1764–1831) and the physicians Edward Jenner (1749–1823) and James Parkinson (1755–1824).

It was during this century that the surgeons of France and England finally managed to cast off the remaining vestiges of medieval restraints, to achieve emancipation and a position of equality with their traditional rivals, the physicians. In France the Royal Society of Surgeons was founded in 1731; in 1743 a royal decree forbade barbers from practicing all except minor procedures in surgery. Two years later in England, the corporation of surgeons was formally separated from the barbers, but it was not until the last year of the century that the Royal College of Surgeons was finally granted a charter.

Among the prominent continental surgeons of this century in France were Jean-Louis Petit (1674–1760), the inventor of the screw tourniquet and of a less lethal procedure for mastoidectomy, and Pierre Desault (1744–95), whose bandage for fractured clavicle is still in use today. In Italy Antonio Scarpa (1752–1832), master anatomist and humanist, devised a successful operation for inguinal hernia, while Giuseppe Flaiani (1741–1808) gave one of the earliest accounts of exophthalmic goiter. The German Lorenz Heister (1683–1758) wrote one of the first systematic illustrated textbooks on surgery (1718) and lived to see this translated into many of the languages of Europe. Indeed an important step toward the final emancipation of the surgeon has sometimes been credited to the fame of this single book—in addition to the successful fistula operation performed by Félix on the grateful Louis XIV.

METHODS OF TREATMENT

IN spite of the startling developments in chemistry, there were few therapeutic advances in the eighteenth century. The ancient practices of cupping, bleeding, and purging persisted as the mainstays of the practitioner, while syphilis and other venereal diseases continued to be treated with massive, often fatal, doses of mercury. Theriac, the cure-all of antiquity, was still in use, as was a famous cinchona bark concoction against fevers of all types originated by John Huxham (1692–1768). A disciple of Boerhaave, Huxham deserves to be better remembered as the first physician to differentiate clearly between typhus and typhoid.

Among the more famous English clinicians of the period were William Heberden (1710–1801), who described angina pectoris, night blindness, and the nodules of osteoarthritis on the fingers which still bear his name, and Caleb Hillyer Parry (1755–1822), whose account of exophthalmic goiter is now considered to have precedence over all others. James Currie (1756–1805) sparked a renewal of interest in sea-bathing and hydrotherapy, and the spas of England and the

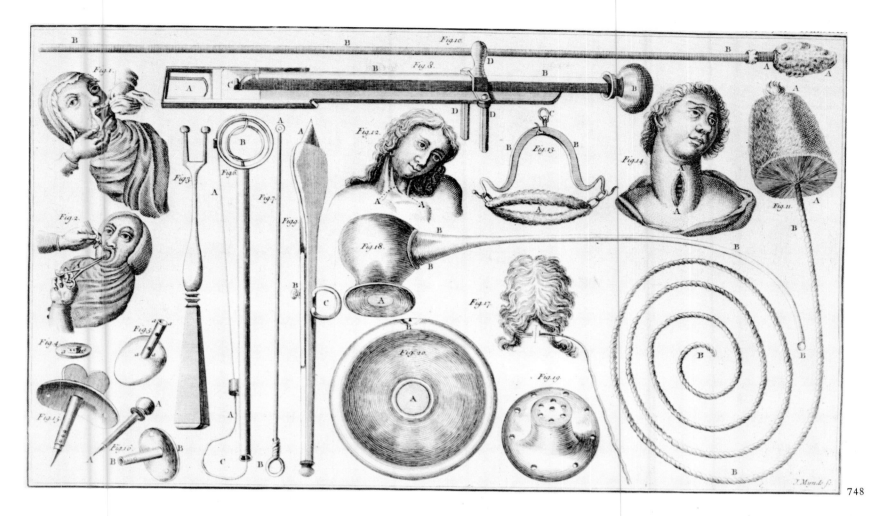

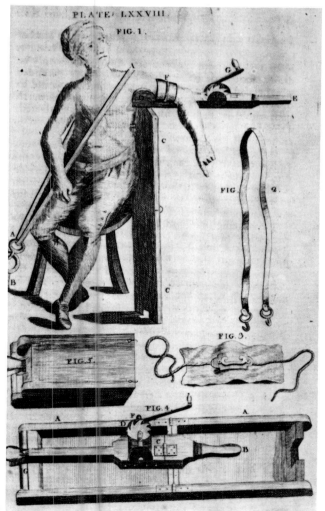

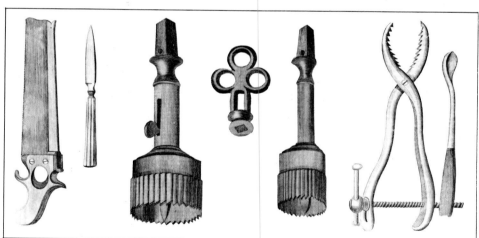

748 *Various instruments and procedures illustrated in a 1743 edition of Lorenz Heister,* A General System of Surgery *(1718), one of the most influential illustrated texts of its time. National Library of Medicine, Bethesda*

749, 750 *Benjamin Bell went even further than Heister in depicting surgical instruments in detail, as this selection from Bell's* A System of Surgery *(1791) demonstrates. National Library of Medicine, Bethesda*

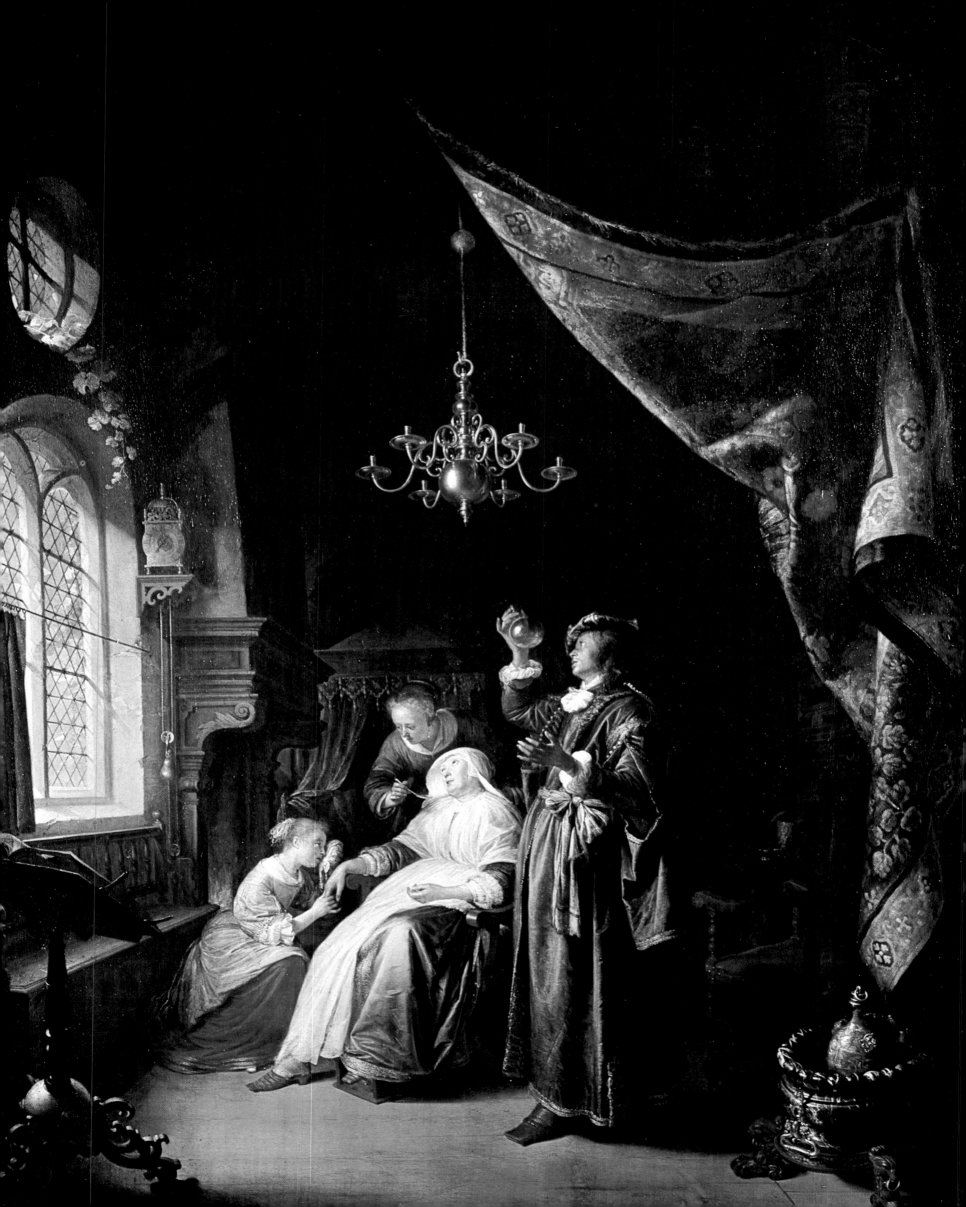

continent became extremely popular with sufferers from gout and other metabolic disorders. Of moderate usefulness were such well-known formulations as Dover's powders, Hoffmann's anodyne of opium, Fowler's solution of arsenic, and Glauber's salt, all of which retained their place in the pharmacopoeias of the world until quite recent times.

DIGITALIS

Undoubtedly the most important drug introduced into the armamentarium of the physician during the eighteenth century was digitalis, whose value in the treatment of dropsy (swelling of the limbs) was announced in 1785 by William Withering (1741–99) after many years of study. Having begun his investigations with a secret folk remedy, Withering quickly identified the active ingredient in the herbal brew as foxglove, *Digitalis purpurea*. This had been used for many years to treat a wide variety of illnesses, but Withering soon discovered that digitalis was not effective in all types of dropsy. At the time, he did not know that dropsy is merely a symptom of different pathological conditions and that only swelling from heart malfunction would respond. Nevertheless Withering did recognize that the drug acted primarily on the heart, was potentially toxic, and had to be administered in gradual doses—essential elements in therapy still observed today.

TREATMENT OF THE INSANE

In keeping with a more sympathetic approach to problems of the masses inspired by the Enlightenment, the decade of the French Revolution witnessed a dramatic change in the care and treatment of the mentally ill. Foremost in this movement was the Frenchman Phillipe Pinel (1745–1826), who pleaded for a more humane regimen for the inmates of the Bicêtre asylum near Paris, where the patients had hitherto been kept chained-up like beasts. An advocate of vitalism, Pinel kept accurate notes of the progress of his mental patients and may well be considered the founder of modern psychiatry.

Of more questionable value to psychiatry were the productions of Franz Joseph Gall (1758–1828), who was diverted from his useful studies on the anatomy of the brain to propound a theory that the strength of certain emotional and intellectual functions associated with localized areas of that organ could be accurately determined by studying the protuberances of the skull. The resulting pseudoscience known as phrenology was to enjoy a wide following for almost a century. Similar in character was the theory developed by the Swiss mystic and physician John Kaspar Lavater (1741–1801), who insisted that from the facial characteristics of an individual one could determine his character and mental capacity.

On the more positive side was the establishment by the English Quaker William Tuke (1732–1822) of the York Retreat for the humane care of the mentally ill. This pioneer institution set a pattern which was soon adopted in many parts of Europe.

QUACKERY AND CULTS

In spite of the significant progress in medical science which marked the eighteenth century, this period may also be considered the Golden Age of duplicity and charlatanism. One of the greatest hoaxes was that perpetrated by Joanna Stephens, who convinced even the great Cheselden that she had discovered a sovereign remedy for dissolving urinary stones, with the result that a gullible public paid five thousand pounds for the secret formula of this worthless concoction. Even more ludicrous was the case of Mary Toft, whose claim of having been delivered of rabbits (vouched for by the king's anatomist and

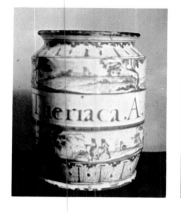
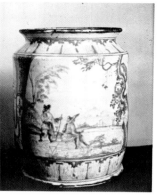

752

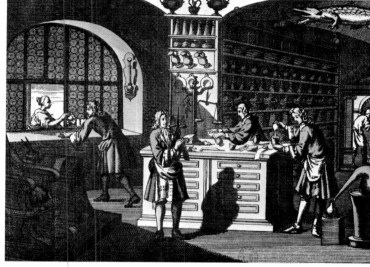

753

751 *The observation of urine (uroscopy) was still one of the basic methods of diagnosis, as Gérard Dou shows in his painting* The Dropsical Woman. *The Louvre, Paris*

752 *Two views of an apothecary jar marked "Theriac" (c. 1700), indicating that the famous cure-all of antiquity was still available for therapy in the 18th century. Deutsches Apotheken-Museum, Heidelberg*

753 *An engraving from* Oeconomus Prudens et Legalis *(1722) showing a pharmacy of the time. Among the drugs frequently dispensed were purges, mercurials, concoctions containing quinine, opium powders, and arsenic solutions. Collection William Helfand, New York*

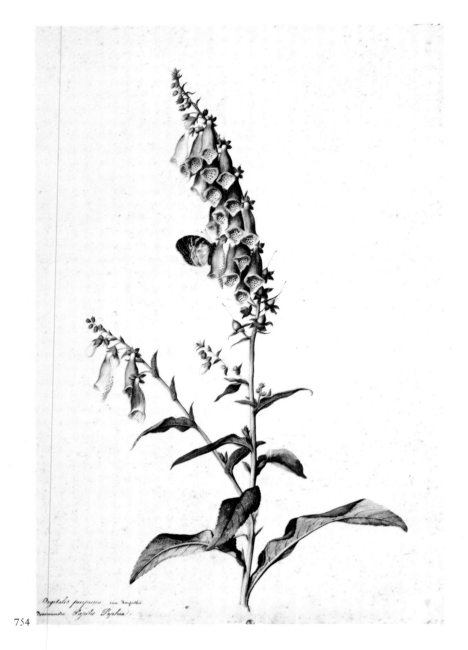

754

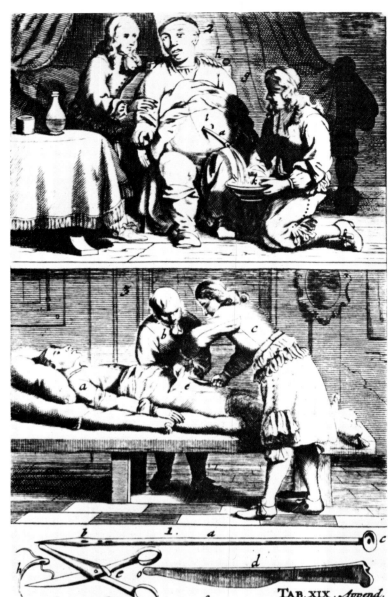

755

754 *Illustration of the plant foxglove* (Digitalis purpurea), *from which William Withering derived digitalis, one of the most important drugs introduced into medicine in the 18th century.* Gabinetto Fotografico, Florence

755 *Treatment of a dropsical patient by tapping the abdomen to remove fluid, as illustrated in a 1741 edition of J. Scultetus,* Armamentarium Chirurgicum (1665). *New York Academy of Medicine*

756 *Phillipe Pinel, innovator in the treatment of mental illness, is shown in this painting of 1793 ordering the chains removed from patients in an institution. World Health Organization, Geneva*

757 *One of William Hogarth's suite,* The Rake's Progress (1763), Bedlam *shows the conditions in London's Bethlehem Royal Hospital, which permitted sightseers to view the insane. National Library of Medicine, Bethesda*

758 *Portrait of Dr. Daniel Hack Tuke, a pioneer in the development of mental hospitals, who established the York Retreat for the humane care of the mentally ill. National Library of Medicine, Bethesda*

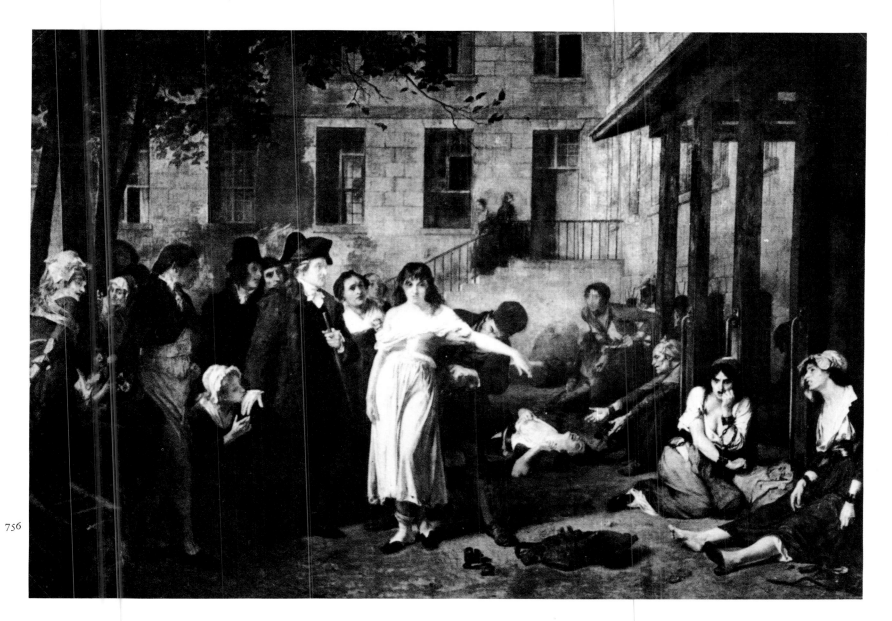

756

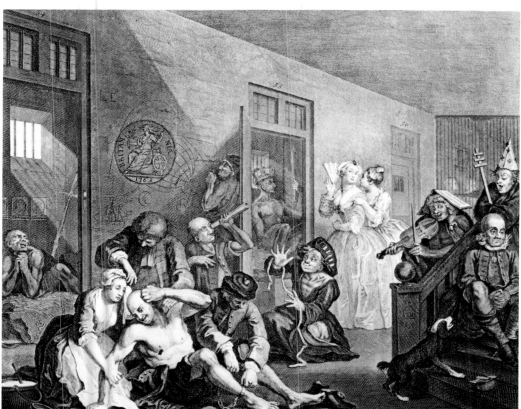

757

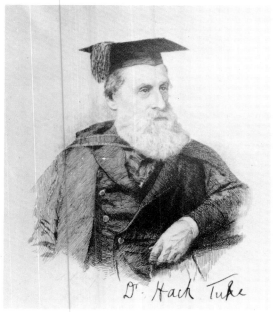

758

De wonderdokter Fop.

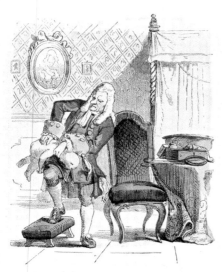

Zoo was er eens een kind heel ziek;
En weet gij, wat ik deed?
Ik brak 't den nek, waardoor het schaap
Geen smart of pijn meer leed.

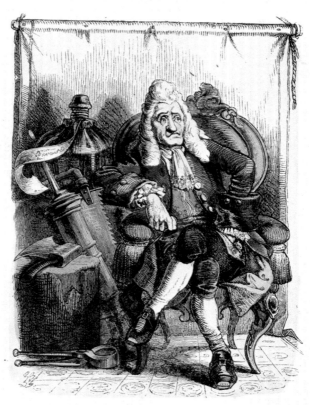

Ik ben de wonderdokter Fop,
De wereld door bekend.
In heel de wereld leeft er geen
Zoo'n hooggeleerde vent.

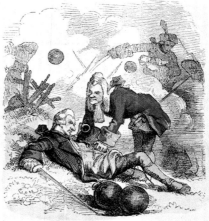

In d'oorlog nam 'k een kapitein
Drie kogels uit de borst;
De man ging dood, en 'k had vergeefs
Mij met zijn bloed bemorst.

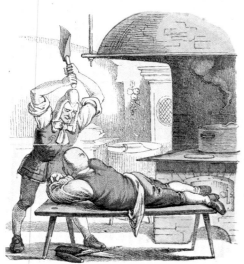

De kok van Zijne Majesteit
Had erge pijn in 't hoofd;
Met éénen bijlslag heb ik hem
Van alle pijn beroofd.

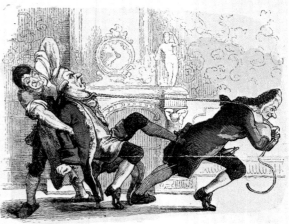

Een rijk heer had een kropgezwel
(Dat was een naar gezicht!)
Ik haalde met een touw 't gezwel
En ook de keel hem dicht,

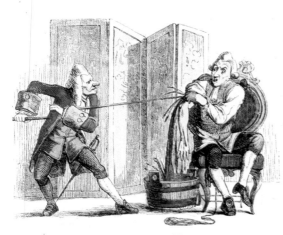

Een man die bang voor pokken was,
Woû zijn gevaccineerd;
Ik entte hem met 't braadspit in,
En heb hem erg bezeerd.

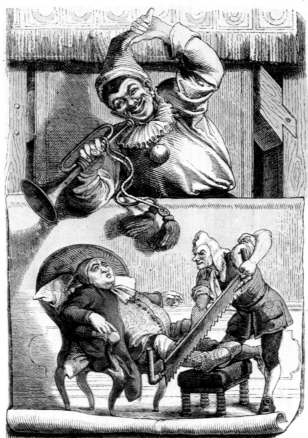

Maar 't grootste meesterstuk deed ik
't Welk braaf wat opzien gaf,
Ik zaagde een heer, die 't pootje had.
Fiksch bei zijn beenen af.

Alzoo genees ik. — Over mij
Klaagt nimmer één patiënt;
Ben ik, de wonderdokter Fop,
Dan geen geleerde vent?

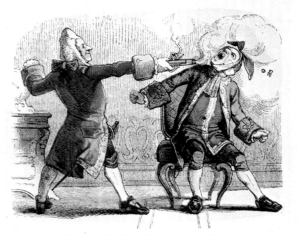

Een man, die kiespijn had, schoot ik
Zijn kies ferm uit den mond;
De man had nooit wêêr kiespijn, en
Was nooit wêêr ongezond.

Munchener platen. Nr. 81 Uitgegeven door **H. van der Moolen** te Geldern.

Druk van Dr. C. Wolf & zoon te Munchen.

surgeon) had all of London, including royalty, in an uproar. Even so sophisticated a personage as the Duchess of Devonshire was a sponsor of the infamous Temple of Health built and supervised by one of the most adroit of quacks, James Graham. Incorporating recent discoveries, Graham's erotic Celestial Bed bristled with a gamut of electrical devices guaranteed to spark even the most worn-out of rakes into renewed vitality.

To their credit it should be pointed out that some quacks became quite expert in certain specialties which legitimate practitioners were perfectly happy to relinquish. The Chevalier John Taylor could boast that he had treated the eyes of all the nobility of England, including George II who had appointed him his personal oculist. The setting of fractures was also relegated to highly skilled men and women; even the great Hans Sloane was perfectly willing to entrust the care of his niece suffering from a "broken back" to Crazy Sal, a famous bone-setter.

In that shadowy no-man's-land which still exists between the charlatan and conventional therapist stood the fascinating figure of Franz Anton Mesmer (1734–1815). A graduate of Vienna, Mesmer soon made his work on animal magnetism the subject of acrimonious debate in every capital of Europe. In Paris his Magnetic Institute attracted hundreds of the idle rich and was castigated as a hotbed of immorality. However, there can be no question that in those darkened rooms Mesmer achieved success in relieving the hysterical symptoms of susceptible young females. Mesmer for a short period had all Paris at his feet; so ardent were his admirers that many followed him to Switzerland after he had been banished from the French capital. That Mesmer's inadvertent use of hypnotic suggestion led the way to Bernheim and Freud is now well recognized by scholars.

PUBLIC HEALTH

In the eighteenth century only the very wealthy could be assured of the services of a qualified doctor of medicine, and this of course forced the general public into the hands of mountebanks, quacks, and others poorly prepared to offer rational treatment.

Dispensaries were scarce, hospitals had no organized clinics, and even people not actually impoverished had no place to turn for help. As a result, apothecaries gradually began to fill the void by responding to obvious needs of the public, thus destroying the monopoly of the physicians. The situation led to eventual acceptance of the apothecaries as general practitioners within the medical community, but this uneasy alliance raised many questions of medical ethics. The principal statement in this field was made by Thomas Percival (1740–1804), who adopted a somewhat patronizing attitude toward the apothecaries, but in his own conduct and in his book stressed those principles of professional conduct which are still valid today.

In the quest for amelioration of the public health an important part was played by the Quakers. The appalling infant mortality from diphtheria (then unnamed) led the philanthropic physician John Fothergill (1712–80) to study and publish an accurate description of this treacherous killer: *Account of the Sore Throat Attended with Ulcers* (1748). His disciple John Coakley Lettsom (1744–1815) was also lavish in his contributions to philanthropy and wrote an early paper on the harmful effects of alcohol and drugs among the laboring class. John Howard (1726?–90) so shocked the conscience of the world by his famous account of the dungeons and lazarettos of Europe that there resulted an outcry for more humane treatment of and improved sanitary conditions for the incarcerated.

The military mind also contributed to the betterment of conditions for prisoneres of war. Sir John Pringle (1707–82), a humane and progressive army surgeon, pleaded for decent ventilation for those confined in ship hulks and military prisons, insisting that jail fever and hospital fever were identical. Naval hygiene became the principal concern of James Lind (1716–94), whose insistence

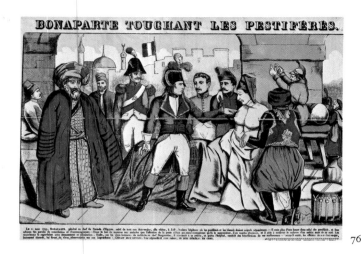

760

759 *Eighteenth-century hand-colored wood engraving in which the methods of doctors are mocked. National Library of Medicine, Bethesda*

760 *Wood engraving showing Napoleon touching a plague victim during his campaign in the Middle East, to reassure his soldiers who were in terror of the epidemic. Collection William Helfand, New York*

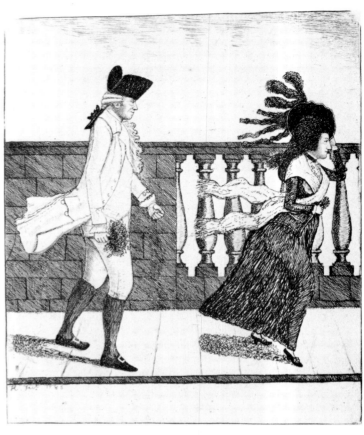

761 *Dr. James Graham, one of the most adroit of quacks, is shown in this engraving (1785) by John Kay following a woman to persuade her to enter his Temple of Health and Hygiene in Pall Mall. Collection William Helfand, New York*

762 *Colored engraving from the 1780s showing treatment by animal magnetism as practiced by Franz Anton Mesmer. "Mesmerism" is now characterized as a form of hypnosis, which Mesmer inadvertently achieved. National Library of Medicine, Bethesda*

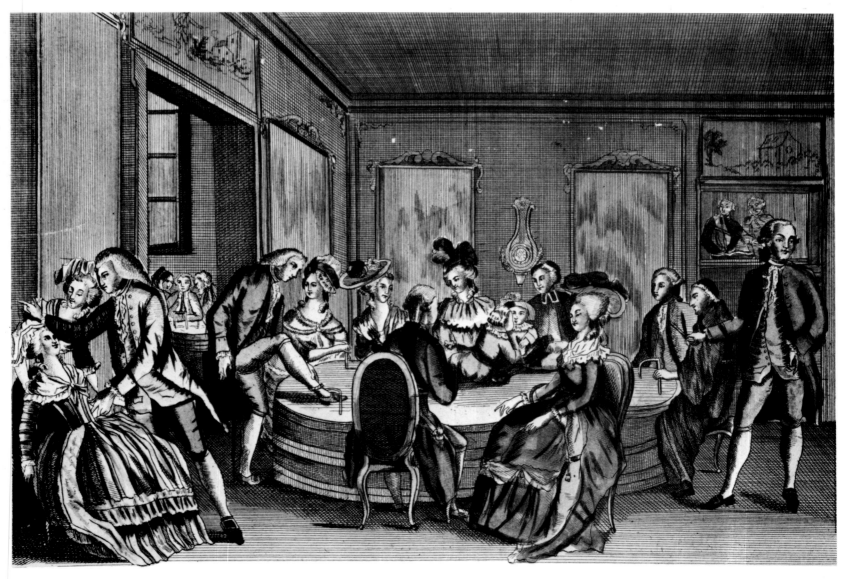

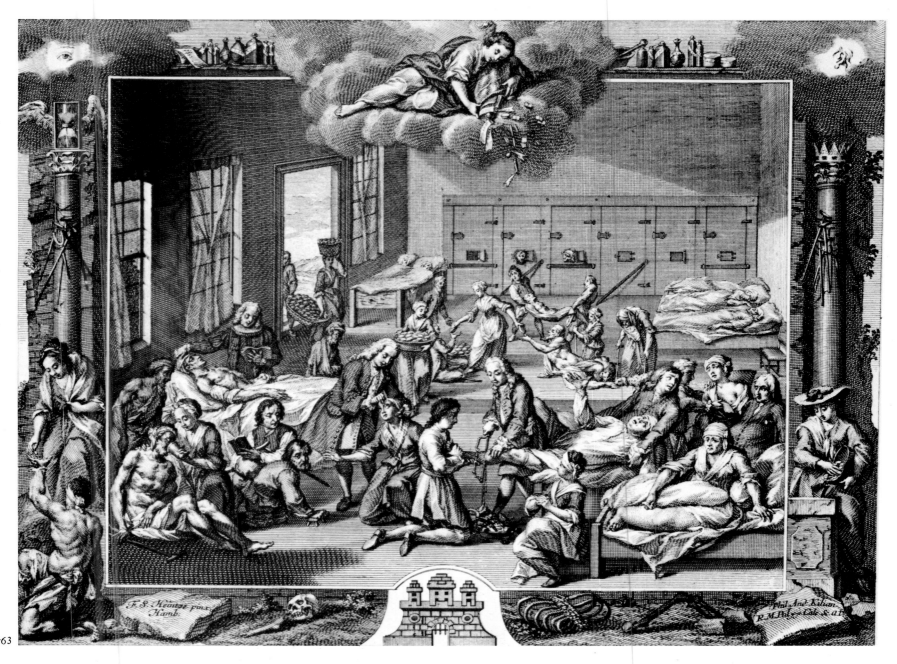

763

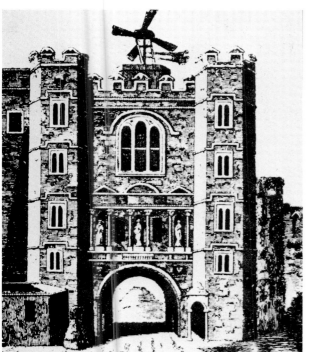

764

763 *An engraving of 1746 entitled* Der Pesthof (The Plague Ward), *illustrating conditions in a Hamburg hospital, where a doctor amputates a leg amidst a variety of medical activities. Germanisches Nationalmuseum, Nuremberg*

764 *Contemporary illustration of the windmill ventilator installed by Stephen Hales on old Newgate Prison in 1752, resulting in a dramatic drop in deaths from typhus inside the prison. British Museum, London*

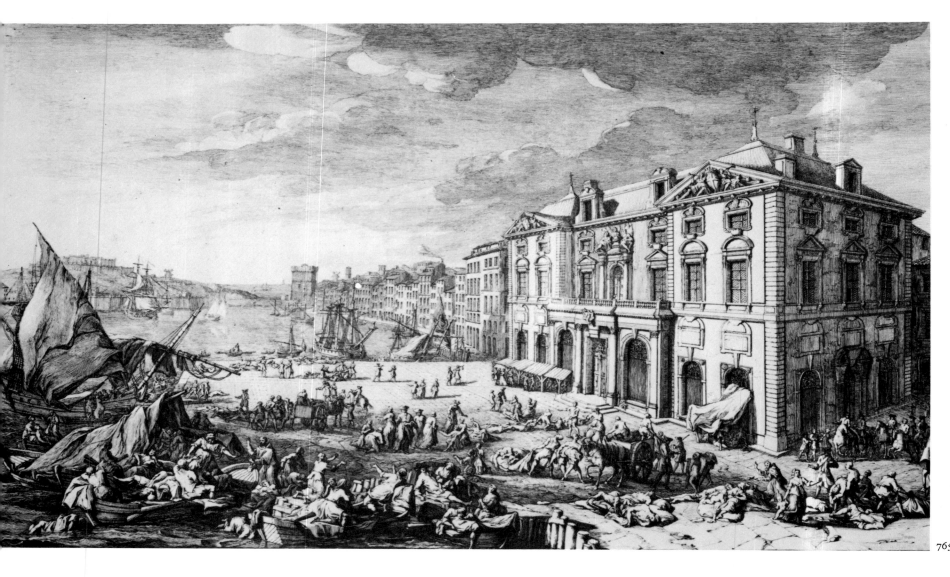

765

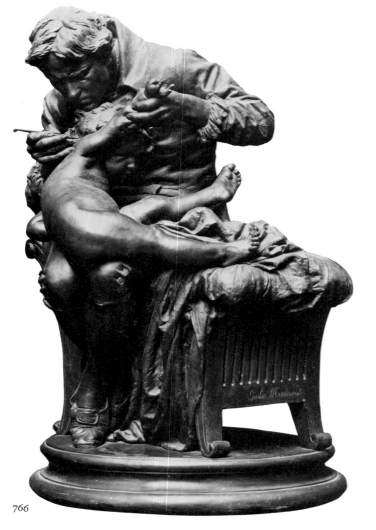

766

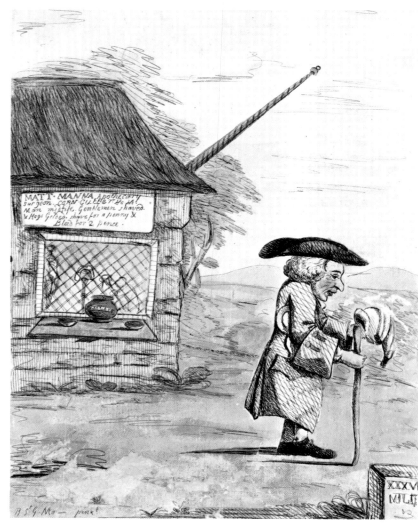

767

on the virtue of lemon juice in preventing scurvy went long unheeded by the Admiralty lords. George Baker (1722–1809) ended the mysterious deaths from "Devonshire colic" when he identified this as lead poisoning caused by drinking apple cider prepared in lead-lined containers.

A modern plan for systematic health coverage was envisaged by Johann Peter Frank (1745–1821). Professor at Pavia and a man of great intellect, Frank conceived a cradle-to-grave supervision of all medical needs not unlike the system now in effect in Great Britain. Although self-medication was frowned upon then as now, the plight of country folk who had practically no access to physicians produced a spate of home medical manuals. Those who did not wish to consult the village dame could turn to *Primitive Physick* (1747), a product of the pen of John Wesley (1703–91). Avowedly empiric this small book supplied prescriptions for many simple disorders, sold for one shilling, and achieved an enormous success. On a somewhat higher level was the *Domestic Medicine* of the Scottish physician William Buchan (1729–1805), which went through innumerable editions and was shelved next to the Bible in many a frontier home.

THE DISCOVERY OF VACCINATION

Although somewhat less lethal than in earlier centuries, bubonic plague, typhus, malaria, and diphtheria still returned with distressing regularity to take heavy tolls. But it was smallpox which remained the single most deadly killer of the period. This scourge, always endemic, frequently assumed epidemic proportions in the cramped medieval towns where refuse and even human excrement clogged the narrow streets and inadequate sewers. It is said that one-third of all the inhabitants of London bore pit marks of smallpox. Early in the century Lady Mary Wortley Montagu (1689–1762) brought back to England the Asian technique of variolation which she had observed in Turkey. This consisted of pricking serum from the sore of a person with smallpox into another's skin to produce a resistance resulting from a mild case of the illness. After two princes of royal blood had been successfully inoculated (1722), the practice became quite popular for a short period but soon lost acceptance as the inherent dangers became increasingly apparent. Inoculation also lost favor in the American colonies and was outlawed by several states until the eve of the Revolution. Debate continued on the value of variolation until Edward Jenner (1749–1823) electrified the world with his famous paper in 1798 on cowpox and the benefits of inoculating humans with the fluid from the sores of vaccinia, a disease of cattle. Vaccination had none of the potential dangers of the earlier inoculation of material from smallpox itself.

Thus the eighteenth century was not merely a period of consolidation or systematization. Overwhelmed as they were by the revolutionary discoveries of the previous century, physicians of the period struggled bravely to absorb and utilize the mass of new science. We can now better assess the considerable contributions of the eighteenth century and observe how closely these can be correlated with the advances which were imminent.

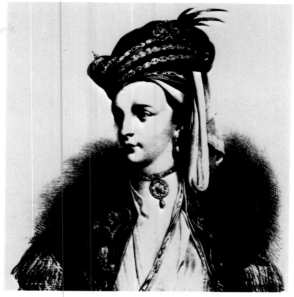

768

765 *Engraving by Jacques Rigaud after a painting by Michel Serre from a drawing made on the spot, showing the Marseilles town hall with citizens attempting to flee the plague of 1720. British Museum, London*

766 *Bronze sculpture by Giulio Monteverde showing Edward Jenner inoculating his son with cowpox liquid as a prevention against smallpox (1873). Galleria Nazionale d'Arte Moderna, Rome*

767 *Colored engraving by R. St. G. Mansergh entitled* Matthew Manna, a Country Apothecary, *dated 1773. The sign reading "Apothecary, Surgeon, Corn Cutter, Etc., Etc., Man midwife . . ." indicates the manifold functions of the apothecary, who moved in to fill the void left either by the unavailability of physicians in the country or by their unwillingness to engage in manual activities. Collection William Helfand, New York*

768 *Portrait of Lady Mary Wortley Montagu, who introduced into England the Asian technique of inoculating for smallpox by variolation (pricking into the skin fluid from a smallpox blister). New York Academy of Medicine*

THE
NINETEENTH
AND TWENTIETH
CENTURIES

The Nineteenth Century

The Beginnings of Modern Medicine

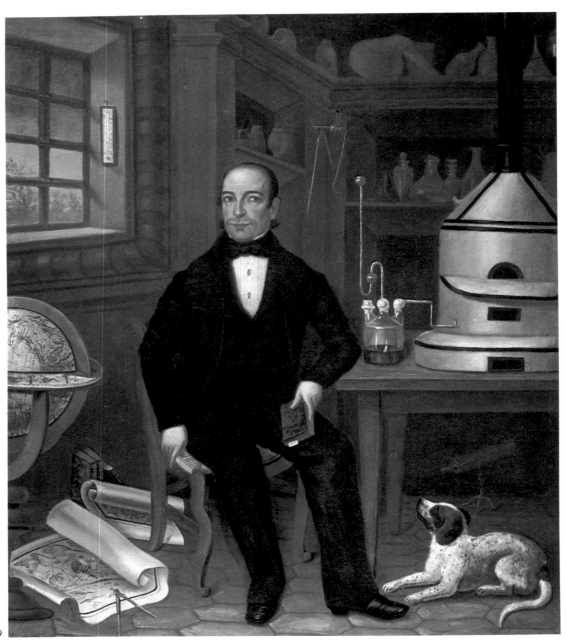

769

A LTHOUGH the early decades of the nineteenth century were a virtual continuation of medical developments in the previous century, two particular advances (anesthesia and the discovery of microorganisms as causes of disease) so altered the course of medical history that concepts of illness, methods of treatment, and hygienic practices at the end of the century bore only slight resemblance to what they were at the beginning. Of course there were other highly significant contributions which advanced the understanding of the structure and function of the living organism, such as the demonstration of the cell as the fundamental anatomical unit, the enunciation of the physiological principles relating to the internal environment of the body, and the introduction of new diagnostic tools into clinical methods. The effects of these other advances were more cumulative, producing their greatest impact in the following century.

Public Health

On the other hand, the organization of physicians, hospitals, and public health activities arose out of the nineteenth century itself, owing much to the alterations wrought by the Industrial Revolution. The rapid changes that followed the building of factories and the expansion of cities led to extreme shifts and crowding of populations. The conditions of factory workers, the spread of slums, and the interdependence of communities and nations also affected medical practice.

Before the discovery of bacteria as the causes of disease, the principal focus of preventive medicine and public health had been on sanitation: the provision of potable water and the dispersal of foul odors from sewage and refuse, which were considered the important factors in causing epidemics. The invention of the water closet by John Harrington (1561–1612) facilitated flushing away human waste and helped to keep some dwellings clean, but the flow from these indoor privies ran into cesspools and ultimately into waterways and wells.

The health of workers in the factories was important to their efficient functioning, and since the spread of epidemic disease was a danger to all segments of the population, the need for remedial measures in public health was urgently appreciated. Johann Peter Frank's *System einer Vollstandigen medicinischen Polizey* (1777–78), using statistics to establish the importance of public health, was a milestone even though its immediate influence was negligible. In 1848, the description by Edwin Chadwick of the sanitary conditions and health of English workers, however, did have a great impact on the upper classes and the governing bodies. His standards for the proper removal of sewage and the protection of water supplies was a stimulus to the government of Britain, as was Rudolf Virchow's militant advocacy of public health measures in Germany.

Epidemics continued to devastate cities and countries. As late as 1854 in London there were 14,000 cases of cholera with 618 deaths. In the United States, cholera ravaged the entire country three times in the nineteenth century. Yellow fever, after striking the northeast from 1793 to 1805, began a series of attacks upon the southern and Gulf of Mexico ports which reached a peak in the 1850s. A sharp decline followed until 1905, when one last explosive outbreak killed over 450 residents in New Orleans. Planned attacks on cholera, typhoid fever, and other pestilences only became feasible after the causes were discovered in the bacteriological era.

The assembling of large numbers of raw troops for the American Civil War was accompanied by inevitable outbreaks of communicable diseases. On both sides little attention was paid to camp sanitation, housing and food were atrocious, and confusion was rampant. No one anticipated the enormous casualties in the first few battles, and seriously wounded men often lay where they had fallen for several days. Many wounded died for want of immediate care, but the North, which lost control of the battlefields in the early fighting, took the heaviest casualties.

Gradually both sides evolved effective ambulance systems and hospitals,

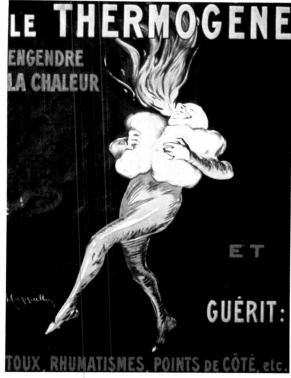

769 *As the century opened,* The Man of Science, *as visualized by Moritz Krantz in 1839, was broadly interested in many disciplines. He was to become more specialized as information and complex instruments proliferated. Gift of Edgar William and Bernice Chrysler Garbisch, National Gallery of Art, Washington, D.C.*

770 *Medications, at that time unregulated, could promise everything. "Le Thermogéne" was advertised to engender heat and cure rheumatism, and other ailments. Collection William Helfand, New York*

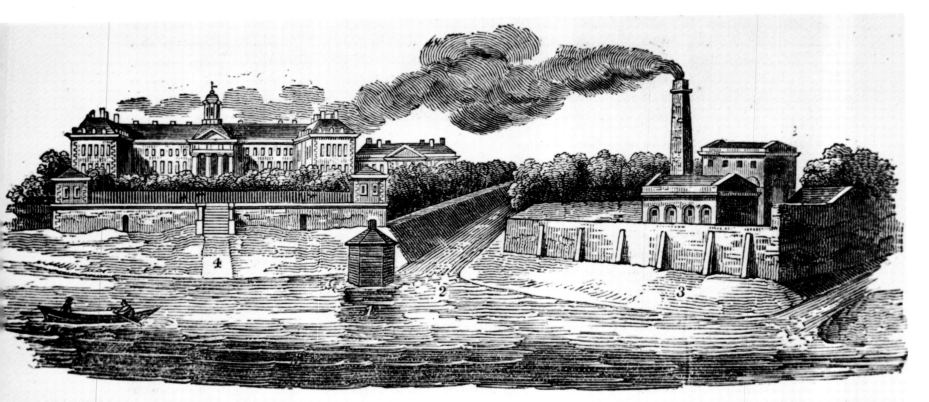

No. 1, is the Dolphin, or spot from which the Company derive their Supply.
2, is the mouth of the great Ranelagh Common Sewer.
3, is the Company's Steam-engine, which draws up the daily supply.
4, is Chelsea Hospital. At low water, the Dolphin is about three yards from the shore.

771

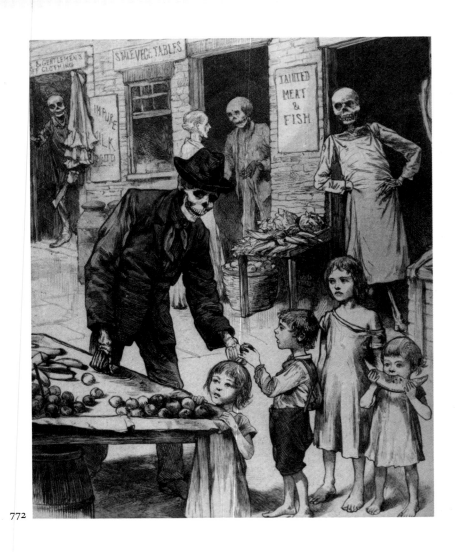

772

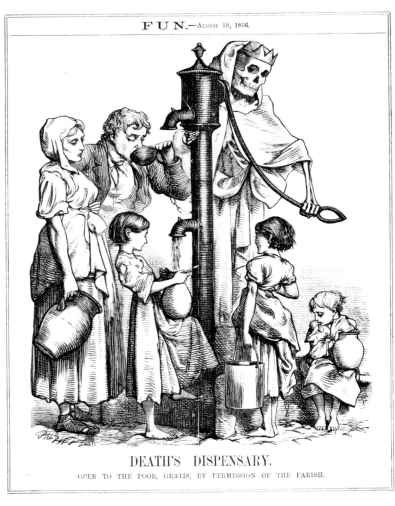

DEATH'S DISPENSARY.
OPEN TO THE POOR, GRATIS, BY PERMISSION OF THE PARISH.

773

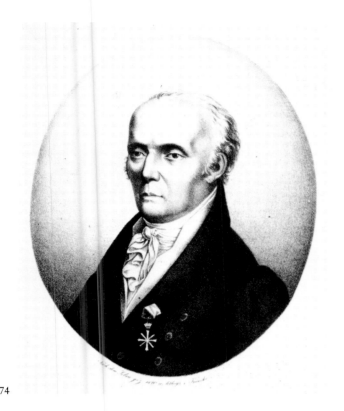

771 *Illustration from an 1828 report showing how sewage got into the water supply of Chelsea Hospital, London. National Library of Medicine, Bethesda*

772 *"A hint to the Board of Health on how the city invites the Cholera" (1864). Department of Health, City of New York*

773 *Satirical woodcut (1866) indicating that pollution was an acknowledged source of disease even before bacteria were discovered to be the cause. Collection William Helfand, New York*

774 *Johann Peter Frank used statistics to establish the importance of public health measures. New York Academy of Medicine*

775 *Not only was garbage collected in open dumps, it was freely picked through by scavengers, as shown in this engraving from* Harper's Weekly *(Sept. 29, 1866). National Library of Medicine, Bethesda*

774

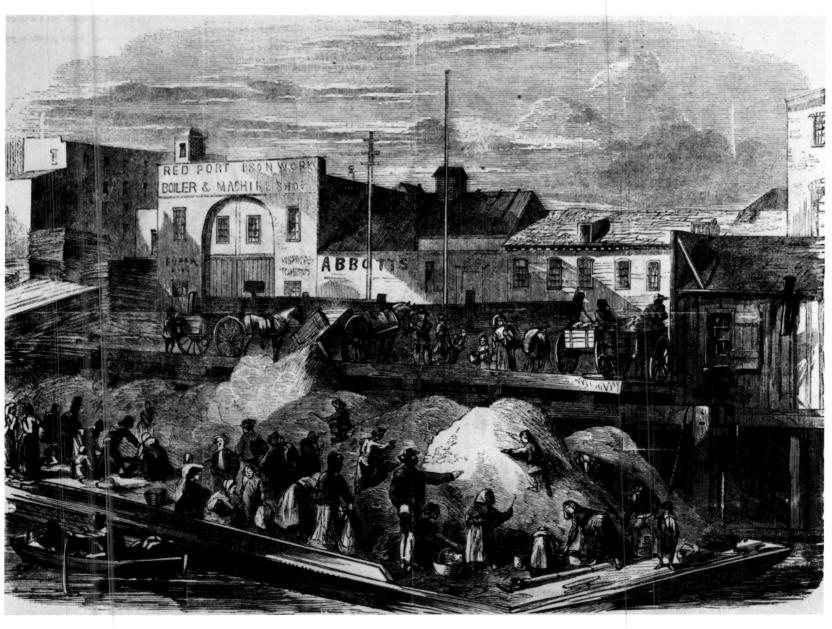

775

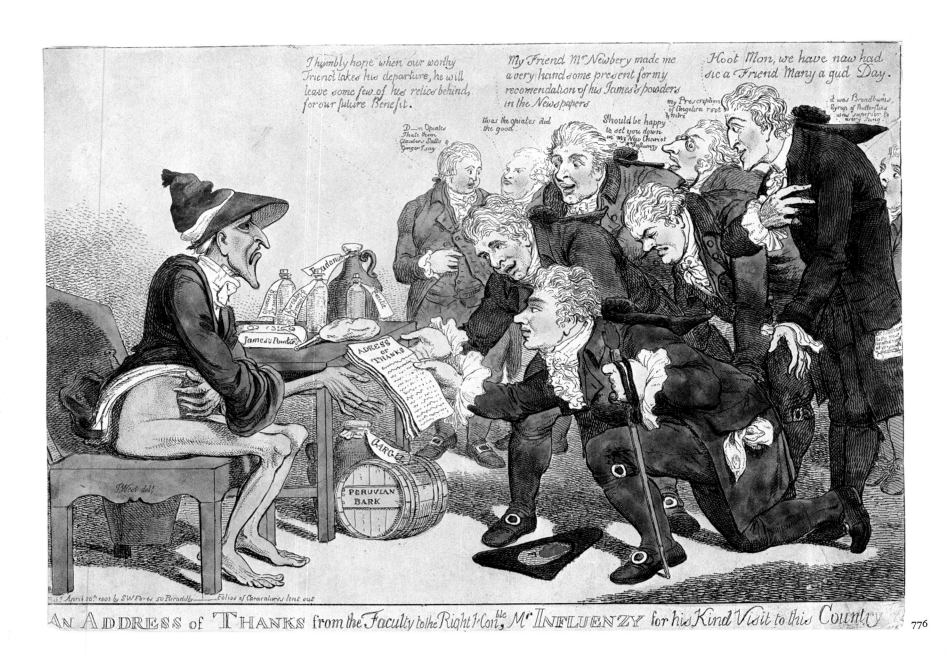

AN ADDRESS of THANKS from the Faculty to the Right Hon.ble M.r INFLUENZY for his Kind Visit to this Country

776

776 *Colored woodcut (1803), after James West, making a sarcastic comment on the increase in doctors' business when an epidemic strikes. Collection William Helfand, New York*

777 *An early effort at public health measures was the distribution, in "unsavory neighborhoods," of disinfectants, but still there were open piles of garbage on walks and streets in 1864. Department of Health, City of New York*

778 *An unofficial public health measure was the action of mobs to prevent the landing of possible carriers of cholera, which had struck the United States in epidemics three times in the 19th century. Museum of the City of New York*

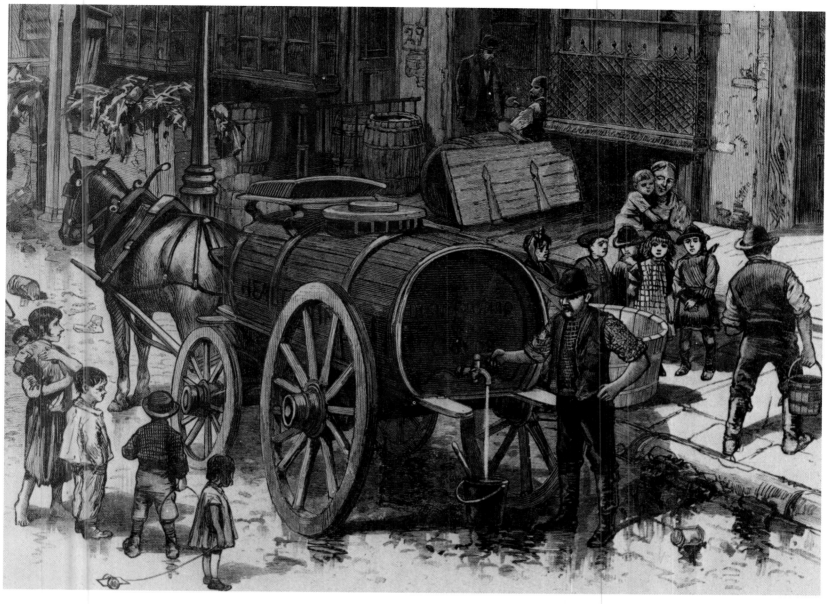

777

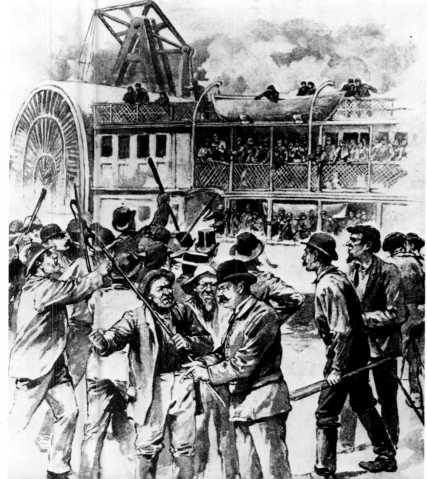

778

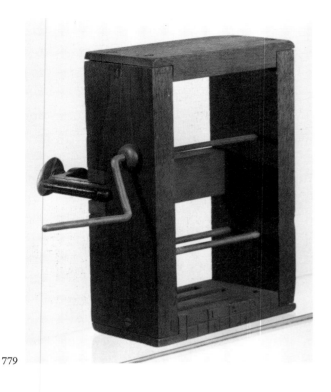

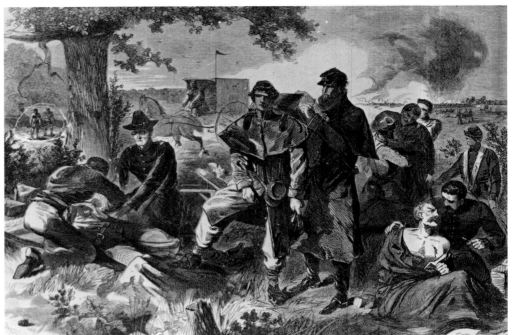

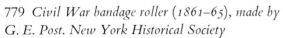

779

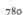780

779 *Civil War bandage roller (1861–65), made by*
G. E. Post. *New York Historical Society*

780 *This wood engraving, after Winslow Homer*
(Harper's Weekly, *July 12, 1862), shows a*
military surgeon treating patients at the rear, during
the Civil War. National Library of Medicine,
Bethesda

781 *Ambulance train shown returning from the*
trenches with wounded, during the campaign in
Charleston harbor (Harper's Weekly, *Sept. 12,*
1863). The Civil War raged for two years before
effective ambulance systems and hospitals evolved.
National Library of Medicine, Bethesda

782 *Photograph by Mathew B. Brady of wounded*
veterans of the Civil War in the Armory Square
Hospital, a distinct improvement over earlier
facilities. Harris Brisbane Dick Fund, Metropolitan
Museum of Art, New York

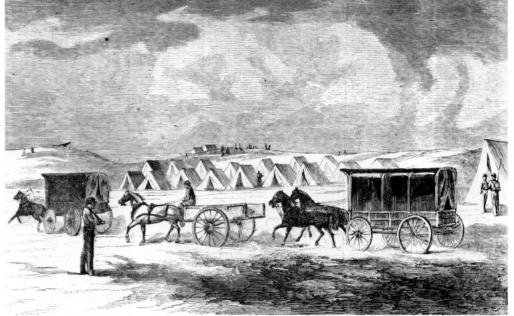

781

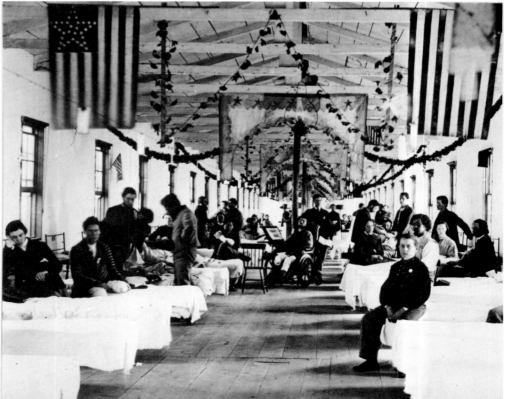

782

procured adequate medical supplies, and developed well-trained surgeons. Yet it was not until the Battle of Gettysburg (July, 1863) that the Union forces were able to remove their wounded from the field at the end of each day's fighting. It had taken two years of bloodshed and suffering to develop a good medical corps.

The man largely responsible for reforming the Union Medical Corps was Surgeon General William A. Hammond, a bright, energetic individual whose much-needed reforms irritated enough regular army officers and politicians to lead to his dismissal in November, 1863, and his subsequent court-martial. The South was more fortunate in that a capable and intelligent surgeon general, Dr. Samuel Preston Moore, took over at the beginning of the war and was able to develop a sound medical corps with a minimum of interference. The South, however, lacked an effective transportation system, did not have as many well-trained surgeons, and was hard put to provide adequate medical supplies. Despite these handicaps, Moore was able to tender southern troops medical care comparable to that given the Union forces. Not until the transportation system began to break down toward the end of the war did the South have any significant medical problems.

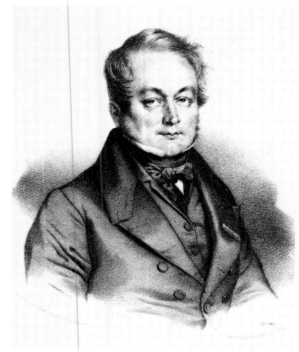

PHYSIOLOGY

As the century began, France held the lead in medicine. François Magendie (1783–1855) was one of the early French leaders who painstakingly tried to keep his observations simple and free of speculation. He is especially remembered for his experimental proofs that the posterior roots of the spinal canal carry sensory nerve fibers (receiving impulses to the cord) and the anterior roots are motor nerves (transporting impulses away from the cord to the muscles). The priority of this accomplishment was challenged by Charles Bell, among others, and the principle is now called the "Bell-Magendie law." Magendie's analyses of the actions of drugs also made him a founder of the discipline of pharmacology. Never holding an academic position, he was nevertheless a typical investigator of the early nineteenth century in combining the careers of medical practitioner and laboratory experimentalist.

On the other hand, Claude Bernard (1813–78), the virtual founder of experimental physiology, was entirely a man of the laboratory. He further developed the precepts of his teacher Magendie, postulating questions that could be answered only through experimental vivisectional techniques, which he perfected into elegant experiments. One of his influential concepts was the principle of homeostasis, which stated that the "internal environment" is constant in warm-blooded organisms and that physiological mechanisms resist any external factors which tend to alter this internal state.

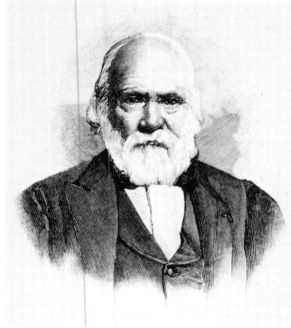

Among other exceptional accomplishments, Bernard clarified the multiple functions of the liver, studied the digestive activity of the pancreatic secretions and the association of the pancreas with diabetes, and pointed out the connection of the nervous system with the constriction and dilation of the smaller arteries. In his *Introduction to the Study of Experimental Medicine* in 1865, he set down the standards for future experimentalists. An imaginative thinker, he had a firm attachment to objectivity, as indicated by his admonition, "Put off your imagination as you take off your overcoat, when you enter the laboratory. . . ."

Another French contributor to physiology who was a practitioner of medicine as well as an investigator, Charles Édouard Brown-Séquard (1817–94), the son of an American sea captain and a French mother, is sometimes considered the founder of endocrinology, although Bernard had actually opened the field. In the course of his many travels, he lectured in either French or English on a variety of topics which included some of his own discoveries. Brown-Séquard taught that the adrenals, thyroid, pancreas, liver, spleen, and kidneys had secretions (later to be called hormones) which entered the bloodstream and could be used in treatment. He also believed that injections of extracts of the testis would produce rejuvenation.

783 *François Magendie, who called himself a ragpicker in science—i.e., perceiving and isolating individual bits of information—was actually a significant pioneer in physiology and pharmacology. New York Academy of Science*

784 *A clinician as well as an investigator, Charles Édouard Brown-Séquard is sometimes considered the founder of endocrinology. Musée d'Histoire de la Médecine, Paris*

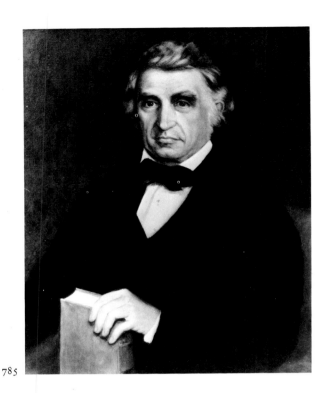

785

785 *William Beaumont, an obscure U.S. Army surgeon, took advantage of an unprecedented opportunity to make a classic study of gastric physiology when a patient was left with a permanent exterior opening to his stomach. National Library of Medicine, Bethesda*

786 *Photograph of Ivan P. Pavlov, Russian physiologist, carrying out an experiment to demonstrate the proof of his theory of conditioned reflexes. World Health Organization, Geneva*

787 *Painting (1889) by Louis Lhermitte showing the great physiologist Claude Bernard, who illuminated many functions of the internal organs, at work on experimental vivisection. Palais de la Découverte, Paris*

Germany's role in medicine was in a large measure due to the influence of Johannes Peter Müller (1801–58), who started out as a romantic "nature-philosopher" but later developed a more objective view of biological functions. His work focused on morphology (structure) rather than experiment, but he inspired numerous students who were to contribute to knowledge in physiology.

Lacking laboratories and the communities of scholars essential for much of the work in the basic sciences, America contributed little to physiology and histology, but there was one notable exception. William Beaumont (1785–1853), an obscure army surgeon who had learned medicine through an apprenticeship, took advantage of a rare opportunity to pave the way for the present understanding of the gastric process. In 1822, while serving in Fort Michilimackinac in northern Michigan, he was called to treat a French Canadian who appeared to be dying from a shotgun blast at close range. The lower chest and abdomen were torn open and the left lung, diaphragm, and stomach were badly lacerated. The wound was filled with blood, bone splinters, lead shot, wadding, bits of clothing, and the contents of the stomach. Although it seemed obvious that the wound was fatal, Beaumont cleaned and dressed it, and tried to make his patient comfortable. Miraculously, after a lengthy convalescence, Alexis St. Martin, the patient, survived, but he was left with a permanent gastric fistula giving direct access to his stomach. Notwithstanding strong objections from St. Martin and other difficulties, Beaumont conducted a long series of experiments which he summarized in 1833 in his classic work, *Experiments and Observations on the Gastric Juice and the Physiology of Digestion.* While his achievement received only limited recognition in America, European scientists hailed it as a major accomplishment.

In England, many physiologists illuminated the functions of the nervous system in the nineteenth century. Marshall Hall (1790–1857) may be mentioned for his work on shock and his discovery that some reflexes could be elicited without going through the higher centers. William Sharpey described the clearing action in mucous membranes by microscopic, mobile hairs, the cilia.

A far-reaching influence on physiology and on subsequent attitudes toward behavior came from the experiments on animals by Ivan Pavlov (1849–1936) in Moscow. After having studied in the laboratories of Ludwig and Heidenhain in Germany, he became professor of pharmacology and then of physiology at the Military Medical Academy in Russia. He made detailed investigations on the heart, liver, pancreas, and alimentary tract, but his most influential work was on the conditioned reflex. For instance, he showed that one could condition a dog to salivate and its stomach to secrete in response to an outside stimulus even in the absence of food, by repeatedly linking the stimulus to the providing of food.

CHEMISTRY AND PHARMACOLOGY

Just as correlations were made between bedside findings and changes in the organs, so too was the chemistry laboratory brought to bear on understanding the functional alterations caused by disease. By the middle of the nineteenth century, examinations of blood and urine were routine.

One of the most significant accomplishments was the synthesis by Friedrich Wöhler (1800–82) of urea, a natural product of the body, from an inorganic compound, ammonium carbonate. After that, the separation between the organic and the inorganic was no longer distinct. Organic chemistry would become merely the chemistry of carbon compounds. In applying the techniques of inorganic chemistry to the study of the chemical mechanisms of the body, Felix Hoppe-Seyler (1825–95) opened the field of physical chemistry. His discovery in 1862 of hemoglobin (the oxygen-carrying substance in the red cells of the blood) was a milestone in medicine.

As advances in physiology and chemistry proceeded, it became possible to isolate drugs in pure form and thus examine their actions in animals and humans.

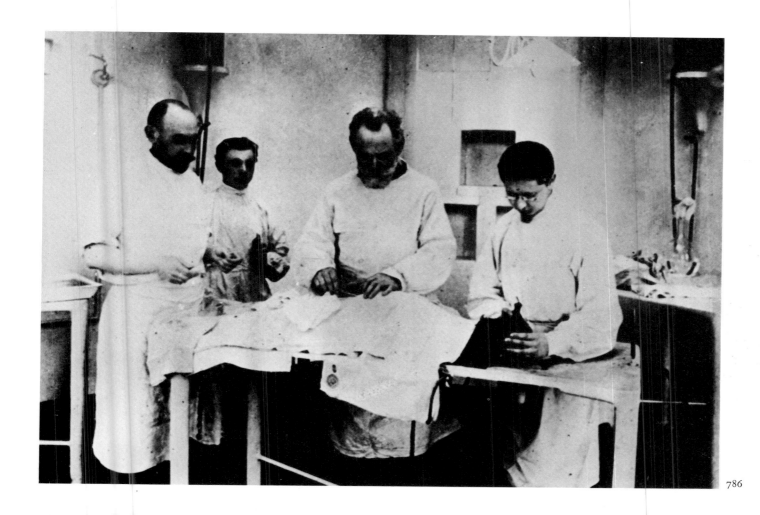

786

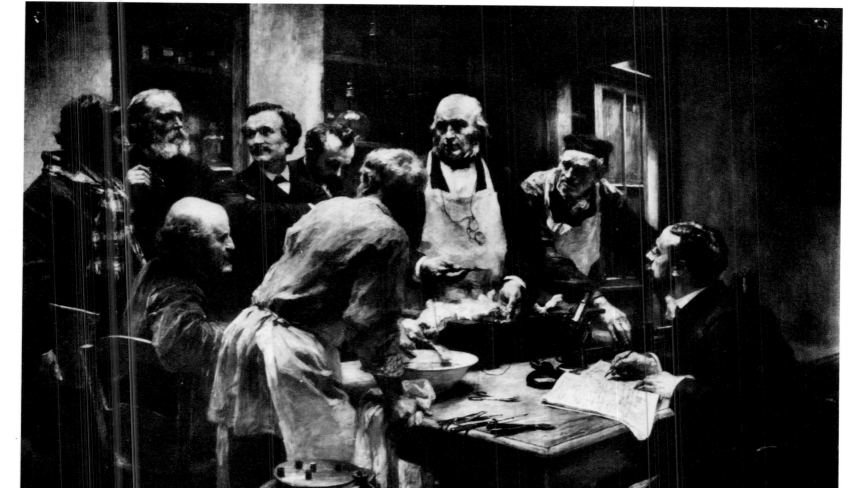

787

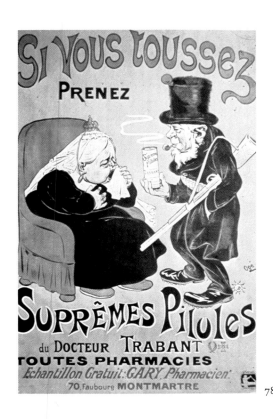

788

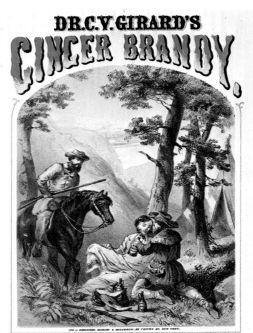
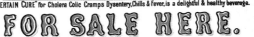

789

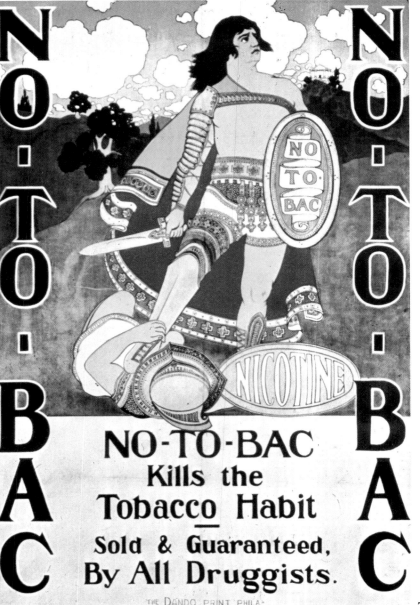

790

788–793 *Colorful 19th-century advertisements for patent medicines and cure-alls, from a time without government regulation of ingredients or verification of claims. Ginger Brandy lithograph, courtesy of the Library of Congress, Washington, D.C.; all others, Collection William Helfand, New York*

791

Thus the discipline of pharmacology was developed. On the basis of preliminary investigations in France by J. F. Derosne in 1803 and A. Seguin in 1804, F. W. A. Sertürner in Germany isolated morphine in 1806. Pelletier and Caventou in 1818 did the same in France with strychnine, quinine, and other drugs. Pierre Robiquet was another of the many pharmacist-chemists in France and Germany who discovered and isolated the new plant alkaloids so important to medicine—among them atropine, colchicine, and cocaine.

Pharmacology became an independent subject for the first time through the efforts of Rudolph Buchheim (1820–79) in Dorpat and his pupil Oswald Schmiedeberg (1830–1920) in Strassburg. Schmiedeberg's teachings on experimental pharmacology were brought to America by John J. Abel (1857–1938), who further enlarged upon the earlier activities of H. C. Wood and Silas Weir Mitchell of Philadelphia. Abel became head of materia medica and therapeutics at the University of Michigan in 1891, and later, at Johns Hopkins, he occupied the first chair in the United States in the new discipline of pharmacology. Other schools soon established departments of pharmacology, but the schools of pharmacy were relatively late in introducing this specialized discipline.

In England Alexander Crum Brown (1838–1922) and Thomas Frazer advanced the discipline by correlating the actions of drugs with their chemical composition. As more and more drugs were isolated and their chemical nature understood, it became possible to create therapeutic compounds by building them from basic units. Alkaloids and antipyretics (fever-lowering compounds) were among the first drugs synthesized.

Cell Theory

Matthias Schleiden (1804–81) and Theodor Schwann (1810–82), the latter a student of Johannes Müller's, developed one of the most important conceptions of modern biology. Although it had been previously known that parts of plants were cellular, Schleiden was the first to state explicitly that each plant was a community of cells with each cell having a separate existence. Schwann generalized Schleiden's conclusions to all life—animal and plant. Much of the information that led to the understanding and elaboration of the cell theory depended on technical advances in microscopes. It was not until the 1830s when Amici and Chevalier produced the achromatic lens that the finer structure of cells could be examined.

Even when the idea was accepted that all living creatures are composed of living cells, the question arose of how the cells originated. Schleiden proposed that the cell and its components formed as a result of a chemical precipitation out of an undifferentiated mass. It was another student of Müller's, Rudolf Virchow, who overthrew the speculative explanations and firmly established the proposition (in which he was joined by many other investigators) that cells arise only from preexisting cells. At first the view proposed by Schleiden was embraced by many outstanding scientists, including Karl Rokitansky, a great pathologist of the time, but the concept of Virchow finally gained full acceptance.

Microscopic Anatomy and Embryology

Among the pupils of Johannes Müller who contributed to an understanding of the microscopic structure of organs was Jacob Henle (1809–85), who was also responsible for early ideas concerning microorganisms as causes of disease. Albert von Kölliker (1817–1905) wrote what may have been the first organized textbook on histology. He explained the development of the embryo on the basis of the new cell theory. The spermatozoan had been known for centuries, but Karl Ernst von Baer (1792–1876) gave the first description of the ovum (egg) of mammals. Robert Remak (1815–65) classified tissues according to their embryological origin into three primary systems (germ layers): ectoderm, mesoderm, and entoderm. The

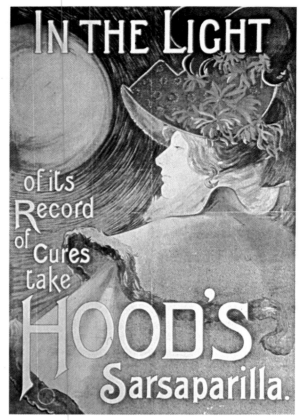

792

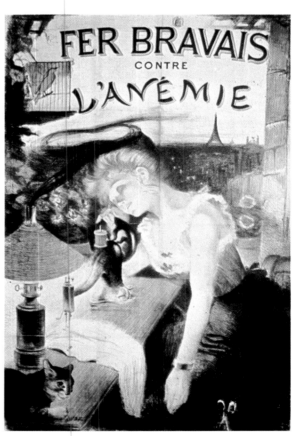

793

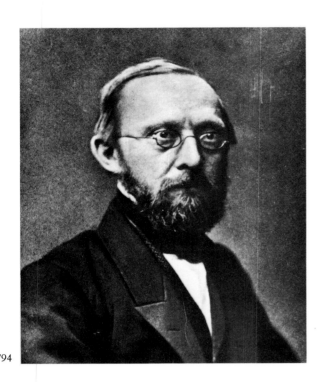

794

794 *Rudolf Virchow was the dominant figure in European medicine in the second half of the 19th century and is considered to have been one of its greatest pathologists.* World Health Organization, Geneva

795 Vaccinating the Poor, *a wood engraving (1873) after Solomon Eytinge, Jr., illustrates an increasing understanding that public health measures were a duty of government.* National Library of Medicine, Bethesda

796 *Photograph (c. 1890) of medical students at work on a cadaver. Anatomical dissection had become essential to proper medical training.* Minnesota Historical Society, St. Paul

mechanism of cell division, the means by which the embryo enlarges, organs increase, and tissues regenerate was reported by Walter Fleming in 1882. Wilhelm Waldeyer (1836–1921) named the chromosome in the nucleus of the cell and put forth in 1891 the theory that the basic unit of the nervous system is the nerve cell, the neurone. He also pointed out that cancerous growths arise from epithelial cells in the ectodermal tissue layer.

PATHOLOGY

In keeping with the spirit of correlating the clinical manifestations of illness with the pathological findings in organs, autopsies were the major focus in medicine. In the French and British schools the availability of corpses for pathological examination was quite limited, whereas in Austria and Germany medical institutions were often the centers in which autopsies were performed, usually by one prosector and his pupils. Moreover, in France and Britain the principal pathological studies were made by the clinicians.

Carl Rokitansky (1804–78), a Czech who worked in Vienna at the Institute of Pathology, was an example of the nonpracticing physician, a type that was to become common in the nineteenth century. In his day he was the most outstanding morphological pathologist in the world, performing together with his assistants almost 60,000 autopsies in less than fifty years. His classifications of the changes in organs produced by disease set standards acclaimed by all. However, Rokitansky's reliance on humoral theories (he tried to reconcile the ancient concepts with modern anatomical knowledge) led to devastating criticisms by the young Virchow which shook his standing, but he remained an honored pathologic anatomist throughout his life.

Rudolf Virchow (1821–1902), one of Müller's students in Germany, was called the "Pope" of medicine in Europe because of the eminence of his scientific influence. He strove to integrate clinical medicine, morbid anatomy, and physiology. His dictum, "all cells come from other cells," radically altered the direction of medical thinking toward the concept that disease was produced by disturbances in the structure and function of the body cells. Such ideas had occurred before, but Virchow was so thorough in proofs and so convincing in argument that the medical world readily accepted his pronouncements. Henceforth the target of treatment would be the cell. Among his other major contributions were the discovery of the disease entity leukemia and his studies on the nature of thrombosis, embolism, and phlebitis, which promulgated principles still valid today.

Virchow's indefatigable energy and voracious mind took him into a variety of fields besides pathology: anthropology, archaeology, history, politics, public health, and sociology. His zeal for reform encompassed proposing that social conditions were a primary culprit in epidemics and advocating a reorganization of medical education and licensure.

However, with all his extraordinary gifts, Virchow was not above human frailties. His attacks on Rokitansky and on Karl August Wunderlich, the influential German clinician, while soundly based, contained elements of personal acrimony. Nor did he readily accept the bacterial theory of disease, pointing out that the presence of a bacterium in a diseased area did not of itself signify that it was the cause of the disease. His emphasis on the reaction of the body's cells to an invading organism rather than the organism itself is consonant with present views that the host's response to a noxious agent—bacterial, viral, or chemical—is as significant as the invader. Yet, Virchow did make too little of the role of microorganisms, and in the frustrating battle for asepsis by Semmelweis (described later) Virchow did not give his support.

But throughout his long life Virchow's scientific interests and influence never waned. By the time of his death, he had been acclaimed throughout the world. If medicine consists essentially of endeavors related to concepts of illness, methods of

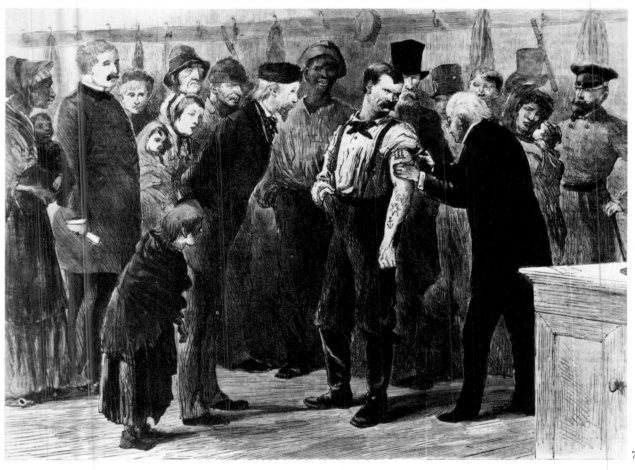

795

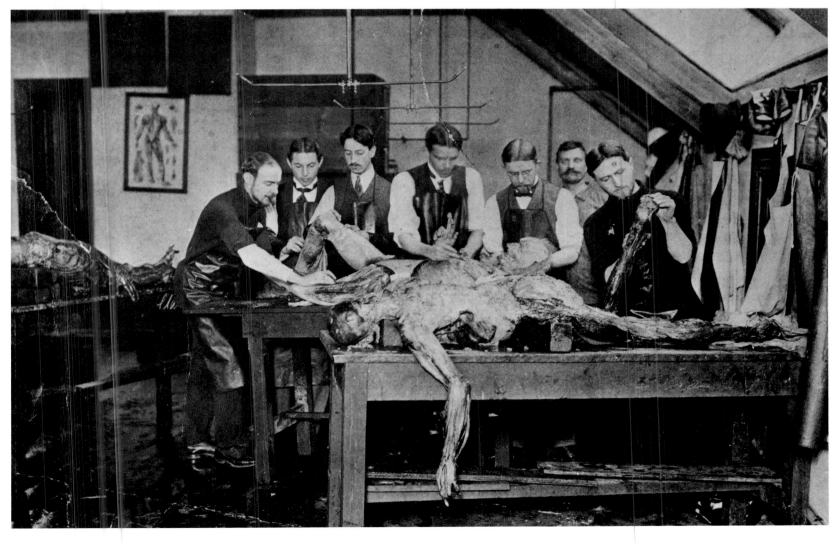

796

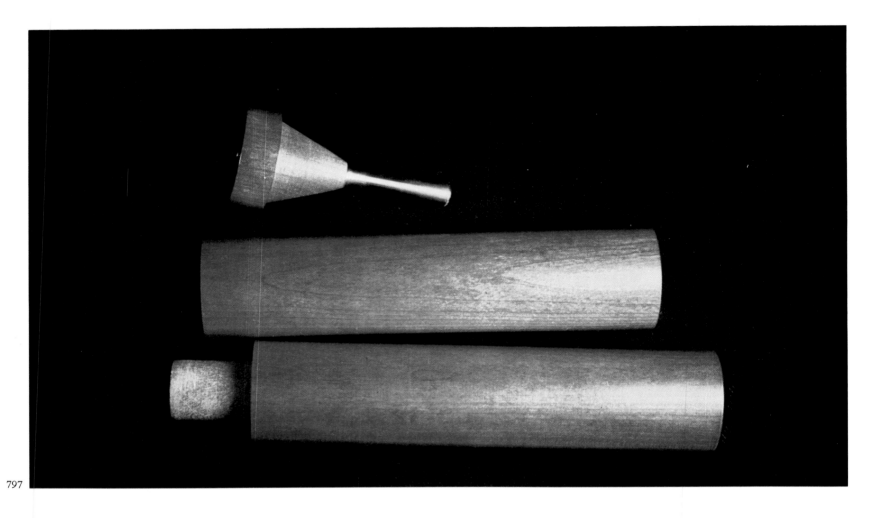

797

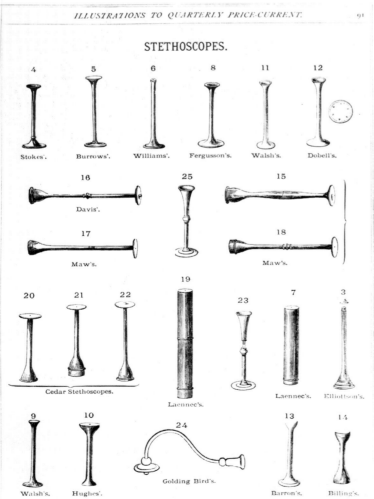

STETHOSCOPES.

4   5   6   8   11   12

Stokes'.   Burrows'.   Williams'.   Fergusson's.   Walsh's.   Dobell's.

16   25   15

Davis'.

17   18

Maw's.   Maw's.

20   21   22   19   23   7   3

Cedar Stethoscopes.

Laennec's.   Laennec's.   Elliottson's.

9   10   24   13   14

Walsh's.   Hughes'.   Golding Bird's.   Barron's.   Billing's.

798

STETHOSCOPES, CHEST, TONSIL, THROAT, MOUTH, NOSE AND EAR INSTRUMENTS.

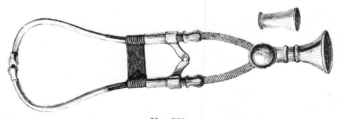

No. 220.

Camman's Double Stethoscope...$3 00

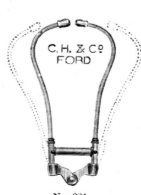

No. 221.

Camman's Double Stethoscope, with covered spring, $5 00. Ditto, with open spiral spring, $4 00.

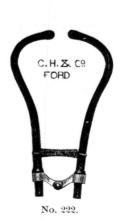

No. 222.

Camman's Double Stethoscope, hard rubber, $3 00.

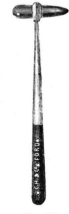

No. 227.

Flint's Hammer, 75c.

799

510

treatment, education and organization of the healing professions, and measures directed toward preventing disease and maintaining health, then Virchow was indeed the complete man of medicine.

CLINICAL SCHOOLS AND THE CLINICIANS

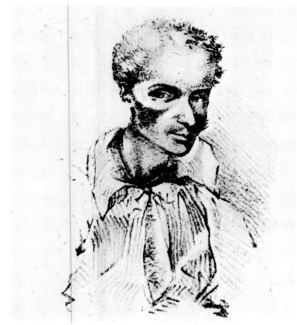

THE outstanding characteristic of nineteenth-century medicine was the correlation of discoveries in the laboratory and autopsy room with observations at the bedside, and it was principally the hospital where such investigations and interconnections were pursued. In the first half of the century, leadership in clinical science resided in France, but it later passed to the British Isles, and then to the German-speaking countries.

PARIS

An important factor in the emergence of Paris as the leading clinical school was the French Revolution. As the old regime was swept away, so were ancient ideas and inhibitions, opening the way to new approaches by experiment, an emphasis on pragmatism rather than theory, and bedside observation instead of reasoning by concept. The hospital became more important as the focus of medical activity, public health measures were seen as a duty of government, and medical practice was open to all classes. The wounds sustained in the savage turmoil of the Revolution and after had increased the need for surgery, and since physicians appeared to have little effect on illnesses and epidemics surgeons gained an equal status. Nevertheless, as surgery and medicine coalesced into one profession, specializations began to occur as the new discoveries accumulated.

Philippe Pinel (1745–1826) was representative of both the eighteenth and nineteenth centuries. His concern for the classification of disease was a holdover from the past, and his concentration on objective clinical study in a special field fitted the trend toward specialization. Pinel's close observation of people with mental illness and his astute evaluation of the results of treatment led him to advocate a change in insane asylums from forcible restraint to gentleness, persuasion, and a cheerful environment which benefited from the influences of family and friends.

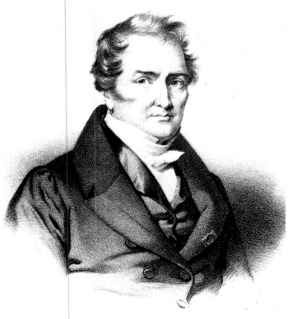

René-Théophile-Hyacinthe Laënnec (1781–1826) was one of the greatest clinicians of all time. He made outstanding contributions to the pathological and clinical understanding of diseases of the chest—notably emphysema, bronchiectasis, and tuberculosis—but he is best remembered for his invention and use of the stethoscope.

Before Laënnec, the sounds of the lungs and heart were studied by holding one's ear against the chest, a technique with numerous disadvantages. After observing two children transmit scratching noises to each other's ear via a wooden board, Laënnec got the idea of rolling up a sheaf of papers to aid him in listening to a patient's chest. His next step was to construct a wooden cylinder, and he was amazed to discern sounds he had never heard or hardly appreciated before. Using the new information, Laënnec was able to illuminate the clinical picture of many diseases. His monaural stethoscope was further improved and eventually became the binaural device used today as a regular tool of every clinician.

As an adherent of the hated royalist cause, Laënnec did not reach the popularity or influence that was achieved by his contemporary François-Joseph-Victor Broussais (1772–1838), whose physical vigor, brilliant personality, and devoted espousal of progressive social attitudes made him virtually the most influential physician in France. In agreeing with the Parisian school on the importance of matching the clinical picture with abnormalities (lesions) in the organs of the body, Broussais vigorously ridiculed attempts to classify diseases according to symptoms. In his view, proper treatment must focus on the pathologic changes

797 *Laënnec's type of wooden stethoscope. Collection Dr. Philip Reichert, New York*

798, 799 *Catalog illustrations (1869 and 1880) of various types of stethoscopes. National Library of Medicine, Bethesda*

800 *René-Théophile-Hyacinthe Laënnec, drawn and lithographed by himself in 1820, four years before he died of tuberculosis. Bettman Archive, New York*

801 *François Broussais rejected the humoral theory of disease, but favored extensive bleeding as therapy. New York Academy of Medicine*

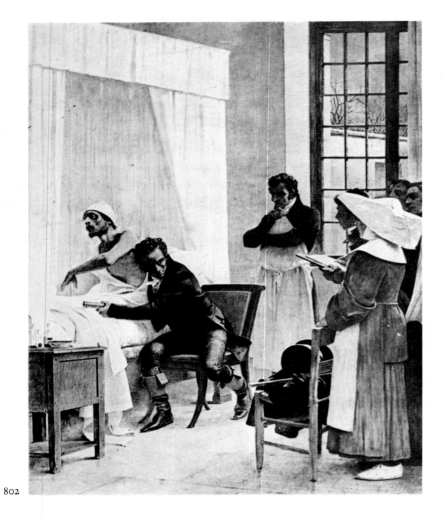

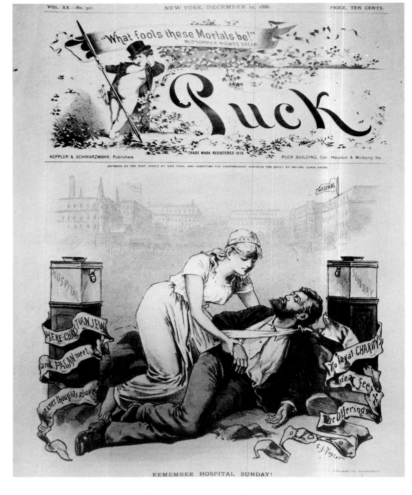

802

803

802 *In 1816, T. Chartran painted Laënnec listening with his ear against the chest of a patient at Necker Hospital. National Library of Medicine, Bethesda*

803 *A plea on the cover of* Puck *(Dec. 22, 1886) for public support of voluntary hospitals: "Remember Hospital Sunday!" Mt. Sinai Hospital Archives, New York*

804 *Tranquilizing chair (1810) suggested by Benjamin Rush, whose treatise on insanity was an outstanding systematic study. National Library of Medicine, Bethesda*

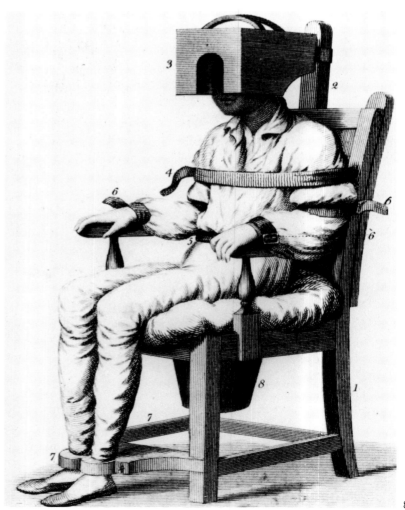

804

in tissue, not on the outmoded doctrines of the humors. The remarkable numbers of intestinal lesions which he saw, especially of typhoid fever, led him to conclude that the gastrointestinal tract was the primary source of most illnesses, especially those with fever. Believing Brown's doctrine that irritation was the basic property of living tissues, he considered changes in tissue heat the fundamental determinant of health and illness. From the congestion he saw in the intestines, he reasoned that disengorgement to reduce heat was necessary. He therefore used an accepted method of removing the plethora of blood: bloodletting. Instead of the cumbersome maneuver of venesection, he employed an easier means—applying leeches. So convincing were his teachings that the physicians of France imported in a single year over forty million leeches.

One of the most effective techniques of evaluating the efficacy of treatment is statistics, although circumspection and objectivity in collection and analysis are required. The very introduction of numerical analysis of bloodletting results by Pierre-Charles-Alexandre Louis (1787–1872) was not only a fatal blow to venesection but a major force leading to the scientific evaluation of all therapies.

Although Pierre Bretonneau (1778–1862) preceded Louis in establishing typhoid fever as a specific entity, Bretonneau's complex term "dothienenteritis" was replaced by Louis's simpler "typhoid." On the other hand, Bretonneau's "diphtheria" (*diphthérie*) had a more permanent place in history.

Among other outstanding names of the French school were Armand Trousseau (1801–67), who contributed masterful and perceptive treatises on illness; Jean-Baptiste Bouillaud (1796–1881) (evidently the model for Balzac's Dr. Bianchon); Pierre-Adolphe Piorry, a pioneer in the use of an instrument for percussion of the chest (the pleximeter); François-Olive Rayer, a contributor to clinical and laboratory knowledge who inspired Bernard in physiology, and Davaine and Villemin in their work on infection. Guillaume B. A. Duchenne (1806–75) and Jean-Martin Charcot (1825–93) were the virtual founders of neurology in France. Duchenne, who started as a country practitioner, made use of the new electrical current reported by Michael Faraday (1791–1867) to treat patients with rheumatism and to study the actions of muscles. Charcot became world-famous through his clinical teachings at the Salpêtrière Hospital of Paris where he made an extraordinary number of original contributions to different fields of medicine, most of them related to the nervous system. He was the eponym for several syndromes, including "Charcot's joint" (the joint derangement of locomotor ataxia caused by syphilis). His reputation and his writings on hysteria and hypnotism attracted the young Freud in Vienna, who went to Paris specifically to observe the work of Charcot.

Surgery in Paris was comparatively well-developed, especially in the first half of the century, with much of the advance due to the bloody events of the Revolution and Napoleonic wars. Perhaps the most personally popular of all surgeons was Dominique-Jean Larrey (1766–1842), so highly respected and admired by friend and foe alike that Napoleon called him the most virtuous man he had ever known. Although Larrey was famous as a surgeon (he is said to have performed over two hundred amputations during a twenty-four-hour period in the Russian campaign) and also as a clinician (he wrote vivid descriptions of "trench foot," scurvy, contagious eye infections, and a method of feeding through a stomach tube), perhaps his most influential contribution was the creation of "flying ambulances," wagons for stretcher use during battle. Unheard of until then, Larrey's vehicles and transport system went into operation as the action started, affording a tremendous boost to morale and a much greater opportunity for effective treatment. Moreover, his attention to the wounded of both sides in battle was, in a sense, the harbinger of the principles of the Red Cross, which was formed later in the century.

While Larrey was adored, his colleague Guillaume Dupuytren (1777–1835) was actively disliked, though still admired. A spellbinding lecturer, incisive bedside teacher, indefatigable worker, enormously successful practitioner, and brilliant

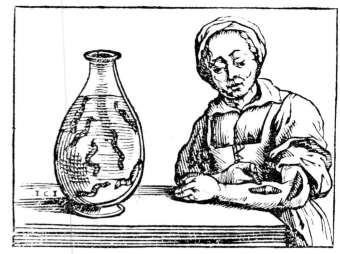

805

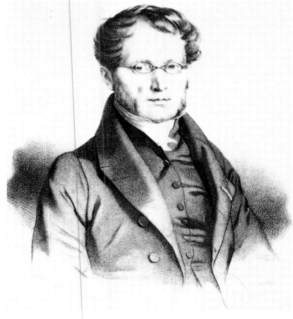

806

805 *Woodcut from Willem van den Bossche,* Historia Medica (1638) *showing the use of leeches as a preferred method of bloodletting, a technique so favored in the 19th century that 40 million leeches were imported into France in a single year. National Library of Medicine, Bethesda*

806 *Pierre-Charles-Alexandre Louis, through the use of statistics, proved that bleedings were harmful rather than beneficial to healing, and argued that all therapies should be open to scientific evaluation. New York Academy of Medicine*

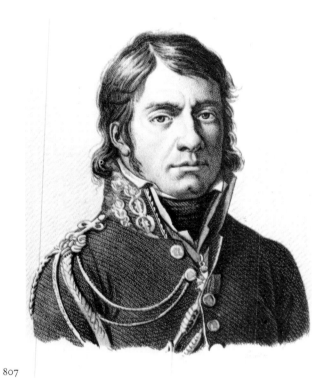

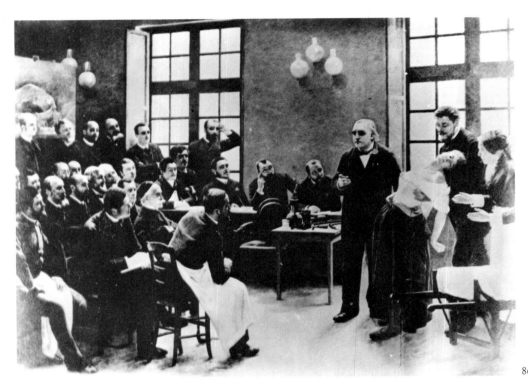

807

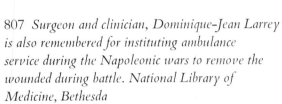

808

807 *Surgeon and clinician, Dominique-Jean Larrey is also remembered for instituting ambulance service during the Napoleonic wars to remove the wounded during battle. National Library of Medicine, Bethesda*

808 *One of the founders of neurology in France, Jean-Martin Charcot is shown in this painting by Pierre-André Brouillet (c. 1887) demonstrating a patient with hysteria at the Salpêtrière. National Library of Medicine, Bethesda*

809 *Improvised stretcher photographed in 1876. W. H. Over Museum, Vermillion, South Dakota*

810 *Meath Hospital, Dublin, site of the famous "Irish School" of clinicians, which included Cheyne, Stokes, Graves, Corrigan, and Colles, all eponyms for diseases they identified. New York Academy of Medicine*

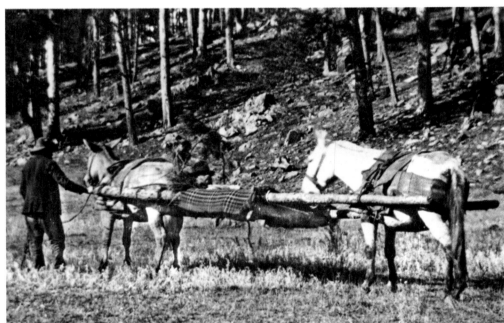

809

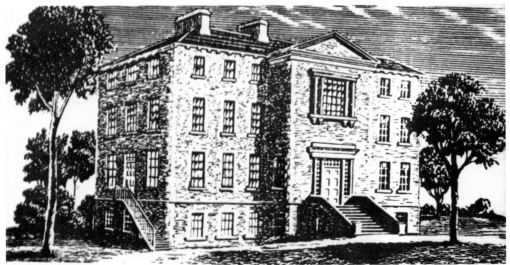

810

contributor to surgical knowledge, he nevertheless alienated colleagues and acquaintances by his cold, abrasive manner and devious machinations against others. He was innovative in devising instruments and bold in performing daring operative feats with successful outcome. Pierre-François Percy (1754–1825), a surgical colleague, called him "the first of surgeons and the least of men."

There were many other surgeons in Paris who were pioneer contributors: Récamier, who may have been the first to remove the uterus; Roux, the thyroid; Lisfranc, the rectum. Pravas introduced the syringe. Lembert contributed to intestinal surgery, Menière to the medical and surgical aspects of ear diseases. Pierre-Paul Broca (1824–80) firmly established, on the basis of clinical and pathologic evidence, that the speech function is located in a distinct area of the brain, now called "Broca's area." He was also a pioneer in anthropology, a discipline opposed by the government and by churchmen who felt that the concept of the anatomical localization of the mind in the brain was too materialistic. Paris continued to be a great school for surgical teaching and learning throughout the century, although the principal centers of influence shifted in the later decades to Britain and the German-speaking countries.

DUBLIN

Simultaneous with the great tradition that developed in Paris, a spirit of clinical investigation also arose in Dublin at Meath Hospital, both self-generated and influenced by Parisian principles. As in London, many of the clinicians in Dublin were Scottish in either origin or training. One may say that a strong Scottish thread ran through the fabric of medicine in England, Ireland, and the United States.

John Cheyne (1777–1836), although born and trained in Scotland where he published a book on diseases of children, made his greatest contributions in Dublin as an influential member of a group often referred to as the "Irish School." His detailed accounts of a variety of diseases and his writings on education gained him a worldwide reputation as a great teacher and practitioner. The term "Cheyne-Stokes respiration," a type of irregular breathing, has remained in medical parlance.

William Stokes (1804–78) was born in Dublin, but he too studied and wrote in Scotland (*The Use of the Stethoscope*) before returning to Dublin in his early twenties to become a highly popular lecturer and bedside teacher. Two of his books, *Diseases of the Chest* and *Diseases of the Heart*, were to become important standard texts for generations. In addition to the breathing abnormality which linked his name with Cheyne's, there is a type of dysfunction of the heartbeat first described by Robert Adams in the same century called "Stokes-Adams" heart block. Although he mistakenly believed that typhoid and typhus fevers were the same disease, he understood and emphasized the importance of public health and preventive measures.

The most famous teacher of the Dublin group was Robert James Graves (1796–1853), whose bedside rounds were widely known as superb instructional exercises. He is the eponym ("Graves' disease") for that combination of thyroid enlargement, nervousness, sweating, and pronounced stare referred to as "toxic exophthalmic goiter." It was Graves who overturned the past dietary restrictions for patients with fever by urging a full, nutritious diet for all ill patients. He suggested that his own epitaph could well read, "He fed fevers."

Another influential clinician of the Dublin school was Dominic John Corrigan (1802–80). He is best remembered for his description of the pathologic cause and characteristic pulse, called "Corrigan's pulse," of a disease of the aortic valves of the heart. Abraham Colles (1773–1843) described so thoroughly the principles and methods of treating a fracture of the wrist that it has continued to be known as the "Colles fracture."

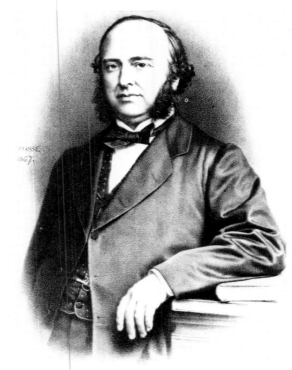

811

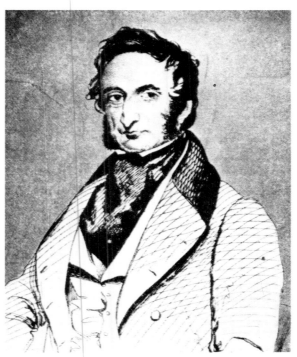

812

811 *Pioneer neurosurgeon Pierre-Paul Broca, who reported the localization of speech control in the frontal area on one side of the brain. New York Academy of Medicine*

812 *Robert James Graves, after whom overactive thyroid disease was named, condemned the ancient medical policy of restricted diets during illness. New York Academy of Medicine*

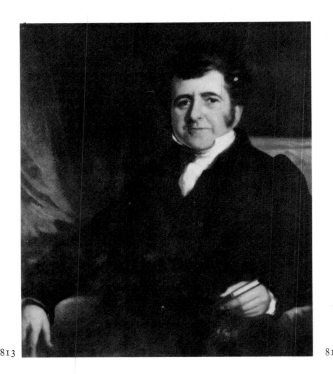

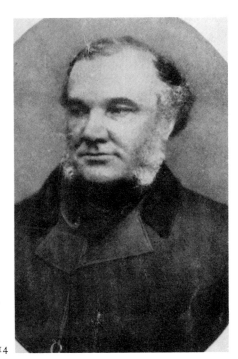

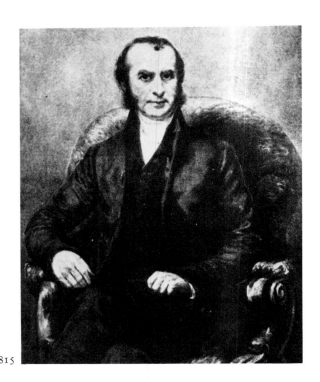

813   814   815

LONDON AND EDINBURGH

One of the most influential teaching institutions of the century, Guy's Hospital and Medical School, built in 1724 through the sponsorship and financial support of Thomas Guy, a publisher and investor, became world-famous as a center for practice and study. The "great men of Guy's"—Bright, Addison, Hodgkin, all physicians, and Cooper, a surgeon—were the leading lights of London and all were products of the Edinburgh Medical School.

One of the many innovations of Richard Bright (1789–1858) was the assignment of a special clinical ward with all the supporting facilities for the express purpose of studying one particular group of diseases, a forerunner of the subspecialty organization of the twentieth century. His masterful reports on the clinical and pathological nature of diseases of the kidneys led to the name "Bright's disease."

Perhaps the most imposing of the leaders at Guy's was Thomas Addison (1793–1860), whose severe, pompous manner, precisely chosen words, and physically impressive appearance struck fear into students. His thorough examinations and perceptive analyses earned him the awestruck respect of his colleagues. Pernicious anemia and adrenal insufficiency are both still referred to as "Addison's anemia" and "Addison's disease of the adrenals."

The third member of the medical triumvirate, Thomas Hodgkin (1798–1866), was a man of exceptional generosity and modesty. A practicing Quaker, he dressed in the characteristic clothing of the sect and devoted much of his time to charity, eventually leaving clinical activities to engage in philanthropic work, travel, and study. "Hodgkin's disease," a term introduced by Samuel Wilks in 1865, is a clinicopathologic syndrome described by Hodgkin in 1832 which is characterized by enlargements of the spleen and lymphatic system.

Another famous member of the staff at Guy's Hospital was William Withey Gull (1816–90). He especially condemned prescriptions containing multiple drugs and composed many widely quoted epigrams: "Savages explain; science investigates." "Nursing, sometimes a trade, sometimes a profession, ought to be a religion."

Many other physicians made contributions in the early half of the century. James Parkinson (1755–1824), for instance, gained recognition for his description of a neurological disorder now known as "Parkinson's disease," but he was also an important writer on paleontology. John Hughlings Jackson (1835–1911) and

William Richard Gowers (1845–1915) advanced further the idea that functions of the brain and spinal cord are localized in specific areas, as had been established in the Paris school.

BRITISH SURGERY

The fourth of the "great men of Guy's" was Astley Cooper (1768–1841). Bettany wrote, "No surgeon, before or since, has filled so large a space in the public eye." Although his financial position was secure because of his wife's fortune, he slaved day and night—examining, operating, studying, demonstrating, lecturing, dissecting, and writing. In each of his many endeavors he was brilliant, thorough, and communicative. An elegant, careful operator (before the days of ether anesthesia!), he took pains to enable his students to witness clearly every step of the procedure. "Cooper's fascia" and "Cooper's hernia" are only two of the designations for his work.

Since he had a passion for dissection and lost no opportunity to pursue his anatomical studies, he had dealings, out of necessity, with people who obtained corpses surreptitiously—the so-called "resurrectionists." He helped to defend them with argument and money. Those who were imprisoned he rewarded by supporting their families. Despite the clear antagonism of the populace to "body-snatching," Cooper remained unassailable in position and esteem. His life from beginning to end seemed to be an unbroken upward path of success.

Mention may be made of an entirely different fate that befell Robert Knox (1791–1862) in Edinburgh, a contemporary of Cooper's and one of the most famous teachers of anatomy at the time. When the nefarious activities of Burke and Hare, who murdered to obtain the bodies sold for dissection, were brought to light, Knox was falsely accused of complicity. Although later completely exonerated, he was vilified by the people, and his prestige was so irretrievably lowered that he never again achieved a position of influence.

The surname Bell, important in nineteenth-century surgery, was held by two unrelated families of Scotland. Benjamin Bell (1749–1806), a prominent, popular, practicing surgeon in Edinburgh trained in Paris and also in London, wrote a multivolume system of surgery that rivaled the influential text by Heister. His sons George and Joseph, grandson Benjamin, and great-grandson Joseph continued the highly respected surgical tradition into the twentieth century.

The second separate family of Bells contained even more famous members in the persons of the brothers John (1763–1820) and Charles (1774–1842), who were among the leading surgeons of Britain. Although Charles Bell was a highly competent surgeon, he became better known as an anatomist—especially of the nervous system. The priority of his experiments proving the motor function of the anterior nerve roots emerging from the spinal canal and the sensory characteristics of the posterior roots has been challenged by scholars who suggest that Magendie in Paris gave the first definitive proofs. Bell did discover that the fifth cranial nerve has both sensory and motor bundles and that the seventh cranial nerve could produce a paralysis now called "Bell's palsy."

John Bell, who also wrote and illustrated books on anatomy, is best remembered for his writings on history, vascular surgery, and wounds, and he may have been the model for Conan Doyle's arch-detective Sherlock Holmes. The bitter, personal controversies which surrounded John Bell, at one time forcing him to leave Edinburgh for London, were typical of the acrimonious feuds which involved other surgeons of the English-Scottish schools.

Robert Liston (1794–1847) was probably the most dexterous operator in England, introducing innovative techniques and successfully removing tumors deemed by others to be unresectable. He was also the first in Britain to employ ether anesthesia. His colleague and antagonist James Syme (1799–1870) developed procedures which permitted the excision of joints, thus preserving the limb from

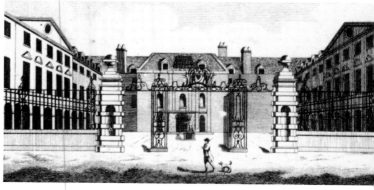

816

813 *Richard Bright, innovator of the method of studying and treating a specific group of diseases in a specialized ward. His accurate observations and reports on kidney diseases led to the name "Bright's disease."* New York Academy of Medicine

814 *Thomas Addison, whose outstanding contribution was in the study of pernicious anemia and of adrenal insufficiency, each of which is referred to as "Addison's disease."* New York Academy of Medicine

815 *Thomas Hodgkin was responsible for describing a syndrome characterized by enlargements of the spleen and lymphatic system, which is now called by his name.* New York Academy of Medicine

816 *Guy's Hospital, built in the 18th century by the publisher Thomas Guy, was a center for some of the most famous and influential clinicians in England.* New York Academy of Medicine

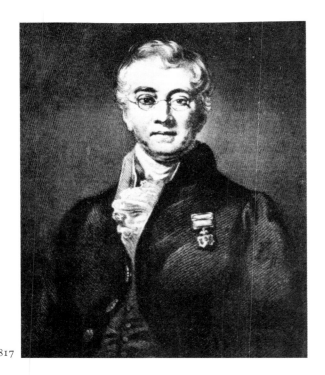

817

817 *One of the leading surgeons of Britain, Sir Charles Bell was better known as an anatomist, especially of the nervous system. "Bell's palsy" is named after him. New York Academy of Medicine*

818 *A selection of instruments illustrated in Benjamin Bell,* A System of Surgery *(1791), a multivolume text prepared by the first of a different line of prominent physicians named Bell. National Library of Medicine, Bethesda*

819 *Print showing the execution of William Burke, who murdered to obtain bodies for sale to anatomists. New York Academy of Medicine*

820 *Engraving of St. Bartholomew's Hospital, London, which was founded in the 12th century and became one of the great teaching hospitals of England. New York Academy of Medicine*

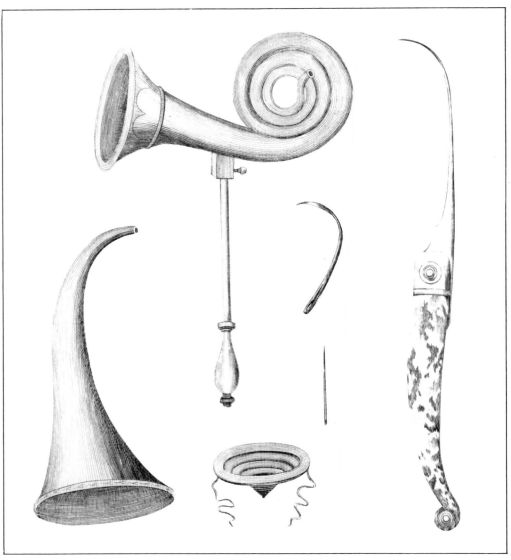

818

amputation. A contemporary later wrote of Syme, "He never wasted a word, or a drop of ink, or a drop of blood."

Benjamin Brodie (1783–1862), William Fergusson (1808–77), and James Paget (1814–99) were also outstanding surgeons of London. Brodie, a versatile and generous man, was a busy practitioner, physiologist, philosophic writer, and medical statesman, but the immensely popular Fergusson may have exceeded him in variety of interests. Not only did he write a highly reputed system of surgery and a book on the history of anatomy and surgery but he also invented instruments, did expert carpentry and metalwork, played the violin well, fished, danced, and enthusiastically supported budding writers and students.

Of the three, however, Paget's name is best known to succeeding generations, partly because of the eponymic "Paget's disease" of the nipple (an eczema which heralds the presence of carcinoma) and "Paget's disease" of the bones (a deformity produced by an error in calcium metabolism). He discovered the trichina infestation in human muscles, wrote brilliant essays, gave painstakingly prepared, eloquent lectures, and at St. Bartholomew's Hospital gained the reputation of being the best surgical diagnostician in Britain, with fabulous prescience in deciding what operation to do. "Go to Paget to find out what is the matter, and then to Fergusson to have it cut out" was a popular saying.

James Young Simpson (1811–70), perhaps the most famous obstetrician and gynecologist in Britain, born, trained, and nurtured in Scotland, introduced chloroform as an anesthetic. In his quest for a more pleasant and more controllable agent than ether, he had tried a drug suggested to him by a Liverpool chemist which had just been named "chloroform" by J. B. Dumas in Paris, but it had been

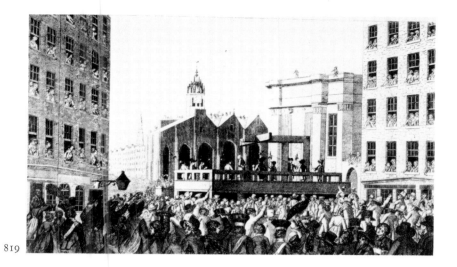

819

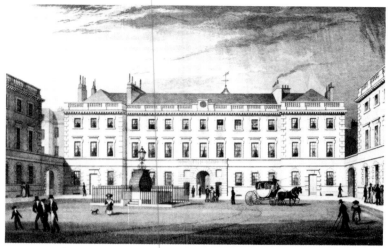

820

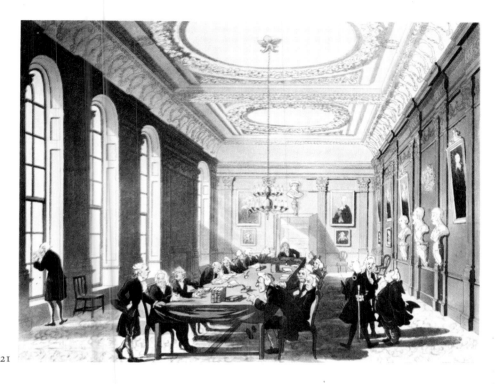

821

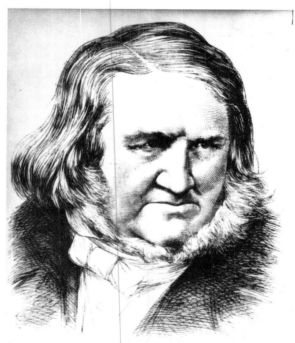

822

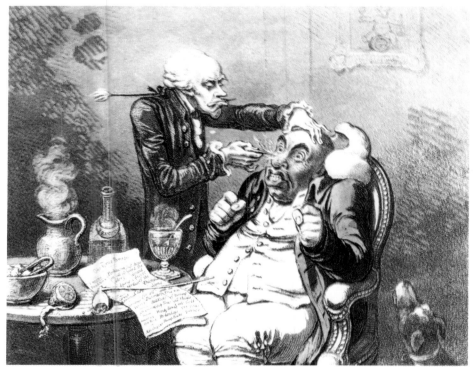

823

821 *Colored etching by Thomas Rowlandson and Augustus Pugin of* The College of Physicians *(1808). Smith, Kline, and French Collection, Philadelphia Museum of Art*

822 *James Young Simpson introduced chloroform anesthesia to obstetric delivery and suppported women's rights in medical education and practice. New York Academy of Medicine*

823 *Quackery mocked in* Metallic Tractors . . . *(1801) by James Gillray. National Library of Medicine, Bethesda*

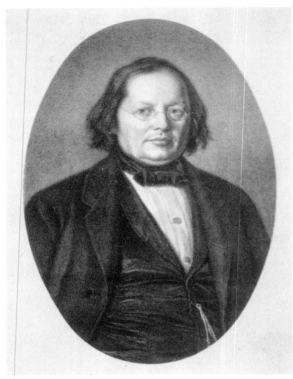

824

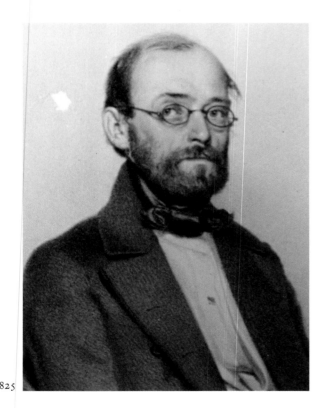

825

824 *Joseph Skoda was a nihilist in all therapy, but he especially condemned bleeding and purging.* New York Academy of Medicine

825 *Preeminent in the medicine of Vienna, Karl Rokitansky was one of the greatest pathologists of the time.* National Library of Medicine, Bethesda

discovered earlier, in the 1830s, by each of three independent investigators: S. Guthrie in the United States, Soubeiran in France, and Liebig in Germany. One evening Simpson and friends inhaled the substance at home and found they all had been rendered unconscious. Impressed by its effectiveness and pleasant smell, he tried it for operations and deliveries. For the next half-century, chloroform was the most frequently used anesthetic in Great Britain. Simpson also made many other contributions to obstetrics and gynecology. Although he was a highly principled man, supporting women's entrance into medicine, his personal animosity toward James Syme spilled over to include the teachings of Joseph Lister, Syme's son-in-law.

NEW VIENNA

In the German-speaking countries *Naturphilosophie* was still prominent at the same time as the scientific-minded were advancing the cause of observational medicine. If the British and French schools were skeptics in therapy, the Vienna school was virtually nihilistic, placing little if any reliance on drugs. The leading man in medicine in Vienna was Karl Rokitansky, but he was entirely a pathologist. The outstanding clinician and perhaps the most nihilistic of all was Joseph Skoda (1805–81), a pupil of Rokitansky's. Skoda refined Laënnec's ausculatory and percussive techniques to explain the physical bases for the various sounds produced by pathological lesions in the chest, showing that it was not the disease itself but the alterations in the physical conditions in the organ which produced the properties of pitch and timbre. An objective evaluator of treatment, he saw little use for medications or active interference in sickness, even giving placebos to patients with pneumonia to demonstrate that the illness ran its course unaffected by any therapy. At the time, this nihilism was probably more beneficial than the bleedings, emetics, and purgings that were still part of medical treatment.

Ferdinand Hebra (1816–80), one of the first to specialize entirely in skin diseases, began his career on Skoda's service for chest diseases but, with his teacher's support, founded a division of dermatology. He based his classification on the gross and microscopic changes in the tissues instead of on symptomatology or on general disease categories. His treatment was therefore directed toward the local problem rather than abnormalities in the humors which were still considered the primary causes. He discovered that the destruction of the itch-mite parasite cured scabies, a condition he recognized as transmissible from person to person.

There were other exceptional leaders in Vienna, one of whom, Joseph Hyrtl (1810–94), originally from Germany, became a famous teacher and historian of anatomy. Perhaps the most noteworthy historical figure in Vienna was Ignaz Semmelweis, whose important contributions and tragic career are described in the chapter on infection.

GERMANY

The theorizing, mystical *Naturphilosophie* which enveloped scientific and medical thinking in Germany in the early part of the century gradually gave way to direct observation and experiment, with the establishment of laboratory studies on body functions led by Johannes Müller and his followers.

Meanwhile a clinical school was emerging all over Germany, not in just one or two cities; possibly this was because Germany at the beginning of the century was a conglomeration of divided, independent political units, with no one central city representing the focus of feeling or governmental organization. Johann Lukas Schönlein (1793–1864), erected a classification of diseases, as a Natural History school, which turned out to be so arbitrary and artificial that it did not outlast him. But his intensive use of percussion and auscultation, incisive lectures and clinical demonstrations, and emphasis on the newest methods, including examination of the blood and urine, made him a leader in clinical medicine. His name was given to

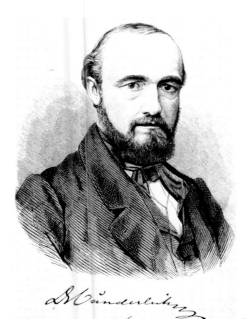

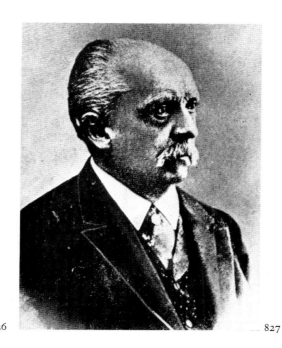
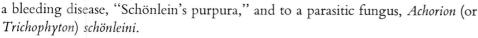

826

827

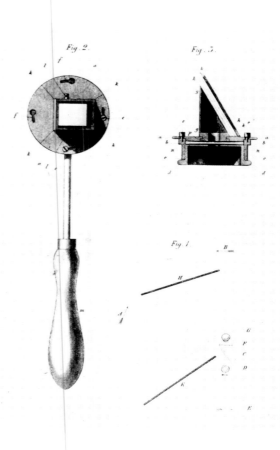

828

a bleeding disease, "Schönlein's purpura," and to a parasitic fungus, *Achorion* (or *Trichophyton*) *schönleini*.

Hermann von Helmholtz (1821–94) was one of the great geniuses of medicine, who entered the profession only because a career in physics appeared to offer little chance of a livelihood. Eventually he did become a physicist and professor of physics in Berlin in 1871, but the thirty years spent in medical practice and investigation were never forgotten. "Medicine was once the intellectual home in which I grew up; and even the immigrant best understands and is best understood by his native land."

Even while a young army surgeon he had maintained his interest in physics and mathematics, and in 1847 he published a treatise of far-reaching importance to physics and physiology, *Uber die Erhaltung der Kraft* (*The Conservation of Energy*), which formulated the law (also independently developed by J. R. Mayer in 1842) that although energy could be transformed into different forms its total amount was constant—whether in the universe or in a living organism. In his later years as a physicist Helmholtz also added to the knowledge of electrodynamics, and his assistant Heinrich Hertz (1857–94) discovered the waves on which the electromagnetic transmission of the twentieth century is based.

Helmholtz made his greatest impact on medicine through quantitative determinations in the physiology of sight, sound, and nerve impulses. Taking the original work of 1801 by Thomas Young, an English ophthalmologist, he confirmed and broadened the studies to develop an explanation of color vision, the Young-Helmholtz theory. Intent on trying to look inside the eye of a living person, he devised an instrument consisting essentially of a concave mirror with a hole in the center which shone light into the pupil and enabled the viewer to see the reflected image of the retina. Helmholtz reported "the great joy of being the first to see a living human retina." From then on, abnormalities in the eye were open to the diagnostic gaze of the physician.

Another influential member of the German clinical school, Karl August Wunderlich (1815–77), was in large measure responsible for popularizing the thermometer in clinical practice. Although Wunderlich went too far in believing that each disease entity had its own characteristic fever graph, his studies on fever made practitioners realize how important the temperature curve was. Wunderlich also wrote extensively on his reactions to what he saw at various clinics abroad. It was he possibly more than anyone else who brought back to Germany many of the principles and methods of the Paris school. He emphasized the need for more intensive study of therapy, which had been virtually left out in the French and Austrian institutions.

826 *Karl August Wunderlich popularized the thermometer in clinical practice and introduced into Germany many new concepts from other countries. New York Academy of Medicine*

827 *Hermann von Helmholtz, a physician whose chief interests lay in physics and mathematics, made his greatest discoveries through work in the physiology of sight, sound, and nerve impulses. World Health Organization, Geneva*

828 *Engraving of the ophthalmoscope devised by Von Helmholtz that made the inner eye visible to an examining diagnostician. National Library of Medicine, Bethesda*

829 *Electromagnetic generator in hand-held cylindrical electrode, widely used in the mid 1800s for relieving pain. Museum of Electricity in Life at Medtronic, Minneapolis*

830 *Stimulating coil for electrotherapy (c. 1855) and "electric egg" (c. 1880), ancestor of the light bulb. Both devices were used in electrophysiological investigations. Museum of Electricity in Life at Medtronic, Minneapolis*

831 *Reproduction of a sketch by Dr. Alban Gold Smith recreating the scene of Dr. Ephraim McDowell performing the first successful abdominal operation on the ovary for a huge cyst, in December, 1809. Medical Communications, Inc.*

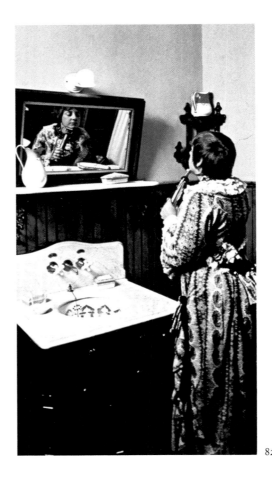

829

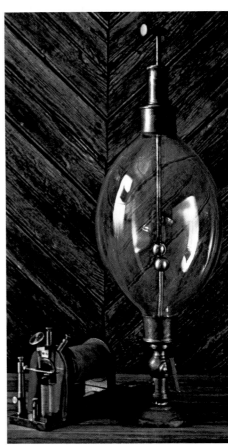

830

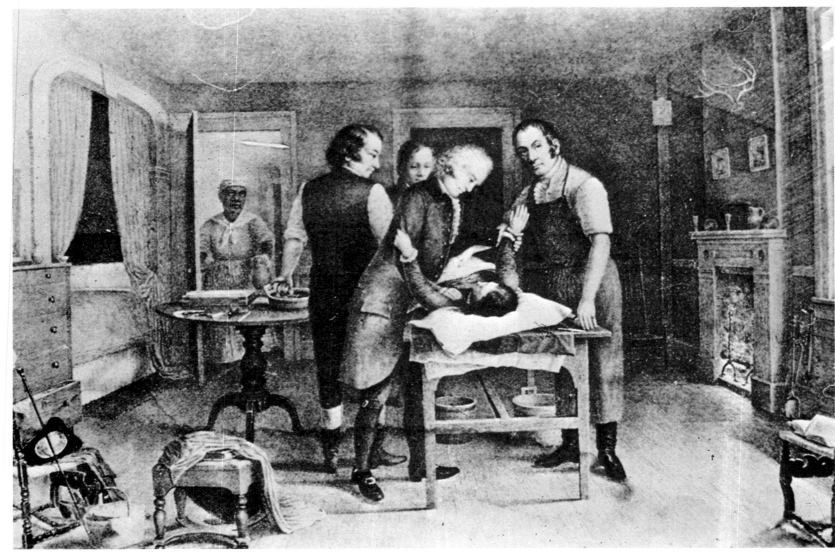

831

Although American medicine throughout the nineteenth century continued to depend upon Western Europe for innovations, individual American physicians demonstrated both intelligence and initiative. Ephraim McDowell (1771–1830), a physician practicing on the Kentucky frontier, was confronted in 1809 by a patient suffering from a large ovarian cyst. Fortunately for the patient, McDowell was a well-trained practitioner who had studied at the University of Edinburgh. He informed his patient that an operation to remove the cyst was considered almost certain death, but if she were willing to travel the sixty miles to his office in Danville he would attempt the operation. The patient, in the midst of winter, made the long trek on horseback and placed herself in his hands. McDowell recorded that while she recited psalms, he opened her abdomen and removed a diseased ovary weighing almost twenty pounds. Twenty-five days after the operation the patient returned home to live for another thirty-one years. McDowell successfully removed several more ovarian cysts before publicizing his work and gaining international recognition.

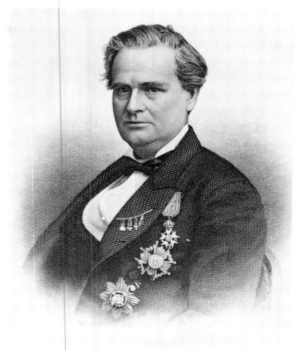

Obstetrical and gynecological problems are common to all peoples, and this may explain why still another American physician, equally far removed from the centers of medical learning, also pioneered in this area. J. Marion Sims (1813–83), a Southerner, acquired his medical education at the Charleston Medical School and Jefferson Medical College in Philadelphia—an education, he later wrote, which taught him nothing about the practice of medicine. He subsequently began practicing in Alabama, where he discovered a penchant for surgery. In this capacity he was called in to help with a young slave girl who had been in labor for seventy-two hours. Using forceps he delivered the child, but the mother had suffered so much injury that she was left with an opening between the vagina and urinary bladder—a condition considered hopeless. Encountering other cases of this type, he determined to help them. He assembled several slave women suffering from this condition, vesicovaginal fistulas, and at his own expense began four years of experimentation.

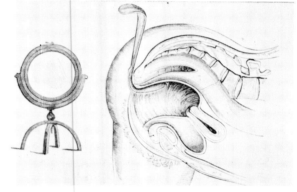

He despaired of success until one day he made a startling discovery. While treating a middle-aged woman for a retroversion of the uterus, he remembered the advice of a professor to place the patient in a knee-elbow position and to push the uterus back into position by using one finger in the rectum and another in the vagina. Reluctant to add to his patient's discomfort by introducing a finger into the rectum, he sought to correct the situation by means of two fingers inserted in the vagina. In the process of turning his hand, the womb seemed to disappear and the patient was suddenly relieved. As she rolled over on her side, she was embarrassed by an explosive sound of air. Sims realized that in turning his hand he had permitted the external air pressure to push the vagina back into normal position, and he could scarcely wait to get back to the hospital to apply his findings. He placed one of his fistula cases in the same position, opened the vagina, and heard the air rush in. He wrote later: "Introducing the bent handle of a spoon I saw everything, as no man had ever seen before. The fistula was as plain as the nose on a man's face." After the discovery of the knee-elbow (Sims') position (later modified to a side position), he devised a special (Sims') speculum and catheter, learned the value of silver sutures, and developed new surgical techniques which finally enabled him to restore his patients to health. In the process he laid the basis for the specialty of gynecology.

Many other American physicians and surgeons deserve mention: Dr. Philip Syng Physick (1768–1837), generally credited with establishing surgery as a specialty in America; Drs. Joseph and John Warren of Revolutionary War fame and their descendants who provided leadership in New England medicine for several generations; Daniel Drake (1785–1852), stormy petrel of American medical education; and Oliver Wendell Holmes (1809–94), poet, essayist, teacher, and medical practitioner. Holmes, best known as a literary figure, was the first to

832 *James Marion Sims, pioneer investigator of gynecological and obstetrical disorders, laid the groundwork for the specialty of gynecology and founded the Woman's Hospital of the State of New York, the first institution of its kind. National Library of Medicine, Bethesda*

833 *Early model of Sims' speculum, with a reflecting glass to direct light. Medical Communications, Inc.*

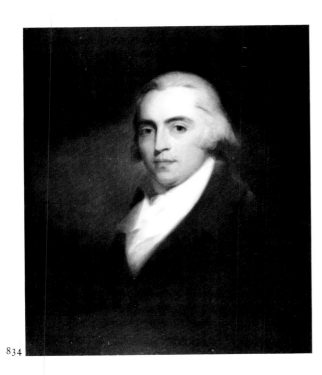

834

834 *Philip Syng Physick, a surgeon at Pennsylvania Hospital, is sometimes credited with establishing surgery as a specialty in America. National Library of Medicine, Bethesda*

recognize the contagious nature of childbed or puerperal fever. Holmes's observations antedate by four years those of Ignatz Semmelweis, the man generally credited with this discovery.

In the second half of the century, one of the most famous physicians was William Osler (1849–1920), who was born and educated in Canada and held professorships not only there but in England and the United States, notably at the Johns Hopkins Hospital and Medical School in Baltimore. Although he was a pragmatic practicing physician who made outstanding contributions to clinical medicine, his main influences were as a beloved teacher of a long line of pupils destined to make lasting contributions to medicine; as a writer of an encyclopedic medical text which was a standard for generations; and as the model of a cultured, articulate, insatiably curious, highly principled physician. He also gave a significant impetus to the study of the history of medicine in the United States.

METHODS OF TREATMENT

IN the early years of the nineteenth century, the principal therapies open to European and American physicians were general regimens of diet, exercise, rest, baths and massage, bloodletting, scarification, cupping, blistering, sweating, emetics, purges, enemas, and fumigations. There were multitudes of plant and mineral drugs available, but only a few rested on sound physiological or even empiric foundations: quinine for malaria, digitalis for heart failure, colchicine for gout, and opiates for pain. Many physicians continued to use compounds of arsenic for such diverse complaints as intermittent fever, paralysis, epilepsy, edema, rickets, heart disease, cancer, skin ulcerations, parasites, indigestion, and general debility. Antimony, which had its heyday in a previous century, was also still much in use, possibly sometimes aiding patients with parasitic infestations. For the most part, leading European practitioners, as well as some in America, permitted illnesses to run their course without interference, for careful observers noted little benefit from the therapies available. On the other hand, others believed that "desperate diseases require desperate measures" and favored the use of drastic drugs and procedures. In the United States, by the 1830s and 1840s, the influence of "heroic" medicine (such as bloodletting and strong drugs) was mitigated somewhat by the Louisiana Purchase in 1803, which introduced a large French-speaking population into the U.S. including French physicians who generally preferred assisting nature to battling the disease. Their close contacts with the Paris clinical school also taught them (and educated physicians in the northeast) the advantages of correlating clinical diagnoses with pathological changes in the organs.

MEDICAL SYSTEMS

Claude Bernard wrote, "Systems do not exist in Nature but only in men's minds." Nevertheless, numerous systems of therapy and explanations for illness flourished in the nineteenth century, a few of which may be mentioned. Some now seem close to quackery, but generally these theories of disease and treatment were sincere attempts to reconcile the symptoms of an illness with current knowledge.

Perhaps the most influential system was homeopathy, a creation of Samuel Hahnemann (1755–1843) in Germany, which taught that drugs which produced symptoms in a person resembling those of a specific illness would cure the patient if used in smaller amounts. However, the homeopathic system used such infinitesimal doses that they could hardly have had any effect, and, furthermore, the homeopaths were uncritical in their evaluation of results. But while their methods may have denied patients the therapeutic benefits of the few available specifics like quinine and digitalis, the homeopaths did spare their patients the harm of bleeding and purging. The doctrine spread throughout the world and was especially popular in the United States, where schools of homeopathy were founded, notably in

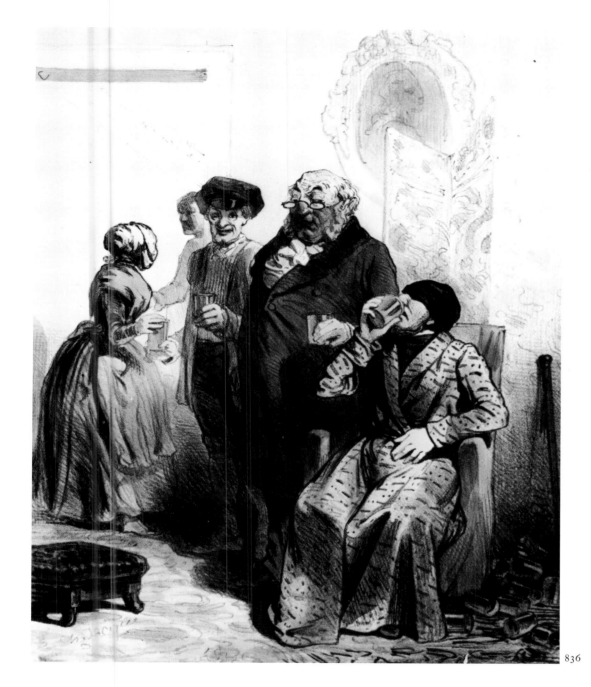

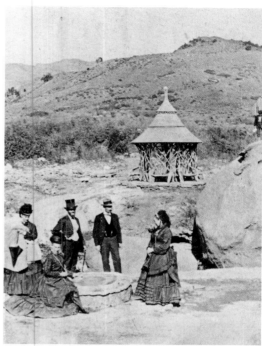

835 *Hydrotherapy, an all-purpose treatment that attempted to rid the body of all excesses by infusing water in every conceivable way, was caricatured by Charles-Émile Jacque in* The Hydropaths. First Treatment *(c. 1880). National Library of Medicine, Bethesda*

836 *Photograph of visitors "taking the waters" in the 1870s at Navajo Soda Springs, Manitou Springs, Colorado. Denver Public Library*

Philadelphia and New York. As newer knowledge in physiology, pharmacology, bacteriology, and pathology developed and as more useful therapeutic agents appeared, homeopathy lost much of its appeal.

Hydrotherapy, an all-purpose therapy, was based on the ancient concepts of the humors—the necessity for expelling excesses. Vincenz Priessnitz (1799–1851), the principal proponent, administered water in every conceivable way, but his regimen also included simple, nourishing food and exercise. This system, which achieved great popularity, led to the founding of hydropathic institutions in Europe and the United States. The opposite view—using only dry foods and substances—also had advocates, but they were few. The Thomsonians, who emphasized herbal medicines and steam baths, were one of a diverse group of practitioners—prominent especially in the U.S.—who stressed "Nature's remedies and folk medicine."

Another medical therapy, which arose in the eighteenth century but had a strong impact throughout the world in the following century, was cranioscopy. Also called phrenology, the doctrine was promulgated by Franz Joseph Gall (1758–1828), a clinician born in Germany and educated in France and Austria, who practiced and lectured in Paris for over twenty years. He taught that the shape and irregularities of the skull were projections of the underlying brain and consequently

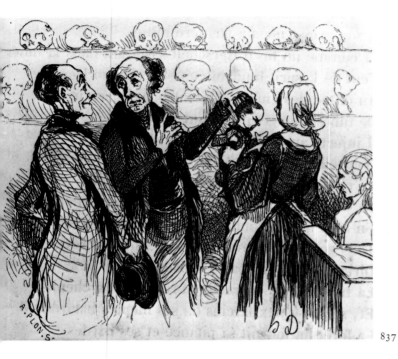

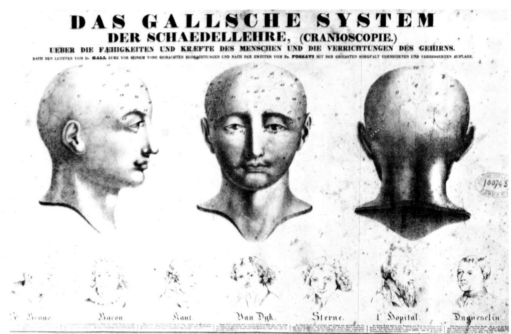

837 *Woodcut after drawing by Honoré Daumier published in Antoine-François Fabre, Némésis Médicale Illustrée . . . (1841), showing a mother bringing her baby to have his head "read" by a phrenologist. National Library of Medicine, Bethesda*

838 *The phrenological system of Franz Joseph Gall claimed to be able to analyze correctly the personalities of well-known figures of the time. National Library of Medicine, Bethesda*

indications of a person's mental characteristics—a conclusion with no basis in fact. Gall's concept of localizing mental processes was a good idea, but his uncritical exaggerations carried it too far. However, the very notion that the brain is a composite of discrete but interrelated functions anatomically confined to specific areas, an old but incompletely realized concept, was a principle that was to become the basic tenet of brain physiology.

In the United States, Andrew Taylor Still (1828–1917), who had attended medical lectures in Kansas City, organized a doctrine of medicine in 1892 which he called osteopathy. Concluding that drugs were ineffective in producing cures, he set up a system with two basic tenets: the living human body contains within itself all the remedies necessary to protect against disease; the correct functioning of the body requires a proper alignment of the bones, muscles, and nerves. Considerable dispute developed between osteopaths and regular practitioners, but over the decades osteopathic physicians so modified the original principles that they became almost indistinguishable in their methods from traditional physicians. They took up drugs, accepted vaccines, and utilized surgery. Many schools of osteopathy in the United States now have virtually the same curricula, educational standards, and practices as the regular schools.

Another healing system which ascribes disease to derangements in structure and function of the vertebrae is chiropractic, founded in 1895 by Daniel D. Palmer (1845–1913), who had earlier practiced magnetic healing. Proper adjustments of the spinal column are supposed to cure the ailments of the internal organs—a doctrine physicians generally regard as without foundation. In 1968 the U.S. Secretary of Health, Education, and Welfare reported to Congress that the claims of chiropractic were invalid, were not subjected to research evaluation, and should not entitle its practitioners to be reimbursed under the Medicare law. Nevertheless, the U.S. National Center for Health Statistics estimated that in 1965–66 approximately two percent of the population consulted chiropractors for treatment of back problems and other ailments.

Another healing cult which is more religious than medical is Christian Science. In the eighteenth century, Phineas P. Quimby (1802–66), a mesmerist, attributed his cures to the faith of the patient. Mary Baker Eddy (1821–1910), one of his patients though not his direct disciple, in mid-nineteenth century founded the Christian Science church, which views health and recovery from disease as dependent entirely on following God's divine laws. Confrontations between Christian Science and physicians have occurred when an operation or other

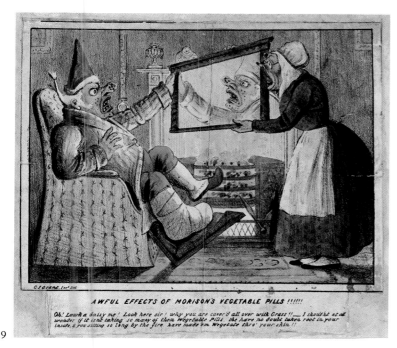

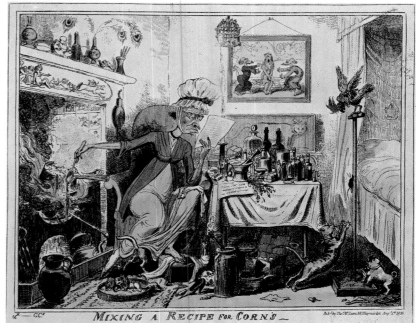

treatment deemed necessary has been refused by a church adherent.

There were also numerous quack cults whose objective was to amass money by hoodwinking the public, eager as it was to find more convincing cures than were offered by orthodox physicians. James Morison's "Hygeian" system in England held out the glowing prospect of a medical doctrine applicable to all types of illnesses—the cure of disease and the maintenance of health by freeing the blood of all impurities through the use of secret-formula pills (which later analysis showed to be a combination of strong laxatives). Although many reputable public figures within and outside the medical profession condemned Morison as a charlatan, and although newspapers lampooned the "Universal Pills," Morison's business thrived through widespread testimonial advertising and clever salesmanship in which the medical profession was castigated. Sales, which spread into France, the United States, Germany, and other countries, continued through the nineteenth century even after Morison's death in 1840. Even exposure of the fraud in notorious court cases failed to dampen the enthusiastic embrace of the public, which sent several petitions to Parliament containing ten to twenty thousand signatures condemning orthodox medicines and extolling the virtues of Morison.

Another cure-all of great popularity was "Dr. James's Fever Powder," which was developed in the eighteenth century and still used into the twentieth. Its principal ingredient was antimony. The good reputation of Dr. James and his apparently sincere belief in the efficacy of his nostrum, together with the extravagant promotional activities by James and the bookseller John Newbery, succeeded in spreading the powder's fame.

Since there was virtually no regulation of secret nostrums in most countries, the popularity of patent medicines depended entirely on the effectiveness of their advertising. Strong opposition to self-medication and proprietary drugs did not develop until the twentieth century. Indeed some nineteenth-century preparations were introduced by physicians themselves, and the government even allowed advertising on the very tax stamps levied on these products.

ANESTHESIA

Surgery made steps forward very slowly, limited as it was by lack of effective pain control during operations and by devastating postoperative infections. Both of these obstacles were substantially lifted by the discovery of anesthesia and the proof that germs caused infection.

839 *Lithograph by C. J. Grant showing the Awful Effects of Morison's Vegetable Pills! ! ! ! ! (1835). Nothing reputable physicians said to debunk Morison's pills as merely laxatives could convince the public to stop using them as cure-alls. Collection William Helfand, New York*

840 *George Cruikshank satirizes home remedies as well as patent medicines in this lithograph of 1822. Collection William Helfand, New York*

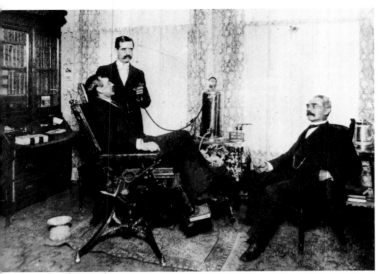

841

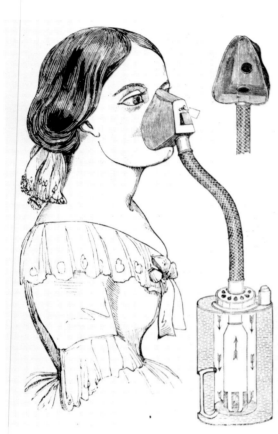

842

Although effective anesthesia was first discovered and put to surgical use in the United States, soporific, narcotic, and analgesic agents such as opiates and plants containing hyoscyamus and mandragora had been put to such use for thousands of years. Alcohol also had been resorted to for centuries to make a patient oblivious enough to pain to permit surgical procedures on the surface of the body or on the bones. Abdominal operations, including Caesarean section, were indeed performed at various times and places, but the systematic invasion of body cavities and internal systems was not feasible until the patient could be put to sleep deeply and safely enough to permit unhurried operative maneuvers.

In 1772, Joseph Priestley discovered nitrous oxide gas. Later, whiffs of nitrous oxide (soon called "laughing gas") were indulged in at "revels" for social amusement and the euphoria produced. Noting a reduced sensitivity to pain in these "revelers," Humphry Davy (1778–1829) suggested that "laughing gas" might be useful to surgery, but no one followed up his suggestion.

Other means of preventing pain through the loss of consciousness were also put forth from time to time. Henry Hill Hickman in 1824 produced a state of "suspended animation" in animals through asphyxia achieved by inhalation of carbon dioxide, which permitted him to perform operations without causing pain. He recommended this technique for use on humans but could not convince scientists.

Mesmerism, or "animal magnetism" (although branded quackery it was an early form of hypnotism), also played a part in opening minds to the possibilities of making people insensitive to pain. Although James Esdaile in India, stimulated by the publications of John Eliotson, performed seventy-three painless operations of different types using mesmerism, the medical profession worldwide remained unconvinced. Indeed, upon John Eliotson (1791–1868), the principal advocate of mesmerism, the brunt of denunciation fell. The hostile reception that his demonstrations and writings received led to his virtual ostracism. A well-trained, energetic investigator and practitioner, he seems always to have been eager to embrace new ideas, though sometimes with insufficient critical evaluation. For instance, his vigorous espousal of phrenology was one of the reasons for opposition to his reports. On the other hand he had been among the first to take up Laënnec's stethoscope, a step so unusual at the time that it also counted against him among his colleagues.

Unrecognized as a psychophysiological phenomenon (James Braid introduced the term "hypnotism" in 1843) and therefore misinterpreted by both proponents and opponents alike, mesmerism occupied the attention of doctors and the public for years. When the mesmerists learned of ether anesthesia they applauded its discovery, claiming that their own contributions had prepared the minds of the time to accept a sleep-induced state for operation. In England, Liston's remark on using ether for the first time, "This Yankee dodge beats mesmerism hollow," indicates that mesmerism's analgesic effects had been implicitly realized even by the antimesmerists.

As anatomical knowledge and surgical techniques improved, the search for safe methods to prevent pain became even more pressing. The advent of professional dentistry added a new urgency to this quest because of the sensitivity of mouth and gums. Although death as an alternative frequently drove patients to the surgeon, few people were known to die from toothache. The urge to see a dentist was easily resisted, so it may be more than coincidence that dentists seized the initiative in the quest for freedom from pain.

By 1831 all three basic anesthetic agents—ether, nitrous oxide gas, and chloroform—had been discovered, but no medical applications of their pain-relieving properties had been made. In all likelihood the first man to apply his social experiences with laughing gas to surgery was Dr. Crawford W. Long (1815–78) of Georgia. In 1842 he performed three minor surgical procedures using sulfuric ether. Apparently not realizing the significance of what he had done, Long made no effort

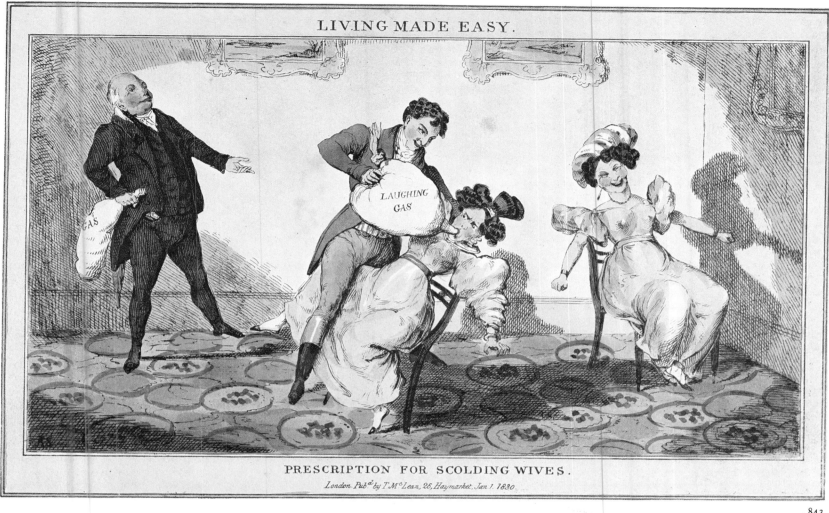

843

to publicize his discovery until several years later when anesthesia had been hailed as a major breakthrough.

A Connecticut dentist, Dr. Horace Wells (1815–48), on learning of the peculiar properties of nitrous oxide in 1844, tested them by having one of his own teeth removed while under the influence of the gas. Delighted with the results, he administered it to several patients, and then demonstrated his procedure before Dr. John C. Warren's medical class at Harvard. For some inexplicable reason, the patient cried out, and Wells was booed and hissed. Following Wells's failure, his friend and fellow dentist William T. G. Morton (1819–68) began experimenting with sulfuric ether. Encouraged by its effectiveness in his dental practice, he, too, contacted Dr. Warren and in 1846 gave the first public demonstration of surgery without pain. News of this momentous event spread rapidly throughout the Western world, and a new era for surgery began. Until Oliver Wendell Holmes supplied the name "anesthesia," the Boston medical community had been at a loss for a term to describe the condition brought on by this new agent.

After ether was widely accepted, James Simpson in Edinburgh abandoned it for chloroform because of its disagreeable odor, irritating properties, and long induction period. For about a century, chloroform continued to be the choice agent in Britain until its unmanageable toxicity and delayed damage to the liver was appreciated. In Germany, even when in 1894 the superior safety of ether over chloroform had been clearly shown (a more than five times higher mortality for chloroform), chloroform remained the favored anesthetic for almost twenty-five years.

In Britain, Simpson's advocacy of anesthesia in childbirth was vehemently condemned by the Calvinist church fathers as contrary to the Biblical admonition that a woman must bring forth her child in pain. However, the employment of chloroform by John Snow (1813–58) for Queen Victoria during her delivery helped

841 *Photograph made in 1884 showing Dr. Joseph C. Hunter administering nitrous oxide at his office in Boulder Hot Springs, Montana. The use of gas had become commonplace, even far from the large centers of medical treatment. Montana Historical Society, Helena*

842 *Chloroform inhaler illustrated in* On Chloroform and Other Anaesthetics *(1858) by John Snow, who was influential in making anesthesiology a specialty of medicine. National Library of Medicine, Bethesda*

843 *"Laughing gas" (nitrous oxide) was not taken seriously at first, as this print of 1830 indicates, nor thought of as an anesthetic until the 1840s. National Library of Medicine, Bethesda*

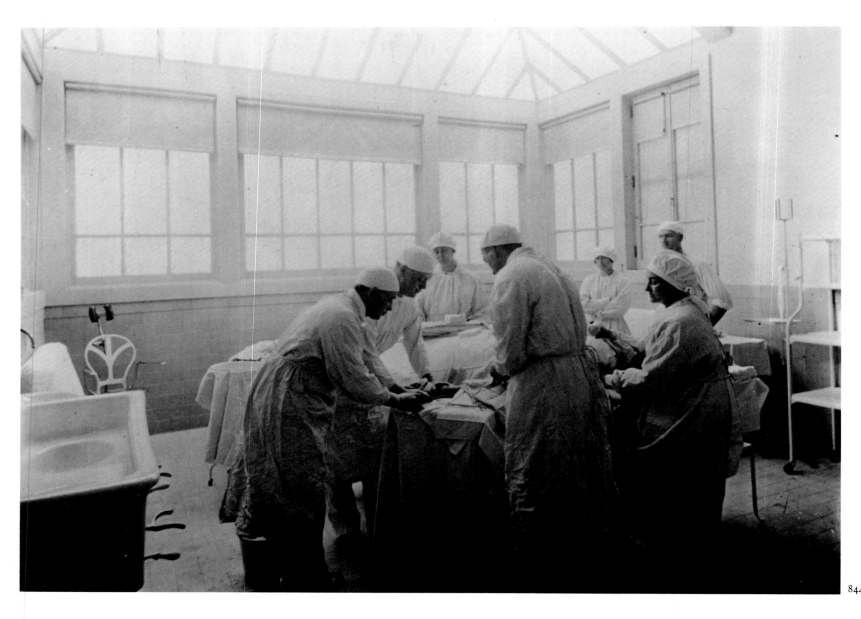

844

844 *Photograph (c. 1919) of an operating team shows the nurse anesthetist giving anesthetic by dripping it on a gauze mask over the patient's face. National Library of Medicine, Bethesda*

disarm the opponents. The development of anesthesiology as a specialty of medicine owes much to Snow, who devised techniques and analyzed the physiological effects of different agents.

Ether was taken up by many other countries shortly after its introduction: notably France, Sweden, Portugal, Spain, Cuba, and South America. Even in Germany, where chloroform held first position, some preferred ether. Johann Friedrich Dieffenbach (1795–1847), a pioneer in plastic surgery, wrote, "The wonderful dream that pain has been taken away from us has become reality. Pain, the highest consciousness of our earthly existence, the most distinct sensation of the imperfection of our body, must bow before the power of the human mind, before the power of ether vapor."

Other anesthetic agents were introduced near the end of the century. Ethyl chloride was sprayed locally to induce insensitivity. Cocaine by topical application to the eye was reported by Carl Koller in 1884. Sigmund Freud had earlier studied the anesthetic properties of cocaine but did not pursue the work. The injection of cocaine into nerve trunks to block sensation was investigated by William Halsted in the United States. Cocaine was also the first drug injected into the spinal canal in 1898 to produce anesthesia, but once its dangers were realized other less toxic and nonhabituating agents were developed. Numerous methods of administering anesthetics were tried, and the rectal route was introduced by Pirogov in Russia. Oré of France originated the intravenous method in 1874. After Fischer in 1902 had synthesized veronal, this barbiturate and other safer and more manageable agents for intravenous use were developed.

The "open" method of dripping the anesthetic on a gauze mask was replaced by "closed" systems in which an airtight mask could deliver a precisely measured amount of vapor and remove the exhaled carbon dioxide through absorption by a calcium compound. Advantages were also perceived in the insertion of tubing through the mouth and voice box into the trachea, thereby preventing the aspiration of secretions and controlling the patient's respiration. The twentieth century saw refinements in endotracheal anesthesia which permitted an anesthetist to control the flow of air, oxygen, and other gases into the lungs and thus have complete mastery over breathing during an operation. Muscle-relaxing drugs were also put to use in placing the anesthetist in control of respiratory movements and the surgeon in a position to perform manipulations through a totally relaxed abdominal wall.

At first, physicians and surgeons administered anesthesia in addition to their own specialties. As techniques became more complex and knowledge increased, special nurses and technicians were assigned the task. Even well into the 1940s many highly reputable hospitals continued to employ nurse-anesthetists rather than physicians specializing in anesthesia. In 1935 Frank Hoeffer McMechan, supported by his wife Laurette Van Varsevold McMechan, spoke for anesthesiology: "The safety of the patient demands that the anesthetist be able to treat every complication that may arise from the anesthetic itself by the use of methods of treatment that may be indicated. The medical anesthetist can do this, the technician cannot."

SURGERY

When anesthesia had become commonplace and the limitations of pain had disappeared, surgical procedures multiplied in number and complexity. No longer did the operator have to place the first emphasis on speed and to limit his manipulations mainly to surface areas of the body and the skeletal system. Yet the potential benefits of surgery were overshadowed by the frequent, devastating infections which often resulted in death. Outstanding surgeons everywhere were continually plagued by the dread complications of postoperative purulent infection and gangrene. Only when the bacterial origin of disease had been discovered and the necessity for keeping germs away from the operative field had been proved, notably by Lister, could surgery enter with safety the interior regions of the body. Every country participated in the new age of surgical progress, but the German-speaking countries were early at the forefront.

In the late nineteenth century, perhaps the outstanding surgical innovator in Europe was Albert Christian Theodor Billroth (1829–94). Born a German and educated in Berlin, he made his principal contributions in Zurich and, especially, in Vienna, where he was the first to successfully perform extensive operations on the pharynx, larynx, and stomach. Billroth's honest, forthright nature was shown by his unprejudiced reports of results, good and bad, a practice he insisted on for all of his staff. His teaching abilities, prominence as a writer on surgery, and personal influence were such that his students filled many of the prestigious chairs of surgery in Europe. His *General Surgical Pathology and Therapeutics* went through eleven editions, and his *History of the German Universities*, a book-length treatise on almost all aspects of medical education, set down the ideal tenets toward which schools in Europe and the United States aspired.

Throughout the world, the abdomen, neck, chest, cranial cavity, and spinal cord became common sites for surgical therapy. For instance, operations on the esophagus, stomach, and intestines—heretofore seldom dealt with effectively—were enlarged in scope and refined in technique, especially by the group surrounding Billroth. The nature of appendicitis, one of the most frequent surgical ailments, was elucidated only in 1886 when Reginald Heber Fitz (1843–1913) of Boston described the clinicopathologic entity formerly referred to as "typhlitis." In 1878 the gallbladder was opened by J. Marion Sims (1813–83), a founder of modern gynecology. The approaches to tumors of the brain and spinal cord by Victor

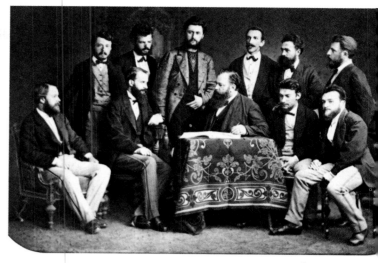

845

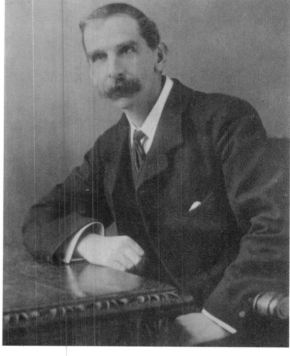

846

845 *Theodor Billroth, photographed with his ten assistants, was the first to perform successful radical operations on the pharynx, larynx, and stomach. National Library of Medicine, Bethesda*

846 *Victor Horsley, neurological surgeon, was the first successfully to remove a tumor of the spinal cord, in 1887. New York Academy of Medicine*

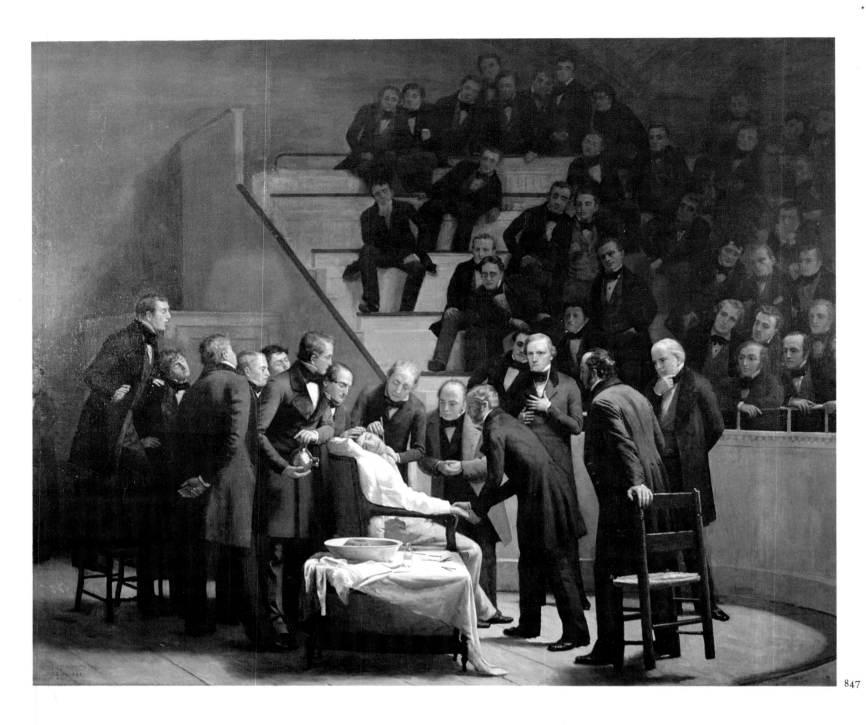

847

847 *Painting (1882) by Robert Hinckley of the
first successful public demonstration of surgical
anesthesia, October 16, 1846, at the Massachusetts
General Hospital. Francis A. Countway Library of
Medicine, Boston Medical Library, Cambridge*

848 *Currier & Ives print (1877) which takes the
doctor's point of view: "How difficult it is to keep
people well if they will persist in eating lobster,
cucumbers, green apples and buttermilk." National
Library of Medicine, Bethesda*

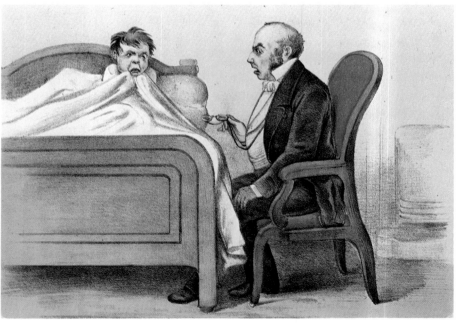

848

Horsley (1857–1916) in England gave impetus to neurological surgery. Newer instruments and techniques were developed by Koeberle, Péan, and Lembert. Ruge introduced the frozen section method of quick pathological examination. The older, standard procedures, such as hernia repair, were modified by Bassini and others to obtain better results. Plastic surgery was improved by Dieffenbach and Thiersch. For every organ and every region, a roster of names could be assembled of surgeons in the nineteenth century who made outstanding contributions.

Especially notable were the advances in operative treatment of the reproductive organs of women. The pioneer work of Ephraim McDowell in 1799 and of J. Marion Sims in 1852 in the United States has already been described. In Europe, Thomas Spencer Wells in 1858, Robert Lawson Tait in 1871, and W. A. Freund in 1878 developed operative procedures on the ovaries, Fallopian tubes, and the uterus. Removal of the baby by Caesarean section became more efficient and safe through the techniques of Porro in 1876 and Saenger in 1882.

So many were the innovations and so far was the domain of surgery extended that by World War I most of the basic operative procedures performed today (with the principal exceptions of thoracic and cardiac surgery) had already been developed. For the most part, the remarkable achievements of surgery in recent decades have been due to increases in physiological understanding, the introduction of safe methods of blood transfusion, the production of antimicrobials, and the improved management of the patient before, during, and after operation.

THE PROFESSION

IN the early half of the century, advances in physiology, pathology, and chemistry were not reflected in medical practice, for the physician's equipment was still limited. Doctors were even considered useless or harmful by large segments of the public conditioned by the failure of bleedings, purgings, and other manipulations to affect illness or stem epidemics and by the extravagant but convincing claims and cures promised by quacks. Attacks on nostrums and patent medicines were unpopular and generally ignored.

A dichotomy existed, especially in England, between those who favored mandatory licensing control over all healers, including physicians, and those who strongly advocated allowing anyone to practice medicine, giving patients a choice from among many practitioners and claimants. Political progressives believed that regulation would lead to domination and self-serving restriction of others by the medical profession; conservatives preached that only official bodies could or should determine who was fit to treat people.

EDUCATION AND LICENSURE

The nineteenth century saw the establishment of more uniform educational and licensure requirements, but even in ancient times there had been some official supervision and rules for medical practice. The certification ordered by Roger II of Sicily in the twelfth century was expanded by Frederic II in the thirteenth century to comprise a nine-year curriculum, an organized system of state licensing examinations, a mechanism for regulating apothecaries, and a sanctioned schedule of fees. Spain and Germany followed with rules of licensure shortly afterward. In 1511, Parliament, during the reign of Henry VIII, created a certifying board which continued to function for about three hundred years.

By the eighteenth century in England, medical education was entirely in the hands of individual doctors, mostly but not exclusively surgeons, who had their own private schools which dealt principally with anatomy and surgery until other subjects were later added. Although the teachers, such as the Hunter brothers, often imparted a high order of instruction, the students received their clinical education by walking around the wards observing the leaders in the great institutions of London: St. Bartholomew's, St. Thomas's, St. George's, Guy's,

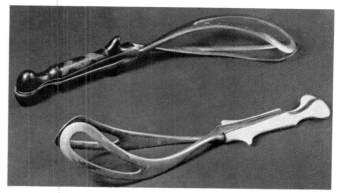

849

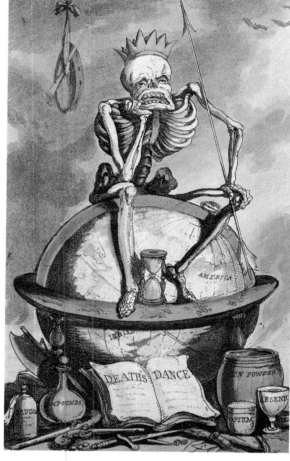

850

849 *Obstetric forceps used in the second half of the 19th century, a time of great advances in the safe handling of deliveries, both for the mother and child. Semmelweis Medical Historical Museum, Budapest*

850 *In this colored engraving, Death's Dance (1835), the satirist suggests that medications prescribed by doctors belong in the category of killing substances. Collection William Helfand, New York*

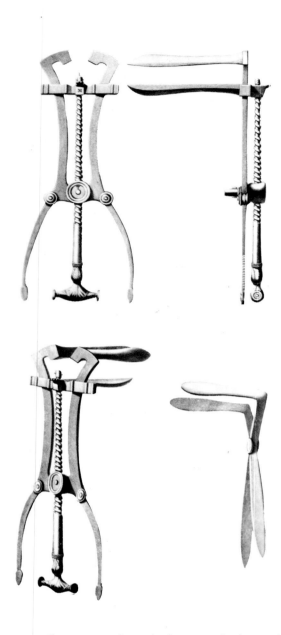

851 *Illustrations of specula from a medical text of 1847, showing the increased refinements in instruments for gynecological procedures. National Library of Medicine, Bethesda*

London, and Middlesex hospitals. In contrast, Edinburgh had a regular medical school, operational since 1736, with formal courses of instruction which included regular lectures and bedside teaching.

Attempts to set up adequate certifying bodies met considerable difficulty. At one time there were three separate medical councils (for England, Scotland, and Wales), and the General Council of Medical Education of 1858 was created to try to produce order in the certifying process. A coordinating body was finally formed by the end of the nineteenth century.

When the nineteenth century dawned, America had only four small medical schools to supply physicians for its burgeoning population, compelling most doctors to acquire their training by apprenticeship. In 1807 the University of Maryland Medical School was organized by a small group of Baltimore physicians as a private venture, and in succeeding years dozens of these proprietary medical schools came into existence. Three or four physicians would apply for a state charter, rent or buy a building, and begin advertising for students. The school year ordinarily lasted from eight to fourteen weeks, and the course work consisted exclusively of listening to lectures. Many proprietary schools granted degrees after one academic year, although they usually required the student to have served a one- or two-year apprenticeship prior to admission. Since these schools were dependent upon student fees for income, few applicants were ever turned down and even fewer failed to graduate. At the initial meeting of the American Medical Association a committee was appointed to examine medical education, and one of its proposals was to lengthen the school year to six months. When the University of Pennsylvania and the College of Physicians and Surgeons in New York followed the recommendation, their enrollments fell drastically, and the lesson was not lost on other schools.

Nearly all efforts to reform medical education foundered on this same rock. Those institutions which raised entrance requirements, lengthened the school year, or increased the amount of course work invariably found themselves losing students to schools with easier requirements. Despite pioneering efforts by Harvard, Michigan, and other schools, it was the end of the nineteenth century before the level of medical education was raised appreciably.

In an effort to bring a measure of unity into the profession, local and state medical societies had gradually come into existence, and these in turn led to the formation of the American Medical Association in 1847. While this organization did not become an effective force until the end of the nineteenth century, it was a strong advocate of improved medical education, fought to establish a code of medical ethics, promoted public health measures, and generally sought to improve the professional status of physicians. While the appearance of the A.M.A. boded well for the future, the public image of the American medical profession as of 1850 was at its nadir.

As the century drew on, a conjunction of circumstances moved American medicine toward professionalization. The most important of these were the fundamental developments in medicine itself. By 1900 the major outlines of human physiology were understood, the role of pathogenic organisms and their vectors was explained, and medicine could operate from a reasonably factual basis. A second factor was the rising American standard of living which brought with it a broadening of education at all levels, and medical schools could scarcely remain untouched.

The first medical school to lead the reform movement was associated with Lind University in Chicago (later Chicago Medical College and presently Northwestern University). In 1859 Lind raised its entrance requirements and lengthened its academic year to five months. The school received no support in its fight to raise educational standards until 1871, when Harvard overhauled its medical school and instituted a three-year graded course, a nine-month academic year, and written and oral examinations. Despite a better than forty percent drop in

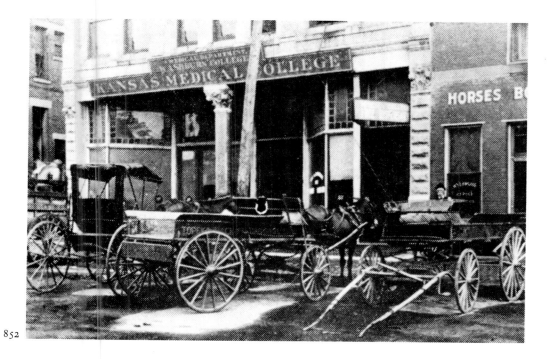

852

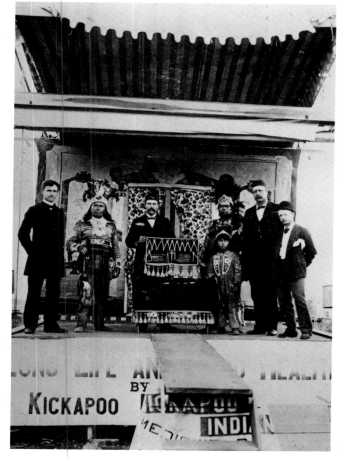

853

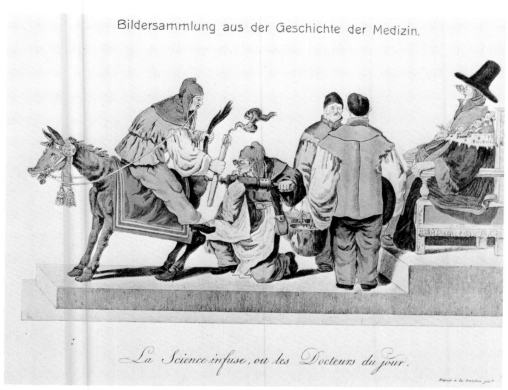

854

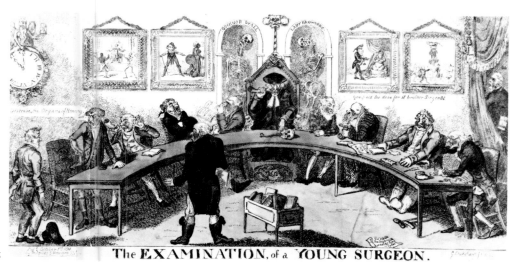

855

852 *Mid-19th-century photograph of Kansas Medical College of Topeka, one of many unregulated schools that sprang up all over the U.S. Kansas State Historical Society, Topeka*

853 *Photograph of Kickapoo Indian Medicine Show taken in Marine, Minnesota, around 1890. The public in many parts of the world was taken in by the claims and cures promised by quacks. Minnesota Historical Society, St. Paul*

854 *German satire on medical methods used by "today's doctors." National Library of Medicine, Bethesda*

855 *The Examination of a Young Surgeon (1811) by George Cruikshank lampoons licensure proceedings. National Library of Medicine, Bethesda*

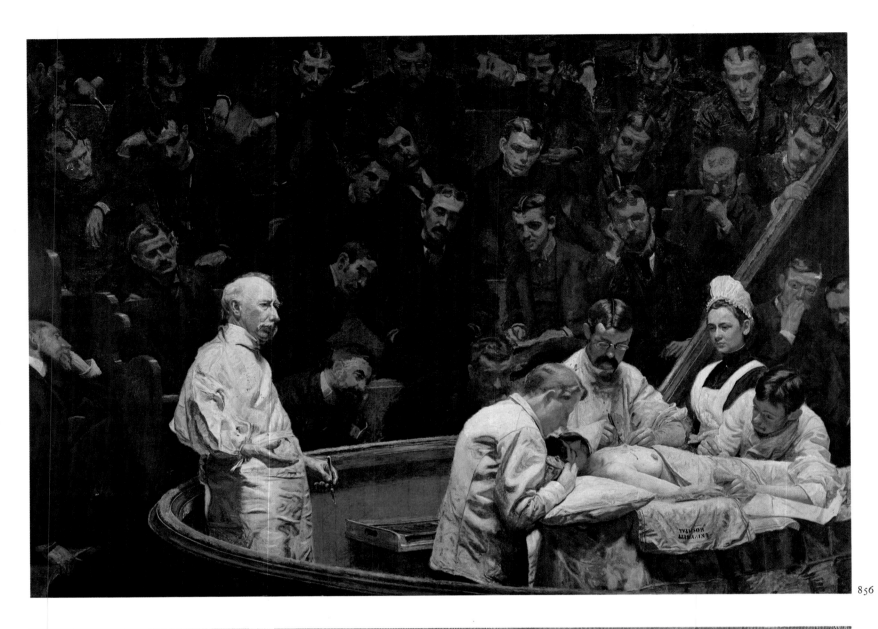

856

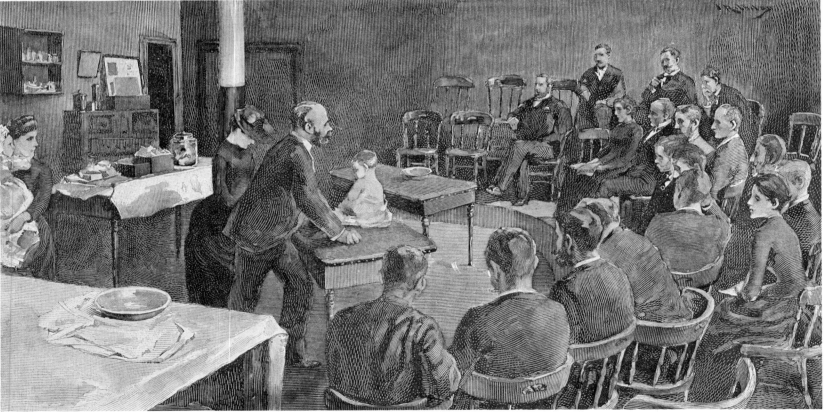

857

enrollment, Harvard persisted, and within a few years Pennsylvania, Syracuse, and Michigan swung into line.

The next major step came with the establishment in 1893 of The Johns Hopkins University School of Medicine, which assembled a remarkable faculty headed by William H. Welch and William Osler. Welch, a pathologist, was among the first to introduce microscopy and bacteriology into the United States, and Osler was a firm advocate of more bedside training for medical students. Under the guidance of these two, assisted by William S. Halsted and other outstanding professors, Hopkins drastically reshaped American medical education and set a pattern which persists today. From its inception, Hopkins required a college degree as a prerequisite for admission, provided a four-year graded curriculum, made extensive use of laboratories for teaching purposes, and integrated the hospital and college facilities to provide clinical training to advanced students.

Hopkins flourished, and within a few years its former students and professors were carrying the Hopkins system to all parts of the United States. Two other steps were still needed to place medical education upon a sound basis. In 1904 the A.M.A. created a permanent committee on education, which two years later became the A.M.A. Council on Medical Education. The council immediately began evaluating schools in terms of the ability of their graduates to pass licensing board examinations. However, the council was too closely identified with medicine, and its members recognized the need for a more objective evaluation. This was achieved by persuading the Carnegie Foundation for the Advancement of Teaching to undertake the task. The foundation employed Abraham Flexner, a man who had already studied American higher education, to survey the field, and the report which ensued was a damning indictment of medical education. More important, the Flexner Report (1910) brought foundation money to the better schools, and, by improving them, forced the weaker ones out of business. In the meantime the Council on Education had begun to classify schools on an A, B, C basis, evaluations which played a key role in standardizing medical education.

In France, the decrees of Napoleon in 1803 categorized those who could practice medicine into doctors of medicine, doctors of surgery, and health officer doctors, each division with its own educational prerequisites and licensing examinations. Schools for apothecaries were built and a system ordered for inspecting the shops of apothecaries, druggists, and spicers. Tuition at all of the four state medical schools was kept low to permit students of limited means to enter the medical profession.

In Germany, the regulations varied in the different principalities. In the Duchy of Nassau, for instance, before it was taken over by Prussia, the physicians and surgeons were in one body under the state, and although strict examinations had to be passed to practice medicine a university degree was not essential. In Prussia, in 1825, three classes of licensed doctors were recognized: graduate physicians (who had to spend four years at a university and pass rigorous state examinations— including an additional test for those who entered surgery); wound doctors, first class (with fewer years of schooling and less difficult examinations); and wound doctors, second class (with even less education and less rigorous examinations). Obstetricians, ophthalmologists, and public health doctors also had separate requirements.

State practice of medicine and social insurance were also seen in the German principalities, where the physicians were paid by the state but were also permitted some private practice. In Prussia, the proportion of doctors who depended on state stipends became less and less. Bismarck finally turned to medical and social insurance as a means of receiving the support of the general populace in his aim of unifying Germany.

In Russia, after 1864, local governmental organizations, the zemstvos, were responsible for medical service to the poor and mentally ill and acted as public health overseers. The feldsher, a combination of male trained nurse and pharmacist

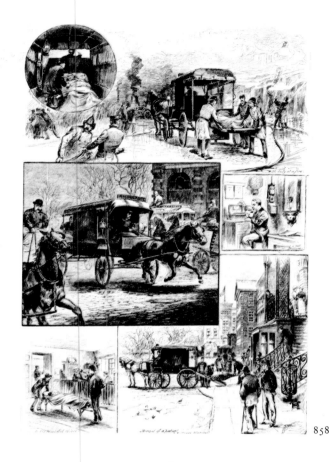

858

856 The Agnew Clinic (1889) by Thomas Eakins reflects the increasing prestige of American medical schools, but it took another twenty years before raised standards became general. University of Pennsylvania, School of Medicine, Philadelphia

857 Sketches from the New York Polyclinic School of Medicine and Surgery (1891), by Irving R. Wiles, demonstrates the integration of hospitals and college facilities to provide clinical training, a factor in the reshaping of American medical education. National Library of Medicine, Bethesda

858 Vignettes of the New York Ambulance Service at work, published in Harper's Weekly, May 24, 1884. National Library of Medicine, Bethesda

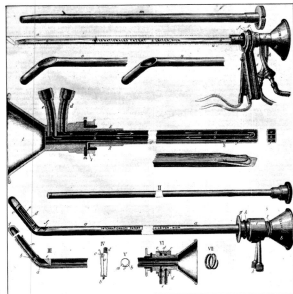

859

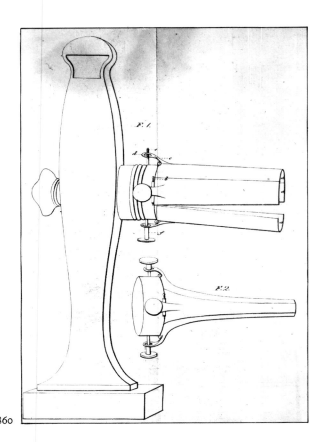

860

859 *Illustration of the first practical cystoscope, developed by Nitze and Leiter in Germany, as it appeared in* Wien Medizinisch Presse (1879). *National Library of Medicine, Bethesda*

860 *One of the early instruments that led to more sophisticated devices was this oral speculum invented by Philipp Bozzini and illustrated in Christoph Wilhelm Hufiland's* Journal der Practischen Heilkunde (1807). *National Library of Medicine, Bethesda*

who went out into the countryside, was also a provider of health care. Regular physicians continued to be trained in the large city universities.

SPECIALIZATION

Specialization in the nineteenth century was at first vehemently opposed by many in the profession who felt that it would be detrimental to the patient. Examples from the past of itinerant charlatans who specialized in pulling teeth, cutting for the stone, or treating only one kind of illness (for instance, venereal disease) caused ethical practitioners, and many lay people also, to regard with suspicion any physician who established himself to treat one group of diseases or one organ system. It smacked too much of the tradesman. Nevertheless, as the pressures of scientific, social, and economic factors became irresistible, specialization became an accepted fact. As medical information grew to be voluminous and new techniques became more complex, one practitioner could not encompass all. The patient was urged to seek a physician who devoted his time and skill to one type of illness or manipulation. Also, the opportunity for commanding higher fees, working less onerous hours, and receiving greater respect were all strong incentives to doctors to specialize. Moreover, the increasingly significant industrial principle of the division of labor also seemed to encourage the compartmentalization of medicine. In some instances the spur was principally the enormous increase in information (as in pathology), while in others it was the newly devised instruments which required special experience (as in urology and laryngology). Another factor was the abandonment of humoral ideas of general disease in favor of a focus on local organs in diagnosis and treatment.

Some examples may be cited. The invention of the head mirror by the country practitioner Adam Politzer in Vienna in 1841 aided specialization on the ear. In Britain, the first surgeon for ear diseases was James Yearsley, who founded a hospital in mid-century devoted entirely to the ear. William Wilde (1815–76), Oscar Wilde's father, helped to establish in Dublin the St. Mark's Hospital for the ear and eye. Operation on the mastoid for infection, which became a common procedure for many decades, was brought into otology by Hermann Schwartze in the 1870s. The first hospital in England specializing in the throat was a contribution of Morrell Mackenzie (1837–92). In the United States the organization of the Metropolitan Throat Hospital and The New York Laryngoscopic Society, both in 1873, were due to the efforts of Clinton Wagner.

Diseases of the eye, ear, nose, and throat were at first combined in one specialty. The first professor of ophthalmology was Joseph Baer in 1812 in Vienna, although a special dispensary for the eye was formed in 1805 in England. The ophthalmoscope invented by Helmholtz in 1851 was an incentive to specialization, as were the refractive principles of Donders and the surgical contribution of Von Graefe.

The itinerant, irregular bladder stone removers of ancient and medieval times were in a sense early urological specialists. The invention of instruments which could be passed into the bladder for observation gave impetus to the specialty. Nitze and Leiter in Germany, by improving earlier inadequate devices, constructed the first practical cystoscope. Since this was before the invention of the electric light bulb, the light source was an exposed platinum wire lit by electric current. After X-rays were introduced by Wilhelm Konrad Roentgen (1845–1923), it took until the 1920s before a feasible technique could be devised for adequately visualizing the urological tract. The intravenous method reported by Swick in 1929 was the forerunner of the later sophisticated angiography (injecting radiopaque dyes into the bloodstream to make the vascular system visible in X-rays). Much of urology was done by general practitioners and surgeons in the nineteenth century. Even in the 1930s, outstanding hospitals and teaching institutions still combined urology and general surgery in the same department.

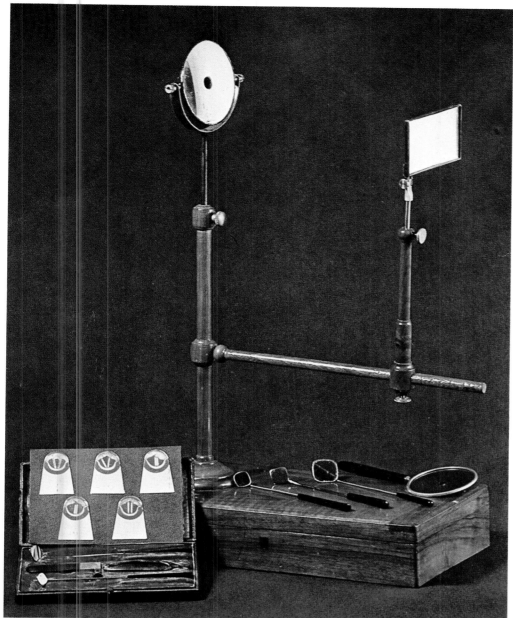

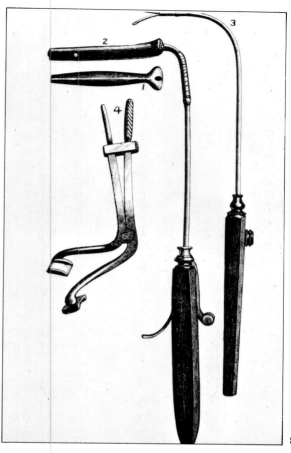

861 *Autolaryngoscope and mirrors for exploring nasal passages, constructed in 1858 by Janos Czermak, Czech medical scientist who held the chair of biology at the University of Pest. Semmelweis Medical Historical Museum, Budapest*

862 *Instruments designed and used by Joseph O'Dwyer, around 1880, for intubation to alleviate the suffocating symptoms of diphtheria. Medical Communications, Inc.*

The spirit of the Enlightenment of the eighteenth century and Rousseau's writings were among the incentives to concentrate on the problems of children. Nils von Rosenstein, George Armstrong, and William Cadogan were pioneers in this specialty. Charles Billard in France and Charles West in Britain were important contributors of the nineteenth century. In the United States Abraham Jacobi, fleeing from Germany because of his espousal of the political and social reforms of 1848, soon found himself giving most of his attention to children's diseases and influencing others to do the same.

Scientific dermatology had its beginnings in Hebra's work in the New Vienna school, but Lorry, Alibert, and Willan had taken the earlier steps. Syphilis was an important part of dermatologic practice until well into the twentieth century, when its protean manifestations brought it into internal medicine. Philippe Ricord and Jean-Alfred Fournier clarified the clinical nature of syphilis and separated it from other venereal diseases.

Neurology was relatively late in becoming a separate specialty, and then it was often combined with psychiatry. Neuropsychiatrist was a common title after Pinel. Psychiatrists such as Janet, Esquirol, Bayle, and Georget gave France the leadership until the reports of Griesinger and others drew attention to Germany. Emil Kraepelin's classification of mental disease into dementia praecox, manic-depressive psychosis, and paranoia was useful to the new specialty.

In the nineteenth and twentieth centuries, specialties and subspecialties became more and more numerous, so that now there is virtually no general branch of medicine or surgery without its subdivisions of specialization.

539

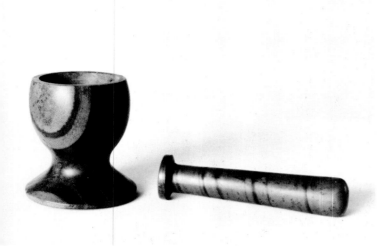

863

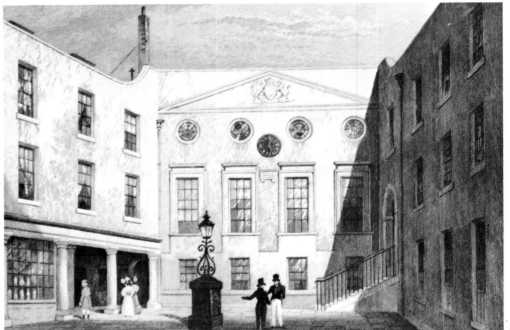

864

863 *The mortar and pestle have been tools of pharmacy for thousands of years, as this set from the Treasury of Persepolis, ancient Persia, demonstrates. Oriental Institute of the University of Chicago*

864 Apothecaries' Hall, Pilgrim St. *(1831), engraved from a drawing by Thomas H. Shepherd, illustrates the increased social and professional status of pharmacists in the 19th century. Collection William Helfand, New York*

865 *The roles of physician and pharmacist had begun to diverge in Europe, but in the U.S., out of economic necessity, some doctors continued to prepare and sell medications—as shown in this photograph of Dr. James Raizon of Trinidad, Colorado, in his drugstore (c. 1880). State Historical Society of Colorado, Denver*

866 *The pharmacist increasingly became a merchant and dispenser of medicines, especially in the U.S., as well as a dealer in confections and cosmetics, as this photograph (c. 1880) of the Moritz Drugstore, Denver, Colorado, shows. Denver Public Library*

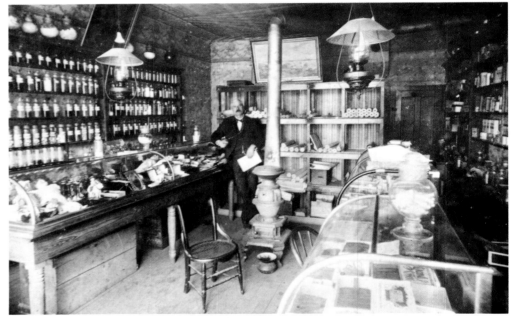

865

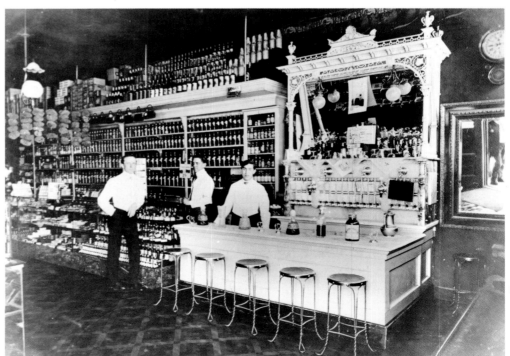

866

PHARMACY

Pharmacy has been a part of medical practice throughout the centuries. The physician frequently compounded and dispensed drugs in addition to practicing medicine, and the apothecary often engaged in medical practice as well as compounding and dispensing. Rivalry between the two groups, which was intense in the seventeenth century, continued into the nineteenth century. The respective roles of the physician and the apothecary or pharmacist gradually became clearer, but in some countries, notably the United States in the nineteenth century, the physician continued to prepare and sell medications out of economic necessity.

The social position of the pharmacist in most places was high, and educational requirements after the seventeenth century became more and more rigorous, especially in Italy. In France the new standards grew to include a university education, special training internships, and even specialized certifications for clinical laboratory analysis, community practice, or industrial pharmacy. In Germany, where the pharmacist seems virtually always to have occupied a high social and professional position, the apprenticeship system evolved into an elaborate progression of examinations leading to a stratification by educational accomplishment.

The pharmacist in recent years, especially in the U.S., is becoming primarily a merchant and dispenser of medicines, owing to economics and the decreasing need for the compounding of prescriptions.

PHARMACOPOEIAS

Lists of drugs to guide therapeutics have existed since ancient times, but the word pharmacopoeia (which means the making of medical substances) was first applied to such a listing in the sixteenth century. However, it was not until the nineteenth century that national pharmacopoeias were developed: Prussia in 1799, Austria in 1812, France in 1818, United States in 1820, Britain in 1864, and Germany in 1872. Many of these standard listings continued for a long time to include some of the bizarre, ancient substances combined in multi-ingredient formulas. For instance, theriac was still in the pharmacopoeia of London in the eighteenth century. Therapeutic agents in practice frequently did not keep pace with advances in general science, biology, physiology, and chemistry.

DENTISTRY

Dentistry really began its professionalization as an independent discipline with the work of Pierre Fauchard (1678–1761), who was the first clearly to devote full time to the teeth. He collated the considerable body of information that had accumulated through the centuries and described the use of tin and lead for filling cavities, but more importantly he established the ethical principle that secret methods should be openly reported in detail so that the results could be evaluated and used by others. Fauchard also emphasized the need for special training of doctors of the teeth and for the examination of candidates by those experienced in the discipline instead of by surgeons. His *The Surgeon Dentist* (1728), which became the authoritative text for generations, was the foundation of subsequent dentistry. Writings by others in France followed rapidly: Devaux (who also collaborated with Fauchard), Gerauldy, Bienn, Mouton (who constructed the first gold crowns and other new prostheses), Bourdet (who devised new instruments), and many others. Duchateau, an apothecary in the region of Sèvres, molded the first porcelain dentures.

In Germany, incidental dissertations on the teeth by physicians and surgeons were replaced by reports from specialists such as the dentist to Frederick the Great, Philipp Pfaff, who in 1755 described how to make plaster models from impressions

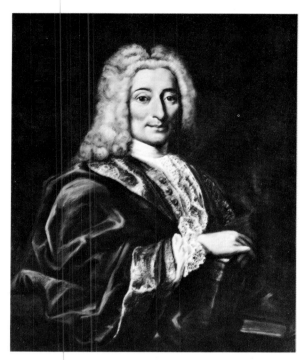

867

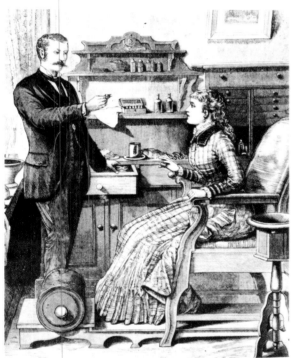

868

867 *Portrait of Pierre Fauchard, founder of modern dentistry. Pierre Fauchard Academy, Minneapolis*

868 *By the 19th century, dentistry was a specialized field, especially in the U.S., where the world's first dental school was established. New York Academy of Medicine*

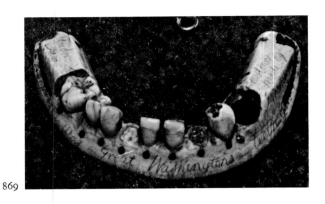

869

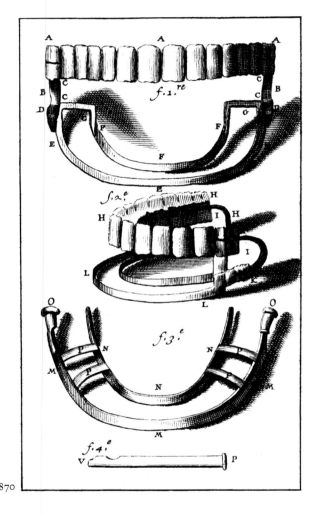

870

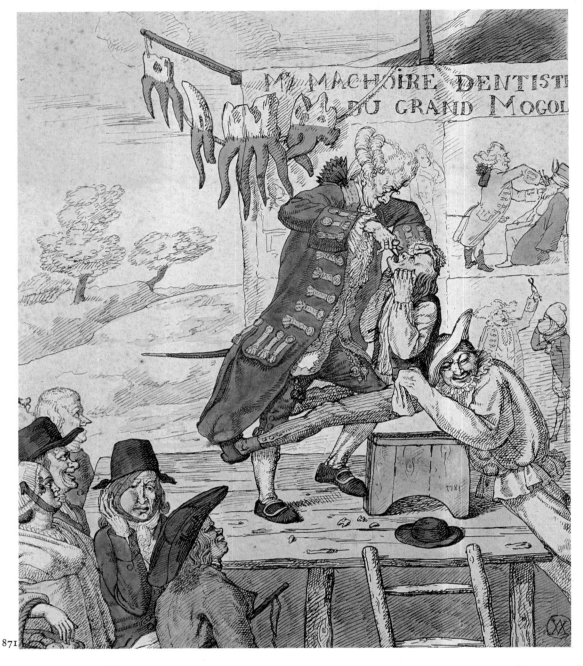

871

in wax. The craftsmen (usually woodworkers) who actually fashioned the prostheses designed by Adam Brunner were the forerunners of dental technicians.

Dentistry gradually became a separate specialty in other countries too, but it was in the United States especially that dentistry reached its fullest development in the nineteenth century and afterward, largely due to the efforts of Horace H. Hayden (1768–1844) and Chapin C. Harris (1809–60). The introduction of anesthesia by dentists was as important to dental procedures as it was to the surgery of other organs.

The first dental school in the world was established in 1839 as the Baltimore College of Dental Surgery. In 1870, although there were 10,000 dentists in the United States, only 1,000 were graduates of a school.

Advances in prostheses, such as the production of vulcanite in 1855 by Charles Goodyear, technical innovations in the management of cavities, improvements in the correction of occlusive derangements, and the elevation of educational standards gave American dentistry world leadership.

Eventually the specialization of dentistry, with its complex techniques, became so complete that it was separated from medical practice. However, in recent decades, the physiology and surgery of the head, neck, and mouth have brought a greater interdependency among physicians, surgeons, and dentists.

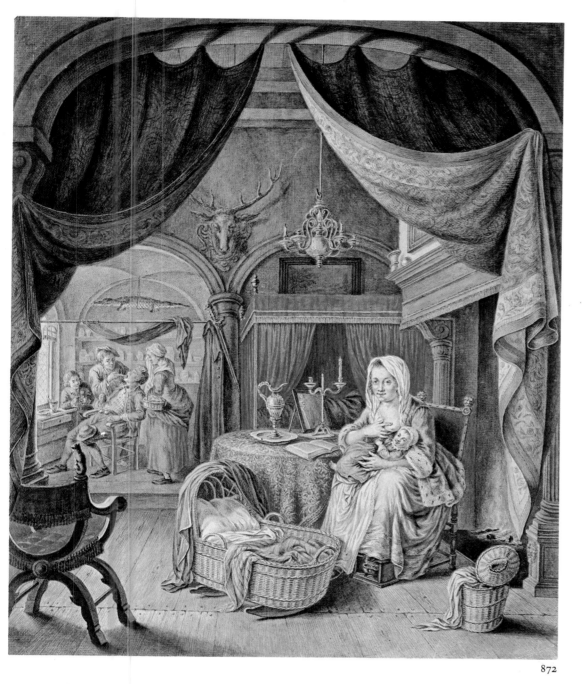

872

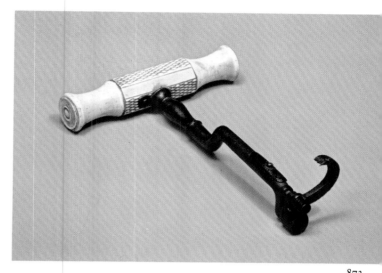

873

869 *George Washington's false teeth. New York Academy of Medicine*

870 *Engraving of dental prostheses, from Pierre Fauchard,* Le Chirurgien Dentiste (1728). *National Library of Medicine, Bethesda*

871 *Caricature,* Sans Efforts, *of the itinerant dentist of the 18th century performing upon a small stage before an audience. National Library of Medicine, Bethesda*

872 *The pharmacist was often a part-time dentist, able to combine tooth-pulling with his other tasks, as shown in this 18th-century drawing after Gérard Dou. National Library of Medicine, Bethesda*

873 *Eighteenth-century tooth extractor, with bone handle. Private collection, Cooper Bridgeman Library, London*

Nursing

Since nursing only became fully established as a profession in the nineteenth and twentieth centuries, we are accustomed to regard nursing care in earlier centuries as rudimentary and unstructured. Yet in India, hundreds of years before Christ, Charaka had summarized four qualifications for a nurse: "knowledge of the manner in which drugs should be prepared or compounded for administration, cleverness, devotion to the patient waited upon, and purity (both of mind and body)." We are also apt to think of nurses as exclusively women, but throughout history males also have attended to the sick in hospitals. During the Crusades, the Hospitalers of St. John, the Teutonic Knights, and the Knights of St. Lazarus performed nursing duties, and male members of the mendicant orders of St. Dominic (the black friars) and St. Francis (the gray friars) also acted as nurses in the Middle Ages.

Nevertheless, women have been the principal performers of nursing duties in every period and every country. The nuns of religious orders, such as the Poor Clares, and secular groups with religious purposes, such as the Tertiaries of St. Francis and the Beguines of Flanders, carried on most of the nursing in medieval and even later times. Perhaps the oldest religious group devoted entirely to nursing was the order of Augustinian Nuns in the Hôtel-Dieu of Paris. Indeed, the idea of

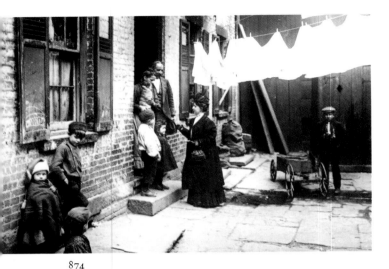

874

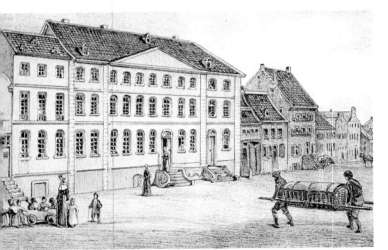

875

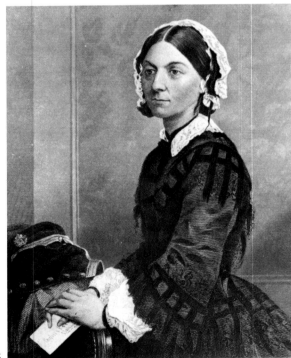

876

attending the sick is so closely associated with the Church that even in hospitals which are totally nonreligious the nurses are often called "sister."

During the Reformation, however, hospitals were generally removed from Church connection or control. The dedicated, free services of the nuns and charitable secular groups were frequently replaced by those of poorly paid workers. Hospitals tended to become filthy, germ-infested buildings where people often died of infection rather than the illness which brought them there. Sick people who could afford it were treated at home. A reactive move toward cleanliness and humanitarianism engendered by the Enlightenment of the eighteenth century was turned back again by the economic and social changes of the Industrial Revolution. The arduous, menial, and sometimes repulsive tasks involved in caring for the sick were certainly no inducement to anyone to go into nursing as a wage-earning activity, especially when industry opened up much more rewarding positions.

John Howard in the eighteenth century had shocked the upper classes with his book *Hospitals and Lazarettos*. Dorothea Lynde Dix (1802–87), in England and the United States, mounted a personal campaign which eventually achieved the transfer of the mentally ill from brutality and negligence in penal institutions to psychiatric hospitals with more appropriate nursing facilities. Elizabeth Gurney Fry (1780–1845), an English Quaker, organized the Society of Protestant Sisters of Charity in 1840, which attempted to send nurses into the homes of the sick whether poor or rich. Theodor Fliedner (1800–64), a Lutheran minister in Germany, and his wife Frederika were influenced by Fry's work. In 1835 they established a modest hospital in Kaiserswerth, staffed without pay by the deaconesses of his church, in which the character, health, and education of nurses achieved a high standard.

Others, too, attempted to better the lot of the sick by upgrading hospitals and nurses, but it was Florence Nightingale (1820–1910), with a virtually single-minded sense of mission to make over nursing, who was the motivating force that led toward a truly professional status for nurses. Her interest was not to establish a feminist movement but, rather, to provide more highly skilled and humane treatment of the ill. She nursed her grandmother through a terminal illness, as well as the tenants on her father's estate, but her first formal exposure to medicine was a three-month course of training at Kaiserswerth, with the deaconesses.

Her experiences in various charitable institutions, during which she wrote critical reports of the needs of hospitals, were finally crowned with the assignment by Sidney Herbert, the secretary of war, to take a contingent of Catholic, Anglican, and secular nurses to Scutari to care for the British wounded in the Crimean War. Miss Nightingale found conditions in the overcrowded military hospitals appalling: miles of dirty beds, no facilities or equipment with which to care for or properly feed the soldiers, and a mortality rate which at times reached over forty percent.

Although most of Miss Nightingale's hours were spent in organizing, directing, and writing, the soldiers quickly responded to her obvious concern for their welfare. "We lay there by the hundreds; but we could kiss her shadow as it fell and lay our heads on the pillow again content." Intense opposition to her by local military officials evaporated gradually in the face of ever-increasing casualties and deaths. Her presence and administrative genius during the years 1854 and 1855 saved the hospital from total demoralization. After the war, in renewing her fight to reform the military system, she was responsible for the establishment of the first military medical school and also for many other innovations which made military barracks safer and more sanitary. She also had many rebuffs and disappointments along with her successes. When Secretary of War Sidney Herbert was about to die in 1861, he said to his wife, "Poor Florence, poor Florence, our joint work unfinished."

In civilian life, hers was also the moving spirit and architectural mind behind the reconstruction of St. Thomas's Hospital and its founding as an educational institution for nurses, whose first class was graduated in 1861. Miss Nightingale's energies and writings were in large measure responsible for the transformation of

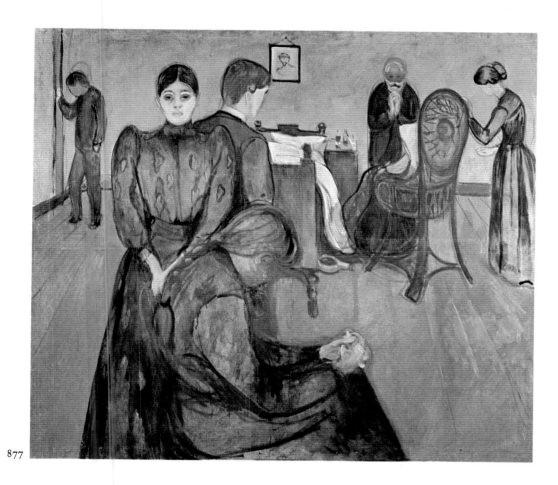

877

874 *Photograph of the Visiting Nurse on her rounds (1895). Department of Health, City of New York*

875 *Kaiserswerth Hospital, Germany (c. 1830), one of the first hospitals to train nurses systematically. Kaiserswerth Institute, Düsseldorf*

876 *Florence Nightingale, the motivating force leading to professional status for nurses. National Library of Medicine, Bethesda*

877 Death in the Sick Chamber *(c. 1892) by Edvard Munch. Nasjonalgalleriet, Oslo*

878 *Engraving from* Harper's Weekly *(1860) showing conditions in Bellevue Hospital, New York. Museum of the City of New York*

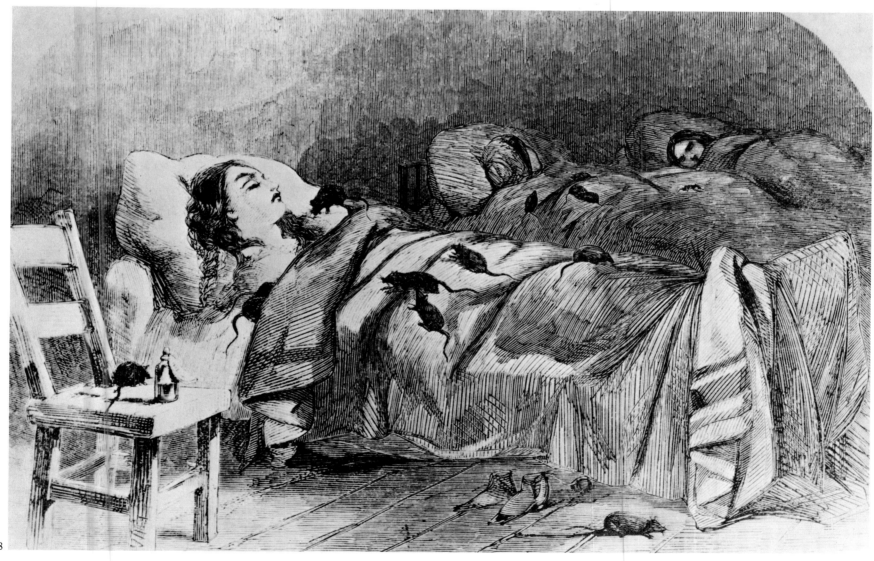

878

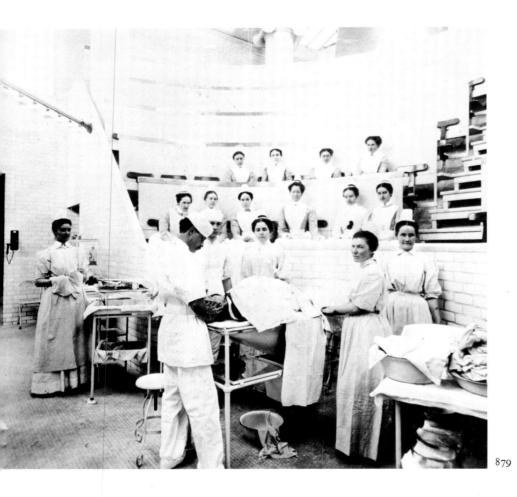

879

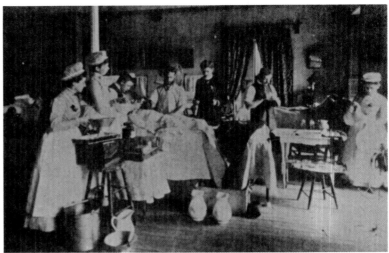

880

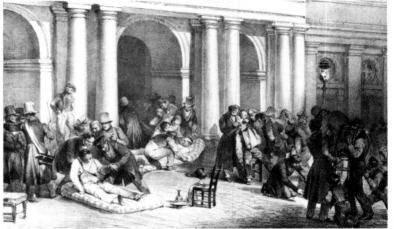

881

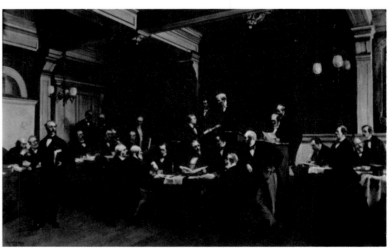

882

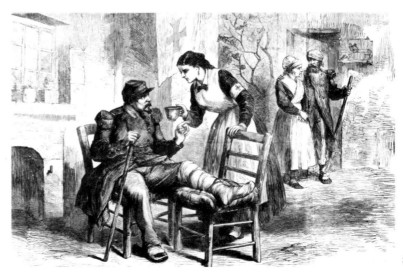

883

879 *Observing an operation was part of a nurse's training at St. Luke's Hospital in 1899. Museum of the City of New York*

880 *Carefully dressed in uniforms introduced in 1876, nurses take part in operation in a ward of Bellevue Hospital (c. 1880). Medical Communications, Inc.*

881 *Emergency treatment in the Court of the Palais Royal, Paris, during the July Revolution, 1830. National Library of Medicine, Bethesda*

882 *Painting by Edouard Armand-Dumaresq of* The Signing of the Geneva Convention for Protection of Prisoners, Wounded, and the Red Cross in Wartime, *1864. American Red Cross Archives, Washington, D.C.*

883 *Wood engraving,* Cared For, *from* Harper's Weekly *(Jan. 21, 1871), illustrating reports on nursing work done by the Red Cross. National Library of Medicine, Bethesda*

nursing from a low, unpopular, almost casual endeavor into a highly respected, essential part of the healing arts. However, her crusade was not without its personal cost. Worn down by resentment, bickering, and exhausting activity, she had a number of illnesses that probably were largely nervous breakdowns. Her health had remained fragile ever since she contracted a serious febrile illness (probably typhus or typhoid) in the Crimea; nevertheless, she continued to write intensively and to exert considerable influence.

Not all of the opposition to Miss Nightingale was merely personal. Even in the twentieth century, some leaders of nursing believe that the Nightingale focus on bedside care to the virtual exclusion of more scientific methods of teaching and practicing is too narrow. Curiously, she was not convinced that bacteria caused disease and continued to hold the ancient belief in "miasmas" as responsible. But she preached the necessity for cleanliness and saw clearly that the separation of maternity patients from sick people in a hospital was essential to their safe care. Her basic tenets are still cogent: "The art is that of nursing the sick. Please mark, not nursing sickness. . . . This is the reason why nursing proper can only be taught at the patient's bedside and in the sick room or ward. Lectures and books are but valuable accessories."

The Red Cross

Since the sixteenth century, many agreements had been mutually arrived at by opposing forces regarding the treatment of prisoners and the wounded, but in practice these rules were rarely followed. During the military action of the combined forces of France and Italy against Austrian troops in 1859, Jean Henri Dunant (1828–1910), a Swiss banker, happened to visit the scene of battle at Solferino in northern Italy after the fighting had ceased. The pitiable condition of the tens of thousands of wounded soldiers still lying unattended on the ground so aroused him that he immediately set about persuading the victorious French commanders to free the captured Austrian military surgeons to help care for the injured of all three nations. Dunant himself pitched in to try to save as many lives as possible. "*Tutti fratelli*" (all brothers) he kept repeating when local civilians resisted helping the enemy wounded. His book, *Un Souvenir de Solverino*, published three years later, shocked European leaders into action. Writers such as Victor Hugo, the Goncourt brothers, and Joseph Ernest Renan took up the cry for international humanitarianism. In the second of two international conferences, the Geneva Convention of 1864, sixteen nations signed a treaty establishing the International Red Cross and specifying the regulations that should apply to the treatment of wounded soldiers, which included the recognition that all hospitals, military and civilian, were to be neutral territory; that medical personnel of any country, and their equipment, were to be free from seizure or molestation. The protective insignia was to be a red cross on a white field (the reverse of the Swiss flag). The new spirit passed its first test in 1866 when a group of volunteer civilian students entered the battlefield to care for the Austrian wounded after the battle of Königgrätz. Austria, which had withheld its signature from the original convention, immediately joined.

Dunant lost his fortune—some say because of lavish expenditures in founding the Red Cross—and in 1867 he was bankrupt. After dropping out of sight for about fifteen years, he was discovered in a small home for the aged in Switzerland, poor in resources and unstable of mind. In 1901 when he received the first Nobel Peace Prize (together with Frédéric Passy), he donated the entire sum to charity.

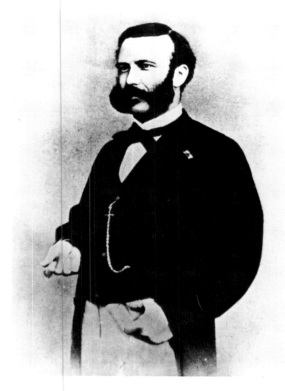

884

884 *Jean Henri Dunant, Swiss national who founded the Red Cross and made its symbol the reverse of his flag. American Red Cross Archives, Washington, D.C.*

Infection

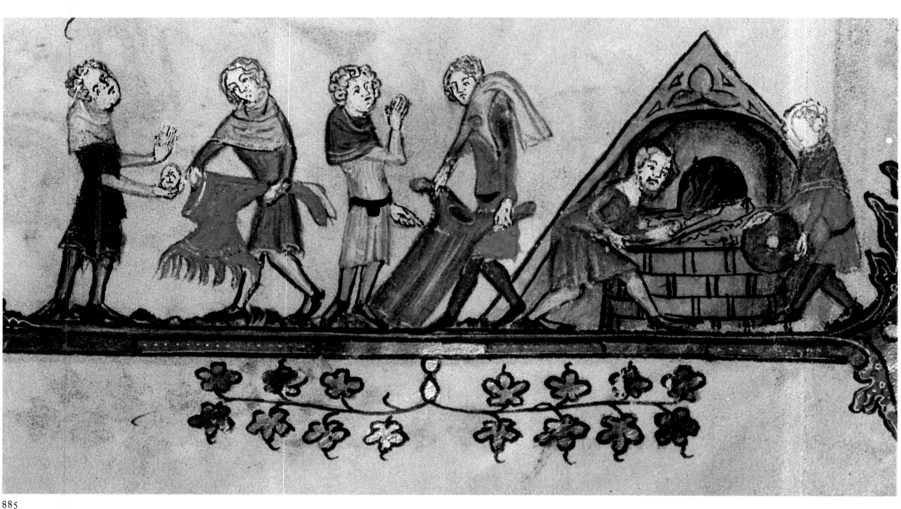

885

THE firm knowledge that bacteria were causes of diseases and were the transmissible agents responsible for contagion was acquired in the nineteenth century, but the idea that there were tiny creatures which could produce illness had been held for thousands of years. Varro, in the first century B.C., had said that swampy land was dangerous because "certain minute animals, invisible to the eye, breed there, and borne of the air reach the inside of the body by way of the mouth and cause disease." In the Middle Ages, shunning lepers, fleeing from areas of pestilence, and segregating the severely ill all represented an awareness that diseases could be transmitted. In the sixteenth century, Fracastoro demonstrated extraordinary perception in his assumption that there were "seeds" in the environment which could multiply in the body and produce disease. His contemporary Giralamo Cardano reasoned that these "seeds of disease" were live creatures. Athanasius Kircher, a Jesuit cleric of the seventeenth century in Rome, saw through a crude, early microscope that vinegar and sour milk contained "worms" and that the blood of people who died of the plague harbored animalcula.

LIVING ORGANISMS

Among the early proofs that living organisms could cause disease was the discovery of harmful parasites and fungi. In 1589 Thomas Moffet made accurate drawings of lice, fleas, and mites. He even described the mite which caused scabies and advised combating it with sulfur, a medication that remained the effective treatment for centuries. Moffet also discovered the disease which infects silkworms hundreds of years before Pasteur, but his reports were ignored.

The discoveries of Leeuwenhoek in the seventeenth century had led to the microscopic observation of other heretofore unseen creatures, but they were regarded as incidental findings. Furthermore, many fantastic tiny creatures were imagined rather than seen under the early microscopes, so the possible association of microscopic animalcula with illness was for the most part shrugged off.

Evidence slowly began to accumulate. When Agostino Bassi of Lodi (1773–1856) in the late eighteenth century linked a disease in the silkworm with a fungal parasite (*Botrytis paradoxa*), he enlarged his views to suggest that many contagious diseases such as smallpox, typhus, plague, and cholera were also due to live organisms—as yet undiscovered. Jacob Henle in the mid-nineteenth century deduced from earlier published reports that living organisms were indeed the causes of infections. In promulgating a series of precise requirements for a specific organism to be considered the causative agent, he antedated by several decades the postulates of his pupil Robert Koch. He even theorized that the parasites which caused the contagious illnesses were probably plants, and bacteria have been so classified until very recently.

The first studies of the pathogenic nature of bacteria were on a relatively large-sized and easily seen bacterium, the bacillus (rod-shape) of anthrax, a fatal disease in sheep and horses. Casimir Davaine and Pierre Rayer in 1850 produced the deadly disease in healthy animals by injecting them with the blood of dying sheep. They subsequently found the anthrax organism in the blood of the sheep so killed. Others were able to repeat and confirm the experiments.

SPONTANEOUS GENERATION

The ancient view that life could arise from inanimate substance was still a widely held concept in the nineteenth century, for it seemed logical to believe that maggots commonly found in decaying matter were hatched through fermentation and putrefaction. When bacteria were seen under the microscope to be ever-present in sour milk and spoiled meat, it appeared rational to assume that they similarly arose as a result of chemical processes. Even though scientists in the seventeenth century had discovered that maggots came from eggs deposited in rotting matter by adult

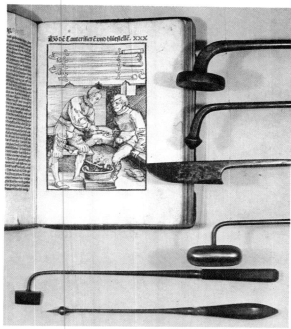

886

885 *Although the nature and causes of infectious diseases such as plagues were unknown before the 19th century, this medieval manuscript illustration indicates an understanding that contagion could be fought by burning the clothes of those infected. Ms. Bodleian 264, fol. 83 r., Bodleian Library, Oxford*

886 *Selection of medical cauterizing instruments used from the end of the Middle Ages to the beginning of the 19th century, shown in front of illustration of usage from Hans von Gersdorff,* Feldtbuch der Wundartzney *(1540). Semmelweis Medical Historical Museum, Budapest*

887

887 *Title page of the poem* Syphilis. Sive Morbus
Gallicus *(1530), by Girolamo Fracastoro, from which
the disease got its name. Fracastoro was the first
clearly to attribute the spread of disease to living
organisms, even summarizing the methods of transmission. National Library of Medicine, Bethesda*

888 *Unwelcome wherever they paused, lepers were
kept moving, announcing their approach with
rattles and begging for support along the way, as seen
in this engraving (1608) by Jan Visscher.
Bibliothèque Royale Albert 1er, Brussels*

889 *Illustration from* Harper's Weekly *(Sept. 11,
1858) showing rioters attacking a quarantine hospital
for "breeding pestilence . . . occasioning every year
yellow fever panics which inflicted severe injury
on the trade of the port." Museum of the City of
New York*

890 *Engraving of a street scene in Jersey City, N.J.,
during a smallpox scare when vaccination was made
compulsory. National Library of Medicine,
Bethesda*

insects, opinion was still strong that they were generated by fermentation and putrefaction. In the eighteenth century, Lazaro Spallanzani clearly proved that no organisms could develop in a sealed flask of liquid heated long enough to destroy any living creature, but belief in spontaneous generation remained rooted in scientific thought. In the early nineteenth century, Theodor Schwann concluded that the chemical processes of fermentation and putrefaction were themselves the result of activity by the live organisms. It is interesting that commercial producers of food and wine made practical use of these ideas long before scientists appreciated their implications.

CONTAGION AND BIOLOGIC PREVENTION OF DISEASE

Although belief in religious and supernatural causes and cures for disease was predominant among ancient peoples, many realized that some illnesses could be transmitted or even prevented by nonreligious means. For instance, the Indians and the Chinese learned that purposely contracting a mild case of some diseases could confer a resistance to subsequent occurrences of the illness. This seemed to indicate that disease could be passed from person to person without divine intervention. Centuries later a battle developed in Europe and the United States between those who believed that diseases were definitely contagious and those who ascribed epidemic illnesses to causes such as environmental change and internal bodily derangements. The controversy reached its height in the eighteenth century.

The anticontagionists, who numbered among them some outstanding scientists and physicians, had noticed that quarantine was not convincingly successful and that an epidemic such as yellow fever was often terminated by a change in the weather. Furthermore, they observed that even people in contact with yellow fever victims did not necessarily contract the disease. (They did not know that mosquitoes were responsible for transmitting the infective agent or that their absence in winter ended the threat of being bitten and infected.) In addition, the apparently spectacular cures of yellow fever with drastic purges reported by Benjamin Rush in the American colonies convinced many that contagious infective organisms could not be the cause. Indeed, had not other completely different causes of disease been proved, such as a dietary insufficiency in scurvy? The fact that epidemics were most frequent in the crowded conditions of slums was interpreted by the anticontagionists as additional evidence that the environment was the prime cause—unhealthy air, poor food, polluted water—rather than living creatures. On the other hand, the spectacular results of inoculations to prevent smallpox were a strong, added argument in favor of those who believed disease to be transmissible. Edward Jenner had introduced the new concept of creating an immunity to a dangerous disease by producing an entirely different mild illness through vaccination. Therefore, as innovative as Pasteur's work was to be and as skeptical as many scientists were, the use of biological methods to prevent disease had already entered the atmosphere of medicine.

ASEPSIS AND SEMMELWEIS

Nevertheless, even those who accepted the principle that disease could be transmitted from person to person apparently failed to see the connection between contagion and the gangrenous complications of surgical wounds or the fatal childbed (puerperal) fever. In the eighteenth century, Charles White of England and Joseph Clarke and Robert Collins of Ireland had sharply reduced the occurrence of postpartum sepsis (infection) by regimens of personal and environmental cleanliness, limited vaginal examinations during labor, and active cleansing of beds and linen. Yet virtually no one seems to have continued these practices. Even when Oliver Wendell Holmes in 1843 attributed puerperal fever to infections carried to the new mother by obstetricians from other infected persons, most physicians regarded this

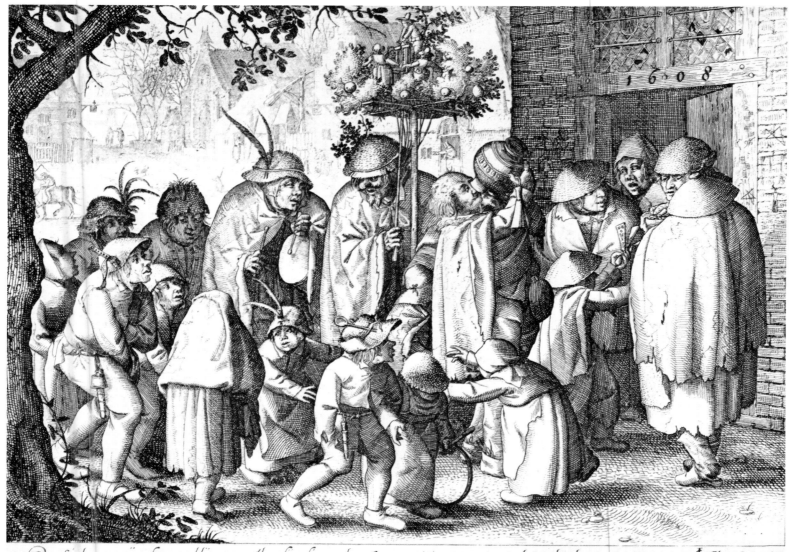

De Sieckgens zijn seer verblijt = Als sy sien de Copper tijt = om te maken de kanne = wan   Visscher. Inventor.
De Trommel sy dan reppen = met de clappen sy cleppen = en spelen oock met Iamie = man   fecit. et excudebat.

888

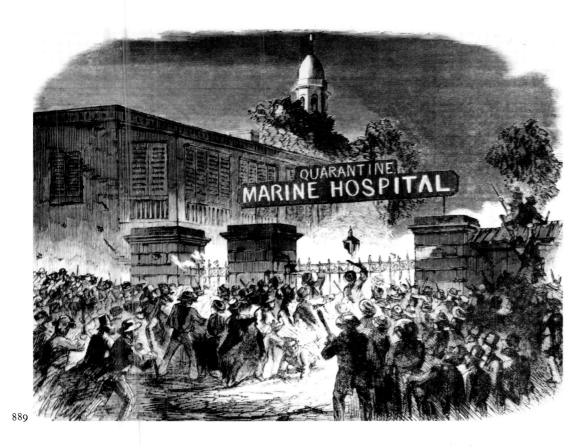

889

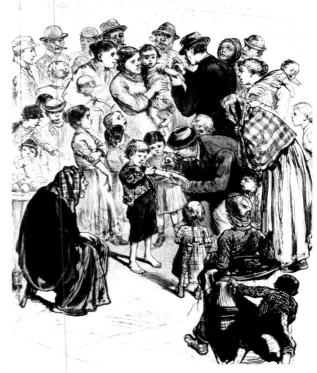

890

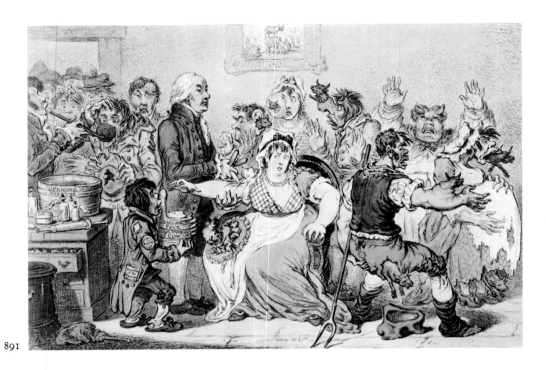

891

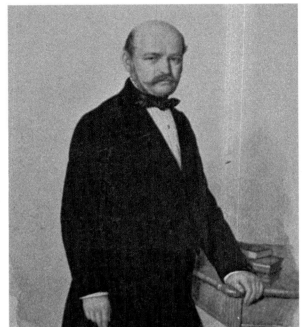

892

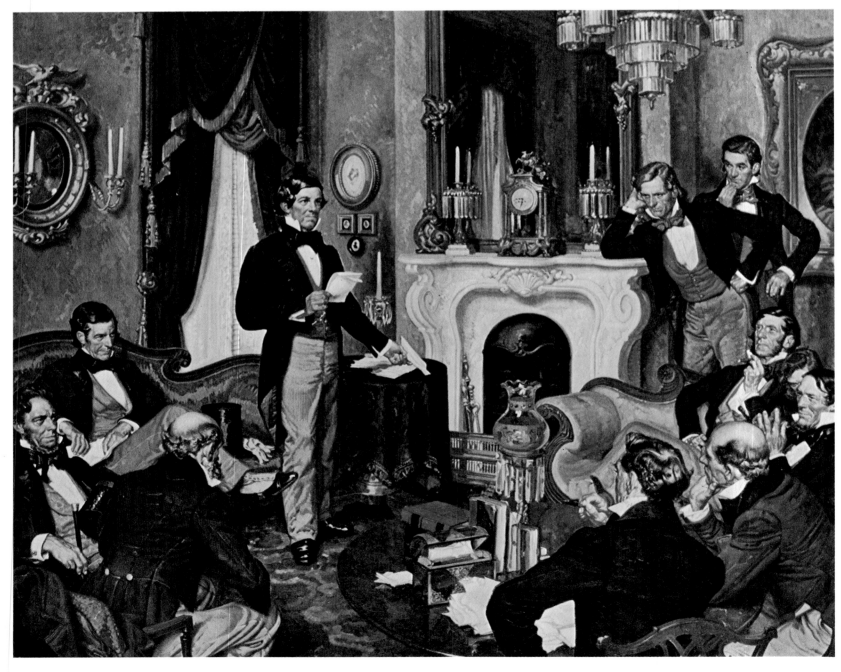

893

as impractical theorizing without proof. It was Ignaz Semmelweis (1818–65), in keeping with the new statistical spirit of the nineteenth century, who assembled the facts and analyzed the happenings on the obstetrical wards of the Allgemeines Krankenhaus in Vienna to prove the contagious nature of postpartum infection.

He noted that the annual mortality rate on one of the wards where medical students were trained was over ten percent and that it reached almost twenty percent during some months—chiefly due to puerperal fever. On the ward where midwives received instruction, the deaths never even reached as high as three percent. Ignoring the seemingly obvious conclusion that staff skills on the second ward were therefore superior, he discovered that the doctors and students usually came to the ward to examine patients directly from the autopsy room. In contrast, the midwives and their teachers on the second ward participated in clinical instruction without attending the autopsies. Furthermore, he noted that the women who came down with infections were usually in a row of beds conforming to the routine of examination that day. The suspicions of Semmelweis were further confirmed when he viewed the autopsy of his colleague Kolletschka, who had died of an infection from a scalpel wound sustained while performing an autopsy on a puerperal fever victim. His friend's organs showed the same changes as seen in the bodies of those dead of postpartum infection.

The next step for Semmelweis was clear: to require the physicians and students under his charge to scrub hands with soap and water and soak them in a chlorinated lime solution before entering the clinic or ward, and to repeat this after each examination. Despite complaints, he persisted in his demands. Over the next few months, the eighteen percent obstetrical death rate declined startlingly to a low of one and two-tenths percent. One might have expected the hospital staff immediately to have embarked upon a similar regimen, or, at the very least, to have tested the conclusions further by repeating the clinical experiment. Instead, the chief of service, apparently for reasons of personal antagonism, condemned Semmelweis, arranged to have him lowered in rank, and further limited his practicing privileges. When he reported his results to the Medical Society of Vienna, his paper was greeted with virulent attacks. Although some outstanding medical scientists and practitioners, such as Rokitansky in pathology, Skoda in medicine, and Hebra in dermatology, supported Semmelweis, he was too deeply hurt to remain in Vienna and returned to Budapest, where his methods effected a marked diminution in mortality rates. Indeed, Semmelweis may be credited with having for the first time constructed a statistically tested system of asepsis (keeping germs away from the patient) before the germ theory had arrived.

When he finally completed a book, *Die Aetiologie der Begriff und die Prophylaxis des Kindbettfiebers*, in 1861, ten years after his original discoveries, the profession hardly took notice, and prestigious scientists like the great Virchow actually opposed his ideas. The brilliant, intense, and sensitive Semmelweis ultimately was broken by the indifference and callousness of his superiors and colleagues. Committed to an asylum, he died in 1865 of a blood infection, virtually the same kind of illness that had stricken the mothers he had tried to save.

ANTISEPSIS AND LISTER

In contrast to Semmelweis, Joseph Lister (1827–1912) had the advantages of a prestigious position in Glasgow, an intellectual climate already modified by works on infection and germs, an ability to present views in a simple manner, and an equanimity that enabled him to continue on his course undeterred by criticism.

Among the variety of substances used on wounds from earliest times, some like wine and turpentine were probably antiseptic in effect while others no doubt contributed to infection. Pus was generally the expected concomitant of wounds, but there was virtually no understanding of how it was produced. Simpson of St. Andrews in the eighteenth century had realized that pus came in some way from

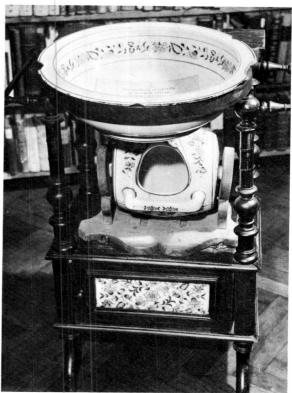

894

891 *The vaccination technique of Edward Jenner did not meet with unalloyed approval, as evident in this print by James Gillray entitled* The Cow Pock—or—the wonderful effects of the new inoculation ! (*1802*). *National Library of Medicine, Bethesda*

892 *Portrait of Ignaz Semmelweis, in 1857, who, 30 years before Pasteur discovered that bacteria caused disease, realized that fatal fevers after childbirth were caused by contamination on doctors' hands. Semmelweis Medical Historical Museum, Budapest*

893 *Artist's visualization of Oliver Wendell Holmes reading his celebrated essay* The Contagiousness of Puerperal Fever *before the Boston Society for Medical Improvement in 1843. Wyeth Laboratories, Philadelphia*

894 *Basin and stand used by Ignaz Semmelweis to scrub his hands before examining each patient, a precaution he required of his staff which lowered the obstetrical death rate dramatically. World Health Organization, Geneva*

895 *Illustration of "air purifier" on ward cart from "On Some of the Causes Which Render the Air in Surgical Wards Impure"* (American Journal of Medical Science, 1867) *by Thomas G. Morton. National Library of Medicine, Bethesda*

896 *Sixteenth-century woodcut by Jonas Arnold showing a Caesarean operation, which for centuries carried a high risk of infection. National Library of Medicine, Bethesda*

897 *Wood engraving from William Watson Cheyne,* Antiseptic Surgery *(1882) depicting use of Lister carbolic spray as antiseptic precaution during an operation. National Library of Medicine, Bethesda*

898 *Thirty-five years after Lister's reports, there was still insufficient concern for sterile conditions in many operating rooms, as can be seen in this photograph (c. 1901) of Dr. John Allan Wyeth operating. Museum of the City of New York*

899 *Photograph (c. 1890) of the operating room at St. Luke's Hospital, St. Paul, Minnesota, showing nurses gowned and capped but no one wearing gloves. Minnesota Historical Society, St. Paul*

900 *Photograph showing William Stewart Halsted, the leading surgical teacher of his time, performing an operation. Halsted was responsible for many innovations, including the wearing of rubber gloves by nurses and surgeons. Medical Communications, Inc.*

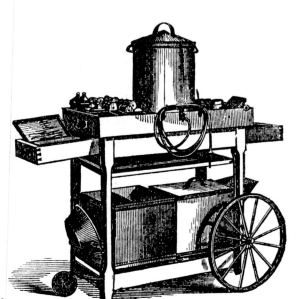

895

capillaries, and Julius Cohnheim (1839–84) later proved that white blood cells (pus cells) indeed migrated out through the walls of tiny blood vessels into inflamed tissues. However, these and other reports gave no hint that the inflammations and putrefactions which brought forth pus could be due to agents passed from person to person.

Lister noticed that broken bones over which the skin was intact usually healed without complication, but fractures where bone was exposed through breaks in the skin commonly developed infections and the drainage of pus. He saw the frequent severe infections attending other operations, such as amputations, as additional evidence that something circulating in the air was responsible—possibly invisible particles which he called "disease dust." When the work of Pasteur in 1860 was brought to his attention by Thomas Anderson, he appreciated the connection between his own observations on wounds and the microscopic bacteria involved in fermentation. Whereas Pasteur used heat to sterilize, Lister sprayed carbolic acid over the patient during an operation to kill any bacteria before they could grow in the wound. In 1867 he published a report in the *Lancet* of his experiences with eleven cases, and he gave full credit to Pasteur's work.

As had happened with Semmelweis, Lister's reports were received with either indifference or open hostility. In the United States, where Lister went to present his views, surgeons remained generally unconvinced as late as the 1880s. Nine years after Lister's publication, Samuel Gross (1805–84), the virtually unchallenged leader of American surgery, could write, "Little if any faith is placed by any enlightened or experienced surgeon on this side of the Atlantic in the so-called carbolic acid treatment of Professor Lister."

Many European and American surgeons failed to see the implications of the revelation that infections in wounds came from something foreign introduced at operation: that these invaders should be eliminated or excluded. Instead they focused on the antiseptic itself (carbolic acid) and the mechanics of its use in sprays and soaks, thereby missing entirely the main concept. Yet, almost subconsciously surgeons had absorbed Lister's principles of keeping out germs. B. A. Watson of New Jersey could later say, "We find scarcely a wound treated in the United States today but what some part of Listerism is adopted."

Perhaps the first prominent support of Lister's theories came from Saxtorph of Copenhagen in 1870. Surgeons in the German-speaking countries also readily recognized the part played by bacteria in infection and saw the importance of asepsis and antisepsis. Among the notable surgeons who followed the methods of Lister were Von Volkmann, Von Langenbeck, Czerny, and Von Miculicz. Billroth, one of the greatest innovators and teachers of surgery, did not believe that bacteria were important in wound infections but was willing to use the Listerian system after seeing that it yielded consistently better results.

French surgeons also subscribed to the new doctrine relatively early, so that in 1876 Lucas Championnière could write, "A few years ago Paris hospitals were reckoned among the very worst, even by some of their own surgeons. Now surgery may be carried out in them as anywhere else." Increasing numbers of surgeons in other countries took up the system. Some who observed strict rules of cleanliness nevertheless denied the role of germs. Lawson Tait in England, while criticizing the antiseptic carbolic methods and denigrating the germ theory of disease, nevertheless observed strict rules of cleanliness in what came to be called the "aseptic" (killing or excluding germs before they enter a wound) system, as opposed to the "antiseptic" (killing or removing germs after they have entered). It was Lister's great contribution to emphasize in the minds of surgeons the necessity for getting and keeping wounds free of contamination.

The employment of rubber gloves in operations was an innovation of the early twentieth century. When William Halsted introduced them to protect the hands of his operating-room nurse (whom he later married), one of his students suggested their use by operators too, since they could be sterilized. At first the

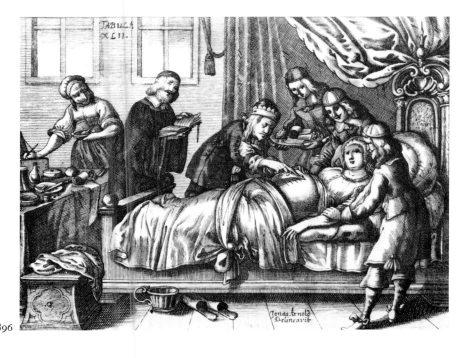

896

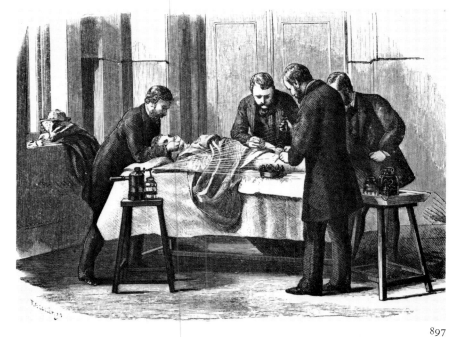

897

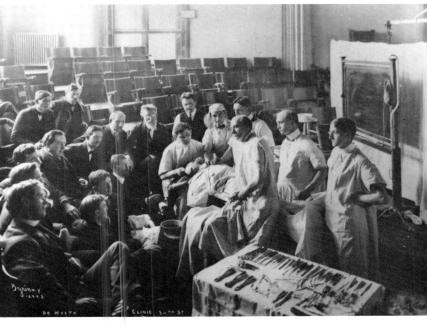

898

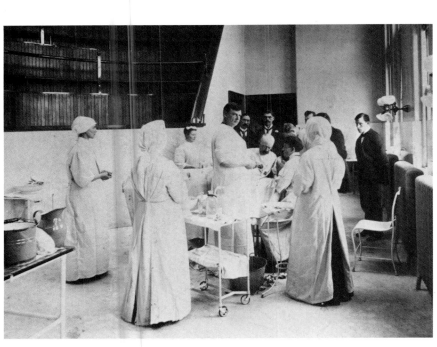

899

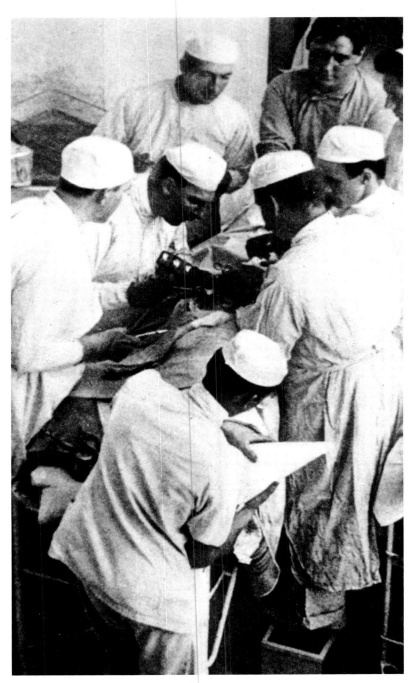

900

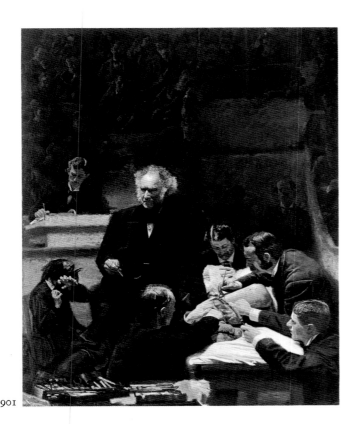

901 The Gross Clinic (1875) by Thomas Eakins
portrays the outstanding American surgeon Samuel
Gross, who put little faith in Lister's principles.
His assistants wear no gowns, and a member of the
patient's family sits nearby. Jefferson Medical
College, Philadelphia

902 Microscopic slides showing (top to bottom):
anthrax bacillus, the first bacterium actually seen and
identified; gas gangrene; diphtheria bacillus;
tubercle bacillus, the cause of tuberculosis; plague;
cholera; typhoid. Drs. Edward J. Bottone and
Bruce A. Hanna, Dept. of Microbiology, Mount
Sinai Hospital, New York

gloves were relatively thick, and many surgeons refused to wear them. Even
when the rubber was made thinner, some operators, especially in Europe, wore
sterile cloth gloves over the rubber. Masks were brought in even later, and as
recently as the 1940s and 1950s many highly placed surgeons left the nose
uncovered, wearing the mask over the mouth only.

LOUIS PASTEUR

It was the monumental work of Louis Pasteur (1822–95) which simultaneously
demolished the theory of spontaneous generation, firmly established the germ
theory of disease, explained the effectiveness of the asepsis and antisepsis of
Semmelweis and Lister, and laid the basis for the biological preventive measures of
the future.

Trained as a chemist, Pasteur found himself ever more involved in biological
phenomena and thus by example demonstrated the interrelation of the branches of
science. Early in his career, at his installation as professor and dean of the faculty of
science at Lille in 1854, he stated, "In the field of observation, chance only favors
prepared minds." His own activities were to be a striking illustration of this
aphorism.

Pasteur's earlier research project in 1851 had been a major step in the
development of stereochemistry, for he proved that there were two types of
tartaric acid crystals. When he discovered that bacteria acted on each type of
crystal differently, he applied these observations to the problems of beet alcohol
production, which he was asked to investigate by a local manufacturer. The result
was not only a solution to the production difficulty but an entirely new focus for
Pasteur's energies, which was to culminate in the germ theory of disease. In rapid
order he proved that microscopic live creatures were responsible for fermentation,
and that some of these tiny organisms grew in the presence of oxygen ("aerobic")
while others lived in the absence of free oxygen ("anaerobic"). He also determined
that heating wine for a few moments at about 60°C. (108°F.) destroyed the
organisms which produced spoilage—a process later called "pasteurization."

When an epidemic in silkworms threatened to devastate the industry, he
discovered that two different diseases were responsible: pebrine, caused by infection
of the eggs, and flacherie, due to an infective intestinal organism. Weeding out the
affected eggs and removing the source of infection in the food saved the silkworm
industry not only in France but also throughout the world.

Suddenly he suffered a stroke from which he recovered only slowly and
incompletely. Having already accomplished myriad far-reaching innovations—
enough to earn him a place among the greatest scientists of history—he might well
have declared a moratorium on further work. But the most famous and useful of
his contributions were yet to come.

His next step was to study the fatal illness in sheep called anthrax ("splenic
fever"). He was able to isolate the anthrax bacillus, confirming Koch's earlier work,
but he could not see a way to prevent or treat the disease. Therefore, when he was
called to investigate the cause of chicken cholera after serious losses to poultry
farmers, he could not have foreseen that his study would lead to a means of
preventing anthrax and, more importantly, to a discovery that would
revolutionize preventive medicine.

On returning from a vacation, he found that cultures of the chicken cholera
organism prepared before he left were harmless when injected into healthy fowls,
but subsequent injections of fresh virulent cultures into the same hens failed to
produce the disease. Armed with this new knowledge, Pasteur treated cultures of
the anthrax bacillus in various ways until he found that microbes grown in a
particular temperature range became harmless without losing their capability of
producing resistance in injected animals. To test the validity of his discovery, a
public demonstration was arranged by the Melun Agricultural Society in 1881.

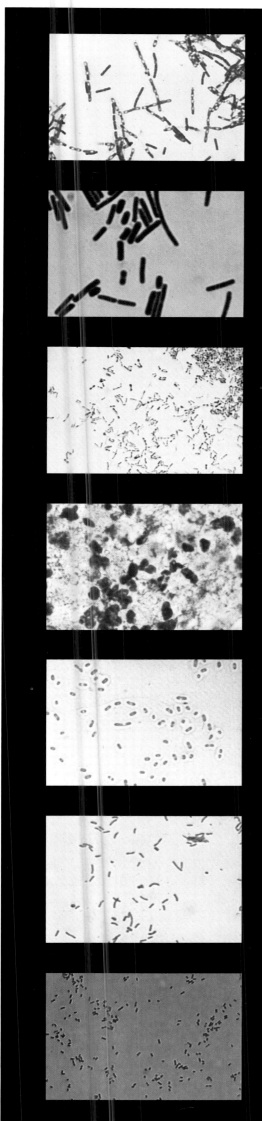

While a skeptical assemblage of physicians, veterinarians, curious citizens, and reporters looked on, virulent cultures of the anthrax bacillus were injected into normal sheep and into an equal number of sheep previously inoculated with attenuated, harmless cultures. In the next few days, all of the unprotected sheep died and all of the prepared sheep remained well. The principle of immunity was thus publicly and dramatically launched. Whereas Jenner had obtained the same protection from smallpox by producing another illness, vaccinia or cowpox, Pasteur established the fundamental principle that attenuated cultures of an organism could afford protection against the disease caused by the organism. Just as Lister had given recognition to Pasteur for his importance to antisepsis, so now Pasteur paid tribute to Jenner's work by calling his own method "vaccination."

Although it had been known that the "poison" of rabies (hydrophobia) was in the saliva of afflicted animals, Pasteur reasoned from the symptoms that it must also reside in the central nervous system. Working with the spinal cords of rabbits he confirmed his suspicions, and, extending his findings with attenuated cultures of anthrax, he developed an extract containing the offending agent of rabies in a nonvirulent form. Having developed a system of protecting rabbits by injections of extracts of more and more virulence, he awaited the chance to apply the method to humans.

In 1885 a young boy named Joseph Meister, who had been bitten by a rabid dog, was brought to him. Pasteur first consulted two physicians who agreed that the boy's outlook was hopeless. One can well understand his caution, for today such a course of action with an untried medication containing dangerous constituents would be unthinkable. But Pasteur proceeded. As the virulence of the injections was increased, he watched ever more closely for signs of rabies, which would have developed in three to six weeks. When the boy remained well after the final inoculation with an extract that ordinarily was rapidly fatal to rabbits, Pasteur knew that his hypotheses and experiments had been correct. The success of the antirabies inoculation gained him widespread public acclaim, for it represented the first time that Pasteur's methods had been applied directly to humans.

From then on, bacteriology and immunology followed an ever-widening course. Pierre-Paul-Émile Roux (1853–1933), Pasteur's pupil, reported finding a filterable virus (one that passes through the finest filters). Together with Alexandre-Émile Yersin (1863–1943) he isolated the diphtheria bacillus and developed an antitoxin. More and more bacteria were discovered, numbers of vaccines and antisera were produced, and the mechanisms of prevention became increasingly clarified.

ROBERT KOCH

While practicing as a country physician, Robert Koch (1843–1910) used his spare moments to begin studies on microorganisms. By the time of his death, he had revolutionized bacteriology, established the sporulation and pathogenic character of the anthrax bacillus, developed and refined techniques of culturing bacteria, advanced the method of steam sterilization, discovered the causes of many diseases (including wound infections, cholera, Egyptian ophthalmia, and sleeping sickness), and introduced effective preventive measures in typhoid fever, plague, malaria, and other diseases. Perhaps his two most influential contributions were the isolation of the tubercle bacillus, the cause of tuberculosis, and the establishment of the essential steps ("Koch's postulates") required to prove that an organism is the cause of disease. His studies with tuberculin (a filtrate from the culture of the tubercle bacillus) convinced Koch and the world that he had found the means of curing tuberculosis, but its subsequent failures were a severe blow to him. However, Koch's tuberculin is still used as a diagnostic tool.

Ferdinand Cohn (1828–98) of the University of Breslau helped to establish the science of bacteriology through his techniques and concepts, including a definitive

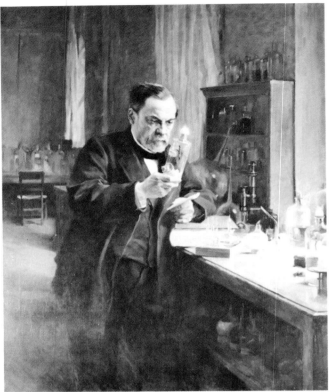

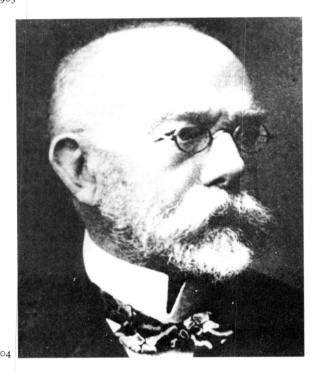

903 *Portrait by Albert-Gustaf Edelfelt of Louis Pasteur in his laboratory. Pasteur demolished the theory of spontaneous generation, explained the basis for contagion, and introduced rational planning for developing immunity. Musée Pasteur, Institut Pasteur, Paris*

904 *Photograph of Robert Koch, 1905 Nobel Prize winner for his discoveries in relation to tuberculosis. World Health Organization, Geneva*

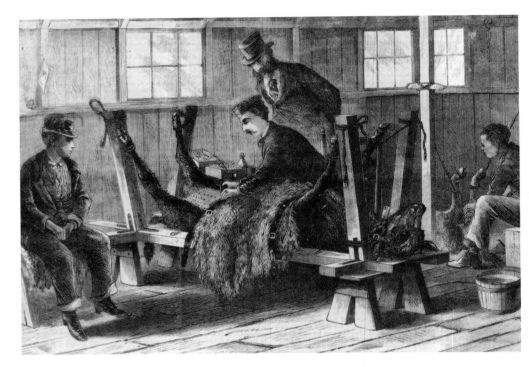

classification of bacteria. He also gave vigorous support to Davaine, Koch, and others who worked in the field. So many other contributors to microbiology have followed in the nineteenth and twentieth centuries that merely listing the names would fill a volume.

In the last decade of the nineteenth century, two especially important additions were made to the understanding of infections: the development of antitoxins and the discovery of viruses.

After Yersin and Roux had found that the toxins produced by the bacteria of diphtheria—not the microorganism itself—could cause the damage to the body that made up the clinical picture, other bacterial diseases were similarly studied. The independent proofs by Von Behring and Kitasato that the body manufactured circulating substances which acted against the toxins prompted Von Behring to obtain neutralizing antitoxic sera from the blood of animals injected with intermittent doses of the toxins. This use of antitoxic sera in treating diseases was called "passive immunization" by Paul Ehrlich, in contradistinction to "active immunization" by inoculating attenuated cultures of the pathogenic organism or its toxin to call forth protecting antibodies. Jenner's vaccination against smallpox and Pasteur's antirabies inoculations were examples of the active production of immunity.

The recognition of antibodies in the blood of a person sick with an infection became useful in diagnosis: finding the specific antibody against a particular germ in the blood determined which organism was the cause. Because of the obvious part played by the circulating toxins and antitoxins, the importance of biologically produced chemical substances appeared to overshadow the role of cells in fighting disease until Elie Metchnikoff (1845–1916) proved that some cells destroyed bacteria by engulfing them (phagocytosis) and by elaborating antibodies against them, for which he was awarded a Nobel prize in 1908. The realization that humans could be carriers of the pathogenic germs of cholera, diphtheria, typhoid fever, meningitis, and dysentery without being ill themselves was also a forward step in understanding host resistance to disease and was also a significant contribution to public health.

Most of the germs responsible for illness could be seen under the microscope to be bacteria. The organisms for smallpox and rabies had not been seen, but the presence of their "poisons" had been appreciated and utilized in immunization. When Loeffler and Roux reported that there were pathogenic organisms (in a disease of cattle) which were so small that even fine filters allowed them to flow through, a new field of investigation, virology, was opened. Subsequently, other

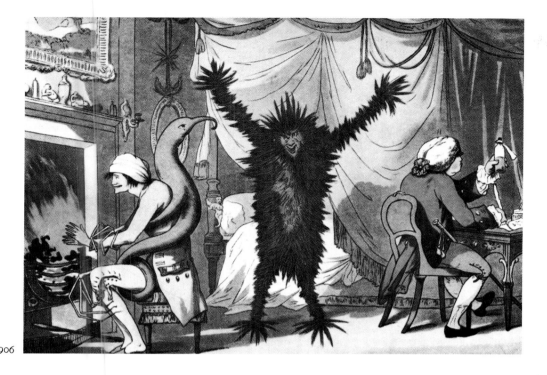

906

905 *Illustration of the method of obtaining anti-smallpox vaccine from blisters on the abdomen of a calf (1872). Department of Health, City of New York*

906 *Colored etching by Thomas Rowlandson entitled* Ague and Fever of Malaria *(1792), in which the patient is depicted in the grip of one beastly aspect of this fluctuating disease while the next waits to take hold of him. World Health Organization, Geneva*

907 *As far back as the 15th century, insects were associated with the transmission of maladies, as is indicated in this illustration from* Hortus Sanitatis *(1491). National Library of Medicine, Bethesda*

research revealed that there were also tiny microbes of a size between bacteria and viruses (named rickettsia for Howard Ricketts [1871–1910], who found the cause of Rocky Mountain spotted fever). Larger protozoan organisms were also found to produce diseases (for example, the plasmodium of malaria).

Intermediate Vectors of Disease

Studies by veterinarians and zoologists showed that some disease-producing organisms underwent life cycles in animal hosts, in the course of which they could infect humans: for instance, lice in typhus, ticks in filariasis, and the tsetse fly in sleeping sickness. The role of these intermediaries in the transmission of disease was suggested by a number of investigators, notably Patrick Manson, Theobald Smith, and F. L. Kilborne.

The mosquito as an insect vector in malaria was partially understood in the eighteenth century by Lancisi and clearly perceived by several observers in the nineteenth century—Beauperthuy of Venezuela, King in the United States, Laveran in France, Flügge and Koch in Germany. In 1880 Charles-Louis-Alphonse Laveran (1845–1922) actually demonstrated the causative organism, a protozoan, but the mechanism of transmission was not proved until fifteen years later by Ronald Ross (1857–1932), who found the parasite in the stomach of an anopheles mosquito which had imbibed the blood of a person with malaria. He was able to transfer the disease from malarial birds to healthy birds through the bites of mosquitoes. This was subsequently proved in 1898 by Grassi and collaborators in Italy also to be the mechanism of transmission to humans.

Although Beauperthuy had stated in 1853 that a mosquito carried yellow fever, Carlos Finlay (1833–1915), a Cuban physician, clearly enunciated the proposition in 1881 that the *Aëdes aegypti* was the insect vector responsible for communicating yellow fever from person to person. When yellow fever became a major problem to the United States following its occupation of Cuba after the Spanish-American War, the army sent a group to seek a solution. Walter Reed (1851–1902), the chairman, James Carroll, Jesse Lazear, and Aristides Agramonte devised human experiments to test Finlay's theory. Members of the commission itself, soldiers of the occupying force, and civilian employees volunteered as subjects. Lazear, an accidental victim of the disease, died during the investigation. The others recovered.

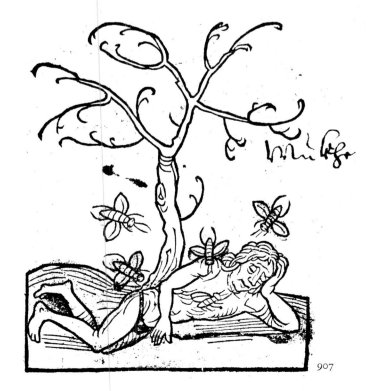

907

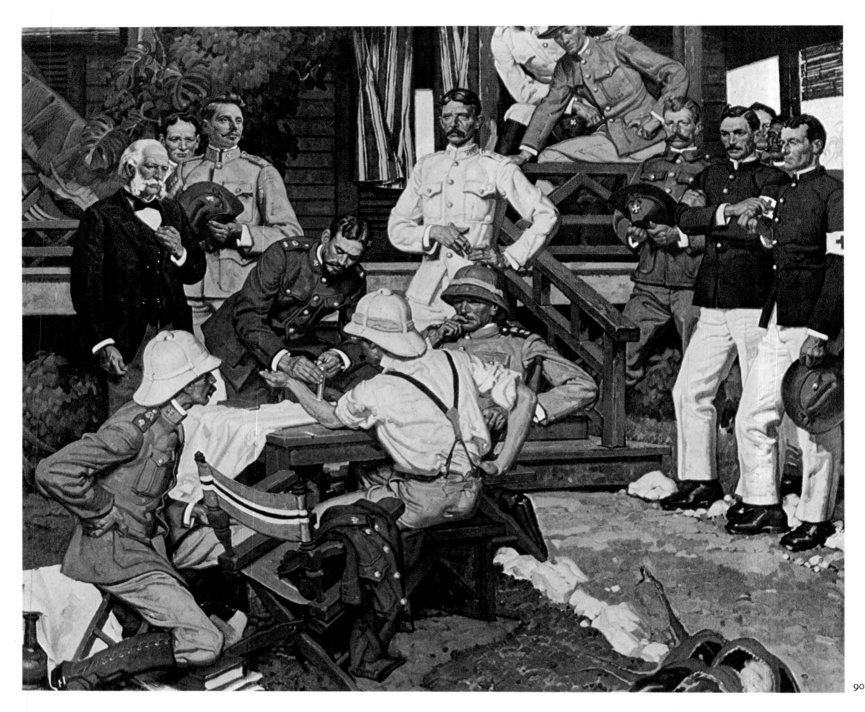

908

908 *Painting by Dean Cornwell showing Drs. Jesse Lazear, James Carroll, Carlos Finlay, and Major Walter Reed investigating the theory of mosquito-borne disease in Cuba following the Spanish-American War, Wyeth Laboratories, Philadelphia*

909 *Colored lithograph from* Puck *magazine showing "The kind of 'Assisted Emigrant' we cannot afford to admit." Collection William Helfand, New York*

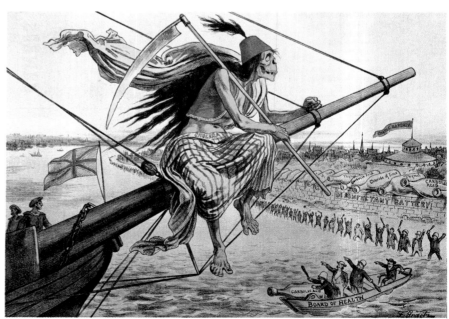

909

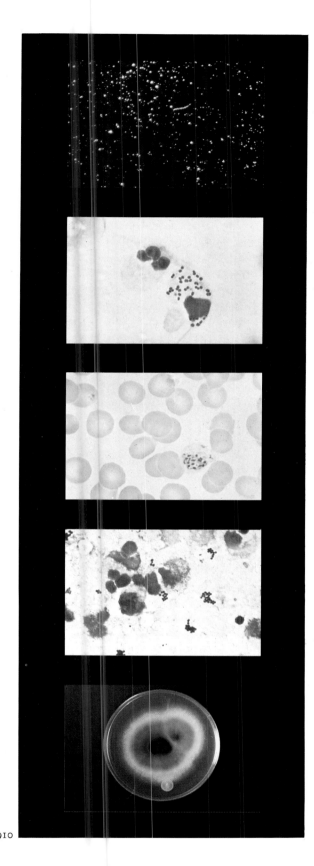

The commission reported in 1901 that the mosquito was an intermediate host of the disease, transmitting the offending organism from person to person through its bite; that the causative organism in the blood of infected humans was a filterable virus; and that the disease could be transferred only through the mosquito's bite and not by direct contact between persons. The resulting public health measures—directed to removing mosquitoes and protecting humans against the insects—eliminated yellow fever from Havana in less than a year. William Crawford Gorgas (1854–1919) was the leader of the sanitary engineering force which achieved the results.

Ehrlich and the Beginnings of Antimicrobials

The most important impetus to discovering ways of fighting microorganisms was given by the ideas and works of Paul Ehrlich (1854–1915). Through the centuries, of course, there had been a few relatively effective anti-infective agents in use, but the establishment of a discipline to seek agents against bacteria and to construct criteria for evaluating effectiveness was accomplished almost single-handedly by Ehrlich.

As a student he examined the methods of making cells visible under the microscope, and he wrote his doctoral thesis on histologic stains. From earlier investigators he took the relevant information which enabled him to develop a theory of specific affinity of cells for dyes: George Hayem's techniques of coloring living cells (vital staining); Hermann Hoffmann's stains of bacteria; the visualization by Carl Weigert of bacterial cocci in tissues. His demonstration of the staining characteristics of the white blood cells with aniline dyes allowed others to understand better the abnormalities of blood cells, thus contributing to the foundations of hematology. He also improved the methods of identifying the tubercle bacillus microscopically. Through techniques of neutralizing toxins with antitoxins in the test tube he illuminated the detection of antibodies by showing that some were heat-resistant and others heat-susceptible. His "side-chain theory," abandoned for many years, nevertheless led others to investigations of importance to immunology. Moreover, in recent decades this theory has been revived by contemporary immunologists, albeit in a more sophisticated form.

As he gained recognition, he enlarged his scope of activities even further. When Fritz Schaudinn in 1905 proved the cause of syphilis to be the *Treponema pallidum*, Ehrlich synthesized chemicals which would destroy the causative organism while sparing the patient. Salvarsan, the arsenical which he made in his laboratory in 1910 (the 606th compound tried), became the standard effective therapeutic agent. Other less toxic arsenic compounds, such as neoarsphenamine, also arose out of his work. For the first time in history the patient with syphilis had a good chance to survive and be cured.

About three decades later, the advent of the sulfonamides for the treatment of bacterial infections was a direct, though delayed, outgrowth of Ehrlich's demonstration that dyes could be antibacterial agents. When penicillin was introduced, Ehrlich's drugs against syphilis were abandoned, but he had set in motion the activities of the twentieth century that were to revolutionize the therapy of microbial diseases.

910 *Microscopic slides showing* (top to bottom): *the germs of syphilis; gonorrhea; and malaria; staphylococci, which cause abscesses;* Trichophyton rubrum, *the genus that causes scalp ringworm and athlete's foot. Drs. Edward J. Bottone and Bruce A. Hanna, Dept. of Microbiology, Mount Sinai Hospital, New York*

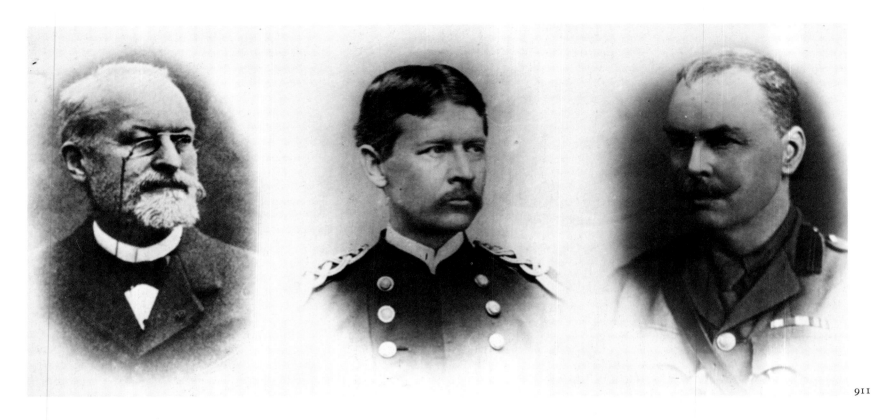

911 *Photographs (left to right) of Alphonse Laveran, who demonstrated the causative organism of malaria; Walter Reed, who proved that the mosquito was the carrier of yellow fever; Sir Ronald Ross, who identified the carrier of malaria as an Anopheles mosquito. National Library of Medicine, Bethesda*

912 *Photograph, 1905, of the fumigation of mosquito-infested sheds in New Orleans, to kill yellow-fever-carrying insects. National Library of Medicine, Bethesda*

913 *General William C. Gorgas photographed at the construction site of the Panama Canal, where his knowledge and skill in sanitation rid the area of mosquitoes. National Library of Medicine, Bethesda*

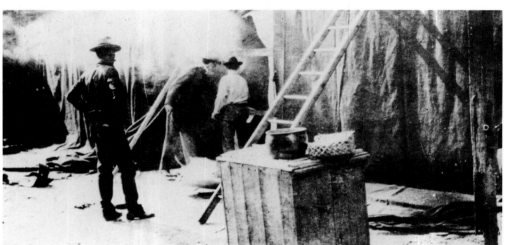

912

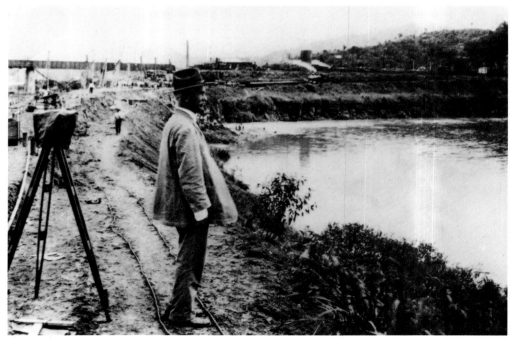

913

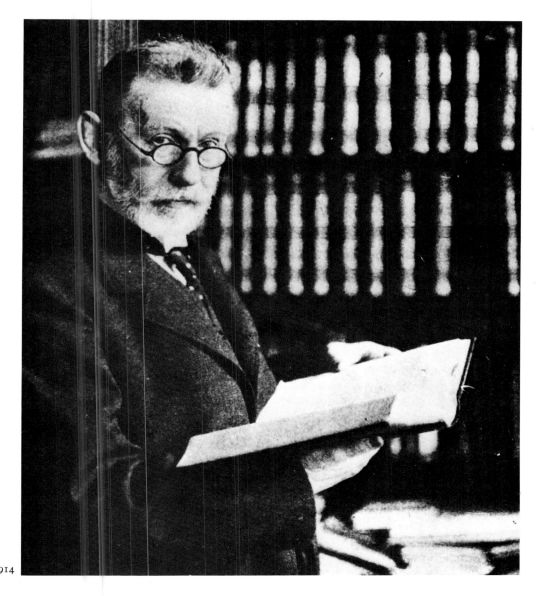

914

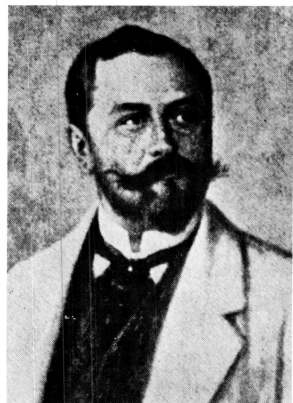

916

914 *Paul Ehrlich, 1908 Nobel Prize winner for his work in immunology, perceived that various chemicals had a special affinity for bacteria, a discovery that led to chemotherapy for infection and began the era of antimicrobials. World Health Organization, Geneva*

915 *Enlarged photograph of the yellow-fever-carrying mosquito* Aëdes aegypti, *which the Cuban physician Carlos Finlay in 1881 identified as the insect vector responsible for transmitting yellow fever from person to person. American Museum of Natural History, New York*

916 *Portrait of Fritz Schaudinn, who discovered* Treponema pallidum, *the causative agent of syphilis. World Health Organization. Geneva*

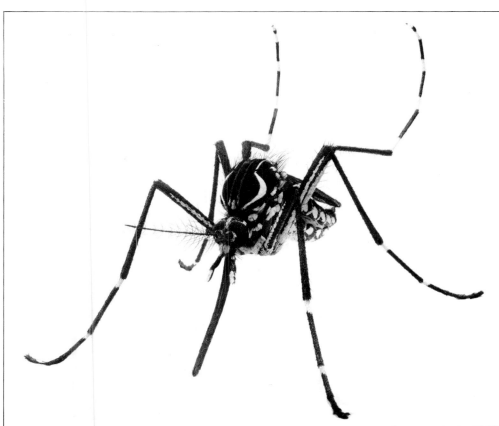

915

Women in Medicine

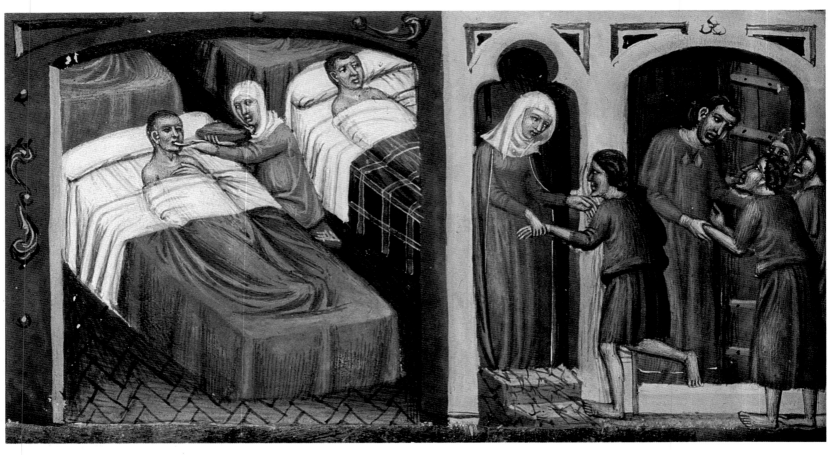

917

WOMEN finally were accepted as full-fledged medical practitioners in the nineteenth and twentieth centuries, but not without a struggle.

Of course women had been highly regarded as comforting healers for a long, long time; there probably were female practitioners in ancient Sumeria, Babylonia, Egypt, Greece, Rome, and in Pre-Columbian America. In the Middle Ages the chief medical activities of women were as midwives, but there were also skillful female doctors practicing secretly or openly. Many of the women in medicine were the wives or daughters of lower-order wound surgeons, and in Christian religious orders women treated the sick throughout the medieval period. Although we may observe a part played by women in medicine throughout history, we may also note that their activities often were undertaken to the accompaniment of disapproval and at times of outright antagonism from the populace—not only from male physicians.

During most of the world's history licensure was not required, so it was principally public acceptance that would enable someone to perform medical functions regularly. When in the fourteenth century examinations began to be required for anyone to practice medicine, both sexes were theoretically equal. At the end of the fourteenth century in Germany, there were fifteen licensed female practitioners. In the fifteenth century the number had increased markedly, but only because the emperor had hired women to treat the indigent sick since male physicians were not available on the same terms. Although the advance of women into medicine was inexorable, it was slow.

In one field alone throughout history were women always accepted and even preferred: midwifery. Among the outstanding midwives to have received historical attention was Mme Boursier in seventeenth-century France, who may have been the first midwife to publish a scientific book on her specialty. For her services to Marie de Médicis (1573–1642), the second wife of Henry IV, she collected handsomely although she never received the pension the king promised. In England Elizabeth Cellier, after examining statistics on deaths after childbirth and abortion, concluded that two-thirds of the deaths were due to the midwife's lack of knowledge. She persuaded James II to agree to a special hospital for women, but her outspoken criticisms of many people (including the king himself) landed her in the pillory and her books on the bonfire. Other volumes on training midwives continued to appear, but they were usually written by men.

Women continued to find it well-nigh impossible to be accepted for training and practice as full-fledged doctors, except perhaps in Italy where women had received medical education for centuries and had even occupied prestigious university chairs.

The career of Dr. James Barry (1797–1865), a medical officer in the British army who enjoyed a high reputation for fifty years as a skillful surgeon, may serve to reflect the prevailing attitudes. Of slight stature, squeaky voice, and beardless face, Barry evidently aroused no suspicion—possibly because of an aggressive manner and a reputation as an accurate marksman. When an autopsy revealed that Barry was a woman, the war department and the medical association were so embarrassed that the findings were hidden and Dr. Barry was officially buried as a man.

THE UNITED STATES

As in Europe, American medical schools were also closed to females. In colonial days, although many women were midwives, nurses, and apothecaries, some actually practiced medicine. On the other hand, the attempt by Harriot Hunt (1805–75) to attend school lectures in Boston was thwarted even by the students themselves. When her application to Harvard Medical School was submitted by Oliver Wendell Holmes, who was then dean, the faculty agreed but the students objected. They drew up resolutions of rejection:

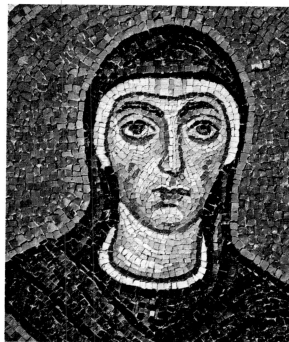

918

917 *In the Christian religious orders of the Middle Ages, women played the major role in caring for the sick and disabled, as is shown in this 13th-century manuscript illustration. Ms. lat. 8846, fol. 106, Rc C 2237, Bibliothèque Nationale, Paris*

918 *Detail from a mosaic of the 5th–6th century portraying St. Felicity of Carthage, the patron saint of sick children. Archiepiscopal Chapel, Archbishop's Palace, Ravenna*

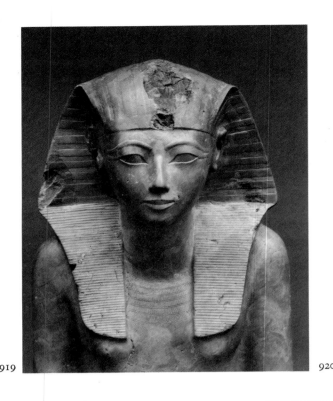

919

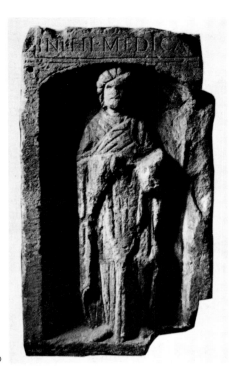

920

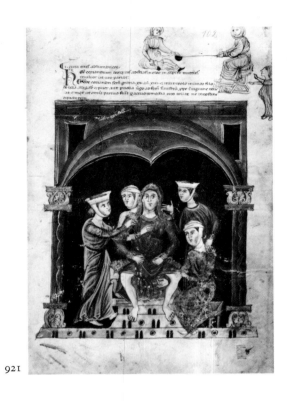

921

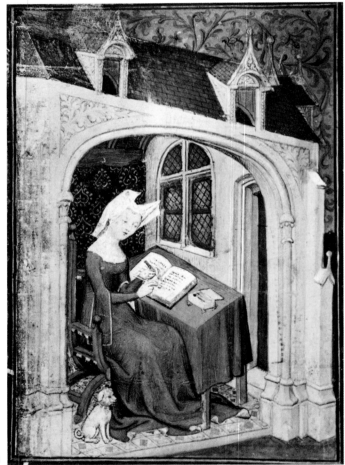

922

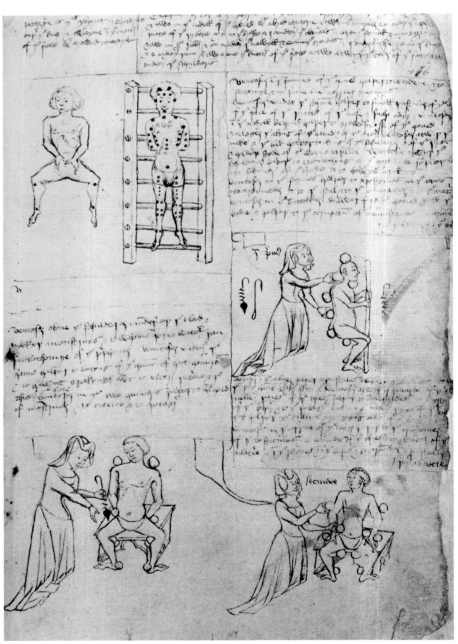

923

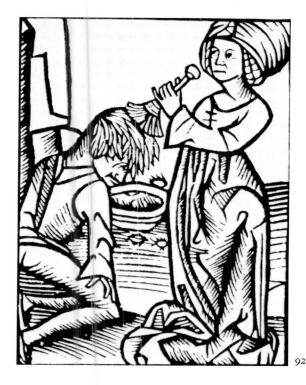

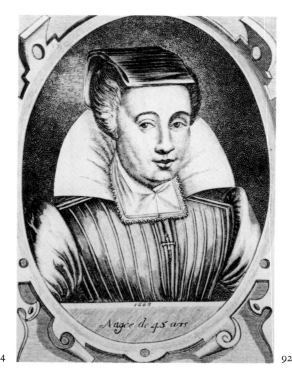

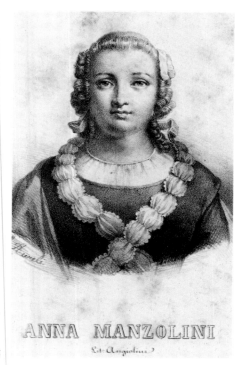

924

925

 ANNA MANZOLINI

926

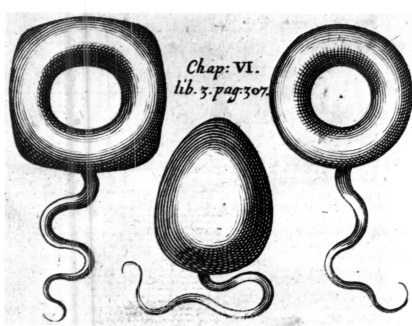

927

919 *Head of Egyptian queen Hatshepsut (c. 1485 B.C.), who was thought to have had medical knowledge. Metropolitan Museum of Art, New York*

920 *Funeral stele of a Gallo-Roman woman doctor, indicating that women were physicians in Roman times. Musée Central, Metz*

921 *Miniature from the* Herbal of Pseudo-Apuleius *(c. 10th–11th century) showing midwives using coriander to accelerate childbirth. Codex Vindob 93, fol. 102 v., Österreichische Nationalbibliothek, Vienna*

922 *Daughter of a physician, Christine de Pisan, shown here in a 14th-century manuscript, was tutored in medicine and championed women's rights. Ms. Harleian 4431, British Library, London*

923 *Page from a 14th-century treatise by John Arderne, surgeon of Newark, showing various treatments by women. Ms. Sloane 6, fol. 177, British Museum, London*

924 *Illustration of a woman delousing a man, from* Hortus Sanitatis *(1491). New York Academy of Medicine*

925 *Portrait of Loyse Bourgeois Boursier, midwife to French royalty, from her textbook* Observations Diverses sur la Sterilité *(1626). New York Academy of Medicine*

926 *Portrait of Anna Morandi Manzolini, 18th-century professor of anatomy at the University of Bologna. Wellcome Institute for the History of Medicine, London*

927 *Engraved plate showing pessaries to correct dropped wombs, from François Mauriceau,* The Accomplished Midwife *(1673). National Library of Medicine, Bethesda*

928 *The Sisters of Charity of Antwerp Nursing the Sick by Jacob Jordaens. Koninklijk Museum voor Schone Kunsten, Antwerp*

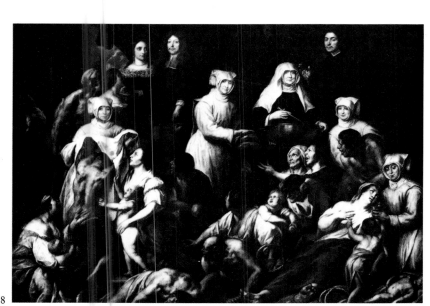

928

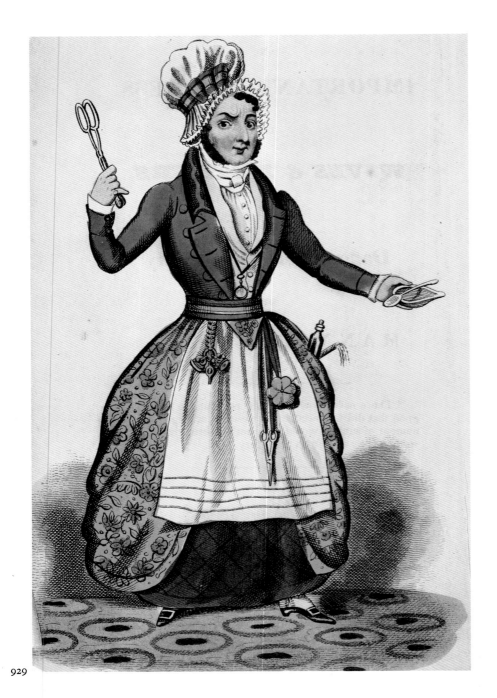

929

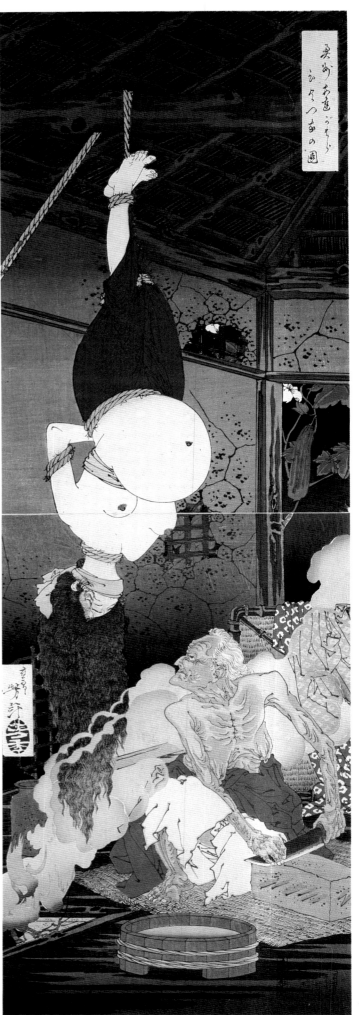

929 *Frontispiece lampooning a male midwife from* An Important Address to Wives and Mothers on the Dangers and Immorality of Man-midwifery (1830). *New York Academy of Medicine*

930 *Japanese woodblock print (c. 1887) by Yoshitoshi, showing a scene from a demon story, with an old crone about to "operate" on a pregnant woman. Collection Walton Rawls, New York*

930

Resolved, that no woman of true delicacy would be willing in the presence of men to listen to the discussion of subjects that necessarily come under consideration of the students of medicine.

Resolved, that we object to having the company of any female forced upon us, who is disposed to unsex herself, and to sacrifice her modesty by appearing with men in the lecture room.

Ultimately, Mrs. Hunt was able to thread through a maze of oppositions elsewhere and obtain an M.D. degree in Syracuse as a homeopathic physician. She even became a professor of midwifery and of diseases of women and children at Rochester College. Later she emigrated to London and devoted herself to phrenology.

There were a few others, but the outstanding breakthrough for a woman was achieved by Elizabeth Blackwell (1821–1910). Summarily turned down by a number of schools, Miss Blackwell persisted until she gained admission to a small school in upstate New York, The Geneva College of Medicine—through a fluke! To show his liberalism the dean had presented the application directly to his students: should a woman be allowed to enter the classes? Having stipulated a unanimous decision, he was confident of a negative verdict. The students, thinking it a great joke, voted unanimously to admit her. The people of the town were so appalled that they snubbed Miss Blackwell throughout her stay. Although some authorities and faculty members predicted unruly incidents at the lectures, the classes were orderly and a genuine, respectful affection sprang up between the students and their female colleague. For instance, Miss Blackwell was asked to be absent when the anatomy of the male reproductive system was to be presented, and the students supported her refusal. Throughout the two years of her schooling (the standard course at the time) she conducted herself with dignity and courtesy, applying herself so diligently that she passed the qualifying examination with the highest average. In 1849, along with the other members of the graduating class, she received her M.D. degree.

Of course even with that the battle was hardly begun. Acceptance by the profession and the public was still far off. When visiting London Dr. Blackwell was hailed by doctors and prominent laymen who had heard of her successful fight and was given access to lectures and hospitals. However, English women, with a few exceptions, were no closer to gaining admission to medicine than before. In Paris Dr. Blackwell found even more opposition to women; the only way open to broadening her training in France was in a school for midwives. Despite the reduced status associated with this enterprise, Dr. Blackwell persisted because of the opportunity to learn obstetrics in an institution which took care of thousands of pregnant women each year. Pursuing her duties she contracted a severe eye infection which incapacitated her for weeks and permanently damaged the eye (which had to be removed years later). The French medical hierarchy, now sympathetic and regretful, reversed its stand and gave her full permission to visit any hospital, clinic, or lecture. Similar invitations were offered when she returned again to London. There she met Florence Nightingale (1820–1910), who impressed Dr. Blackwell with her ideas and goals. Altogether she made several trips abroad but based herself in New York City, where she established a clinic that became The New York Dispensary for Poor Women and Children.

Dr. Blackwell's sister Emily had similar difficulties, for although she was able to enter Rush Medical College in Chicago the Illinois State Medical Society prevented her from continuing. Nevertheless, she was able to finish a second year of training at The Cleveland Medical College, where she and another woman were given degrees, since not all practitioners and faculties resisted women's participation in medicine. Sir James Simpson, for instance, the famous obstetrician in Edinburgh who introduced the use of anesthesia in childbirth, later welcomed Emily Blackwell as a student and praised her lavishly.

Marie Zakrzewska ("Dr. Zak") (1829–1902), who came to the United States

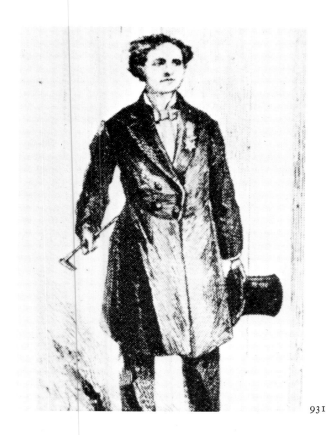

931

931 *Dr. Mary Walker, an assistant surgeon in the Civil War, was an early feminist who dressed as a man and designed a rape-proof costume for women. Medical Communications, Inc.*

932 *Obstetric case with instruments (c. 1870). Smithsonian Institution, Washington, D.C.*

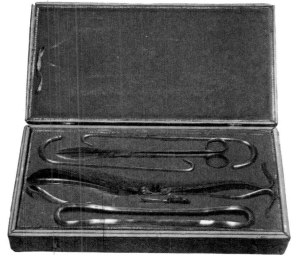

932

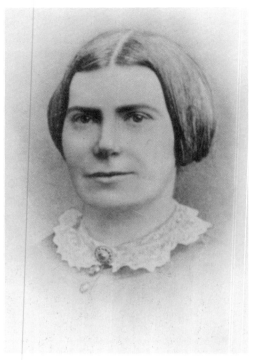

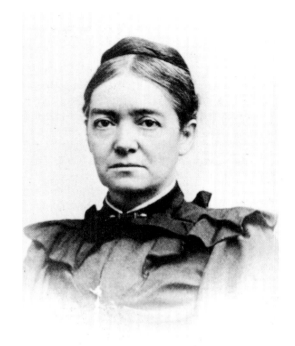

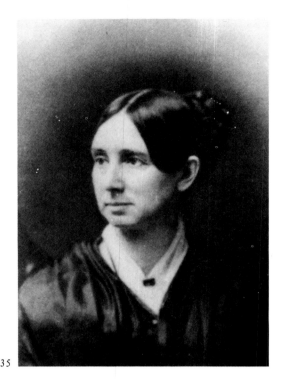

933

934

935

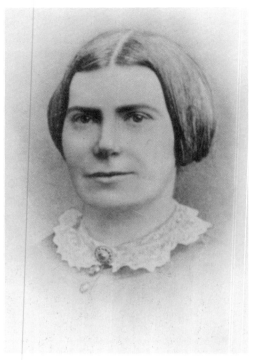

936

933 *Dr. Elizabeth Blackwell, the first woman medical graduate of an American university. New York Infirmary*

934 *Dr. Mary Putnam Jacobi won Harvard's coveted Boylston Medical Prize and established a pioneering pediatric clinic at Mount Sinai Hospital, New York. National Library of Medicine, Bethesda*

935 *Dorothea Lynde Dix, champion of humane treatment of the mentally ill, founded the Pennsylvania Hospital for the Insane at Harrisburg. National Library of Medicine, Bethesda*

936 *Women medical students shown during dissection, training that was thought unseemly for for their sex in the 19th century. Medical Communications, Inc.*

from Berlin where she had been a hospital's chief midwife, also had to fight her way into medicine. Together with the Blackwell sisters she founded the New York Infirmary for Women and Children in 1857. This institution gave the few women who had managed to enter the profession an opportunity to obtain the additional hospital training so necessary to their attainment of practical skills.

Among others in the United States who managed to slip through the educational sieve was Mary Putnam Jacobi (1842–1906). In 1863 she became the first woman to be graduated from the New York College of Pharmacy. Even though she also received a degree from The Female Medical College of Pennsylvania (the first approved, legal medical school for women in the world) and thereafter interned at The New England Hospital for Women and Children, she sought the prestige of a diploma from a great university. After considerable maneuvering and industrious study she achieved the near impossible, a medical degree from the highly reputed University of Paris. Back in New York City, she assisted Elizabeth Blackwell by teaching at the newly established Women's Medical College of The New York Infirmary, remaining there for almost two decades. While attending meetings of The New York County Medical Society and The New York Pathological Society she met Dr. Abraham Jacobi, whom she married in 1873. Her subsequent activities seemed to multiply. She won Harvard's coveted and highly competitive Boylston Medical Prize for a paper submitted anonymously. Her time was filled to overflowing by private practice, teaching at two schools (one of which was for men), writing, and with her husband establishing a pioneering pediatric clinic at The Mount Sinai Hospital.

The dogged persistence and demonstrated excellence of the pioneering women in American medicine gradually led to the opening of all medical schools to females, but it was not done without help from some men. The establishment of the first women's medical school in 1850, The Female Medical College of Pennsylvania (later The Women's Medical College of Pennsylvania), was due in large measure to the efforts of Quaker physicians and other medical men of Philadelphia. Since there were virtually no women doctors available, the faculty positions were filled by men. And courageous, principled men they had to be, for their unpopular participation was held in contempt by most of their colleagues and especially by the medical societies. Additional schools for women soon followed in other cities, notably Boston, New York, Baltimore, and Cleveland.

The university medical schools, however, were slow and even resistant to

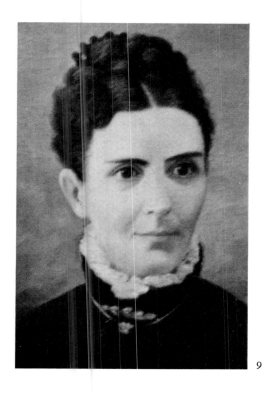

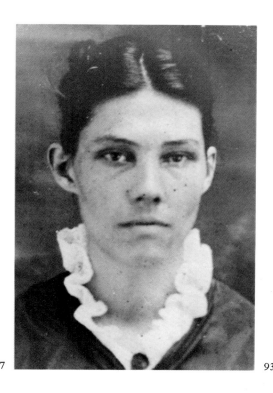

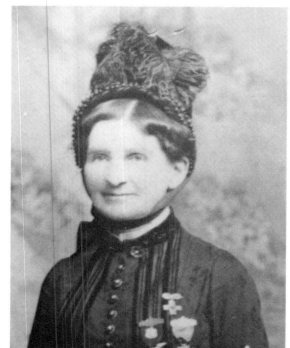

937   938   939

permitting females to enter, but by the last decade of the nineteenth century about thirty-five schools had finally withdrawn their objections. After the turn of the century, separate medical colleges for women became less necessary.

Nevertheless, the national, state, and county medical societies continued to oppose the membership of women. Some of the antagonism was due to the association of many female doctors (for lack of other opportunities) with the homeopathic and eclectic sects that were anathema to the recognized regular practitioners and teachers. However, in addition there were general prejudices against women in medicine resulting from social traditions which placed women on a separate moral plane. It was thought that medicine (especially its concern with sexual matters) was an unseemly subject for women to delve into, but it was not only in medicine that resistance was shown. In the *Transactions of the American Medical Association* of 1871, a noted pathologist merely echoed a view prevalent at the time:

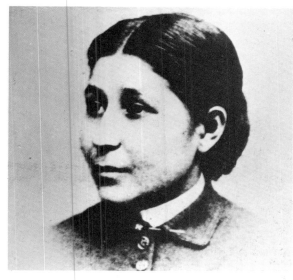

940

> Another disease has become epidemic. "The woman question" in relation to medicine is only one of the forms in which the *pestis mulieribis* vexes the world. In other shapes it attacks the bar, wriggles into the jury box, and clearly means to mount upon the bench; it strives, thus far in vain, to serve at the altar and thunder from the pulpit; it raves at political meetings, harangues in the lecture-room, infects the masses with its poison and even pierces the triple brass that surrounds the politician's heart.

The Montgomery County Medical Society of Pennsylvania may have been the first local group to admit a woman, but it was not until well into the twentieth century that other societies followed suit. In 1915 women were given full membership in the American Medical Association, the same year the Medical Women's National Association was formed. The American Medical Women's Association came later.

EUROPE

Meanwhile a parallel course had been taken in Europe. The same England that had accepted the American Elizabeth Blackwell as a practitioner in the Official Medical Register was rigidly opposed to the training of Elizabeth Garrett (1836–1917).

937 *Dr. Ellis Reynolds Shipp, member of the Deseret (Utah) Hospital Board, headed a nurses home which produced some 500 women graduates. Utah State Historical Society, Salt Lake City*

938 *Dr. Georgia Arbuckle Fix, photographed in 1876, engaged in active practice in Nebraska. Nebraska State Historical Society, Lincoln*

939 *Dr. Hettie K. Painter, graduate of Pennsylvania Medical University, was active in the Civil War and afterward opened the Lincoln Infirmary. Nebraska State Historical Society, Lincoln*

940 *Dr. Susan LaFlesche Picotte, daughter of an Omaha Indian chief, was a graduate of the Woman's Medical College of Nebraska. Nebraska State Historical Society, Lincoln*

941 *Opposed and lampooned on every side, as in this caricature of 1865, Elizabeth Garrett Anderson finally received a doctor's degree, a license to practice, a position in a reputable hospital, and membership in the British Medical Association. New York Academy of Medicine*

942 *Wood engraving from* Harper's Weekly *(July 23, 1870) showing "Miss Garrett before the Board of Medical Examiners at Paris," where she received the M.D. degree in 1870. National Library of Medicine, Bethesda*

943 *Madame Marie Curie, twice winner of the Nobel Prize (the first time anyone had been so honored), shown in her laboratory, from a photograph taken around 1905. Bettmann Archive, New York*

944 Children's Doctor *painted by Andrew Wyeth in commemoration of Margaret Handy (1889–1977), beloved pediatrician, who devoted her life to unselfish care of other people's children. Private collection*

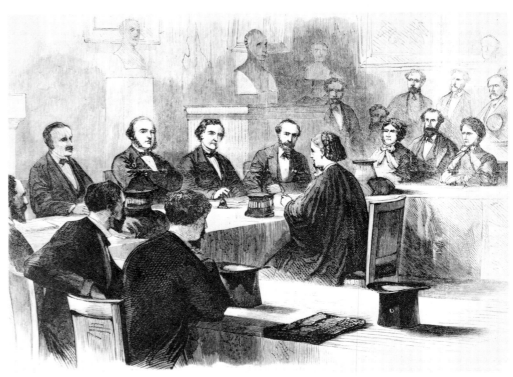

942

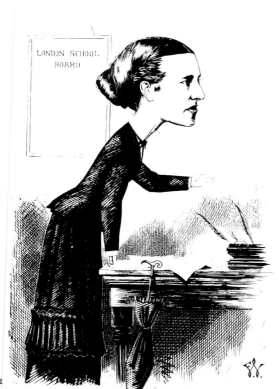

941

Although at first not certain she aspired to a medical degree, Miss Garrett received encouragement from Elizabeth Blackwell. Entering the teaching hospital of Middlesex as a student nurse, she wheedled permission to attend lectures, charmed her way into the clinical courses, and applied herself so diligently that she received outstanding grades. On the threshold of full recognition, she was abruptly asked to leave. She tried to continue elsewhere in getting a degree, but Oxford, Cambridge, and the University of London rejected her.

She next embarked on a different course, aiming at the degree of Licentiate of the Society of Apothecaries, which would accredit her to practice medicine. She satisfied the required apprenticeship with Joshua Plaskit, her former teacher at Middlesex, but official university matriculation was also required. Since England's universities were closed to her, she tried Scotland. Through technicalities, St. Andrews kept her out as an official candidate despite heated debate and threatened lawsuits. However, she did gain an important benefit in adding to her slowly mounting documents a certificate for a semester of private work. Rejected as well at Edinburgh, she obtained further training there by studying with the prestigious Sir James Simpson, a consistent supporter of the women's movement.

Again back at Middlesex in London she received permission from individual practitioners to attend ward rounds. By these diligent methods she had finally by 1865 accumulated the required proofs of training demanded at her first application to the Society of Apothecaries in 1861. When the society still refused to recognize her candidacy, her father decided at whatever cost to bring suit. The apothecaries retreated and allowed her to take the examination, which she passed with ease, becoming the first woman Licentiate of the Society of Apothecaries entered on the Medical Register. Elizabeth Garrett was officially a physician.

If her odyssey had ended there, her achievement would have represented an extraordinary accomplishment. But she went much farther. She built up a large private practice and at the same time established the St. Mary's Dispensary for Women in the slums, where she worked unstintingly. When she sought to obtain a position on the staff of a reputable hospital, she not only succeeded in convincing a reluctant board of directors but also so impressed one of its members, the wealthy James Anderson, that he married her two years later. Not content to remain merely a licentiate she persuaded the Paris faculty, through contacts with the British ambassador, to admit her to the examination for a diploma without having to reside in Paris. She received the M.D. degree in 1870.

Thereafter her activities increased even further. She may have been the first woman to perform an oophorectomy (removal of an ovary), and in the London School of Medicine for Women she served as dean for twenty years. In keeping with the erratic course of her life, it was through an oversight that the British Medical Association—which had never admitted a woman—made her a member. In spite of outraged objections the inadvertent but legal election was not overturned, but the association took care not to open its rolls again to a woman until 1892, when general attitudes toward women in medicine were softened.

As if all this were not enough for one woman's lifetime, after her husband's death in 1907 Dr. Elizabeth Garrett Anderson was elected Mayor of Aldeburgh. Apparently all along the rough, winding, painful road of her career she remained poised, quiet, charming—and persistent.

Of an entirely different personality was Sophia Jex-Blake (1840–1912), a vigorous, outspoken activist who led the struggle in Britain, finally achieving the rights to medical training for herself and other women, but not without numerous frustrations and harassments. When Miss Jex-Blake and her followers found their way blocked to entering classes in the University of Edinburgh despite their official matriculation, she publicly castigated the professor of toxicology for having incited the male students to use physical force. After losing the resulting libel suit (the penalty levied was one farthing), she retaliated in 1873 by bringing legal action against the entire university to force permission for women students to enter the courses and to be examined for a medical degree. Although the case was won, a superior court overturned the decision on a close vote.

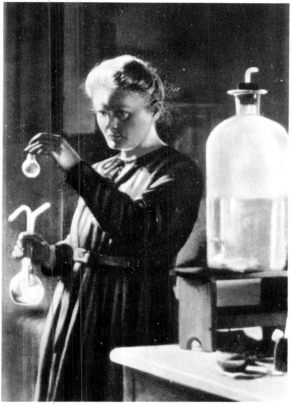

943

Since about the only way left to obtain a medical education was the creation of a special school, Miss Jex-Blake found cooperative physicians, especially Dr. Francis Austie, with whom she was able to found the London School of Medicine for Women (1874). But even after the women were graduated there were no reputable hospitals open to them and no official examining bodies which would certify them for licensure. The New Hospital for Women was therefore established, with vigorous support from Russell Gurney, a member of Parliament. By 1876 public opinion had altered enough to permit Parliament to pass a bill, introduced by Mr. Gurney, which gave women the right to take qualifying examinations.

When the Royal Free Hospital the next year allowed students of the London School of Medicine for Women to receive training on the wards, other hospitals and schools followed in such short order that by the end of the nineteenth century virtually all the great British universities were open to women for education and training in medicine. In Switzerland, Sweden, Denmark, Norway, Finland, Russia, Belgium, Australia, Mexico, Chile, Brazil, and other countries throughout the world, women were also admitted to medical training and practice in the last decades of the century. Holland, like Italy, apparently never restricted women from entering universities or practicing medicine, but it seems that no woman in the Netherlands availed herself of the opportunity until Aletta Jacobs (1849–1929) went through the full formal course and was licensed in 1878. Germany and Austria, among the last to liberalize their attitudes, finally also lifted restrictions at the turn of the century.

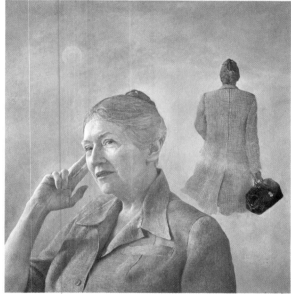

944

However, while women became more and more accepted in the sciences, there were still pockets of resistance. Marie Curie (1867–1934), who together with her husband had captured the attention of the scientific world and received the Nobel Prize in physics in 1903, was refused admittance into the French Academy of Sciences. Her husband Pierre (1859–1906) had also been refused about seven years earlier, but neither of the Curies had then achieved wide renown. When the Academy decided by one vote to reject Marie Curie's application, her pioneer work had already been hailed by distinctions which included the Legion of Honor (which she turned down). The Academy's refusal, which could only have been because of

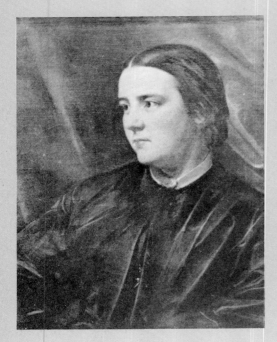

945 *Dr. Sophia Louisa Jex-Blake, an aggressive feminist, painted by Samuel Lawrence. National Library of Medicine, Bethesda*

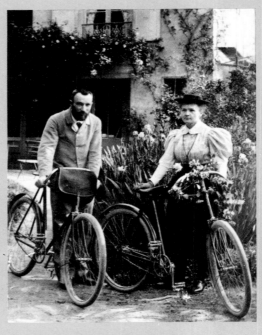

946 *Marie and Pierre Curie before their house at Sceaux near Paris. Musée d'Histoire de la Médecine, Paris*

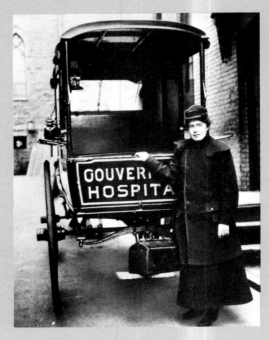

947 *Dr. Emily Dunning Barringer, the first woman ambulance surgeon. New York Times*

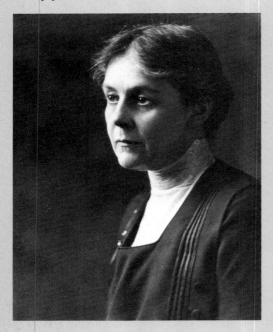

948 *Dr. Alice Hamilton, one of the first women to hold a professorship at Harvard. National Library of Medicine, Bethesda*

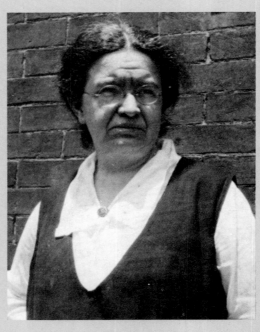

949 *Dr. Florence Rena Sabin gained worldwide fame as a teacher, physician, and researcher. National Library of Medicine, Bethesda*

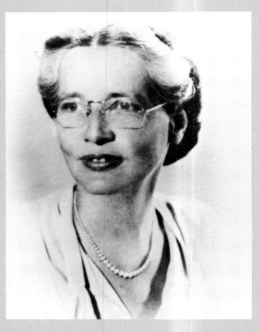

950 *Dr. Helen Brooke Taussig conceived the idea of surgically correcting cardiac abnormalities. National Library of Medicine, Bethesda*

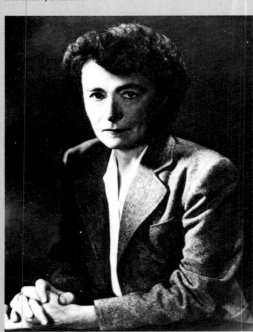

951 *Dr. Gerti Theresa Cori, first woman to win the Nobel Prize in medicine or physiology. National Library of Medicine, Bethesda*

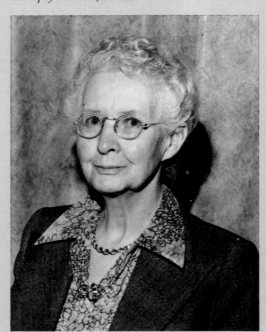

952 *Dr. Mary J. Ross, named outstanding general practitioner for New York State in 1953. United Press International, New York*

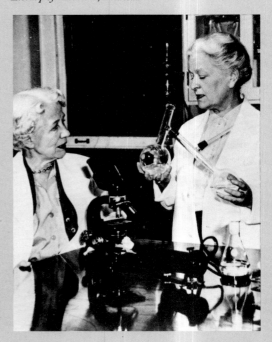

953 *Drs. Elizabeth L. Hazen and Rachel Brown, found and isolated nystatin. United Press International, New York*

her sex, became the more ludicrous when Madame Curie was given a second Nobel Prize, now for chemistry, the first time anyone had been so honored.

Marie Curie's achievements also demonstrated to the world that a woman could shine intellectually and perform brilliantly while fulfilling a warm, loving marriage and bringing up two children. Her notes of 1921 included a passage which revealed the remarkable character of both Curies (her husband died in 1906), who had accomplished their tasks in the face of physical hardship, callous indifference, and monetary deprivation:

> A great number of my friends affirm, not without reasons, that if Pierre Curie and I had guaranteed our rights, we should have acquired the financial means necessary to the creation of a satisfactory radium institute, without encountering the obstacles which were a handicap to us, and which are still a handicap for me. Nevertheless, I am still convinced we were right.
>
> Humanity certainly needs practical men, who get the most out of their work, and without forgetting the general good, safeguarded their own interests. But humanity also needs the dreamers, for whom the disinterested development of an enterprise is so captivating that it becomes impossible for them to devote their care to their own material profits.

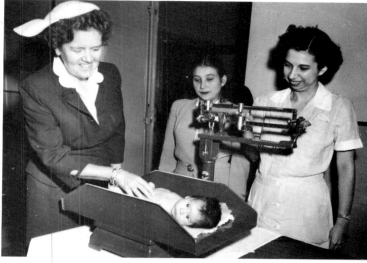

954

TWENTIETH CENTURY

Since then, so many women have entered the medical profession and made outstanding contributions that one hardly takes notice of which worker or investigator is female and which male. Maude Abbott, whose exceptional, thorough classification of congenital heart defects opened the way to the future of cardiac surgery, is remembered as a pathologist, not as a woman pathologist. Nor does one consider for long that it was a woman, Helen Taussig, who conceived the idea, which her colleague Alfred Blalock embarked upon, of surgically correcting cardiac abnormalities. Women now enter medical schools, are chosen for residency training, engage in clinical practice, hold professorships in teaching institutions, and receive grants for research on equal footing with men. In veterinary medicine women have been entering schools and practicing in ever greater percentages (in some schools comprising half the class). In Finland at least half of the dentists are female, and in the Soviet Union a high percentage of the doctors are women.

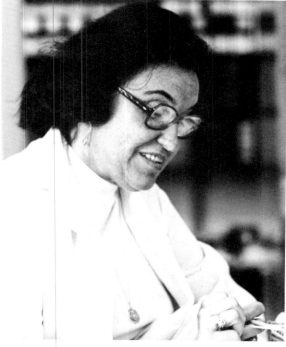

955

But it would be less than accurate to say that females are fully accepted in all fields of medicine. Whereas obstetrics, gynecology, and pediatrics have been the recognized concerns of women throughout the ages, the fields of surgery, orthopedics, and urology have not attracted many women, possibly as much because of a presumption of not being accepted by patients of both sexes as professional resistance. Furthermore, in most countries there are few women in high academic medical directorships except in schools for women.

In 1947, a woman first won the Nobel Prize in the category of medicine or physiology. Gerti T. Cori received this recognition together with her husband, Carl F. Cori, for proving an important concept in genetics, that an enzyme deficiency could be inborn and responsible for a disorder of metabolism. Thirty years later, 1977, Rosalyn Yalow was the second female Nobel laureate in medicine. With Solomon Berson, she developed the radioimmunoassay technique, which opened up new investigations in a variety of fields. Ironically, Dr. Yalow was steered away from graduate school, where women were infrequently admitted in the 1940s, but by getting a job as secretary in the physics department she was able to take the courses that led to her doctorate.

Today, the road is open and the future journey seems clear. The first woman to become president of a state medical society may attract attention, but before long others will follow and, like their male counterparts, hardly be noticed.

954 *Dr. Leona Baumgartner, New York City Health Commissioner from 1954 to 1962, the first woman to hold this position. Wide World Photos, New York*

955 *Dr. Rosalyn Yalow, who in 1977 became the second female Nobel laureate in medicine. Together with Solomon Berson, she developed the radioimmuneassay technique. Mount Sinai Hospital Archives, New York*

The Twentieth Century

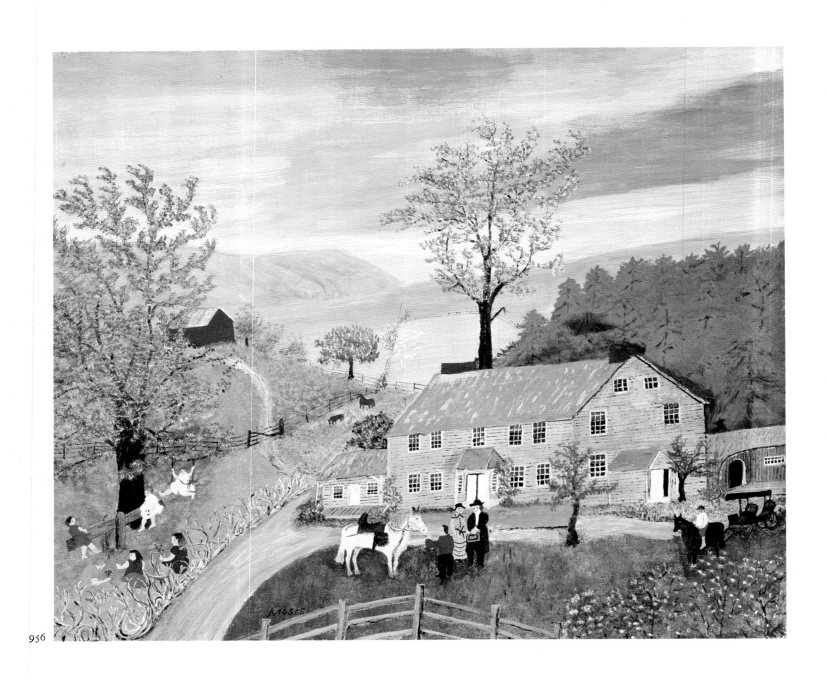

956

IN surveying the state of the healing arts today, one is surely impressed by the contrasts with earlier centuries. Horrible scourges like smallpox, cholera, and diphtheria which devastated populations even as late as the nineteenth century are now rare or nonexistent in most parts of the world; visualization of previously hidden parts of the body is a commonplace of diagnostic methods; many formerly hopeless infections are readily susceptible to a host of antimicrobial medications; the surgeon's techniques have invaded the cranium, chest cavity, heart, and blood vessels; irreversibly diseased organs are replaced by grafts and transplants of healthy structures or are substituted for by mechanical devices. Furthermore, the inner workings of the cell, the basic unit of the body, have been opened to scrutiny by physical and chemical means. But most of these extraordinary innovations, when viewed historically, are chiefly remarkable extensions and elaborations of past contributions and attitudes.

Among the many changes which stamp the twentieth century, we have chosen some to illustrate this stage of medical knowledge in its development from past to future.

CONCEPTS

HUMAN GENETICS

Jean Jacques Rousseau said that when nature finished with him, it broke the mold in which he was cast. But all of us could say the same thing. Mathematicians have calculated that the chances of any two parents producing another one of us exactly as we are, physically, mentally, physiologically, and with the same inborn susceptibilities and resistances are one in several hundred trillion. Yet, research in genetic engineering has progressed so far that it is feasible to challenge the essentially nil possibility of ever having two people exactly alike in terms of their genetic endowment. However, scientists and philosophers are now engaged in considerable debate on whether further research on the transference of genetic substances should not be halted. On one hand, disease and deformity could be defeated before they got started; on the other hand, the possibilities for abuse and accident could lead to havoc and even the destruction of the human species.

The intensive research on inborn or genetic errors started in the 1940s was followed by ever-multiplying investigations that included observing cells in tissue culture. In the 1950s, methods were devised for the accurate study of chromosome numbers and, for the first time, it became clear that the normal human chromosome count is forty-six. Soon, a number of numerical aberrations were discovered, the most common of which is an extra twenty-first chromosome, the cause of Down's syndrome or mongolism. These studies have recently become so refined that individual portions of chromosomes can be identified with various banding techniques which have allowed the accurate description of chromosomal aberrations, leading to more accurate genetic counseling and prevention.

In the late 1960s, techniques were developed for prenatally diagnosing genetic diseases by culturing cells obtained from the amniotic fluid. This has permitted the detection of abnormal fetuses and has expanded the options to include selective abortion of such affected fetuses. Due to these technological advances, the science of human genetics has now become a practical clinical specialty which is capable of proper diagnosis, counseling, and prevention of many serious diseases.

Recent experimental work indicates that at some time it may even be possible to introduce genetic material into defective cells so that they would essentially cure themselves.

IMMUNOLOGY

Immunology began as a rational science in close association with the study of infectious diseases in the latter part of the nineteenth century. Scientists explained

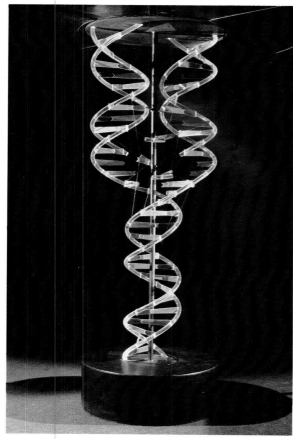

957

956 The Doctor (1950) by Grandma Moses. At the turn of the century, as the world of medicine entered a period of brilliant breakthroughs and technological advancements, the country doctor was still making his rounds on horseback. © copyright 1973 by Grandma Moses Properties, Inc. Galerie St. Etienne, New York

957 Model of the double-helix configuration of the DNA molecule in the process of replication. Xerox Corporation

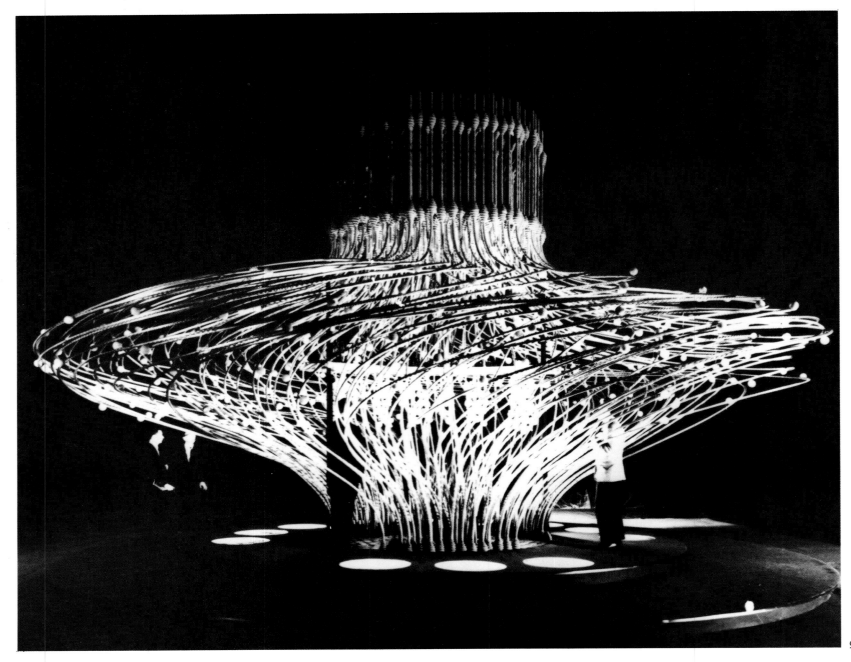

958 *Chart showing the chromosomes of a normal male. New York Academy of Medicine*

959 *Model of a gene more than a quarter of a million times true size, showing some of the genetic processes that go on inside the chromosomes of the cells of all living organisms.* Upjohn Company, Kalamazoo

Normal male.

958

959

why persons who had recovered from certain infections (e.g., smallpox) were often resistant to these same infections during subsequent exposure—an observation long known in antiquity. Even more important, the experimental results led to ways of inducing such resistance *before* the disease occurred.

In the late nineteenth century, Pasteur, Koch, Behring, Kitasato, Ehrlich, and others placed the principles of immunologic protection on a scientific basis, but successes were not universal. For instance, despite much study and experiment, Koch's attempts to produce a vaccine against tuberculosis failed. Furthermore, a reaction was observed in animals and later in humans which occurred during second or third attempts at immunization. Instead of an increased resistance to the disease or chemical, the inoculated individual had an immediate, severe attack ("anaphylaxis") which often resulted in death by asphyxiation.

At the end of World War II, immunology entered a phase which eventually permitted a molecular biological explanation for many of the immune phenomena associated with infectious diseases and which showed that many other biological activities, not directly related to infectious diseases, actually have an immunological basis. In the 1930s it had been discovered that the factors in blood which carry out the immune activity are in the gamma globulin fraction of the blood serum. Later studies showed these factors to be protein molecules, called immunoglobulins, which are capable of a wide range of interacting functions (e.g., with polio virus, tetanus toxin, diphtheria toxin, ragweed pollen).

Another significant advance has been the recognition that our bodies make a strong immune response against "foreign" material such as the agents which cause infectious diseases. Directly related to this is the recent recognition that the common failure of attempts to graft organs (such as the heart or liver) is due mainly to the biological fact that a recipient's body will react just as strongly against the grafted organ as it would an infecting virus or bacterium. Thus the immune system in general has come to be understood as a mechanism which attempts to distinguish between "self" and "nonself" to protect the former from the latter. Much of contemporary immunological research is directed at understanding the biological mechanisms that regulate this capacity. If the immune system can be specifically and adequately controlled, we might vastly increase the possibility of carrying out successful organ and tissue transplants from one individual to another. In addition, if we learn more about how the immune system deals with cancers, we may be able to understand, and prevent, those instances when the system breaks down and fails to destroy fatal growths.

VIROLOGY

For the first thirty years of the twentieth century viruses could be studied only by their pathogenic effects on the animals they infected. They were too small to be seen by the best light microscopes. Then came technical developments such as the invention of the electron microscope in the late 1930s that made it possible to examine the structure of viruses in great detail and to study their relationships and reactions with the cells they infect. Methods were invented for growing cells in culture and for making monolayer cultures which aided exact quantitative studies of viral multiplication and the action of specific antibodies on virus growth. It also permitted accurate observation of the factors involved in the genetics and mutation of viruses.

Advances in biochemistry, biophysics, physical chemistry, and immunology since the 1930s have also contributed greatly to our knowledge of the biology of viruses, and their structure and their relationship to host cells, including their methods of entry, reproduction, and release from them. The practical results of the advances in virology in the twentieth century have had beneficial effects on the health of mankind second only to that of the discovery of antibiotics. Some of these benefits may be cited here. The virus that causes infantile paralysis

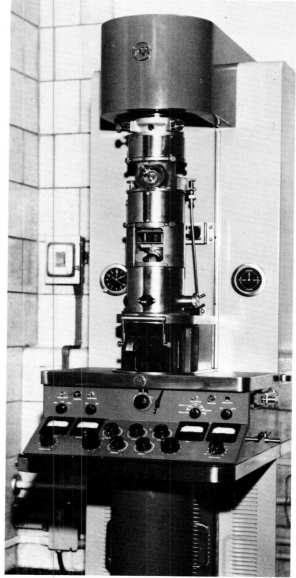

960

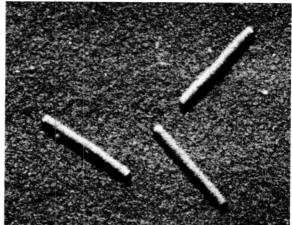

961

960 *The electron microscope, invented in the 1930s, has made it possible to study the structure of viruses in great detail. E. R. Squibb Company*

961 *Image through electron microscope of tobacco mosaic virus, the first virus recognized to transmit a disease, magnified 90,000 times. University of California, Berkeley*

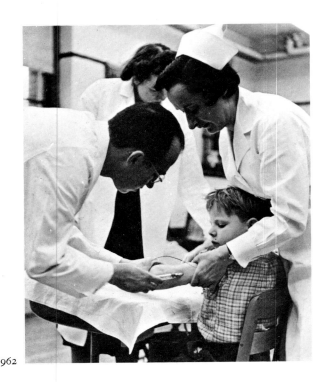

962

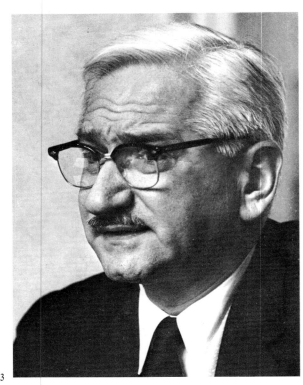

963

962 *Dr. Jonas E. Salk, who, with associates, devised a noninfectious vaccine for poliomyelitis, is shown giving a shot during the mass inoculation trial in 1954. World Health Organization, Geneva*

963 *Dr. Albert Sabin developed a "live, attenuated" oral polio vaccine which has almost entirely re-placed Salk vaccine in the U.S. World Health Organization, Geneva*

(poliomyelitis) was first isolated by Landsteiner and Popper in 1909. A noninfectious vaccine for poliomyelitis was devised by Salk and associates and given a nationwide field trial in 1954. In the year before the Salk vaccine was made available commercially (1955) there were 55,000 cases of paralytic poliomyelitis in the United States. Three years later there were fewer than 200. At present, a "live, attenuated" polio vaccine, developed by Albert Sabin, which is taken by mouth and affords long-lasting immunity, has almost entirely replaced the Salk vaccine in the United States.

Another virus disease, German measles (rubella), is rarely accompanied by serious complications and is practically never fatal in children or adults. However, it has been discovered that if a woman contracts rubella while pregnant, her baby might be infected with the rubella virus and might suffer severe and permanent damage or death. A rubella vaccine made with an attenuated tissue-culture-grown strain of virus is now in general use as part of the routine immunization given to infants in the United States, as are vaccines against regular measles (rubeola) and mumps. The measles vaccine has virtually eliminated this serious disease in vaccinated children. Some success has also been achieved in the prevention of influenza, and vaccines are in use which are from seventy-five to ninety percent effective.

Researches on liver diseases conducted during the past twenty years have led to the discovery of two viruses that cause hepatitis (infection of the liver). An experimental clinical trial is being conducted to determine whether antigen from the protein coat of one of these viruses can immunize persons against the virus (hepatitis B virus).

CANCER

Cancer has been known and feared since antiquity, but its incidence could only be speculatively inferred until fairly recently. Indeed, as knowledge of the disease grew in the nineteenth and twentieth centuries, fear increased when people became more aware of cancer without corresponding assurances of an available cure. Even after surgeons were able to extirpate tumors from previously inaccessible body interiors, cancers were still held in terror. Moreover, the overall mortality and rate of survival after treatment were not accurately known until the twentieth century. Statistics reported in this century from all over the world indicate that cancer steadily has been increasing in frequency. For example, the incidence in 1975 was seventy-five percent higher than in 1933, and, furthermore, the organ pattern has been changing. Before 1900, lung cancer was rare; now it is one of the leading causes of death. There are over one-hundred varieties of malignant tumors, but about half of the cancer deaths now are due to growths in the lung, colon, and breast.

Epidemiologists are closely examining the geographic distribution of cancer occurrence for clues to causation. They have discovered that in Japan and Scandinavia stomach cancer is relatively frequent, whereas its incidence in the U.S. is declining and that of pancreatic growths has increased. Carcinomas (cancers) of the colon, breast, and prostate are infrequent in Japan but common in America; yet, Japanese living in the U.S. show a pattern of occurrence resembling that of their neighbors.

Attempts were made as early as the eighteenth century to understand cancer and its causes, but the first major contributions to knowledge came from the microscopic studies of malignant tumors by Müller, Rokitansky, Virchow, and others in the early nineteenth century. Later investigators learned how to transplant tumors, keep malignant cells alive in the laboratory, and induce tumor growth through chemical and biological stimulation. From a great body of experimental and clinical studies, several possible cancer causes have been implicated.

Near the end of the nineteenth century, Julius Cohnheim suggested that cells

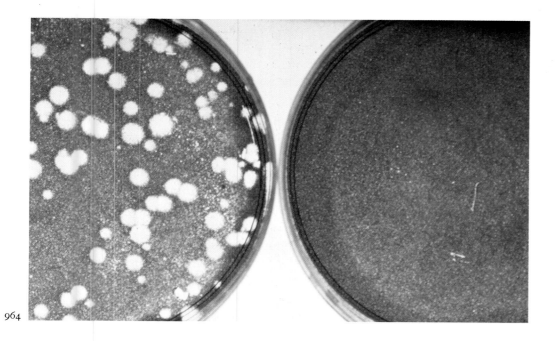

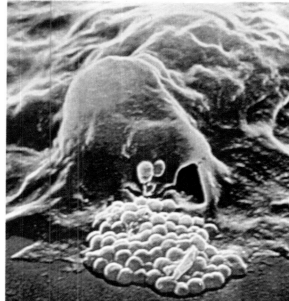

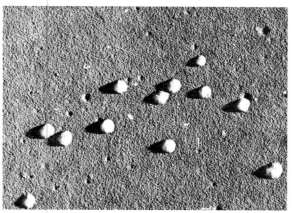

left over in adulthood from the developing embryo were responsible for later malignant growths, but this could account for only one type of rare tumor, the teratoma. Other scientists of the time considered bacteria, molds, and one-celled organisms to be causative agents, but this concept was short-lived. Later, viruses were shown to cause tumors in animals (notably by Peyton Rous in chickens), but no virus has been proved etiologically related to malignant tumors in humans—even though viruses have been found in association with human malignancies.

Genetic makeup has also been regarded as a causative factor in cancer, and, indeed, some families seem to show a propensity for growths and for certain precancerous conditions followed by a high incidence of cancer. Hormones were thought to have some relation to cancer when it was discovered that removal of the ovaries benefited women with advanced breast cancer and that castration arrested and sometimes caused regression of prostatic cancers. Hundreds of chemicals have produced cancers in laboratory animals, and dozens of environmental and occupational carcinogens (cancer-producing substances) have been implicated in malignant growths in humans. However, it is not known whether these agents directly stimulate cell growth, reactivate dormant viruses, or trigger some intermediate mechanism affecting the cell's biochemical activity.

In the past few decades, the cell has been found to include a multitude of smaller components with definite functions in maintaining the life and activity of the cell itself. Study of these intracellular structures, called "organelles," is bringing us closer to the essential fundamentals of protoplasm and to the ways in which malignant aberrations might begin. There is some evidence of cellular immunity to abnormal, potentially malignant cells, which are perceived as "foreign" and therefore destroyed by white blood cells through both direct engulfment and the elaboration of antibodies. Since a breakdown in this surveillance system seems to permit abnormal cells to multiply and become a malignant growth, attempts have been made through antibacterial vaccines and other protein derivatives to increase the body's general immunity in order to enhance resistance to the growth of cancerous cells. There is also a theory that nutriments, including vitamins and possibly other food elements, detoxify and protect the body cells against carcinogenic agents present in food and the environment.

Quite early in the twentieth century, it was learned that X-ray radiation was hazardous when the discoverer Roentgen himself and other pioneer roentgenologists developed skin malignancies. The effects of exposure to radium salts used to paint fluorescent watch dials were seen in the malignant bone tumors

964 *Polio virus. The decolored areas represent the virus, which has destroyed the tissue culture cells (stained with crystal violet). Drs. Edward J. Bottone and Bruce A. Hanna, Dept. of Microbiology, Mount Sinai Hospital, New York*

965 *Defense cells migrate toward a bacterial colony in this scanning electromicrograph.*

966 *Influenza virus magnified 40,000 times. University of California, Berkeley*

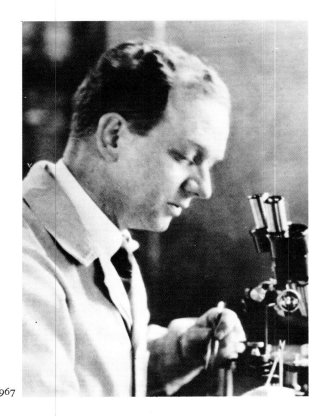

967

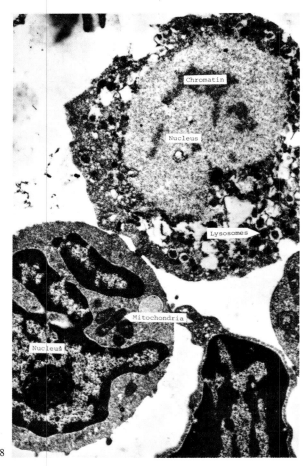

Chromatin

Nucleus

Lysosomes

Mitochondria

Nucleus

968

of factory workers who licked their brushes to get a properly shaped point. The association of radiation and cancer was most dramatically highlighted by the increase of leukemias and other malignancies in people exposed to the Hiroshima atom bomb blast. The potential danger of radiation has been so emphasized lately that the safety of even regular diagnostic X-ray procedures has been challenged.

The proof that an abnormal change in an organ is malignant has rested on the microscopic characteristics of a piece of tissue (biopsy) since the nineteenth century. However, other general diagnostic methods developed since then have also increased the chance of detecting cancer: X-rays; visualization of the interior through intubations of orifices; body scanning with radioactive tracer substances and ultrasonic waves; and chemical analyses of the blood. A highly significant contribution to diagnosis was made in 1928 by George Papanicolaou (developer of the Pap test), who reported that he could identify malignant cells among the normal cast-off vaginal cells of women with cancer of the cervix. His observations grew out of studies of animal menstrual cycles, and from then on the technique of exfoliative cytology (the study of cast-off cells) was used to investigate virtually every hollow organ and secreted fluid.

For centuries, virtually the only definitive treatments of cancers were physical and chemical cauterizations, surgical removal of tumors on the surface of the body, and amputation. Surgeons of today are able to remove affected organ systems and even entire regions of the body with relative safety because of advances in physiology, anesthesia, transfusions, and anti-infective agents; however, the mutilations consequent to extensive resections (especially of the voice box, rectum, urinary bladder, limbs, and breast) have stimulated efforts toward rehabilitation, including self-help clubs, clinics, and special training for professionals. Along with observations that X-rays could cause severe damage came the realization that this power could be used to destroy cancerous tissue. As delivery system improvements permitted more effective and less hazardous doses of radiant energy, cures were reported of cancers of the mouth, voice-box, uterus, and, recently, other malignant conditions formerly with very low survival rates.

Another twentieth-century weapon against cancer is chemotherapy. Although arsenic compounds had been used to combat cancer as early as the eighteenth century, nothing new had been added to the armamentarium until it was discovered in World War I and confirmed in World War II that sulphur mustard (mustard gas) and similar chemicals could arrest malignant growths for a short time. Another group of anticancer compounds was added in 1947 when Sidney Farber, following the lead of biochemist Y. Subbarow, found that a derivative of folic acid (an essential nutrient) competed with folic acid and inhibited acute leukemia in children. Michael Heidelberger later synthesized 5-fluorouracil, a chemical agent still much in use today in chemotherapy. Since then a host of chemical agents have been developed from plants and microbes, each acting at different stages in the transformation and growth of malignant cells. Their principal limitations rest on the degree to which they also injure normal cells. The goal of chemotherapy is to find agents with absent, minimal, or controllable toxicity which act selectively on malignant tumors. Slowly and steadily since World War II tumor-growth diseases which were virtually hopeless in the past have become controllable, retarded, or cured by chemotherapy acting alone or in combination with surgery, radiation, immunity stimulation, and other forms of treatment.

The realization that combinations of different chemical agents could halt or cure cancer had significant influences on medical practice, including the emergence of a new specialty, oncology, and an alteration in therapeutic attitudes. Patients formerly given no hope by the medical profession, who in desperation gravitated toward unorthodox "cures" such as krebiozen and laetrile, now attract the full attention of physicians who see the opportunity of improving the chances for survival of patients with advanced malignant growths or at least of enhancing the quality of their remaining lives.

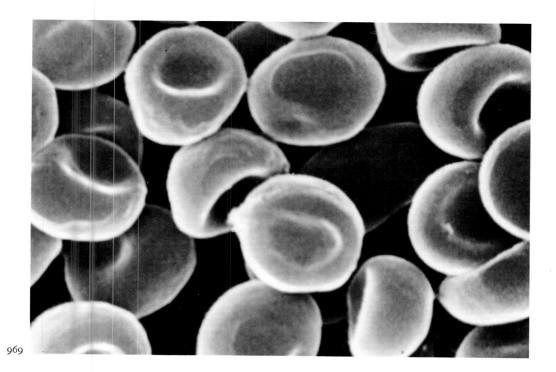

969

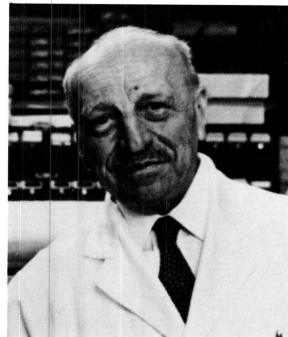

970

PATHOLOGY

The earliest pathologists in contemporary terms were those eighteenth- and nineteenth-century doctors who felt compelled to perform an autopsy ("see for oneself") in an attempt to find physical reasons for the manifestations of disease. Among them, Giovanni Battista Morgagni was the first to arrange and analyze his observations systematically. Rudolf Virchow was the pioneer in fully utilizing microscopic studies in the complete autopsy and set the pattern for the full development of pathology as a distinct specialty.

In the first half of the twentieth century, the techniques and concepts of autopsy pathology soon passed from the realm of general information to that of immediate practicality. It became obvious that samples of tissue, some only a few millimeters wide, could be obtained for microscopic study from a variety of organs, and the interpretations of the pathologist could determine not only the diagnosis and course of therapy, but the ultimate prognosis itself. The techniques for processing tissue for microscopic study were cumbersome and took many days in the early years of the century, but now, if immediate diagnosis is required for urgent therapy, the pathologist is able to prepare tissue samples by freezing and can render a diagnosis within minutes after surgical excision.

Pathologists also began to study the chemicals of the body in their investigations of disease. Small research laboratories were started in many hospital basements, often adjacent to the autopsy room, and it was from these beginnings that the fields of clinical and experimental pathology developed. Disease processes were generated in laboratory animals to provide opportunities for extensive inquiry into the basis, nature, and therapy of similar conditions that occurred in humans.

In the late 1950s pathologists eagerly embraced the electron microscope as a means of expanding their potential for the study of disease. However, it has proved to be useful in the diagnosis of only a small proportion of the diseases that afflict man. Other techniques for the study of subcellular chemistry developed soon after electron microscopy, and both approaches have allowed pathologists to gain new insights into the mechanisms of normal and abnormal cells. In the last decade, many pathologists have sought to define the molecular basis of disease. There is little diagnostic application for these techniques at present, but methods for studying components and products of the cell may prove to be of inestimable value in the care of the patient of the future.

967 *Peyton Rous, whose important work, using chickens, developed evidence that viruses can cause tumors in animals. National Library of Medicine, Bethesda*

968 *White blood cell, magnified about 6,000 times, which has the capability of destroying abnormal, potentially malignant cells. Grant Heilman Photography, Lititz, Pennsylvania*

969 *Red blood cells magnified 6,000 times by electron microscope, one of the techniques developed for the study of subcellular chemistry. Grant Heilman Photography, Lititz, Pennsylvania*

970 *Dr. George Papanicolaou, who, in working on uterine cancer, developed a technique (called the "Pap test") which is widely used as a routine screening for incipient cancer. New York Hospital–Cornell Medical Center*

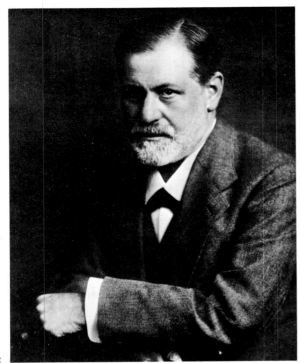

971

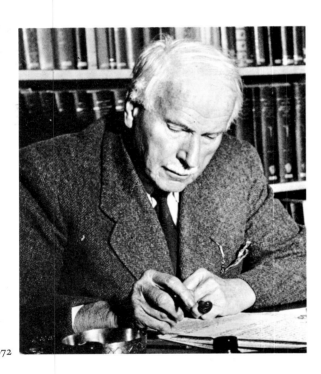

972

971 *Dr. Sigmund Freud, creator of psychoanalysis for the treatment of emotional illness. National Library of Medicine, Bethesda*

972 *Dr. Carl Gustav Jung, a disciple of Freud, who later broke with his mentor's teachings. National Library of Medicine, Bethesda*

PSYCHIATRY

An account of the development of psychiatry in the present century can begin neatly with the year 1900, when Sigmund Freud published *The Interpretation of Dreams* and induced a revolution in the field of psychiatry. Earlier, he had studied under Charcot in Paris, who aroused his interest in the problem of hysteria and the uses of hypnosis. In 1895 he had published, with Joseph Breuer, *Studies in Hysteria*. From these works and the large body of writings which followed, Freud created psychoanalysis. Among its basic concepts are that human behavior is heavily influenced by unconscious mental processes, that childhood experiences play a crucial role in development, and that internal psychological conflict is of central importance in mental life. Early in the development of psychoanalysis, two of Freud's leading collaborators, Carl Jung and Alfred Adler, broke with him and pursued conceptual paths of their own. At a later point, the psychoanalyst Karen Horney also split with the main body of psychoanalysis, as did Harry Stack Sullivan, who wrote extensively on the therapy of schizophrenia.

Another school of psychiatry developed in America during the early decades of the century under the leadership of Adolf Meyer, whose concepts (psychobiology) saw mental illness as the interaction of developmental (i.e., childhood), social, and psychological forces. Nevertheless, psychoanalysis was warmly received, particularly in the United States, and during the 1920s and 1930s a small but active "movement" developed in a number of centers. The impact of psychoanalysis on general psychiatry remained limited, however, until World War II. Prior to the war, psychiatric patients were housed chiefly in large state hospitals which afforded little beyond custodial care. The teaching of psychiatry in medical schools was, by contemporary standards, limited in scope and content, but the war changed all this dramatically. Medical officers on the draft boards, in training camps, and in combat learned at firsthand how prevalent emotional illnesses were and how the theories of psychoanalysis could be adapted to effect therapies for some of the "combat neuroses."

The "marriage" of psychoanalysis with general psychiatry as taught and practiced in medical schools and centers after the war gave rise to a brand of treatment called "dynamic" psychiatry, which depends on some form of "psychotherapy" as its chief method of treatment (i.e., an attempt to influence the patient's psychological state by verbal interaction, in which the relationship of the patient to the therapist usually plays a large role).

Two other streams should be recognized in the flow of twentieth-century psychiatry. Some workers see little or no value in the ideas of psychoanalysis or in the "dynamic" concepts derived from it, for they believe that emotional disturbances are caused "organically," i.e., by actual physical changes in the body (especially the brain). Another group feels that social and environmental forces are crucial in the causation of emotional illness and that these forces are not given sufficient weight by either the "dynamicists" or the "organicists." Regardless of theoretical viewpoints, there is considerable overlap in the therapeutic approaches used by psychiatrists who hold the varying viewpoints.

Beginning with the introduction of thorazine in the 1950s, the use of psychologically active drugs has become firmly established. Electro-convulsive therapy, commonly called "shock therapy," has now convinced many of its earlier opponents (who condemned its indiscriminate use) that it has a helpful role in severe depressions and in some acute attacks of schizophrenia. For about ten years during the 1940s and 1950s "psychosurgery" had a vogue, especially lobotomy, which involved cutting certain nerve fibers in the frontal portion of the brain. In the past few years there has been a renewed advocacy of brain surgery (of a more sophisticated kind) as a way of changing behavior, but opposition is strong, involving issues of civil rights and medical ethics.

In 1960, a report by a U.S. commission initiated the era of "community

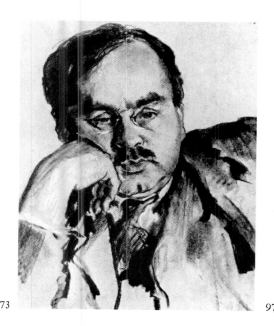

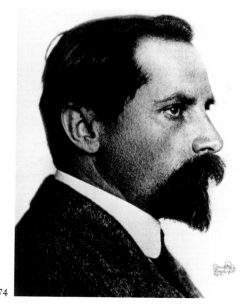

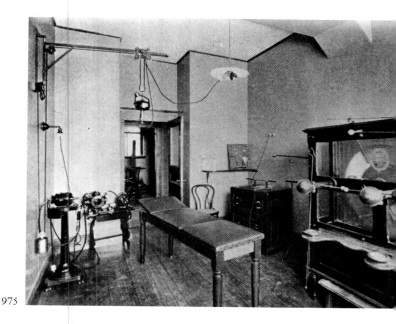

973

974

975

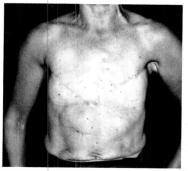

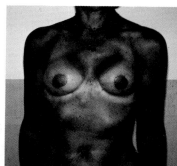

976

psychiatry," which advances notions that the mentally sick should be hospitalized in their communities, that psychiatric centers should offer a broad range of therapies under one roof, and that psychiatric professionals should go into the field and work with groups within the community.

The past decade or more has also seen the growth of psychotherapies loosely grouped under the heading of "behavior therapy" that aim to modify or eliminate neurotic symptoms by techniques which will condition the patient in such a way as to lead to the desired result. The treatment of patients in small groups of up to eight or ten members has long been recognized as highly useful, but during the 1960s offshoots from group therapy began to appear in the form of "sensitivity training groups," "encounter groups," and "marathon groups" extending through an entire weekend. Psychiatrists have generally condemned these offshoots because of the potential for harm in exposing some people to prolonged, intense emotional stress.

The 1960s and the 1970s have witnessed a virtual explosion of research in psychiatry and in fields relevant to psychiatry, notably in neurophysiology and neurochemistry, which offer small but encouraging glimmerings of the correlation between psychological processes and the physical structure of the brain. Additionally, there has been progress in the genetics of schizophrenia and manic-depressive illnesses.

As psychiatry began the twentieth century it came under the powerful influence of psychoanalysis, an influence which remains strong, though subject to many challenges. Today, the swelling tide of research may remind us that Sigmund Freud, even as he developed his psychological theories, predicted that one day all these processes would be explained in biochemical terms.

REHABILITATION

The concept of "rehabilitation" arose in 1918 out of society's compassion for the mutilated veterans of World War I. Training schools, hospitals, and various institutes were founded on a relatively modest scale, but programs were slow to develop despite laws and efforts by volunteer organizations. It took a second destructive world conflict to prompt governments, notably in the U.S., to develop facilities and programs for rehabilitating the limbless, paralyzed, blind, deaf, and "shell-shocked" war victims. Howard Rusk, as head of the American Air Force Convalescent Training Program, was a strong leader in organizing these programs and in extending them beyond the restoration of disabled persons to the reconditioning of military personnel suffering from any illness or injury.

973 *Dr. Alfred Adler, another of Freud's dissenting followers, who set up his own system. National Library of Medicine, Bethesda*

974 *Dr. Adolf Meyer, who saw mental illness as the interaction of developmental, social, and psychological forces. National Library of Medicine, Bethesda*

975 *The Electric Room (photographed in 1904), with equipment for electrotherapy, in the Adams Nervine Asylum, Boston. National Library of Medicine, Bethesda*

976 *Rehabilitation by plastic surgery after radical mastectomy. A sac of Silastic was implanted beneath the skin and a nipple was tatooed on the skin surface to create the form and appearance of a breast. Drs. Bernard Simon and Saul Hoffman, New York*

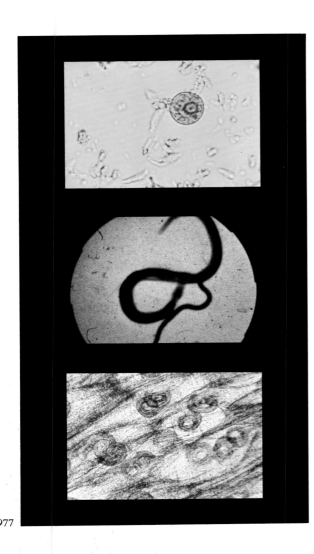

977

977 *Microphotographs* (top to bottom):
Entamoeba histolytica, *egg in stool of person with amoebic dysentery, which can spread rapidly through food and water contamination; schistosome parasite* (worms), *a devastating infestation in Asia and Africa, as usually seen, with male and female together; trichina parasite, which is transmitted through infected pork and encysts in muscles of the body. Drs. Edward J. Bottone and Bruce A. Hanna, Dept. of Microbiology, Mount Sinai Hospital, New York*

Now, virtually every medical school and hospital of size has a department devoted to rehabilitation, often as a special concern of the department of physical therapy. For a long time the main focus of these activities was on physical infirmities resulting from amputation, stroke, spinal injury, and limb destruction. In recent decades, rehabilitative techniques also have been applied to disabilities resulting from surgery, such as laryngectomy, colostomy and ileostomy, and breast excision. Self-help groups have sprung up through the efforts of disabled patients themselves and are indispensable aids in restoring people to full, cheerful living. These clubs often are instrumental in educating the healing professions in the proper management of patients and in altering the negative attitudes of the public to the handicapped and maimed.

PUBLIC HEALTH

The industrial revolution and the urbanization of nations created both problems and incentives to governmental entrance into the field of public health (a term introduced to government by John Simon, chief medical officer of the Privy Council in London).

In much of Europe, public health measures were mainly centralized, the principal hospitals and schools were state owned, and the delivery of medical care was through a relatively uniform system. By contrast, in America local autonomous bodies of the states and cities were the centers for public health activity, the influential hospitals and teaching institutions were voluntary and philanthropic, and the delivery of medical services was pluralistic and noncompulsory. In eastern Europe, health care delivery organization has been in the category of social service, with health centers at the core and their regulation authoritarian in line with the political and economic system. Since World War II, more and more governments have embarked on public health programs, placing their emphases on those aspects of health and disease which are most in need of improvement in their respective countries.

Coordinated international action on matters of health and disease had been taken from time to time for a specific, limited purpose, such as to contain an epidemic, but broad, organized, cooperative efforts to study and control illness in populations began in 1851 when twelve nations sent representatives to Paris for an International Sanitary Conference. During the next fifty-six years, other conferences led to a more permanent organization in 1907, L'Office International d'Hygiène Publique. Twenty-one countries of North and South America established an International Sanitary Bureau in 1902, later to be called the Pan American Health Organization. In 1948, the Paris-based group, the Health Organization of the League of Nations, and the United Nations Relief and Rehabilitation Administration merged into the World Health Organization (W.H.O.), of which the Pan American Health Organization later became an affiliate. As an agency of the U.N., W.H.O. now exchanges epidemiological and statistical information among its approximately 140 members, publishes technical journals and books, offers advisory services and consultants to countries on request, helps to standardize drugs and techniques, and generally acts as a coordinating body among the countries of the world to maintain the health of the world's population.

As infectious diseases are increasingly brought under control, the health of the aged has begun to enter the focus of public health agencies, with interest centered on the causes, prevention, and management of diseases such as cancer, arteriosclerosis, arthritis, and stroke. Social and occupational influences have also become a concern to those associated with "social medicine," a term introduced by Alfred Grotjahn (1869–1931). Physicians and surgeons have had to adjust to changing roles. As technicians they have had to learn the advancing mechanical techniques of diagnosis and therapy; as healers they have become increasingly involved in managing the psyche as well as the body; as scientists they must face an enormous expansion of physical, chemical, biological, and mathematical

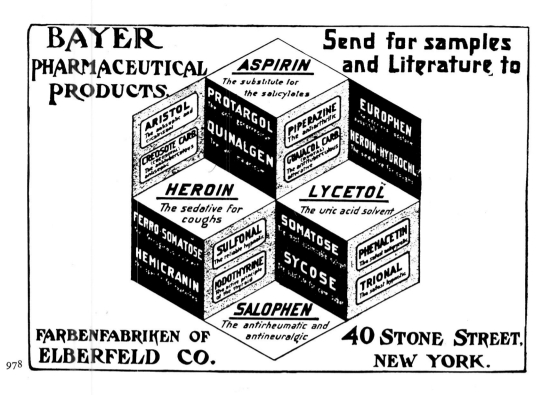

978

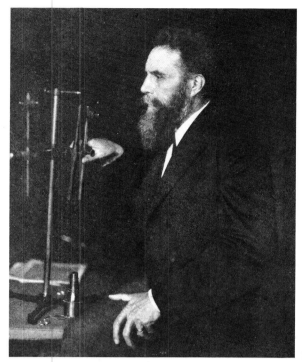

979

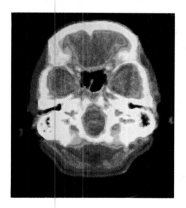 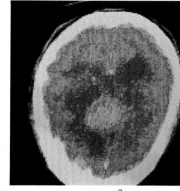

980

information. Now they may have to be sociologists as well, involved in the life styles of their patients, the affected families, and the surrounding population.

DIAGNOSIS AND THERAPY

RADIATION

The Victorian age merged into the twentieth century with the outstanding discoveries of X-rays by Roentgen and radium by the Curies. Even in the early years of the century radium proved useful for the treatment of cancer, and the X-ray became a powerful tool for the diagnosis of disease and later for the therapy of tumors. The first obvious use of the X-ray for diagnosis derived from its ability to show broken or deformed bones. Then the shadows began to reveal other abnormalities, in the chest and the gastrointestinal tract, bringing rational diagnosis to the practice of medicine.

In 1897 and 1898, Walter B. Cannon discovered that when he fed bismuth or barium mixtures to geese and other animals these radiopaque suspensions clearly outlined the animals' gullets on an X-ray plate. Today, similar suspensions make the entire alimentary tract accessible to routine radiological examinations.

X-ray facilities in hospitals and even in offices became centers of diagnostic activity. Tuberculosis became detectable early, and cancers were found more readily at stages when they could be surgically removed. Evarts Graham and Warren Cole developed a method of visualizing the gallbladder, and Moses Swick brought the kidneys into X-ray view by employing special iodide compounds. These workers and others thus took the first steps toward visualization of the blood vessels, heart, and other structures by techniques which used X-rays.

While developments in diagnosis proceeded, treatment with X-rays similarly advanced to the stage where high-voltage machines were able to cure some cancers, like those of the larynx and uterus. However, most of the therapeutic uses of X-rays were palliative, shielding the cancerous patient from his pain. Advances in radiation were most marked in World War II. Some of these derived from the availability for both diagnosis and treatment of artificial radioactive isotopes (man-made chemicals emitting radiation) which could be inserted directly into tumors. Fission products from splitting the atom of uranium, and isotopes from bombardment in nuclear reactors, began to replace radium and electronically generated X-rays just after World War II.

978 *Heroin advertised by Bayer Pharmaceutical Products in 1900. Synthesized by C. R. Wright in 1874, by 1898 it was considered the ideal non-addictive substitute for morphine and codeine. New York Academy of Medicine*

979 *Wilhelm Konrad Roentgen, the discoverer of X-rays. New York Academy of Medicine*

980 *Computerized Axial Tomography, or CAT-SCAN, of a normal brain at the base of the skull (left), and CAT-SCAN of the upper part of the brain showing a tumor (green area near the center). Mount Sinai School of Medicine, New York. Dr. Bernard S. Wolf*

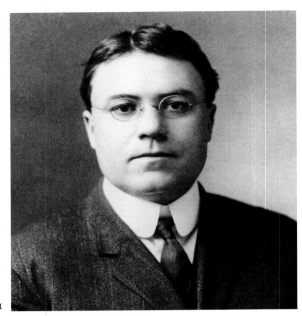

981

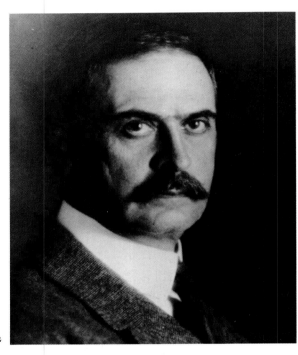

982

981 *Dr. Walter B. Cannon discovered that radio-paque suspensions could be fed a patient to make the alimentary tract visible on an X-ray plate. National Library of Medicine, Bethesda*

982 *Dr. Karl Landsteiner, in 1901, described the major red blood cell types A, B, O, and later AB, enabling blood to be matched for safe transfusion. National Library of Medicine, Bethesda*

983 *Exchange transfusion of a baby's blood, which had antibodies transmitted by its mother that acted against its own blood cells, with new blood. Dr. Richard Rosenfield, Mount Sinai Hospital, New York*

Meanwhile, a new concept developed in the early 1970s: diagnosis by computer processing of many beams of irradiation cast into the body from different directions (computerized axial tomography or CAT-SCAN), which provides insight into the interior of the body far exceeding the capabilities of conventional X-ray machines.

A new development from the use of internally deposited radioactive materials arose after World War II. Radioactive chemicals were injected into the body, and their varied distribution determined by a detector of radioactivity ("scanning") has been able to show abnormalities in the lungs, tumors in the brain, growths in bones, and masses in the thyroid, liver, and other organs.

TRANSFUSION

The achievement of safe blood transfusions in humans was a major step in the treatment of hemorrhage and anemia and opened the way for surgical procedures otherwise too dangerous.

Injections into the bloodstream are known to have been performed as early as the seventeenth century. Wine was often instilled into hunting dogs to treat illness, and Johann Daniel Major of Padua gave medications intravenously through thin silver cylinders. He also suggested that blood could be given into the veins, as did others, but there is no clear evidence that he ever did this in humans. Richard Lower in the seventeenth century was probably the first to make an actual transfusion from animal to animal through tubings, and, according to Samuel Pepys, he also administered sheep blood to a young man to try to change his character (results unknown). Nevertheless, Jean-Baptiste Denis is generally credited with the first successful human transfusion. In 1667 he gave three pints of sheep blood to a person with no apparent ill effects, but his subsequent attempt to give calf blood to a dissipated young man—to mollify his fiery nature—led to a severe reaction and death. Although Denis was exonerated in a trial, the Paris faculty forbade future transfusions. Ten years later Parliament declared transfusions to be illegal. The government in Rome also outlawed the transfusion of blood from person to person, but the Royal Society of London maintained its approval.

In the eighteenth and nineteenth centuries, experimental studies on transfusions in animals, and even humans, demonstrated that exsanguinated animals could be restored, that oxygen was transported by the blood, and that blood made incoagulable by whipping out its fibrin content could be administered to animals. Although it finally became clear that the passage of blood from animals to humans was prohibitively dangerous, the hazards of transferring blood from human to human were more slowly realized. Blundell, Ponfick, Landis, Arthur, and Pager reported on some of the physiological and chemical effects of transfusions, but the contributions to immunology by Ehrlich, Bordet, Gengou, and others were the significant openings that led to the clarification by Karl Landsteiner of the existence of blood groups and to the safe incorporation of blood transfusion into medical practice.

In 1901 Landsteiner described the major red blood cell types A, B, O, and later AB. A person with substance (antigen) A in his blood cells had antibodies against B in the liquid part of his blood (plasma), and type B blood cells were associated with plasma containing antibodies against A. The "universal donor," a term first coined by Ottenberg in 1911, had no antigen in the cells but did have antibodies to both A and B in the plasma or serum (plasma without cells or fibrin). Incompatible transfused blood could cause disastrous reactions, including kidney damage and death, but it was not until 1908 that Ottenberg tested the blood of donor and recipient before every transfusion. Despite the virtual absence of previous testing, serious reactions had not occurred more frequently because, with mathematical distribution of blood types, about two-thirds of random transfusions will have no ABO incompatibilities. Even with the precautions of typing and cross-matching, the severe reactions that sometimes did occur anyway were not explicable until other methods of testing and other human red cell types were discovered.

Initially, the transfusionist drew blood from a donor by multiple syringes and injected it into a patient's vein, but by the end of the nineteenth century Alexis Carrel and George Crile were connecting a donor's artery directly to the recipient's venous system. Crile, Ottenberg, Ellsberg, and others later improved on this by developing special needle-cannulas to permit easier vessel-to-vessel connections. Unger eventually devised an apparatus with a four-way stopcock by which blood could be transferred positively from donor to recipient—the first efficient direct transfusions. However, the system was cumbersome and required that the patient and compatible donor be brought together at the same time. This problem was solved by the exceedingly useful discovery that drawn blood could be kept incoagulable by a nontoxic chemical (sodium citrate) and later transfused as needed. Now blood banks containing stored blood are essential parts of every hospital, and techniques have been developed to test blood and to render its components safe for administration.

For many years, blood transfusions and intravenous injections of various solutions were often accompanied by febrile reactions attributed to the inherent nature of the process. Finally, in the 1920s and 1930s, these reactions were proved to result from previously undetected bacteria in the intravenous apparatus and solutions. When rigorous methods were instituted to eliminate such contaminants, febrile reactions caused by bacterial pyrogens disappeared.

ANTIMICROBIALS

Paul Ehrlich's search for a "magic bullet" which would seek out and kill germs in the body without destroying host cells was rewarded by the synthesis of arsenical compounds effective in the treatment of syphilis, but the principles he enunciated did not lead to an effective battle against microorganisms until about thirty years later.

Michael Heidelberger's work on pneumococcus (the bacterium that causes lobar pneumonia) enabled investigators to make a specific antiserum for each type of pneumococcal germ, but these sera were of limited effectiveness. Earlier (1917), Heidelberger and W. A. Jacobs had reported that sulfanilamide, an azo dye, destroyed bacteria, but no investigator followed this lead. In Germany, Gerhard Domagk, also testing the antibacterial activity of a variety of dyes, reported that prontosil, a textile dyestuff synthesized in 1908, acted against streptococci in mice. The introduction of this chemical into therapeutics dramatically altered the outlook of many infections, including "blood poisoning," heretofore almost invariably fatal. Tréfouël in France showed that prontosil caused the body to produce sulfanilamide, the active antibacterial substance in the dye. Subsequent chemical and clinical studies in the United States and elsewhere yielded a variety of other derivatives: sulfapyridine, sulfathiazole, sulfadiazine, sulfaguanidine, and soluble sulfa drugs for treating urinary infections.

Other antibacterial chemical substances were developed, among which isoniazid proved so effective against the tubercle bacillus that the therapy of tuberculosis was revolutionized. Streptomycin had been introduced earlier, but it required injection and also had potentially serious side effects. Hospitals devoted primarily to the treatment of tuberculosis soon ran out of patients, and the formerly uncertain outlook for the tubercular became dramatically better in the course of a few years.

Pasteur and many after him had observed occasional antagonisms between bacteria. Some investigators tried with varying success in the laboratory and in patients to impede the growth of one species of bacteria by cultures or extracts from another, but the results were either uncertain or the products too toxic.

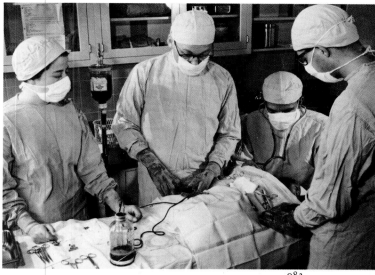

983

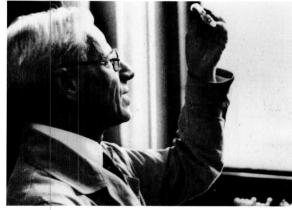

984

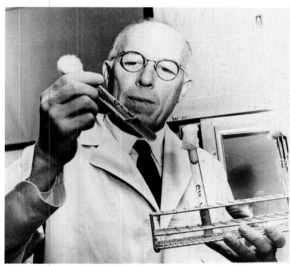

985

984 *Dr. Michael Heidelberger, a pioneer in the chemotherapy of infections and of cancer. National Library of Medicine, Bethesda*

985 *Dr. René Dubos, an important contributor to antimicrobial research. National Library of Medicine, Bethesda*

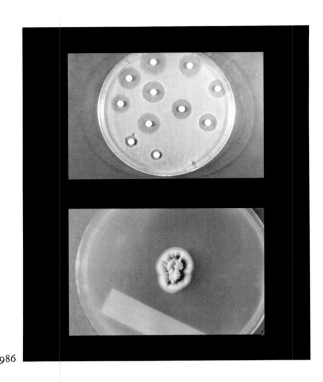

986

986 *Test of organism sensitivity to antibiotics (top); penicillium culture (bottom). Drs. Edward J. Bottone and Bruce A. Hanna, Dept. of Microbiology, Mount Sinai Hospital, New York*

987, 988 *Dr. Ernst Boris Chain and Prof. Howard W. Florey, whose studies established the great therapeutic properties of penicillin. Wide World Photos, New York*

989 *Dr. A. Selman Waksman, discoverer of streptomycin and Nobel Prize winner in 1952. World Health Organization, Geneva*

990 *Huge fermentation tanks used in the production of antibiotics. United Press International, New York*

991 *An intensive care unit, for continuous monitoring of patient's vital signs. Mount Sinai Hospital, New York. Dr. Christopher Bryan-Brown*

992 *Hyperbaric chamber, where increased atmospheric pressure during operation forces oxygen into tissues starved by diminished circulation. Dr. Julius Jacobson, Mount Sinai Hospital, New York*

However, a steady stream of publications appearing in the late nineteenth and early twentieth centuries indicated that the higher bacteria, molds, and fungi also destroyed certain bacteria (a process Vuillemin had earlier named antibiosis). Westling in 1912 named one such effective mold *Penicillium notatum.* Lieske in 1921 and Gratia slightly later proved that a species of penicillium dissolved anthrax bacilli and impeded staphylococci.

In 1929, Alexander Fleming reported in the *British Journal of Experimental Pathology* his observations on the antibacterial action of penicillium, with the suggestion that the mold culture could be used to inhibit bacteria as a help in obtaining their cultural isolation. Whatever Fleming may have thought of the eventual usefulness of what he called penicillin, there was virtually no further research until Howard Florey and Ernst Chain in England made studies in 1941 which convinced them that penicillin had great therapeutic potential. The only difficulty was that penicillin could not be made in quantity in the laboratory, but this was solved by cooperation between the U.S. government and pharmaceutical manufacturers within two years after Florey and Chain had transferred their work to America.

Other types of antibiotics followed in rapid order. Streptomycin was obtained by Selman Waksman from *Streptomyces griseus* in 1944 and proved to be useful against a variety of infections, especially tuberculosis. Other strains of the streptomyces yielded additional therapeutic substances such as chloromycetin and aureomycin. Since 1948 many other similar agents have entered the medical armamentarium, each with a special potency but also with its own limitations. As new substances were used their bacterial targets developed resistance, so researchers have had to enter an ever-quickening race to stay ahead of the adaptation by germs to each new drug. Furthermore, antibacterial agents are limited by their inherent toxicity and newly acquired allergies and sensitivities of patients to the antibiotics.

KIDNEY DIALYSIS

A bold concept almost entirely a product of the twentieth century is the removal of a diseased organ and the transplantation of a healthy organ from another person. The kidney has been the most successful of the organ transplants, but this would not have been possible without a means of keeping the stricken patient alive while awaiting the availability of a suitable kidney donor.

In 1913, John J. Abel, L. G. Rowntree, and B. B. Turner arranged a mechanical system, which they called an "artificial kidney," whereby the blood of a dog could be freed of toxic chemicals by circulating it through collodion tubing that allowed toxins to pass out into surrounding liquid while keeping blood substance inside. For this method to be useful to humans, more efficient tubing had to be developed and a more convenient, safe anticoagulant had to be found to prevent the blood from clotting as it flowed through the apparatus. Both requirements were met in cellophane and in heparin, and Willem J. Kolff from The Netherlands then built an effective though cumbersome apparatus in 1945 which was used successfully in humans. Beginning in 1947, modifications by John Merrell, Karl Walter, and many others finally resulted in smaller and more effective machines. Belding Scribner and other investigators so improved the technique of removing and returning the blood through relatively permanent implanted tubings that patients can now be "dialyzed" for an hour or two as frequently as needed (either in a hospital setting or even at home) on a continuing basis or until a compatible kidney donor is found.

TRANSPLANTATION OF ORGANS

When Christiaan Barnard performed the first heart transplant operation in 1967 at the Groote Schuur Hospital in Capetown, the world realized that a new era of surgery had arrived. Up until that time the public had been minimally aware of the

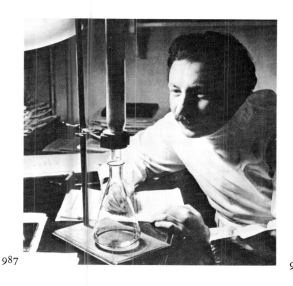

987

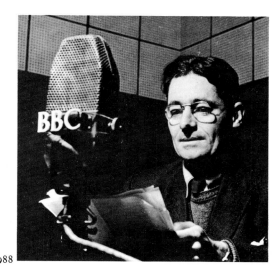

988

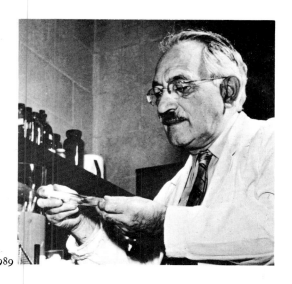

989

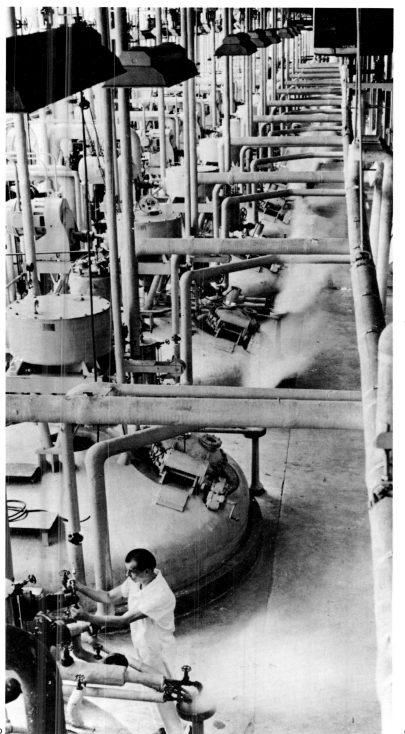

990

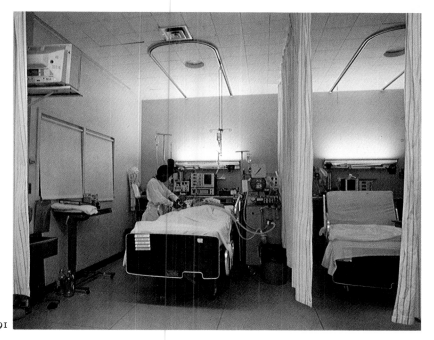

991

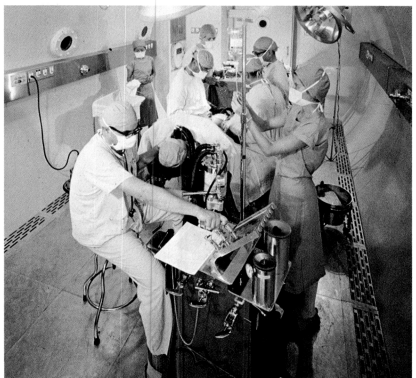

992

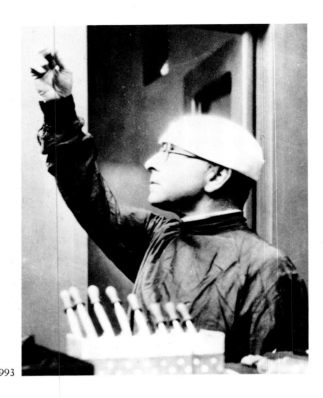

993

993 *Dr. Alexis Carrel, first researcher in America to win a Nobel Prize in medicine or physiology. National Library of Medicine, Bethesda*

994 *New device for heretofore difficult measurement of infant blood pressure. Dr. Leonard Steinfeld, Mount Sinai Hospital, New York*

995 *Artist's visualization of Stephen Hales measuring the blood pressure of a horse. Medical Times, New York*

996 *Scipione Riva-Rocci's sphygmomanometer (1895), the true ancestor of all modern blood pressure devices in clinical use. Dr. Philip Reichert, New York*

advances of kidney transplantation and transplantation research. But when a heart was transplanted the public's emotions ran wild, and newspapers throughout the world proclaimed in headlines daily advances in the transplant world.

The first bonafide report in the medical literature of organ transplantation came from Vienna at the turn of the twentieth century when Emerich Ullmann transplanted a dog's kidney from its normal position to the neck. This autotransplant (from the same individual) worked quite well, but when Ullmann transplanted a kidney from one dog to another dog its function was short-lived. Later, he successfully transplanted a dog's kidney to the neck of a goat, the first xenografting in scientific annals.

Ullmann's work was taken up by Alexis Carrel, who in 1912 was the first researcher in America to win a Nobel prize in medicine or physiology. Carrel realized that a major technical difficulty was the lack of a method of rapidly reestablishing a normal blood circulation to a transplanted organ, and he devised successful surgical techniques for suturing small vessels. Working with Charles Guthrie, he successfully performed a dog kidney autotransplant in 1905, but the recipient eventually died when the kidney failed.

Research in transplantation lay dormant until 1923 when Carlos Williamson concluded that underlying the failures was a fundamental biological principle which had not yet been identified. Examining rejected tissue under a microscope, he described the characteristics of the rejection phenomenon for the first time. In the 1950s, Emile Holman came to the conclusion that rejection of grafts was due to a special antibody for that tissue, that if a host received skin grafts from three different donors each would be rejected by a different antibody formed expressly in response to the genetic makeup of that particular donor. At about the same time, MacFarlane Burnet in Australia and Peter Medawar in England, working separately, achieved a significant breakthrough by discovering the means by which a newborn animal could be permanently induced to tolerate a foreign protein, for which they received a Nobel prize in 1960. However, a number of attempts to transplant kidneys continued to fail because there was still no way to effect tolerance in adult humans to a donor organ. Then, in 1954, a team at The Peter Bent Brigham Hospital in Boston transplanted successfully and permanently a kidney from an identical twin to his brother who was dying of kidney failure. But the transferring of a kidney in nonrelated persons was not successful until researchers were able to prevent the rejection of transplants through drugs that lower the recipient's immunological responses. Thereafter kidney transplantation became feasible on a reasonably large scale.

ORGAN SYSTEMS

CARDIOLOGY

In the early years of the twentieth century, Dutch physicist Willem Einthoven adapted to medical practice a newly discovered instrument for measuring minute electric currents. This instrument, the string galvanometer, provided the first practical tool for recording the electrical activity of the human heart in the electrocardiogram (ECG). By the end of World War I, this instrument had so proved its usefulness in clinical medicine that the science of electrocardiography, especially as developed by Thomas Lewis in England, became a cornerstone of clinical cardiology. With the continued application of basic science to medicine, ECG machines were so improved as to permit not only "spot checks" of cardiac function but continuous recordings of disturbed heart rate and rhythm in acutely ill patients. This led directly to the concept of the coronary care unit, in which prompt recognition of electrocardiographic warnings has significantly reduced the death rate from heart disease.

Studies in the first half of this century of altered pressures and flows in the hearts of animals with natural and induced abnormalities similar to those found in man laid the foundations for modern cardiology and for open heart surgery. In the early 1940s, when André Cournand and Dickinson W. Richards in New York provided a safe and practical method to measure pressures and flows in the human heart, the technique of cardiac catheterization was coupled with advances in thoracic surgery to make use of the earlier knowledge of cardiac abnormalities in experimental animals.

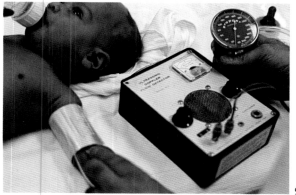

994

Many new drugs have been added to the relatively few effective agents against heart disease discovered in previous centuries. Moreover, newer mechanical and pharmacological methods have often enabled medical and nursing personnel to resuscitate some people stricken with a cardiac catastrophe who heretofore would have been beyond help.

Today we are witnessing yet another phase in the growth of basic knowledge and its application to the cardiac patient. Understanding of the molecular basis for cardiac disease promises considerable benefit in two areas, atherosclerosis (a disease process of complex origins which interrupts the blood supply of the heart and so causes heart attacks) and arrhythmias (disturbances of the orderly beating of the heart which can cause symptoms and even sudden death). Both of these disease processes are now being illuminated by the discoveries of molecular biology (study of the basic chemical structure of living tissues).

HYPERTENSION (HIGH BLOOD PRESSURE)

The first person to measure blood pressure was the clergyman Stephen Hales, who in 1733 inserted a hollow tubing into the neck artery of a horse and was astonished to see the blood rise nine feet in a glass column. This was obviously impractical for regular use with humans, and it took another 143 years before an instrument was invented, by Ritter von Basch, which could measure the blood pressure of a human without breaking the skin. This "sphygmomanometer" was the forerunner of the ingeniously simple device introduced by Scipione Riva-Rocci in 1896, a prototype of the more refined instruments of today. Blood pressure was found to equal the pressure in an inflated cuff, compressing the arm, at a point where the pulse could first be felt as the cuff was deflated. This was called the systolic blood pressure because it coincided with the contraction of the heart. N. S. Korotkoff, in 1905, by using a stethoscope to monitor the pulse not only achieved a more accurate reading but also discovered that the pulse sound disappeared, as the cuff pressure declined, at a point roughly in consonance with the expanding of the heart (diastole) —thus establishing the diastolic pressure.

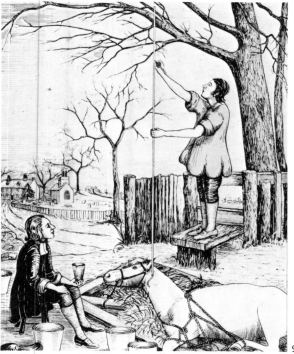

995

Experimental investigations by Harry Goldblatt, R. Tigerstedt, P. G. Bergman, and others first showed that blood pressure could be affected by a substance elaborated in the kidney. Subsequent intensive studies by many researchers, including G.W. Pickering, M. Prinzmetal, I. Page, F. Volhard, D. van Slyke, and Braun-Menendez, have revealed the existence of a complex enzymatic, hormonal mechanism of blood pressure regulation in which the kidneys, adrenals, and nervous system all play an important part.

Numerous treatments have successfully controlled excessively high blood pressure: various diets; operations on the adrenals, kidneys, arteries, and sympathetic nervous system; and many chemical agents. Certain specific causes of high blood pressure have been discovered, such as tumors of the adrenal gland and narrowing of the arteries leading to the kidneys, but causation of the majority of instances of hypertension are yet to be explained.

CARDIAC SURGERY

For a long time the heart was considered outside the limits of surgery. As late as 1896, the usually perceptive historian Stephen Paget wrote, "Surgery of the heart

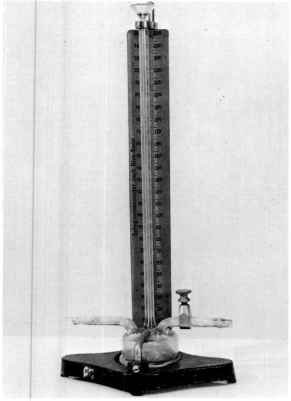

996

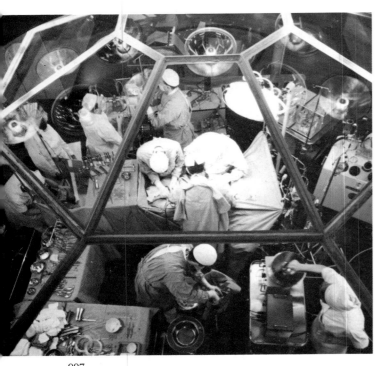

997

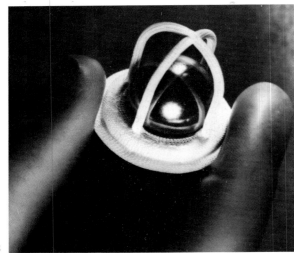

998

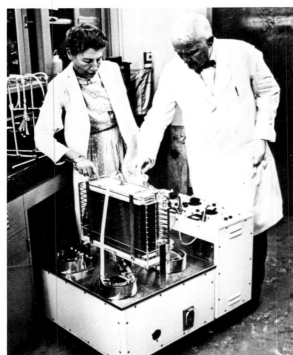

999

has probably reached the limits set by Nature to all surgery; no new method, and no new discovery can overcome the natural difficulties that attend a wound of the heart." Ironically, that same year, Ludwig Rehn successfully repaired a laceration of the heart, and the era of cardiac surgery began.

Later developments in operations on the heart stemmed from several innovations. First, methods were found to enter the chest safely under anesthesia (resulting from Sauerbruch's experiences with his special chamber in 1904) and to introduce anesthetic gases under pressure through intratracheal tubes to keep the lungs inflated. Another development came out of early attempts at sewing together severed arteries. After numerous failures by many investigators, Robert Gross in 1948 succeeded in bridging severed ends of the large main artery (aorta) by tissue and artificial grafts.

In the heart itself, early attempts to correct valve abnormalities were for the most part unsuccessful. The pioneer accomplishment in 1923 by E. Cutler and S. A. Levine of widening a scarred valve inside the heart was followed by numerous failures and only a rare success. Finally, in the 1940s, C. Bailey and D. Haven in the U.S. and H. Sellors and R. Brock in England regularly were able to achieve satisfactory results. When C. Hufnagel in 1952 implanted a synthetic valve, cardiac surgery had reached general acceptance.

An innovation essential to the future of medical and surgical treatment of heart disease came about as Werner Forssmann, a young intern in a German hospital, was trying to work out a technique for emergency injection of drugs directly into the heart. In 1929, while standing behind a fluoroscopic screen and looking into a mirror, he threaded a thin catheter inserted into his own arm vein through the venous channels and into his heart. Daring as this procedure was, it actually had been performed fifteen years earlier by Bleichroeder, Unger, and Loeb without the aid of X-rays. After intracardiac catheterization came into use, investigators were able to perform detailed, quantitative physiological studies, and A. Cournand and D. W. Richards, Jr., were corecipients with Forssmann of a Nobel prize in 1956. Cardiac catheterization also permitted X-ray visualization of the interior of the heart and blood vessels by the injection of radiopaque substances. Another noteworthy innovation was the use of pacemakers to keep the heart beating even though scarring interfered with the transmission of contracting impulses throughout the heart muscle (heart block).

Until mid-century, various remarkable reparative operations on congenital defects and malarrangements of the large blood vessels were performed inside the heart entirely by feel since the heart had to be kept pumping blood. These blind manipulations were based on anatomical dissections by Rokitansky in the nineteenth century and Maude Abbott in the twentieth, who had thoroughly classified cardiac defects. In 1939 Robert Gross reported the first successful cure of a congenital heart anomaly. Acting on suggestions by E. Park and Helen Taussig, Alfred Blalock devised procedures which rearranged the abnormal arterial connections of newborn "blue babies," thus dramatically saving these heretofore doomed children and prompting corrective operations on other congenital defects as well.

However, to permit open, careful procedures on the heart under direct vision, a means was required to keep oxygenated blood circulating, especially to the brain, without action by the heart. After nineteen years of intensive experiment, John Gibbon, his wife, and others constructed a heart-lung machine which accomplished this and enabled him, in 1953, to successfully close a defect inside the heart under direct visualization. Variations of the heart-lung machine subsequently have been used in an increasing number of cardiac operations and to support patients suffering from acute heart attacks. The development of the heart-lung machine and the intracardiac catheter have also made possible recent operations devised to bypass blocked coronary arteries which nourish the heart muscle.

It was to be expected that eventually attempts would be made to replace a hopelessly inadequate heart with a living transplant. Such transplantations in animals, along with intensive study of the physiologic consequences, had been reported in the 1950s and early 1960s, but in 1967 Christiaan Barnard in South

594

Africa actually performed the first cardiac transplantation on a human. During the following five years, well over a hundred heart transplants were tried, with some recipients surviving several years, but as of 1977 there were virtually no long-term survivors and the procedure had been almost abandoned, principally because of an inability to control rejection by the body of the newly transplanted heart.

The use of mechanical devices either to support the damaged heart or to replace it completely (for short periods of time) were first reported in animals by T. Akutsu and W. Kolff in 1958 and later by De Bakey and others. D. Cooley and coworkers in 1969 employed an artificial heart for the first time to keep a patient alive for about two-and-a-half days while awaiting the transplantation of a living heart.

Whether the future course of cardiac surgery will be in the direction of living heart transplantation or mechanical replacement depends in large measure on increased understanding of the immunologic mechanism and on advances in bioengineering.

SURGERY OF THE ARTERIES

Modern vascular surgery began near the end of the last century when Matas of New Orleans developed the first operation directly on an arterial aneurysm. About the same time, the famous Russian physiologist Eck performed a vascular connection between the portal vein and the vena cava, two principal venous trunks in the abdomen. After the turn of the century, Carrel developed a scientific method of connecting the ends of blood vessels (applicable to either small or large arteries and veins) which achieved a watertight suture without narrowing the caliber of the vessel. Nevertheless, a long time elapsed before the technique came into clinical application.

The success of early operations on the heart and great vessels stimulated further research throughout the world on surgery of the blood vessels. Robert Gross first used segments of arteries harvested from people who died in accidents to create a shunt between systemic and pulmonary circulations. Dos Santos of Lisbon attempted to recanalize an occluded artery by removal of the thrombus and the sclerotic plaques on its inner lining. Goyanes of Spain was the first to use a segment of popliteal vein to restore the continuity of the popliteal artery (a large artery along the back of the leg) after excising an aneurysm. In 1948, Kunlin of Paris used a segment of the saphenous vein (a long vein in the leg) to bypass a blockage of the main artery in the extremity. In 1950 Oudot of France performed the earliest successful resection of an occluded bifurcation of the aorta (the main artery in the abdomen), bridging the gap with a homograft (another person's artery). The first effective resection of an abdominal aneurysm of the aorta and insertion of a homograft was reported by Dubost of Paris in 1952.

Nevertheless, homografts were difficult to procure and they suffered anatomical alterations over a period of time, so the need for a synthetic graft material became evident. Glass and aluminum tubes had been tried by Carrel and Tuffier in World War I, and vitallium, polyethylene, and siliconized rubber were also used later. However, the only clearly successful and practical graft material appeared to be a synthetic fabric; the first to be used experimentally on dogs was porous vinyon and vinyon "N" cloth, which Voorhees employed in humans in 1953. Later, many other materials were created, but the search for an ideal artificial graft continues.

In 1921, Nylen used a monocular microscope in the performance of an operation on the ear for deafness. A year later Holmgren described the successful employment of a binocular magnifying instrument which became the prototype for all subsequent microsurgical apparatuses in various fields, as for instance by Donaghy and by Jacobson and Suarez in 1964, who reported on microsurgical techniques for joining small blood vessels. In recent decades limbs have been

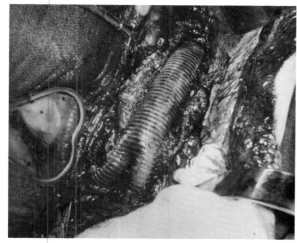

1000

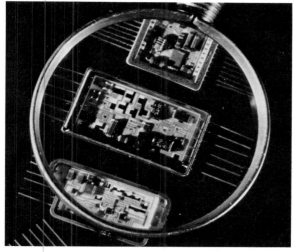

1001

997 *Open heart surgery in progress in a French hospital (1974). World Health Organization, Geneva*

998 *Replacement heart valve. National Heart Institute/World Health Organization*

999 *Dr. John Gibbon and his wife with the first heart-lung machine, which made open heart surgery possible.*

1000 *Artificial aortic graft in place. Dr. Adolf Singer, New York*

1001 *Microminiaturized electronic device for use in a pacemaker. Museum of Electricity in Life at Medtronic, Minneapolis*

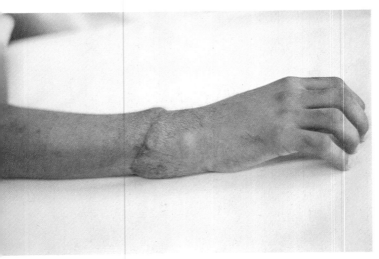

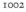
1002

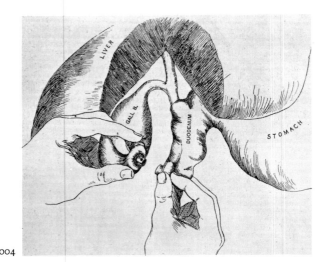
1003

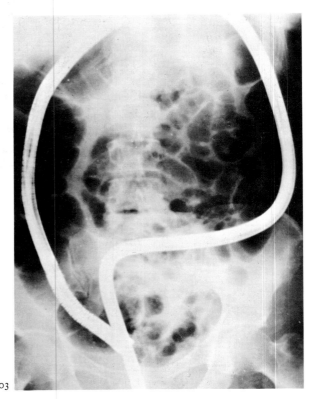
1004

saved from gangrene due to arteriosclerosis of the arteries by procedures which bypass the blocked vessels. Furthermore, through teamwork among several disciplines severed limbs have sometimes been reconnected with survival of the limb and eventual restoration of much of the function.

GASTROENTEROLOGY

A whole field of science rarely develops overnight, but it might well be said that modern gastroenterology was born on the morning of June 6, 1822, when Dr. William Beaumont treated the severe wound of Alexis St. Martin which left his stomach permanently exposed through his abdominal wall. The classic series of experiments conducted by Beaumont proved the presence of hydrochloric acid in the gastric juice, established the intimate relationship between emotional state and gastric secretion and digestion, delineated the details of gastric motor activity, and in many other ways opened the frontiers of physiological research in gastroenterology.

In 1902, the discovery by William Bayliss and Ernest Starling in London that a chemical substance from intestinal tissue (which they called "secretin") was capable of stimulating secretion from the pancreatic gland revolutionized biologic science by proving that organ function could be regulated by chemicals as well as by nerves. Thus the field of endocrinology was born as an offspring of gastroenterology. In 1905, William Hardy's newly coined word, "hormone" (Greek for "I arouse activity"), was first applied in print to the whole class of other postulated chemical messengers like secretin. At the very same time, John Edkins was demonstrating the presence of a stomach-acid-stimulating chemical messenger in the lower half of the stomach of dogs, which he named "gastrin."

Other hormones influencing gastrointestinal function were reported in subsequent years, and today there are over two dozen established and presumed gastrointestinal hormones—with more undoubtedly yet to come. Among the many other noteworthy contributions to understanding the mechanisms involved in diseases of the alimentary tract was the introduction by Dragstedt and Owens of the operation which cuts the vagus nerves for the treatment of peptic ulcer.

In 1965, in a genetics laboratory in Philadelphia, B. S. Blumberg with his colleagues discovered by chance a virus antigen which became the key to the mystery of serum hepatitis (a liver ailment following transfusion), for which he received a Nobel prize in 1976.

In addition to the X-ray techniques for visualizing the alimentary tract, other important technical innovations have included I. J. Wood's gastric suction tube in 1949, an intestinal biopsy tube by Margot Shiner in 1958, the liver biopsy needle by Menghini, and numerous endoscopes which permit visual inspection, tissue sampling, and even surgical manipulation of the esophagus, stomach, duodenum, colon, abdominal cavity, and the ducts of the pancreas and bile system.

One of the outstanding advances in medicine of the twentieth century was the discovery that a correctable nutritional deficiency, associated with the absence of acid in the stomach, was responsible for the fatal disease pernicious anemia. After many years of painstaking animal experiments George Richards Minot reported the cure of a human with the disease by the ingestion of a large quantity of liver. The combined and separate efforts of William Parry Murphy, George Whipple, Edwin Cohn, William Castle, and others were responsible for finally discovering, isolating, and proving that the missing factor was a vitamin (B 12). Minot, Murphy, and Whipple received a Nobel prize in 1934.

ENDOCRINOLOGY

Perhaps the most famous contribution to endocrinology was the isolation of insulin by Frederick Banting and Charles Best in 1921. Over subsequent decades, various types of injectable long-acting insulins were prepared for the treatment of diabetes, and there were other chemical agents synthesized which could be taken by mouth to lower blood sugar.

Clarification by animal experiments of the function of the parathyroid glands, located in the neck, and their relationship to calcium in the blood and bones permitted the effects of parathyroid tumors to be understood. Collip and Hanson in 1925 and Copp in 1962 further illuminated the physiological role of the hormones secreted by these glands.

The discovery in the 1920s of the sex-organ-stimulating principles of the pituitary gland (at the base of the brain) was followed by the introduction in 1928 by Ascheim and Zondek of the first usable pregnancy test ("The A-Z test") based on hormones in blood from the placenta. Soon after, the chemical structures of female sex hormones were delineated and their relationship to the menstrual cycle explained. Based on this understanding, oral contraceptive drugs were later introduced in the 1950s by Gregory Pincus.

The discovery just before 1900 that substances in the inner layer of the adrenal glands (located just above the kidneys) raised blood pressure enabled physicians to recognize the effects of adrenal tumors. Studies on the chemicals secreted by the adrenals, which control the tension of artery walls, led to a clearer understanding of the mechanism of hypertension. The importance of the outer layer of the adrenals to the maintenance of life was only fully appreciated in the 1920s and 1930s, although Addison in the nineteenth century had described the disastrous effects of adrenal disease. Laboratory experiments coupled with clinical observations revealed the interrelationships of the adrenals with the pituitary and the sex organs in health and illness. The isolation and synthesis of hormones from these organs made them available for the treatment of many disease processes (for instance, arthritis, inflammatory conditions, and deficiency states).

The probable functions of the thyroid were learned in 1891 when extracts of the gland helped people with sluggish behavior, increased weight, hair loss, and other symptoms of deficient thyroid activity. In 1910 David Marine and others indicated that goiter (enlargement of the thyroid) represented an iodine deficiency which could be prevented by taking iodine. In the 1940s when investigators succeeded in crystallizing the hormones secreted by the thyroid, the pathologic conditions of the thyroid gland were better understood. Overactive secretions (hyperthyroidism) could be managed by one of several methods: operative removal of a sizable portion of the gland (performed less frequently now); drugs to nullify the effects; and radioactive iodine to diminish thyroid activity.

As more information accumulated, the tiny pituitary gland was seen to be a central control station for virtually all of the endocrine glands. Acting on the sex organs, adrenals, thyroid, and perhaps also directly on other tissues, the pituitary appears to affect many processes, including the growth of bones. Hormones thus represent an important group of chemical messengers by which different organs and tissue systems affect each other.

OPHTHALMOLOGY

At the turn of the century, many of the basic tools of ophthalmology already were known: the slit-lamp microscope to examine with magnification the front structures of the living eye, the ophthalmoscope to see the interior, and the tonometer to measure pressure and thus study glaucoma. The gross and microscopic structures of the eye in health and in disease were well known, but complete details of how the eye functions had not yet been worked out. In terms of treatment, there was a crude operation for removing senile cataracts and pilocarpine drops and some simple procedures for glaucoma. Eyeglasses had been known to Europe since the thirteenth century. However, detached retina was untreatable, and there were no antibiotics or effective drugs against infections and inflammations.

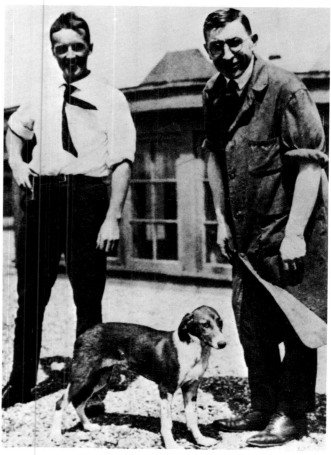

1005

1002 *Severed hand and wrist reattached, one year after reimplantation. Dr. Callisto Danese, New York*

1003 *X-ray showing use of colonoscope to visualize interior of organ. American Cystoscope Makers, Stamford*

1004 *Illustration showing use of the "Murphy button" to achieve simple connection between hollow organs. National Library of Medicine, Bethesda*

1005 *Frederick Banting and Charles Best, photographed in 1921. Working with dog shown, Banting and Best made an outstanding contribution to endocrinology by isolating insulin for the treatment of diabetes. World Health Organization, Geneva*

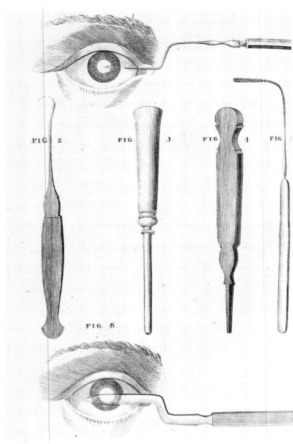

1006

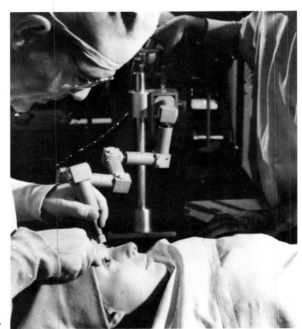

1007

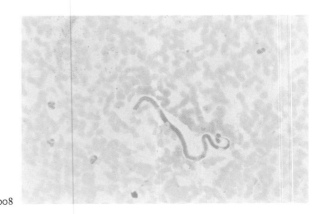

1008

Although special eye doctors had existed since antiquity, there were very few physicians who had the training and equipment to devote themselves entirely to ophthalmology. Treatment of most eye diseases was in the hands of general practitioners, or eye, ear, nose, and throat doctors. Spectacles were often sold over-the-counter or by itinerant spectacle-peddlers after a minimal examination or none at all.

Advances in ophthalmology may be illustrated by the evolution of cataract extraction. By 1900 a reasonably satisfactory operation had replaced the ancient procedure of "couching," whereby the cataract was simply pushed down out of the line of sight. In the early nineteenth century, removal of the lens was made considerably more practical by the advent of local anesthesia (introduced by an ophthalmologist, Carl Koller, in the late nineteenth century) and by sterile techniques. Over the years innumerable small improvements in instruments, suture materials and needles, and operative techniques have made the operation safer and more effective.

In a similar way, the treatment of glaucoma, cross-eyes, and most other major and minor conditions has gradually improved. Innovations also have occurred in eyeglasses, contact lenses, and medications, but perhaps the most dramatic advances have been in antibiotics, operations for detached retina, and the use of corticosteroids, which have transformed some hitherto hopeless diseases into treatable conditions.

Nevertheless, the delivery of the best eye care is not available all over the world. Of the four leading causes of blindness, only one is a problem in knowledge: river blindness, or onchocerciasis, a type of parasitic infestation carried by flies for which neither prevention nor treatment is satisfactory. On the other hand, trachoma is easily preventable and treatable, yet it remains a worldwide scourge simply because the remedies are not always available where they are needed. Similarly, cataracts are also easy to cure, but only if the patient, a trained surgeon, and an operating room can be brought together. A fourth cause of blindness, malnutrition, which promotes degeneration of the eye structures, is also a sociological problem.

We are almost helpless in the face of such degenerative diseases as diabetic retinopathy and senile macular degeneration, a cause of much blindness, and, similarly, we are just beginning to be able to handle some of the inherited diseases. Discoveries in chemical analysis of genetic defects may teach us more about retinitis pigmentosa, retino blastoma, and numerous other causes of disability which are transmitted in the genes.

OTORHINOLARYNGOLOGY

In the ear, nose, and throat specialty (otorhinolaryngology), operations on the ear for infection and for deafness have been among the outstanding contributions of this century. For generations, the disfiguring scar of a mastoidectomy had been a common sight. However, when the antimicrobial agents came into use in the 1940s and 1950s, most ear infections could be managed without major operations, and so mastoidectomy has declined in frequency.

The surgical treatment of otosclerosis, a major cause of deafness, gained its principal impetus from reports by Julius Lempert in 1938 of a fenestration operation which placed the eardrum directly against the labyrinth (an inner ear structure), permitting sound to bypass the usual entrance blocked because of otosclerotic disease. Although Holmgren's introduction in 1923 of the operating microscope (later taken up by other surgical disciplines) had been closely followed by successful fenestration operations in stages, by Sourdille, it was not until Lempert's achievements that otologic surgeons began to take up the operation in earnest.

Samuel Rosen, while performing a fenestration procedure in 1952, noted that freeing the fixed stapes bone immediately improved the patient's hearing.

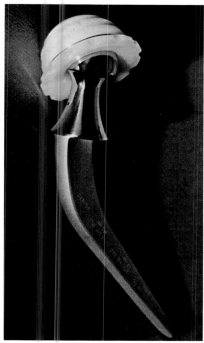

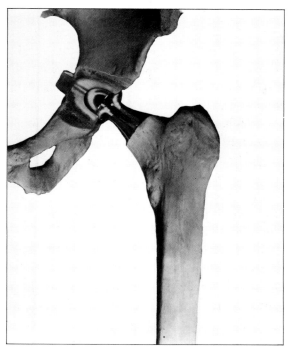

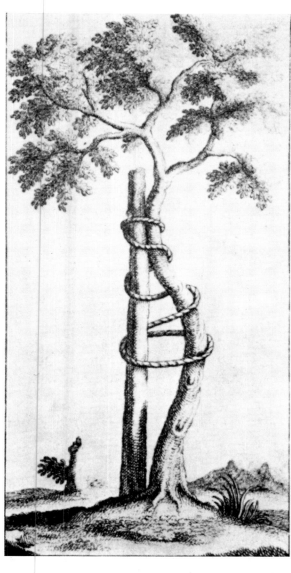

1009   1010

Subsequently, he developed the now popular and effective stapes mobilization operation. Actually, Boucheron in 1888 had reported on sixty operated cases, Miot in 1890 had written up two hundred instances of stapes mobilization, and Faraci in 1899 had summarized his experiences in thirty cases. However, except for an occasional report thereafter, the technique had been forgotten until Rosen's chance rediscovery.

Numerous attempts since 1957 to alleviate total deafness due to nerve degeneration, by implanting electrical devices into the inner ear, have been only partially successful. On the other hand, external hearing aids of great variety and ingeniousness continue to be developed.

ORTHOPAEDICS

In 1741 Nicholas André, Professor of Medicine at the University of Paris, published a book on the prevention and correction of musculoskeletal deformities in children. For its title he created the word "orthopaedic" from two Greek roots, *orthos* (straight) and *paideia* (rearing of children), and his illustration of a staff used to straighten a growing sapling has become the international insignia of orthopaedic societies.

For decades orthopaedists have been physicians or surgeons interested in musculoskeletal deformities and diseases. These were chiefly scoliosis (curvature of the spine), tuberculosis and other infections of the bones and joints, paralysis due to poliomyelitis, and congenital defects such as dislocations of the hip, club foot, and Erb's palsy (birth paralysis of the arm). Eventually it also included fractures, dislocations, and other injuries to the spine and extremities.

Until the twentieth century, most orthopaedic treatment was mechanical, with braces, plaster casts, and manipulation, but some simple operations such as osteotomy (correcting deformed bones by cutting them) and uncomplicated tendon transplants were also done. In 1908, Erich Lexer reported apparently brilliant success with transplantation of total knee joints from one person to another, but this procedure was never taken up by other orthopaedists—possibly because late results did not bear out the early promise. In 1911 Russell Hibbs of New York revolutionized the treatment of scoliosis and spinal tuberculosis by devising a spine fusion operation, which continues to be improved upon and modified.

Fractures of the hip were considered untreatable, and until the present century little was done for them. In the 1930s Smith-Petersen of Boston developed

1011

1006 *Couching knife and needles (1791) for eye surgery. National Library of Medicine, Bethesda*

1007 *Argon laser "light knife" used to obliterate a vascular eye tumor. Bell Laboratories, New Jersey*

1008 *Slide showing microfilaria, the most common cause of blindness in underdeveloped countries. Drs. Edward J. Bottone and Bruce A. Hanna, Dept. of Microbiology, Mount Sinai Hospital, New York*

1009 *Prosthetic device designed to replace hip joint. Richards Manufacturing Co., Memphis*

1010 *Bechtol total hip replacement in place. Richards Manufacturing Co., Memphis*

1011 *Insignia or symbol of orthopaedic societies, taken from Nicholas André, L'Orthopédie (1741). New York Academy of Medicine*

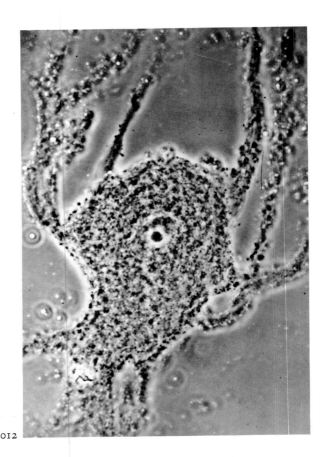

1012

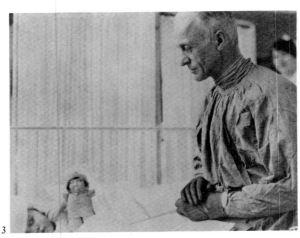

1013

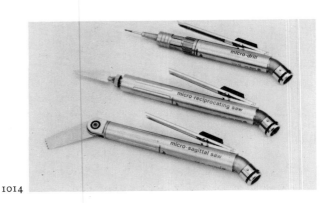

1014

a special nail that could be inserted to hold the fracture fragments together. Shortly thereafter, metal substitutes were devised for the disunited head of the femur. These devices and procedures were improved, especially through the brilliant innovations of John Charnley of England, to the point where a total joint including the socket can be replaced not only for injury but also for some forms of arthritis. At present the procedure appears to be working well for the hip, and something similar is being developed for the knee, ankle, elbow, fingers, and other joints. Joint replacement may become the most important contribution of orthopaedics in this century.

The displaced or "slipped" intervertebral disc, an elastic substance which forms a cushion between each of the vertebrae in the spinal column, was recognized as a common cause of low back ache and sciatica about 1911. A herniated disc was first removed by Mixter and Barr of Boston in 1934. Although this operation has been evaluated with variable enthusiasm, it remains another major contribution of orthopaedics to medicine.

NEUROLOGY

The neurosciences have inherited centuries of accumulated observations—from the experiences of earliest societies with trauma and the trephining of skulls to the pioneering advances of the nineteenth century. One may especially mention the experimental work of Gustav Fritsch and Eduard Hitzig in 1870, which showed clearly that sensory and motor functions could be localized in the cortex of the brain. William Gowers, Hughlings Jackson, and S. Weir Mitchell were at the forefront in establishing clinical methods for evaluating neural disorders.

The structure and function of the nerve cells and fibers had also been clarified by the significant investigations of Camillo Golgi and Santiago Ramón y Cajal before the twentieth century had finished its first decade. The methods of tissue culture which Ross Harrison devised in 1907 to determine how nerve fibers regenerated after injury became an essential tool for research in other fields, among them vascular surgery and virology. Charles Sherrington and Edgar Adrian received a Nobel prize in 1932 for their investigations on reflexes, nerve impulses, and the mechanism of sensation. In recent decades, investigators have shown that while some electrical principles may operate in the conduction of nerve impulses, chemical transmitters, linkages between cells, and feedback mechanisms are integral parts of the functioning of the nervous system and sense organs. For their discoveries on the physiology of vision, George Wald and Ragnar Granit were awarded a Nobel prize in 1967.

Information derived from many disciplines concerning the detailed makeup and activities of cells has also been utilized to help understand and treat neural dysfunction with drugs and operations. Numerous investigators are illuminating hidden recesses of mental function through studies on consciousness, speech, memory, and sleep.

Surgery of the nervous system owes much to the pioneer work in the nineteenth century of Victor Horsley, often called "Father of Neurosurgery." The first person successfully to remove a tumor of the neural substance in the spinal cord, in 1887, Horsley also performed many significant animal experiments and successful cranial operations on humans. However, neurosurgery received its greatest impetus from Harvey Cushing, who was responsible for major advances in surgery of the pituitary gland, management of increased intracranial pressure, and treatment of brain tumors. Not the least of his contributions was the training of outstanding neurosurgeons from all over the world. Walter Dandy, one of his brilliant pupils and later his personal antagonist, advanced neurosurgery through innovations in surgical technique and diagnostic procedures.

In the last twenty years, neurosurgical operations have been extended not only to the removal of growths and aneurysms of the nervous system but also to the relief of pain by severing nerve tracts, the palliation of tremors and abnormal behavior, and the beneficial modification of hormonal mechanisms in the treatment of cancer.

ASSOCIATED HEALING PROFESSIONS

DENTISTRY

In 1840, the world's first dental school was founded in Baltimore, Maryland. A few years later, dental schools were established in Europe. As in medicine, the dental college course was gradually lengthened from a few months to four years in addition to the required minimum predental training. By the mid-nineteenth century, licenses were being issued by various states. In England, the first licenses were issued in 1859, but the dental profession remained under medical control. In Europe there is still some conflict as to whether dentistry is a specialty of medicine or a profession unto itself.

Prior to the twentieth century, dentistry concerned itself primarily with dental caries (cavities), malposition of teeth, and diseases of the supporting tissues of the teeth. Prevention was largely neglected until techniques were developed in this century to conserve and restore teeth and to prevent and arrest disease. In addition, fluoridization of the water supplies to prevent dental caries has been one of the most successful public health measures ever advocated. Dentistry has now developed the following subspecialties: oral surgery, periodontics (diseases of the supporting structures), pedodontics (children's dentistry), prosthodontics (replacement of missing teeth), orthodontics (correction of malposed teeth), public health, oral pathology, and endodontics (root canal therapy).

The materials used to fill cavities in the teeth during the Middle Ages were waxes and resins, followed by gold leaf and lead in the mid-fifteenth century. Today's amalgam fillings, essentially a mixture of silver and mercury, were developed in the early nineteenth century, but other materials have also been introduced. To restore lost or damaged teeth, newly developed synthetic resins and acrylics were adapted to dentistry, and the use of fused porcelain for false teeth became a highly sophisticated art. Other inert materials were also introduced as implants in the jawbones to substitute for lost structures. Some temporary success has even been achieved in the reimplantation of teeth dislodged from their sockets. Experiments have also succeeded in transplanting a tooth from one part of the jaws to another more useful site.

High-speed drilling with water-cooling and the judicious use of local and general anesthetics have for the most part controlled the pain experienced and feared for centuries by patients in the dental chair. The advances in antibiotics, X-ray techniques, and other disciplines in medicine have been taken up by dentistry just as the contribution of general anesthesia by American dentists became the property of medicine.

NURSING

Since the days of Florence Nightingale, the emphases in training and practice have shifted from purely clinical bedside nursing to include more academic and supervisory subjects. Hospital-based nursing schools, while still prominent in Europe, have become fewer in the U.S., where education has moved more and more to academic institutions. Advanced degrees beyond R.N. (Registered Nurse) have extended into many special fields, such as maternal and child care, geriatrics, psychiatry, cardiovascular illness, medical and surgical subspecialties, cancer care, and public health administration.

The earliest activities in medical social service in the U.S. were those performed by nurses who tried to involve patients in occupational therapy. Under

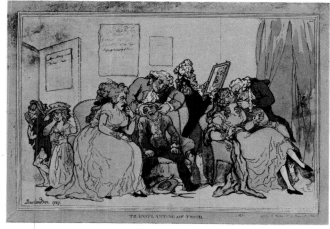

1015

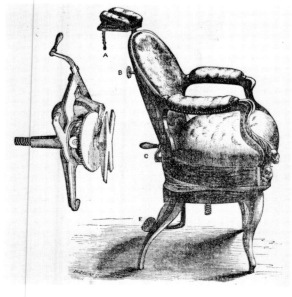

1016

1012 *Slide showing freshly isolated nerve cell. Prof. Holger Hyden, Dept. of Histology, University of Göteborg*

1013 *Dr. Harvey William Cushing, photographed in 1928, famed neurosurgeon responsible for major advances in surgery of the pituitary gland, management of increased intracranial pressure, and treatment of brain tumors. National Library of Medicine, Bethesda*

1014 *Precision surgical tools, which 20th-century technological advances have made possible. Amsco/Hall Surgical Co., Santa Barbara*

1015 *Colored engraving by Thomas Rowlandson,* Transplanting of Teeth *(1787), an operation considered farfetched in the 18th century but which may become a reality in the 20th. Collection William Helfand, New York*

1016 *"Latest model" dental chair advertised in* Dental Cosmos *(1859). National Library of Medicine, Bethesda*

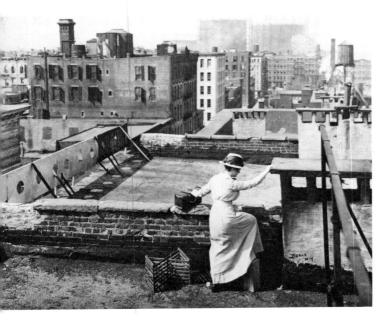

1017

1017 *The Visiting Nurse, taking a shortcut over tenement roofs (1908). Museum of the City of New York*

1018 *Chaldean pedigree chart (c. 4000 B.C.), which indicates that selective breeding of horses was going on 6,000 years ago. World Health Organization, Geneva*

1019 *Comparison of the speech organs of the cat and rabbit, from Giulio Casserio,* De Vocis Auditusque Organis Historia Anatomica *(1601). Careful and detailed studies performed on animals were often responsible for advances in human medicine. National Library of Medicine, Bethesda*

1020 *Slide showing the hookworm egg, a parasite formerly affecting large segments of the population of lands where people walked barefoot on contaminated ground. Drs. Edward J. Bottone and Bruce A. Hanna, Dept. of Microbiology, Mount Sinai Hospital, New York*

medical direction, nurses also gave physical therapy treatments. A visiting-nurse training school founded by Lillian Wald in 1893 was the forerunner of those institutions which train the public health nurse, who goes into homes to oversee the sick and disabled and to educate families in the fundamentals of health and hygiene.

In Britain and other countries, nurses have often had considerable responsibility for the management of patients, which sometimes included duties that in the U.S. devolved upon junior physicians. Recently, however, in intensive care units of hospitals, the specialized nursing staffs have been involved in clinical decisions as well as in administrative planning. Moreover, nurse-clinicians as independent practitioners have begun to appear.

While the professional and economic status of nurses has risen, their intensive, experiential training in individual care has become less based on the bedside. Some deplore this lessening of personal patient care, whereas others point to the advantages of improving the nurse's expertise and usefulness in overall care.

VETERINARY MEDICINE

Regular physicians and specialists in animal illnesses have cared for the flocks and herds over many centuries. However, it was not until the nineteenth and twentieth centuries that the veterinarian became a fully recognized, certified professional with clear-cut education and training accompanied by sophisticated methodology.

Veterinary colleges had been established in France, England, and Scotland in the eighteenth century, but it was not until 1875 that the first veterinary college was founded in America, by the Frenchman Alexandre Liautard, in New York. In 1863, Liautard and Robert Jennings had brought together representatives from seven states to launch the first Veterinary Medical Association. Two years earlier, a veterinary school had opened in Ontario, Canada. Since then, schools of veterinary medicine have increased in number all over the world (although there are still only nineteen in the U.S.), journals have multiplied, and specializations within the profession have divided and subdivided.

There are many examples of far-reaching additions to medical knowledge by veterinarians, of which a few may be cited. Bernard Bang of Denmark, who described a blood disease in fowl, leukosis, and explained the causation of an abortion-producing illness of cattle, also was responsible for devising a test using the tuberculin which Robert Koch had developed. The entire field of virology was opened through the discovery by Klaus Loeffler and Paul Frosch in 1898 that a specific infection (foot-and-mouth disease of cattle) was caused by a filterable virus. In the first catheterizations of the living heart, the veterinary J. B. A. Chauveau was Claude Bernard's coworker and also a pioneer in producing attenuated viruses for immunization. F. L. Kilborne, together with the physician Theobald Smith, presented in 1889 the first proof of an insect acting as a vector in disease. The achievement of the chemotherapy of tuberculosis was linked to the work of William Feldman, who also contributed to the treatment of leprosy with sulfone drugs. Antitetanus immunizations and diphtheria toxoid inoculations arose out of the labors of veterinarian Gaston Ramon. Recently a team of veterinary and medical investigators at the Wistar Institute in Philadelphia obtained a simple vaccine against rabies which is ninety-nine percent effective in humans even after a rabid bite. The hypodermic syringe was derived from Tabourin's first crude instrument, and spinal anesthesia was first used in veterinary medicine. Daniel Salmon may be particularly mentioned for making numerous contributions to the control of human disease. Together with Theobald Smith, he established the efficacy of killed microorganisms for making vaccines. Among other fundamental studies, he demonstrated the transmissibility to humans of tuberculosis in cattle. His researches on the paratyphoid bacterium led to its designation with his name as *Salmonella.*

Diseases of animals have always been significant to human health. Approximately 150 infections (the zoonoses) are transmissible from animals to humans. For instance, a severe erysipelas infection, glanders, originally thought to be confined to horses, was found to be transferable to humans. Similarly, psittacosis (a pulmonary disease of birds), equine encephalitis, and botulism have proved to be of serious consequence to humans as well as animals. Hookworm, a parasite formerly affecting large segments of the poorer population in the South, Egypt, and other countries, penetrates the skin of those who walk barefoot on contaminated ground. Maurice Hall and Jacob Schillinger rid large areas of the parasite by using chemicals on dogs that carried the organism. A malignant tumor of fowl (chicken sarcoma) was discovered by Peyton Rous to be caused by a virus, but the importance of this finding to human cancer is still debated. However, the observation has set many investigators to searching for a linkage between viruses and cancer. In recent years, other links to malignant tumors have been discovered, as for instance William Hardy's demonstration that leukemia in cats is caused and transmitted by a virus.

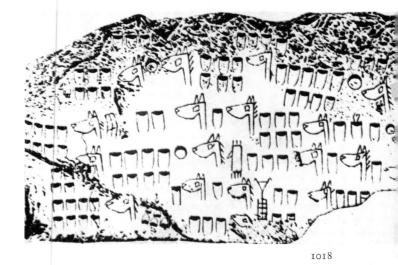

1018

The lessons learned from animal diseases and the experiences of veterinarians in controlling their spread have had considerable impact on public health measures aimed at containing a number of human epidemic illnesses, such as yellow fever, plague, malaria, and cholera. In addition, the danger of mercury poisoning was first detected in cats fed fish from waters contaminated by the metal. Breeders and veterinarians, in noting endocrine derangements in minks who ate domestic chickens, called attention to the potential hazard of administering hormones to fowl raised for human consumption. Recognizing the contributions of veterinarians, health departments have increasingly used their services.

Veterinarians have also played an important part in supervising the activities of research laboratories. Experiments on animal models have been essential to advances in human medicine. The discovery and manufacture of insulin is a prime example. The antipoliomyelitis vaccine is another. Throughout all fields of medicine, new mechanical procedures and operative innovations have usually required testing first on animals. There have been vigorous confrontations between research laboratories and antivivisection groups, but a measure of accommodation in recent decades has led to acknowledgment by one side of the essential role of experiments and agreement by the other to stricter regulation of the care of animals in research institutions.

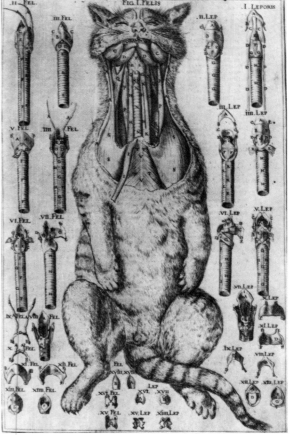

1019

Veterinary medicine has been important to the quantity and quality of food, the prevention of the spread of disease in all living forms, the application to humans of information derived from animal care, and the maintenance of the health of pets whose presence contributes to the enjoyment and psychological well-being of humans. It is in the capacity of private physician to horses, cattle, and small household animals that most practitioners are to be found. Increasingly, the veterinarian has come to be regarded as a teammate of the physician in the study, care, and treatment of living creatures.

What lies ahead? Soon this century's ideas and activities will be reviewed by the next century's historians and scientists—with occasional admiration, we hope; with amused tolerance, perhaps; with astonished dismay, in all likelihood. But we need feel no embarrassment, because each period will take its turn being evaluated by its successors. We enter the future facing backward, seeing only the road on which we have just traveled. We would do well to view today's medicine as merely a marker between the past and future.

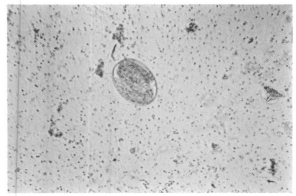

1020

SELECTED BIBLIOGRAPHY

Ackerknecht, E. H. "Anticontagionism between 1821 and 1867." *Bull. Hist. Med.* 22 (1948): 562–93.

———. "Malaria in the Upper Mississippi Valley, 1760–1900." *Bull. Hist. Med.*, suppl. 4 (1945).

———. "Natural Diseases and Rational Treatment in Primitive Medicine." *Bull. Hist. Med.* 19 (1946): 467–97.

———. *Rudolph Virchow: Doctor, Statesman, Anthropologist.* Madison: University of Wisconsin Press, 1953.

———. *A Short History of Medicine.* New York: Ronald Press Co., 1955.

———. *A Short History of Psychiatry.* 2d rev. ed. Translated from the German by Sulammith Wolff. New York: Hafner Publishing Co., 1969.

Adams, F. R. *The Genuine Works of Hippocrates.* Translated from Greek, with preliminary discourse and annotations. New York: William Wood, 1891.

Albucasis. *La chirurgie d'Albucasis.* Translated by Lucien Leclerc. Paris: Baillière, 1861.

Albutt, T. Clifford. *Greek Medicine in Rome.* London: Macmillan & Co., 1921.

———. *The Historical Relations of Medicine and Surgery to the End of the Sixteenth Century.* London: Macmillan & Co., 1905.

Alexander of Tralles. *Alexander von Tralles.* Translated by Theodor Puschmann. Vienna: Braumüller, 1878.

Ali, S. A. "Europe's Debt to Muslim Scholars of Medicine and Science." *Studies Hist. Med.* 1 (1977): 36–48.

Amundson, D. W. "Romanticizing the Ancient Medical Profession: The Characterization of the Physician in the Graeco-Roman Novel." *Bull. Hist. Med.* 18 (1974): 320–37.

Anesthesia Centennial. *J. Hist. Med.* 1, no. 4 (1946). Issue devoted entirely to articles on anesthesia by 22 authors.

Aretaeus. *Aretaeus the Cappadocian: The Extant Works of Aretaeus.* Edited and translated by I. E. Drabkin. Chicago, 1856.

Aristotle. *Works.* Translated by D'Arcy W. Thompson. Oxford: Clarendon Press, 1910.

Ashhurst, A. P. C. "The Centenary of Lister (1827–1927): A tale of Sepsis and Antisepsis." *Ann. Med. Hist.* 9 (1927): 205.

Baas, J. H. *History of Medicine.* 2 vols. 1876. Reprint. Translated by H. E. Anderson. Huntington, N.Y.: R. E. Krieger Publishing Co., 1971.

Ball, J. M. "Samuel Thomson (1769–1843) and His Patented 'System' of Medicine." *Ann. Med. Hist.* 7 (1925): 144.

Banting, F. G., and Best, C. H. "The Internal Secretion of the Pancreas." *J. Lab. Clin. Med.* 7 (1922): 251.

Barrow, M. V. "Portraits of Hippocrates." *Med. Hist.* 16 (1972): 85–88.

Baumgartner, Leona, and Ramsey, Elizabeth M. "Johann Peter Frank and His *System einer vollständigen medizinischen Polizey*," *Ann. Med. Hist.*, n.s. 5 (1933): 525; 6 (1934): 69.

Bayon, H. P. "Trotula and the Ladies of Salerno." *Proc. Roy. Soc. Med.* 33 (1940): 471.

Bean, W. B. "Walter Reed." In *Dictionary of Scientific Biography.* 1975.

Beaumont, William. *Experiments and Observations on the Gastric Juice and the Physiology of Digestion.* 1833. Reprint. New York: Dover Publications, 1959.

Bédarida, M. A. "Population and the Urban Explosion." In *The Nineteenth Century*, edited by Asa Briggs. London: Thames & Hudson, 1970.

Bell, E. M. *Storming the Citadel: The Rise of the Woman Doctor.* London: Constable & Co., 1953.

Benison, S. "Speculation and Experimentation in Early Poliomyelitis Research." *Clio Med.* 10 (1975): 1–22.

Best, C. H. "Reminiscences of the Researches Which Led to the Discovery of Insulin." *Can. Med. Assoc. J.* 47 (1942): 398.

Bhishagratna, K. K. L., trans. *The Sushruta Samhitā.* Calcutta: J. N. Bose, 1907–16.

Billings, J. S. "Our Medical Literature." In *Transactions of the International Medical Congress.* London, 1881.

Blake, J. B., ed. *Education in the History of Medicine.* New York and London: Hafner Publishing Co., 1968.

Blalock, Alfred. "Walter Edward Dandy." *Surgery* 19 (1946): 577.

Blanton, W. B. "Washington's Medical Knowledge and Its Sources." *Ann. Med. Hist.*, n.s. 5 (1933): 52.

Boland, Frank Kells. *The First Anesthetic: The Story of Crawford Long.* Athens: University of Georgia Press, 1950.

Bowers, J. Z., and Purcell, E. F., eds. *Advances in American Medicine: Essays at the Bicentennial.* 2 vols. New York: Josiah Macy, Jr., Foundation and National Library of Medicine, 1976.

Breasted, James H. *The Edwin Smith Surgical Papyrus.* 2 vols. With translation. Chicago: University of Chicago Press, 1930.

———. *A History of Egypt.* 2d rev. ed. New York: Charles Scribner's Sons, 1924.

Brieger, Gert H. "Florence Rena Sabin." In *Dictionary of Scientific Biography.* 1975.

Brim, Charles J. *Medicine in the Bible.* New York: Froben Press, 1936.

Brock, Arthur J. *Greek Medicine: Extracts of Medical Writers from Hippocrates to Galen.* London and Toronto: J. M. Dent & Sons, 1929.

Brockington, C. F. "The History of Public Health." In *The Theory and Practice of Public Health*, by W. Hobson, 4th ed. London: Oxford University Press, 1975.

Brothwell, Don, and Sandison, A. T. *Diseases in Antiquity: A Survey of the Diseases, Injuries, and Surgery of Early Populations.* Springfield, Ill.: Charles C. Thomas, 1967.

Browne, Edward G. *Arabian Medicine.* Cambridge: Cambridge University Press, 1921.

Brunel, Jules. "Antibiosis from Pasteur to Fleming." *J. Hist. Med.* 6 (1951): 287.

Brunschwig, Hieronymous. *The Book of Cirugia.* Milan: Lier & Co., 1923.

Budge, E. A. *The Book of the Dead: The Hieroglyphic Transcript of the Papyrus of Ani.* With English translation. New Hyde Park, N.Y.: University Books, 1960.

Bullough, V. L. *The Development of Medicine as a Profession.* Basel and New York: S. Karger, 1966.

Burget, G. E. "Lazzaro Spallanzani." *Ann. Med. Hist.*, 1st ser. 6 (1924): 177.

Burns, C. R. "Comparative Ethics of the Medical Profession outside the United States." *Tex. Rep. Biol. Med.* 32 (1974): 181–87.

———. *Legacies in Ethics and Medicine.* New York: Neale Watson Academic Publications, 1977.

Burroughs, Wellcome & Co. *The History of Inoculation and Vaccination.* London, 1913.

Burton, Robert. *The Anatomy of Melancholy.* Edited by Floyd Dell and Paul Jordon-Smith. New York: Farrar & Rinehart, 1927.

Butterfield, L. H., ed. *Letters of Benjamin Rush.* 2 vols. Princeton: Princeton University Press, 1951.

Cajal, S. R. *Recollections of My Life.* Translated by E. Horne Craigie. 1937. Reprint. Cambridge, Mass.: M.I.T. Press, 1966.

Camac, C. N. B. *Imhotep to Harvey: Backgrounds of Medical History.* New York: Paul B. Hoeber, 1931.

Campbell, Donald. *Arabian Medicine and Its Influence on the Middle Ages.* London: Kegan Paul, Trench, Trübner & Co., 1926.

Carrel, A., and Guthrie, C. C. "Anastomosis of Blood Vessels by the Patching Method and Transplantation of the Kidney." *J. Am. Med. Assoc.* 51 (1908): 1658.

Carstens, Henry R. "The History of Hospitals, with Special Reference to Some of the World's Oldest Institutions." *Ann. Intern. Med.* 10 (1937): 670–82.

Cartwright, F. F. *The English Pioneers of Anaesthesia.* Bristol: John Wright & Sons, 1952.

Caspari-Rosen, B., and Rosen, G. "Autobiography in Medicine; or, The Doctor in Search of Himself." *J. Hist. Med.* 1 (1946): 290–99.

Cassedy, James H. "History of Medicine and Related Sciences in Europe." In "The Status of Medical History in the Universities of North America and Europe." *Bull. Hist. Med.* 43 (1969): 270–83.

Castiglioni, Arturo. *A History of Medicine.* 2d ed. Translated by E. B. Krumbhaar. New York: Alfred A. Knopf, 1947.

Caton, R. *The Temples and Rituals of Asklepios at Epidauros and Athens.* London: C. J. Clay & Sons, 1900.

Cavendish, Richard, ed. *Man, Myth, and Magic.* Pts. 1 and 2. New York: Marshall Cavendish Corp., 1974.

Celsus. *De Medicina.* With an English translation by W. G. Spencer. Cambridge, Mass.: Harvard University Press, 1938.

Chadwick, E. *Report on an Inquiry into the Sanitary Condition of the Labouring Population of Great Britain.* London: W. Clowes, 1842.

Charaka-Samhita. Translated into English by Avinash Chandra Kaviratna. Calcutta: Charkravarti & Kaviratna, 1896–1913.

Charcot, J. M., and Richer, P. *L'art et la médecine.* Paris: Gaultier, 1902.

Cheyne, Sir William Watson. *Lister and His Achievement.* London: Longmans, Green & Co., 1925.

Chick, H. "The Discovery of Vitamins." *Prog. Food Nutr. Sci.* 1 (1975): 1–20.

Chiera, Edward. *They Wrote on Clay.* Chicago: University of Chicago Press, 1938.

Choulant, Ludwig. *History and Bibliography of Anatomic Illustration.* Edited and translated with notes and biography by M. Frank. Chicago: University of Chicago Press, 1920.

Clar, D. *Leopold Auenbrugger.* Graz: Leuscher & Lubensky, 1867.

Clark, George N., and Cook, A. M. *A History of the Royal College of Physicians of London.* Vol. 2. Oxford: Clarendon Press, 1966.

Clarke, E. G.; Bigelow, H. J.; Gross, S. D.; Thomas, T. G.; and Billings, J. S. *Century of American Medicine, 1776–1876.* Philadelphia: H. C. Lea, 1876.

Clark-Kennedy, A. E. *Stephen Hales.* Cambridge: Cambridge University Press, 1929.

Clay, Reginald S., and Court, Thomas H. *The History of the Microscope.* London: Charles Griffin & Co., 1932.

Clendening, Logan. *Source Book of Medical History.* New York and London: Paul B. Hoeber, 1942.

Cohen, M. R., and Drabkin, I. E. *A Sourcebook in Greek Science.* Cambridge, Mass.: Harvard University Press, 1948.

Comrie, John D. *History of Scottish Medicine.* 2 vols. 2d ed. 1932. Reprint. New York: AMS Press, 1976.

Cooper, Sonoma. "The Medical School of Montpellier in the Fourteenth Century." *Ann. Med. Hist.*, n.s. 2 (1930): 163.

Cope, Oliver; Zacharias, Jerrold; and Pifer, Alan. *Medical Education Reconsidered: Report of the Endicott House Summer Study on Medical Education.* Philadelphia: J. B. Lippincott Co., 1965.

Cope, Z., ed. *Sidelights on the History of Medicine.* London: Butterworth & Co., 1957.

Corlett, W. T. *The Medicine-Man of the American Indian and His Cultural Background.* 1935. Reprint. New York: AMS Press, 1977.

Corner, George W. "The Rise of Medicine at Salerno in the Twelfth Century." *Ann. Med. Hist.*, n.s. 3 (1931).

Cosman, M. L. "Medieval Medical Malpractice and Chaucer's Physician." *N. Y. State J. Med.* 72 (1972): 2439–44.

———. "Medieval Medical Malpractice: The Dicta and the Dockets." *Bull. N. Y. Acad. Med.* 49 (1973): 22–47.

Cournand, A. "Cardiac Catheterization: Development of the Technique, Its Contributions to Experimental Medicine, and Its Initial Applications In Man." *Acta Med. Scand.*, 579, suppl. (1975): 3–32.

Cowell, F. R. "The Ancient Life: The Greece and Rome of Everyday." In *The Birth of Western Civilization*, edited by M. Grant. London: Thames & Hudson, 1969.

Cowen, David L. "Liberty, Laissez-faire, and Licensure in Nineteenth Century Britain." *Bull. Hist. Med.* 43 (1969): 30–40.

Cranefield, Paul. *The Way In and the Way Out.* Mt. Kisco, N.Y.: Futura Publishing Co., 1974.

Crellin, J. K. "Ronald Ross." In *Dictionary of Scientific Biography.* 1975.

Cumston, Charles Greene. *An Introduction to the History of Medicine, from the Time of the Pharaohs to the End of the Eighteenth Century.* New York: Alfred A. Knopf, 1926.

Curie, Eve. *Madame Curie.* London: William Heinemann, 1938.

Curley, F. J. "Elisha Perkins' Patent Metallic Tractors." *Synthesis* 2 (1975): 8–21.

Cushing, Harvey. *The Life of Sir William Osler.* Oxford: Clarendon Press, 1925.

Dabry, P. *La Médecine chez les chinois.* Paris: Librairie Plon, 1863.

Daremberg, Charles. *Etat de la médecine entre Homère et Hippocrate.* Paris: Didier, 1869.

———. *Histoire des sciences médicales, contenant l'anatomie, la physiologie, la médecine la chirurgie, et les doctrines de pathologie générales.* Paris: Baillière, 1870.

———. *Oeuvres choisies d'Hippocrate.* Paris: Labe, 1885.

Debus, Allen G. *The Chemical Dream of the Renaissance.* Cambridge: W. Heffer & Sons, 1968.

———. *English Paracelsians.* Chicago: University of Chicago Press, 1968.

———. *Science, Medicine, and Society in the Renaissance; Essays to Honor Walter Pagel.* New York: Neale Watson Academic Publications, 1972.

DeJong, R. N. "The First American Textbook on Psychiatry: A Review and Discussion of Benjamin Rush's *Medical Inquiries and Observations upon Diseases of the Mind.*" *Ann. Med. Hist.* 2 (1940): 195.

De Mondeville, Henri. *Die Chirurgie des Heinrich von Mondeville.* Edited by Julius Pagel. Berlin: A. Hirschwald, 1892.

de Moulin, D. Book review of *Die alexandrinischen Chirurgen: Eine Sammlung und Auswertung ihrer Fragmente*, by Markwart Michler. In *Bull. Hist. Med.* 44 (1970): 385–86.

Denny-Brown, D. et al., eds. *Centennial Anniversary Volume of the American Neurological Association, 1875–1975.* New York: Springer Publishing Co., 1975.

Diepgen, Paul. *Geschichte der Medizin: Die historische Entwicklung der Heilkunde und des ärztlichen Lebens.* Berlin: Walter de Gruyter & Co., 1959.

Dobell, C. *Anthony van Leeuwenhoek and His "Little Animals."* New York: Harcourt, Brace & Co., 1932.

Dos Santos, J. "The Carrel-Guthrie Controversy." *Surgery* 77 (1975): 330–31.

Draper, John W. *The Historical Influence of the Medical Profession.* 1863. Reprint. New York: Scholarly Reprints, 1977.

Dubos, R. J. *Louis Pasteur: Free Lance of Science.* Boston: Little Brown & Co., 1952.

———. *Man, Medicine, and Environment.* New York: Praeger Publishers, 1968.

Duclaux, E. *Pasteur; The History of a Mind.* 1920. Reprint. New foreword by R. Dubos. Metuchen, N. J.: Scarecrow Press, 1973.

Duffy, J. *Epidemics in Colonial America.* Baton Rouge: Louisiana State University Press, 1971.

———. *The Healers: The Rise of American Medicine.* New York: McGraw-Hill, 1976.

———. *Sword of Pestilence: The New Orleans Yellow Fever Epidemic of 1853.* Baton Rouge: Louisiana State University Press, 1966.

Dukes, Cuthberg. *Lord Lister.* London: Leonard Parsons, 1924.

Dulieu, L. *La chirurgie à Montpellier de ses origines au début du dix-neuvième siècle.* Avignon: Presses Universelles, 1975.

Dumesnil, R. *Histoire illustreé de la médecine.* 1935. Reprint. Paris: Librairie Plon, 1950.

Duveen, Denis I. "Lavoisier." *Scientific American* 194 (1956): 84–94.

———, and Klickstein, Herbert S. "Antoine Laurent Lavoisier's Contributions to Medicine and Public Health." *Bull. Hist. Med.* 20 (1955): 164–79.

Ebbell, B. *The Papyrus Ebers: The Greatest Egyptian Medical Document.* With translation. Copenhagen: Ejnar Munksgaard, 1939.

Edelstein, Emma J., and Edelstein, Ludwig. *Asclepius: A Collection and Interpretation of the Testimonies.* Vol. 2, books 1 and 2. Baltimore: Johns Hopkins University Press, 1945.

Edelstein, L. "The Genuine Works of Hippocrates." *Bull. Hist. Med.* 7 (1939): 236–48.
———. "The Hippocratic Oath: Text, Translation, and Interpretation." *Bull. Hist. Med.*, suppl. 1 (1943).
Edman, I., ed. *The Works of Plato.* New York: Modern Library, 1928.
Edwards, Chilperic. *The Hammurabi Code.* London: Watts & Co., 1921.
Edwards, H. "Theodoric of Cervia: A Medical Antiseptic Surgeon." *Proc. Roy. Soc. Med.* 69 (1976): 553–55.
Elgood, Cyril. "Jundi Shapur: A Sassanian University." *Proc. Roy. Soc. Med.* 32 (1939): 1033.
———. *A Medical History of Persia and the Eastern Caliphate.* Cambridge: Cambridge University Press, 1951.
Ellis, Harold. *A History of Bladder Stones.* Oxford: Blackwell Scientific Publications, 1969.
Engel, George L. "Enduring Attributes of Medicine Relevant for the Education of the Physician." *Ann. Intern. Med.* 78 (1973): 587–93.
Esser, A. Albert M. "Pathologie und Therapie der Lider bei Vāgbhata." *Klin. Monatsbl. f. Augenh.* 98 (1937): 216.

Farley, J., and Geison, G. L. "Science, Politics, and Spontaneous Generation in Nineteenth Century France: The Pasteur-Pouchet Debate." *Bull. Hist. Med.* 48 (1974): 161–98.
Fishbein, Morris. *Fads and Quackery in Healing.* New York: Covici, Friede, 1932.
———. *A History of the American Medical Association, 1847 to 1947.* Philadelphia and London: W. B. Saunders Co., 1947.
Fishman, A. P., and Richards, D. W. *Circulation of the Blood: Men and Ideas.* New York: Oxford University Press, 1964.
Flack, I. H. "The Pre-History of Midwifery." *Proc. Roy. Soc. Med.* 40 (1947): 713–22.
Flexner, Abraham. *Medical Education: A Comparative Study.* New York: Macmillan Co., 1925.
Flexner, S., and Flexner, J. T. *William Henry Welch and the Heroic Age of American Medicine.* 1941. Reprint. New York: Dover Publications, 1966.
Foley, J. J. "Marie Curie: The Birth of a Science." *Radiol. Technol.* 47 (1975): 134–40.
Forssmann, W. *Experiments on Myself: Memoirs of a Surgeon in Germany.* Translated by H. Davies. New York: St. Martin's Press, 1975.
Fort, George F. *Medical Economy during the Middle Ages.* New York: Augustus M. Kelley, Publishers, 1970.
Foster, Michael. *Claude Bernard.* New York: Longmans, Green & Co., 1899.
Fracastoro, G. *Hieronymi Fracastorii: De contagione et contagiosis morbis et eorum curatione.* Vol. 3. Translated, with notes by Wilmer Cave Wright. New York: G. P. Putnam's Sons, 1930.
———. *Syphilis; or The French Disease.* Translated by H. Wynne-Finch. London: William Heinemann, 1935.
Frank, Johann Peter. Review of *The People's Misery: Mother of Disease.* In *Bull. Hist. Med.* 9 (1941): 81–100.
———. *Seine Selbstbiographie: Herausgegeben, eingeleitet und mit Erläuterungen versehen von Prof. Dr. Erna Lesky.* Bern: Verlag Hans Huber, 1969.
Franklin, T. J., and Snow, G. A. "An Outline of the Historical Development of Antimicrobial Agents and of Chemotherapeutic Theories." In *Biochemistry of Antimicrobial Action,* 2d ed. London: Chapman & Hall, 1975.
Frazer, James George. *The Golden Bough: A Study in Magic and Religion.* Abr. ed. New York: Macmillan Co., 1963.
French, Sidney J. *Torch and Crucible: The Life and Death of Antoine Lavoisier.* Princeton: Princeton University Press, 1941.
Freud, Sigmund. *An Outline of Psychoanalysis.* Translated by James Strachey. New York: W. W. Norton & Co., 1949.
———. *Totem and Taboo: Some Points of Agreement between the Mental Lives of Savages and Neurotics.* Translated by James Strachey. New York: W. W. Norton & Co., 1952.
Frieden, N. M. "Physicians in Pre-Revolutionary Russia: Professionals or Servants of the State?" *Bull. Hist. Med.* 49 (1975): 20–29.
Friedenwald, Harry. *Jews and Medicine and Jewish Luminaries in Medical History.* Rev. ed. 3 vols. New York: Ktav Publishing House, 1967.
Frye, R. N., ed. *The Cambridge History of Iran.* Vol. 4. Cambridge: Cambridge University Press, 1975.
Fulton, John F. *Harvey Cushing: A Biography.* Springfield, Ill.: Charles C. Thomas, Publisher, 1946.
———. "Robert Boyle and His Influence on Thought in the Seventeenth Century." *Isis* 18 (1933): 77.
———. *Selected Readings in the History of Physiology.* Springfield, Ill.: Charles C. Thomas, Publisher, 1930.

Galdston, I. *Progress in Medicine: A Critical Review of the Last Hundred Years.* New York: Alfred A. Knopf, 1940.
Galen. *Hygiene.* Translated from the Greek by R. M. Green. Springfield, Ill.: Charles C. Thomas, Publisher, 1951.
———. *On the Natural Faculties.* Translated by A. Brock. London: Loeb Classical Library, 1952.
———. *On the Usefulness of the Parts of the Body.* 2 vols. Translated, with introduction and commentary by M. T. May. Ithaca: Cornell University Press, 1968.
Garrison, F. H. *Contributions to the History of Medicine.* New York and London: Hafner Publishing Co., 1966.
———. *An Introduction to the History of Medicine.* 4th ed. Philadelphia: W. B. Saunders Co., 1929.
Gask, G. E. "Early Medical Schools." *Ann. Med. Hist.,* 3d ser. 1 (1939): 128; 2 (1940): 15, 383; 3 (1941): 524.
Gemayel, A. *L'hygiène et la médecine à travers la Bible.* Paris, 1932.
Gerster, Arpad. "On the Hippocratic Doctrine of the Injuries of the Cranium." *Proc. Charaka Club* 1 (1902): 32.
Giere, Ronald N., and Westfall, Richard S. eds. *Foundations of Scientific Method: The Nineteenth Century.* Bloomington: Indiana University Press, 1973.
Gifford, G. E. "Medical History: Curio or Cure?" *Clio Med.* 10 (1975): 304–8.
Gilbert, W. *On the Loadstone and Magnetic Bodies: and, On the Great Magnet of the Earth.* Translated by P. F. Mottelay. London: Bernard Quaritch, 1842.
Glasser, Otto. *Wilhelm Conrad Röntgen.* Springfield, Ill.: Charles C. Thomas, Publisher, 1934.
Godlewski, G. "Carrel: Un grand precurseur." *Bruxelles Med.* 55 (1975): 53–66.
Goodspeed, A. W. "Contributions of Helmholtz to Physical Science." *J. Am. Med. Assoc.* 38, no. 2 (1902).
Gordon, B. L. *Medicine throughout Antiquity.* Philadelphia: F. A. Davis Co., 1949.
Gordon, H. L. *Sir James Young Simpson and Chloroform.* London: T. Fisher Unwin, 1897.
Gorgas, Marie D., and Hendrick, Burton J. *William Crawford Gorgas.* New York: Doubleday, Page & Co., 1924.
Gray, Laman A. "Ephraim McDowell: Father of Abdominal Surgery." Paper read before Filson Club, 8 January 1968, Louisville. Mimeographed.
Greenspan, E. M. *Clinical Cancer Chemotherapy.* New York: Raven Press, 1975.
Grmek, Mirko Drazen. "Santorio Santorio." In *Dictionary of Scientific Biography,* 1975.
Gross, Samuel D. *Auotbiography of Samuel D. Gross, M.D., with Sketches of His Contemporaries.* 2 vols. 1887. Reprint. New York: Arno Press, 1972.
Gruner, O. C. *A Treatise on the Canons of Medicine of Avicenna, with Translation of the First Book.* New York: Augustus M. Kelley, Publishers, 1970.
Gunther, Robert T., ed. *The Greek Herbal of Dioscorides.* Translated by J. Goodyear. 1933. Reprint. New York: Hafner Publishing Co., 1968.
Guthrie, Douglas. *A History of Medicine.* Philadelphia and London: J. B. Lippincott Co., 1946.
Guthrie, W. K. C. "The Revolution of the Mind: Old Gods and the New Reason." In *The Birth of Western Civilization,* edited by M. Grant. London: Thames & Hudson, 1969.

Haagenson, C. D., and Lloyd, W. E. B. *A Hundred Years of Medicine.* New York: Sheridan House, 1943.
Haeser, Heinrich. *Lehrbuch der Geschichte der Medizin und der epidemischen Krankheiten.* 3 vols. Jena: Hermann Dufft, 1875–82.
Haggard, Howard W. *Devils, Drugs, and Doctors: The Story of the Science of Healing from Medicine-Man to Doctor.* New York: Blue Ribbon Books, 1929.
Hahnemann, Samuel. *Organon of the Rational Art of Healing.* London: J. M. Dent & Sons, 1913.
Hall, H. G. "Molière: Satirist of Seventeenth-Century French Medicine: Fact and Fantasy." *Proc. Roy. Soc. Med.* 70 (1977): 425–31.
Hall, W. S. "The Contributions of Helmholtz to Physiology and Psychology." *Am. Med. Assoc.* 38, no. 9 (1902).
Halsted, W. S. "Practical Comments on the Use and Abuse of Cocaine Suggested by Its Invariably Successful Employment in More Than a Thousand Minor Surgical Operations." *N. Y. Med. J.* 42 (1885): 294.
Hamarneh, S. K. *The Genius of Arab Civilization, Source of Renaissance.* New York: New York University Press, 1975.
———. "India's Contribution to Medieval Arabic Medical Education and Practice." *Studies Hist. Med.* 1 (1977): 5–35.
———. *The Physician, Therapist, and Surgeon: Ibn Al-Quff (1233–1286).* Cairo: Atlas & Smithsonian, 1974.
Hamilton, A. *Exploring the Dangerous Trades: The Autobiography of Alice Hamilton.* Boston: Little, Brown & Co., 1943.
Hamilton, Mary. *Incubation.* London: Simpkin, Marshall, Hamilton, Kent & Co., 1906.
Hanlon, J. J. *Public Health: Administration and Practice.* 6th ed. Pt. 1. St. Louis: C. V. Mosby Co., 1974.
Harley, G. W. *Native African Medicine.* Cambridge, Mass.: Harvard University Press, 1941.
Harris, C. R. S. *The Heart and the Vascular System in Ancient Greek Medicine from Alcmaeon to Galen.* Oxford: Clarendon Press, 1973.
Harris, James E., and Weeks, Kent R. *X-raying the Pharaohs.* New York: Charles Scribner's Sons, 1973.
Harris, Marvin. "Riddle of the Pig." *Nat. Hist.* 81 (1972): 32–36; 82 (1973): 20–25.
Harris, Seale. *Woman's Surgeon.* New York: Macmillan Co., 1950.
Harvey, William. *De Motu Cordis: Anatomical Studies on the Motion of the Heart and Blood.* Translated, with annotations by C. D. Leake. Springfield, Ill.: Charles C. Thomas, Publisher, 1941.
Haviland, T. N., and Parish, L. C. "A Brief Account of the Use of Wax Models in the Study of Medicine." *J. Hist. Med. Allied Sci.* 25 (1970): 52–76.
Heaton, Claude E. "The Influence of J. Marion Sims on Gynecology." *Bull. N.Y. Acad. Med.,* 2d ser. 32, no. 9 (1956).
Helfand, W. H. "James Morison and His Pills." *Trans. Br. Soc. Hist. Pharm.* 1 (1974): 101–35.
———, and Julien, P. "Medicine and Pharmacy in French Political Prints." *Pharm. Hist.* 17 (1975): 119–31.
Henle, J. *On Miasmata and Contagia.* Translated, with introduction by George Rosen. Baltimore: Johns Hopkins University Press, 1938.
Herman, John H. *Urology: A View through the Retroscope.* New York: Harper & Row, Publishers, 1973.
Herrlinger, R. *History of Medical Illustration from Antiquity to 1600.* Translated from the German by Graham Fulton-Smith. Munich: Heinz Moos Verlagsgesellschaft & Co., 1967.
Hippocrates. *Hippocrates.* 4 vols. Greek text with English translation by W. H. S. Jones. London: Loeb Classical Library, 1923–31.
Hoff, Ebbe C., and Phebe M. "The Life and Times of Richard Lower, Physiologist and Physician." *Bull. Inst. Hist. Med.* 4 (1936): 517.
Holländer, Eugene. *Anekdoten aus der medizinischen Weltgeschichte.* Stuttgart: Ferdinand Enke Verlag, 1931.
———. *Die Karikature und Satire in der Medizin.* Stuttgart: Ferdinand Enke Verlag, 1921.
———. *Plastik und Medizin.* Stuttgart: Ferdinand Enke Verlag, 1912.
Holmes, O. W. *Medical Essays, 1842–1882.* Boston: Houghton Mifflin Co., 1891.
Homer. *The Iliad.* Translated by W. T. Murray. Cambridge, Mass.: Harvard University Press, 1934.
Hrdlicka, A. "Trepanation among Prehistoric People." *Ciba Symposia* 1, no. 6 (1939).
Huard, Pierre, ed. *La médecine japonaise.* Paris: Editions Roger Dacosta, 1974.
———, and Wong, M. *Chinese Medicine.* New York: McGraw-Hill, 1968.
Hudson, Robert P. "Abraham Flexner in Perspective: American Medical Education 1865–1910." *Bull. Hist. Med.* 46 (1972): 545–61.
———. "Goals in the Teaching of Medical History." *Clio Med.* 10 (1975): 153–60.
Hume, Edward H. *The Chinese Way in Medicine.* Baltimore: Johns Hopkins University Press, 1940.
Hunter, John. *Lectures of Anatomy.* 1837. Reprint. Amsterdam, London, and New York: Elsevier Publishing Co., 1972.
———. *A Treatise on the Venereal Disease.* With additions by Dr. Philip Ricord. Philadelphia: Blanchard & Lea, 1853.
Hurd-Mead, K. C. *A History of Women in Medicine.* 1938. Reprint. Boston: Milford House, 1973.
Hurwitz, Alfred, and Degenshein, George A. *Milestones in Modern Surgery.* New York: Hoeber-Harper, 1958.

Jakobovits, Immanuel. *Jewish Medical Ethics: A Comparative and Historical Study of the Jewish Religious Attitude to Medicine and Its Practice.* New York: Bloch Publishing Co., 1967.
James, C. D. T. "Mesmerism: A Prelude to Anaesthesia." *Proc. Roy. Soc. Med.* 68 (1975): 10–11.
Jarcho, Saul. "The Correspondence of Morgagni and Lancisi on the Death of Cleopatra." *Bull. Hist. Med.* 43 (1969): 299–325.
———. "Giovanni Battista Morgagni: His Interests, Ideas, and Achievements." *Bull. Hist. Med.* 22, no. 5 (1948).
———. *Human Paleopathology.* New Haven and London: Yale University Press, 1966.
———. "The Legacy of British Medicine to American Medicine, 1800–1850." *Proc. Roy. Soc. Med.* 68 (1975): 737–44.
Jayne, Walter A. *The Healing Gods of Ancient Civilizations.* New Haven: Yale University Press, 1925.
Jenner, E. *An Inquiry into the Causes and Effects of the Variolae Vaccinae.* 1798. Reprint. London: Dawsons of Pall Mall, 1966.
Jolly, Julius. *Indian Medicine.* Translated from German by C. B. Kashikar. Poona: C. G. Kashikar, 1951.
Joly, Robert. "Esclaves et médecins dans la Grèce antique." *Sudhoffs Arch.* 53 (1969): 1–14.
Jones, W. H. S. *Malaria and Greek History.* Manchester: Manchester University Press, 1909.
———. *Philosophy and Medicine in Ancient Greece.* Baltimore: Johns Hopkins University Press, 1946.

Karsh, E. "The Conquest of Surgical Pain." In *1978 Medical and Health Annual.* Chicago: Encyclopedia Britannica.
Katz, A. M. "Hippocrates and the Plane Tree on the Island of Cos." *AMA Arch. Int. Med.* 104 (1959): 653–57.
———, and Katz, P. B. "Diseases of the Heart in the Works of Hippocrates." *Br. Heart J.* 24 (1962): 257–64.
Kaufman, M. R. "The Doctor's Image: An Approach to a Study of a Universal Ambivalence." *Mt. Sinai J. Med.* 43 (1976): 76–97.
———. "The Greeks Had Some Words for It: Early Greek Concepts on Mind and Insanity." *Psychiatr. Quart.,* January 1966, pp. 1–33.
Kelly, E. C. *Medical Classics.* Vol. 5. Baltimore: Williams & Wilkins Co., 1905.
Kelly, Howard A. *Walter Reed and Yellow Fever.* New York: McClure, Phillips, 1907.
Kerényi, Karl. *Der göttliche Arzt.* Basel: Ciba, 1948.
Keys, Thomas E. *The History of Surgical Anesthesia.* Rev. and enl. ed. With introduction by Chauncey D. Leake. New York: Dover Publications, 1963.
King, Lester S. "Georg Ernst Stahl." In *Dictionary of Scientific Biography.* 1975.
———. *Growth of Medical Thought.* 1963. Reprint. Chicago: University of Chicago Press, 1974.
———. "Medical Theory and Practice at the Beginning of the Eighteenth Century." *Bull. Hist. Med.* 46 (1972): 1–15.
———. "Medicine, History, and Values." *Clio Med.* 10 (1975): 285–94.
———. "Viewpoints in the Teaching of Medical History: Introductory Comments." *Clio Med.* 10 (1975): 129–32.
Klickstein, Herbert S. *Marie Sklodowska Curie: "Recherches sur les substances radioactives."* With facsimiles of original thesis and English translation. St. Louis: Mallinckrodt Chemical Works, 1966.
Kohn, D. and Shani, A. "A Short History of Medical Thermometry." *Koroth* 6 (1975): 725–29.
Kremers, E., and Urdang, G. *History of Pharmacy.* Rev. ed. Philadelphia: J. B. Lippincott Co., 1976.
Kump, Warren L. "Health Care Delivery Systems in Ancient Greece and Rome." *Pharos,* April 1973, pp. 42–48.

Laignel-Lavastine, Maxine. *Histoire générale de la médecine, de la pharmacie, de l'art dentaire, et de l'art vétérinaire.* 3 vols. Paris: Michel, 1936–49.
———, and Molinery, M. Raymond. *French Medicine.* Translated by E. B. Krumbhaar. New York: Paul B. Hoeber, 1934.
Laín Entralgo, P. *The Therapy of the Word in Classical Antiquity.* Edited and translated by L. J. Rather and J. M. Sharp. New Haven: Yale University Press, 1970.
Lapage, G. *Achievement: Some Contributions of Animal Experiments to the Conquest of Disease.* Cambridge: W. Heffer & Sons, 1960.
Latham, R. G. *Works of Thomas Sydenham.* 2 vols. Boston: Milford House, 1974.
Leake, C. D. *An Historical Account of Pharmacology to the Twentieth Century.* Springfield, Ill.: Charles C. Thomas, Publisher, 1975.
———, ed. *Percival's Medical Ethics.* 1927. Reprint. New York: AMS Press, 1976.
Leibowitz, J. D. "Medical Ethics in Jewish History." *Medica Judaica* 1 (1971): 10–15.
Leroi-Gourhan, A. *Treasures of Prehistoric Art.* New York: Harry N. Abrams, 1967.
Lesky, Erna. "Structure and Function in Gall." *Bull. Hist. Med.* 44 (1970): 297–314.
———, ed. *Johann Peter Frank, seine Selbstbiographie.* Bern: Verlag Hans Huber, 1969.
Levy, H. S. *Chinese Footbinding: The History of a Curious Erotic Custom.* New York: Walton Rawls, 1966.
Lévy-Bruhl, L. *La mentalité primitive.* Paris: Librairie Félix Alcan, 1922.
Lichtenthaeler, C. *Pourquoi un cours d'histoire de la médecine.* Geneva: Librairie Droz, 1966.
Lidz, T. "Adolf Meyer and the Development of American Psychiatry." *Am. J. Psychiatr.* 123 (1966): 320–32.
Lindeboom, G. A. "Hermann Boerhaave (1668–1738): Teacher of all Europe." *Am. Med. Assoc.* 206 (1968): 2297–2301.
Lindskog, G. E. "Oliver Wendell Holmes. *Miscuit utile dulci.*" *Yale J. Biol. Med.* 47 (1974): 277–80.
Lipton, E. L.; Steinschneider, A.; and Richmond, J. B. "Swaddling, a Child Care Practice: Historical, Cultural, and Experimental Observations." *Pediatrics* 35, suppl. (1965): 519–67.

Littré, E. *Oeuvres complètes d'Hippocrate.* 10 vols. Paris: Baillière, 1839–61.
Litwak, R. S. "The Growth of Cardiac Surgery: Historical Notes." *Cardiovas. Clin.* 3 (1971): 6–50.
Long, Esmond R. *Selected Readings in Pathology from Hippocrates to Virchow.* Springfield, Ill.: Charles C. Thomas, Publisher, 1929.
Long, Perrin H., and Bliss, Eleanor A. *The Clinical and Experimental Use of Sulfanilamide, Sulfapyradine, and Allied Compounds.* New York: Macmillan Co., 1939.
Lowie, R. H. *Indians of the Plains.* 1954. Reprint. New York: American Museum of Natural History, 1963.
Lutzker, E. *Medical Education for Women in Great Britain.* Reprint of master's thesis. New York: Columbia University Press, 1959.
Lyons, A. S. "Teaching the History of Medicine—New Approaches." *Trans. Coll. Phys. Phila.*, 4th ser. 40 (1972): 22–39.

McGovern, J. P., and Burns, C. R. *Humanism in Medicine.* Springfield, Ill.: Charles C. Thomas, Publisher, 1974.
McKie, Douglas. *Antoine Lavoisier: Scientist, Economist, Social Reformer.* New York: Henry Schuman, 1952.
MacKinney, Loren. "Early Medicine in Illuminated Manuscripts." Pt. 1 in *Medical Illustrations in Medieval Manuscripts.* Berkeley and Los Angeles: University of California Press, 1965.
———. "Medical Miniatures in Extant Manuscripts: A Checklist Compiled with the Assistance of Thomas Herndon." Pt. 2 in *Medical Illustrations in Medieval Manuscripts.* Berkeley and Los Angeles: University of California Press, 1965.
McMurrich, J. Playfair. *Leonardo da Vinci: The Anatomist.* Baltimore: Williams & Wilkins Co., 1930.
Maimonides, Moses. *Treatise on Hemorrhoids: Medical Answers.* Edited and translated by F. Rosner and S. Muntner. Philadelphia and Toronto: J. B. Lippincott Co., 1969.
Majno, G. *The Healing Hand: Man and Wound in the Ancient World.* Cambridge, Mass.: Harvard University Press, 1975.
Major, Ralph H., ed. *Classic Descriptions of Disease.* 3d ed. Springfield, Ill.: Charles C. Thomas, Publisher, 1945.
———. *A History of Medicine.* 2 vols. Springfield, Ill.: Charles C. Thomas, Publisher, 1954.
Malgaigne, J.-F. *Oeuvres complètes d'Ambroise Paré.* Paris: Baillière, 1840.
Margotta, R. *The Story of Medicine.* Edited by Paul Lewis. New York: Golden Press Publications, 1968.
Marinatos, S. *Crete and Mycenae.* New York: Harry N. Abrams, 1960.
Marks, E. *The Aphorisms of Hippocrates.* New York: Collins, 1817.
Marks, Geoffrey, and Beatty, William K. *Women in White: Their Role as Doctors through the Ages.* New York: Charles Scribner's Sons, 1972.
Marshall, Sir John. *Mohenjo-Daro and the Indus Civilization.* London: Arthur Probsthain, 1931.
Martí-Ibáñez, Felix. *Ariel: Essays on the Arts and the History and Philosophy of Medicine.* New York: MD Publications, 1962.
Mastromatteo, E. "From Ramazzini to Occupational Health Today from an International Perspective." *J. Occup. Med.* 17 (1975): 289–94.
Mather, Cotton. *The Angel of Bethesda.* Edited by Gordon W. Jones. Worcester, Mass.: American Antiquarian Society, 1972.
Meigs, J. W. "Puerperal Fever and Nineteenth-Century Contagionism: The Obstetrician's Dilemma." *Trans. Stud. Coll. Physicians Phila.* 42 (1975): 273–80.
Melicow, M. M. "Percivall Pott (1713–1788): Two Hundredth Anniversary of First Report of Occupation-induced Scrotum Cancer in Chimney Sweepers (1775)." *Urology* 6 (1975): 745–49.
Metchnikoff, Elie. *The Founders of Modern Medicine: Pasteur-Koch-Lister.* 1939. Reprint. Books for Libraries Press, 1971.
Mettler, Cecelia. *History of Medicine.* Edited by Fred A. Mettler. Philadelphia: Blakiston Co., 1947.
Meyer-Steineg, Theodor. *Chirurgische Instrumente des Altertums.* Jena: Verlag von Gustav Fischer, 1912.
———, and Sudhoff, Karl. *Geschichte der Medizin.* 2d ed. Jena: Verlag von Gustav Fischer, 1922.
Middleton, W. S. "John Morgan, Father of Medical Education in North America." *Ann. Med. Hist.*, 1st ser. 9 (1927): 13.
Middleton, William S. "The Practice of Medicine: Past, Present, and Future." *Perspect. Biol. Med.* 15 (1972): 334–50.
Millepierres, F. *La vie quotidienne des médecins au temps de Molière.* Paris: Librairie Hachette, 1964.
Miller, Genevieve. "The Teaching of Medical History in the United States and Canada." *Bull. Hist. Med.* 44 (1970): 482–83.
———. "The Teaching of Medical History in the United States and Canada: Historical Resources in Medical School Libraries." *Bull. Hist. Med.* 44 (1970): 251–78.
———. "The Teaching of Medical History in the United States and Canada. Report on Individual Schools." *Bull. Hist. Med.* 43, nos. 4, 5, 6 (1969): 344–75, 444–72, 553–86.
Mitchell, J. F. "The Introduction of Rubber Gloves for Use in Surgical Operations." *Ann. Surg.* 122 (1945): 902.
Mitchell, S. W. *History of Instrumental Precision in Medicine.* 1892. Reprint. New York: Burt Franklin & Co., 1971.
Moll, A. A. *Aesculapius in Latin America.* Philadelphia and London: W. B. Saunders Co., 1944.
Møller-Christensen, V. *The History of the Forceps.* Copenhagen and London, 1938.
Moodie, R. L. *The Antiquity of Disease.* Chicago: University of Chicago Press, 1923.
Moon, R. O. "The Influence of Pythagoras on Greek Medicine." In *Proceedings of the Seventeenth International Congress of Medicine, London, 1913.* Sect. 23. London: H. Frowde, 1914.
Moore, F. D. *Transplant: The Give and Take of Tissue Transplantation.* Rev. ed. New York: Simon & Schuster, 1972.
Morse, W. R. *Chinese Medicine.* New York: Paul B. Hoeber, 1934.
Muntner, S. "The Antiquity of Asaph the Physician and His Editorship of the Earliest Hebrew Book of Medicine." *Bull. Hist. Med.* 25 (1951): 101–31.

Nathan, H. "Erich Lexer, 1867–1937." *Med. Welt.* 24 (1973): 2088–90.
Naylor, Ronald. "Galileo: Real Experiment and Didactic Demonstration." *Isis* 67 (1976): 398–419.
Needham, J. *Science and Civilization in China.* 7 vols. Cambridge: Cambridge University Press, 1954–76.
Neuburger, Max. *History of Medicine.* Vol. 1. Translated by Ernest Playfair. London: Oxford University Press, 1910.
Neuhof, H. *The Transplantation of Tissues.* With the collaboration of S. Hirshfeld. New York and London: D. Appleton & Co., 1923.
New York Academy of Medicine. *Milestones in Medicine.* 1938. Reprint. New York: Hawthorn Books, 1971.
Nicaise, E. *Chirurgie de Maître Henri de Mondeville.* Paris: Librairie Félix Alcan, 1893.
Nissen, Rudolph, and Wilson, Roger. *Pages in the History of Chest Surgery.* Springfield, Ill.: Charles C. Thomas, Publisher, 1960.
Norris, J. "East or West? The Geographic Origin of the Black Death." *Bull. Hist. Med.* 51 (1977): 1–24.
Northup, G. W. "History of the Development of Osteopathic Concepts, with Notes on Osteopathic Terminology." *J. Am. Osteopath. Assoc.* 75 (1975): 405–9.
Nutton, V. "The Chronology of Galen's Early Career." *Classical Quart.* 23 (1973): 158–71.

Ober, W. B., ed. *Great Men of Guy's.* Metuchen, N. J.: Scarecrow Press, 1973.
Olch, Peter. Book review of *Simpson and Syme of Edinburgh*, by John A. Shepherd. In *Bull. Hist. Med.* 46 (1972): 93–94.
———. "William S. Halsted and Local Anesthesia: Contributions and Complications." *Anesthesiology* 42 (1975): 479–86.
Olmsted, J. M. D. *Charles-Édouard Brown-Séquard.* Baltimore: Johns Hopkins University Press, 1946.
———. *Claude Bernard: Physiologist.* New York: Harper & Bros., 1938.
———. *François Magendie: Pioneer in Experimental Physiology and Scientific Medicine in Nineteenth Century France.* New York: Henry Schuman, 1944.
O'Malley, C. D. *Andreas Vesalius of Brussels, 1514–1564.* Berkeley and Los Angeles: University of California Press, 1965.
———, ed. *The History of Medical Education: An International Symposium Held February 5–9, 1968.* Berkeley: University of California Press, 1970.
O'Malley, Charles D., and Saunders, J. B. de C. M. *Leonardo da Vinci on the Human Body.* New York: Henry Schuman, 1952.
Onians, Richard Broxton. *The Origins of European Thought: About the Body, the Mind, the Soul, the World, Time, and Fate.* 2d ed. Cambridge: Cambridge University Press, 1954.
Oppenheimer, Jane. Book review of *Un grand médecin et biologiste: Casimir-Joseph Davaine (1812–1882)* by Jean Théodoridès. In *Bull. Med. Hist.* 44 (1970): 591–93.
Osler, Sir William. *The Evolution of Modern Medicine.* New Haven: Yale University Press, 1921.
———. "The Influence of Louis on American Medicine." *Bull. Johns Hopkins Hosp.* 8 (1897): 161.

Pachter, Henry M. *Paracelsus, Magic into Science.* New York: Henry Schuman, 1951.
Packard, Francis R. *History of Medicine in the United States.* 2 vols. New York: Paul B. Hoeber, 1931.
———. *Life and Times of Ambroise Paré, 1510–1590, with a New Translation of His Apology and an Account of His Journeys in Diverse Places.* New York: Benjamin Blom, Publishers, 1971.
———. *The School of Salernum: Regimen sanitatis Salernitanum.* English translation by Sir John Harrington. London: Oxford University Press, 1922.
Pagel, J. *Rudolf Virchow.* Leipzig: W. Weicher, 1906.
Pagel, W. *William Harvey's Biological Ideas: Selected Aspects and Historical Background.* New York and Basel: S. Karger, 1967.
Paget, J., ed. *Essays and Addresses by Sir James Paget.* London and New York: Longmans, Green & Co., 1902.
Paget, Stephen. *John Hunter: Man of Science and Surgeon (1728–1793).* London: T. Fisher Unwin, 1897.
Paré, Ambroise. *The Collected Works of Ambroise Paré.* Translated from the Latin by T. Johnson. Pound Ridge, N.Y.: Milford House, 1948.
Paulus Aegineta. *The Seven Books of Paulus Aegineta.* 3 vols. Translated by Francis Adams. London: Sydenham Society, 1844–47.
Pavlov, I. P. "Experimental Therapeutics as a New and Exceedingly Fruitful Method of Physiological Investigation." Translated by Morton H. Frank and Joyce J. Weiss. *Bull. N. Y. Acad. Med.* 50 (1974): 1018–31.
Payne, J. F. *Thomas Sydenham.* London: T. Fisher Unwin, 1900.
Pazzini, A. *Storia della medicina.* Milan: Societa Editrice Libraria, 1947.
Pellegrino, E. D. "Medical History and Medical Education: Points of Engagement." *Clio Med.* 10 (1975): 295–308.
Percival, Thomas. *Percival's Medical Ethics.* 1803. Reprint. Edited, with introduction by Chauncey D. Leake. Baltimore: Williams & Wilkins Co., 1927.
Phillips, S. D. *Aspects of Greek Medicine.* New York: St. Martin's Press, 1973.
Piggott, S., ed. *The Dawn of Civilization.* New York: McGraw-Hill, 1967.
———. *Prehistoric India to 1000 B.C.* Harmondsworth, Middlesex: Penguin Books, 1950.
Pinel, P. *A Treatise on Insanity.* Translated from the French by D. D. Davis. New York: New York Academy of Medicine and Hafner Publishing Co., 1962.
Platt, Walter B. "Fabricius Guilhelmus Hildanus: The Father of German Surgery." *Bull. Johns Hopkins Hosp.* 16 (1905): 7.
Plinius Secundus, C. *The Natural History of Pliny.* Translated by John Bostock and H. T. Riley. London: H. G. Bohn, 1856.
Pomeroy, S. B. *Goddesses, Whores, Wives, and Slaves.* New York: Schocken Books, 1975.
Powell, J. H. *Bring Out Your Dead.* Philadelphia: University of Pennsylvania Press, 1949.
Power, D'A. *The Foundations of Medical History.* Baltimore: Williams & Wilkins Co., 1931.
Poynter, F. N. L. *Medicine and Culture.* London: Wellcome Institute for the History of Medicine, 1969.
Poynter, N. *Medicine and Man.* London: C. A. Watts, 1971.
Preuss, Julius. *Biblisch-talmudische Medizin.* Berlin: S. Karger, 1921.
Priestley, Joseph. *The Memoirs of Joseph Priestley.* London: Johnson, 1805.
Pritchard, J. B., ed. *The Ancient Near East: A New Anthology of Texts and Pictures.* Vol. 2. Princeton: Princeton University Press, 1973.
Puschmann, Theodor. *Handbuch der Geschichte der Medizin.* 1905. Reprint. 3 vols. New York: AMS Press, 1976.
Quen, J. M. "Case Studies in Nineteenth Century Scientific Rejection: Mesmerism, Perkinism, and Acupuncture." *J. Hist. Behav. Sci.* 11 (1975): 149–56.

Radbill, S. X. "Pediatric Dermatology in Antiquity: Part 1." *Int. J. Dermatol.* 14 (1975): 363–68.
Ramazzini, B. *De morbis artificum diatriba* [Discourse on the diseases of workers]. 1713. Rev. ed. of Latin text. Edited and translated, with notes by Wilmer Cave Wright. Chicago: University of Chicago Press, 1940.
Ranke, Hermann. *Medicine and Surgery in Ancient Egypt.* Philadelphia: University of Pennsylvania Press, 1941.
Ranking, George S. A. "The Life and Works of Rhazes (Abu Bakr Muhammad ben Zakaruja ar-Razi)." In *Proceedings of the Seventeenth International Congress of Medicine, London, 1913.* Sect. 23. London: H. Frowde, 1914.
Reichel-Dolmatoff, G. *The Shaman and the Jaguar: A Study of Narcotic Drugs among the Indians of Colombia.* Philadelphia: Temple University Press, 1975.
Rhazes. *A Treatise on the Small Pox and Measles.* Translated by A. Greenhill. London: Sydenham Society, 1848.
Richards, D. W. "The First Aphorism of Hippocrates." *Perspect. Biol. Med.* 5 (1961): 61–64.
———. "Medical Priesthoods, Past and Present." *Trans. Assoc. Am. Phys.* 75 (1962): 1–10.
Richer, P. *Le dèmoniaque dans l'art.* Paris, 1887.
Richter, Paul. "Ueber Uhedu in den aegyptischen Papyri." *Arch. Gesch. Med.* 2 (1909): 73–83.
Ridenbough, Mary Young. *The Biography of Ephraim McDowell.* New York: Charles L. Webster, 1890.
Riesman, David. *The Story of Medicine in the Middle Ages.* New York: Paul B. Hoeber, 1936.
———. *Thomas Sydenham.* New York: Paul B. Hoeber, 1926.
Rieux, J. "La vie et l'oeuvre de J. A. Villemin." *Presse Méd.* 35 (1927): 1273.
Rinkel, M., and Viets, H. R. "The Electron Microscope, in Notes and Queries." *J. Hist. Med.* 6 (1951): 406–8.
Risse, G. B. "The Role of Medical History in the Education of the 'Humanist' Physician: A Reevaluation." *J. Med. Educ.* 50 (1975): 458–65.
Robinson, V. *Pathfinders in Medicine.* New York: Medical Life Press, 1929.
Robinson, Victor. *Victory over Pain.* New York: Henry Schuman, 1946.
Rogers, F. B. *Selected Papers of John Shaw Billings, Compiled with a Life of Billings.* Chicago: Medical Library Association, 1965.
Rogge, C. W. "Ambroise Paré (1510–1590) and the Evolution of the Surgical Instrumentarium." *Arch. Chir. Neerl.* 27 (1975): 1–15.
Rolleston, Sir Humphry. "History of Cinchona and Its Therapeutics." *Ann. Med. Hist.*, n.s. 3 (1931): 261.
Rolleston, J. D. "F. J. V. Broussais (1772–1838), His Life and Doctrines." *Proc. Roy. Soc. Med.* 22 (1939): 405.
Rosen, George. *From Medical Police to Social Medicine: Essays on the History of Health.* New York: Neale Watson Academic Publications, 1974.
———. "Hospitals, Medical Care, and Social Policy in the French Revolution." *Bull. Hist. Med.* 30 (1956): 124–49.
———. *The Specialization of Medicine.* New York: Froben Press, 1944.
Rosenfield, L. C. *From Beast-Machine to Man-Machine: Animal Soul in French Letters from Descartes to La Mettrie.* New and enl. ed. New York: Octagon Books, 1968.
Rosner, Fred. *Biblical and Talmudic Medicine: Selections from Classical Jewish Sources.* New York: Ktav Publishing House, 1976.
———. "The Physician's Prayer Attributed to Moses Maimonides." *Bull. Hist. Med.* 41 (1967): 440–54.
———. *Sex Ethics in the Writings of Moses Maimonides.* New York: Bloch Publishing Co., 1974.
———. "The Spleen in the Talmud and Other Early Jewish Writings." *Bull. Hist. Med.* 46 (1972): 82–85.
Roth, C. *The Jews in the Renaissance.* New York: Harper & Row, 1965.
Rousselot, Jean, ed. *Medicine in Art: A Cultural History.* New York: McGraw-Hill, 1967.
Rufus of Ephesus. *Oeuvres de Rufus d'Ephèse.* Translated by C. Daremberg and C. Emile Ruelle. Paris: Imprimerie Nationale, 1879.
Rush, Benjamin. *The Autobiography of Benjamin Rush.* Edited by George W. Corner. Princeton: Princeton University Press, 1948.
Ryder, R. D. *Victims of Science: The Use of Animals in Research.* London: Davis-Poynter, 1975.

Saffron, M. H. "Salernitan Anatomists." In *Dictionary of Scientific Biography.* 1975.
Saintignon, Henri. *Laënnec; Sa vie et son oeuvre.* Paris: Baillière, 1904.
Sarma, P. J. "The Art of Healing in Rigveda." *Ann. Med. Hist.*, 3d ser. 1 (1939): 538.
Sarton, George. *Galen of Pergamon.* Lawrence: University of Kansas Press, 1954.
———. *Introduction to the History of Science.* 3 vols. Baltimore: Williams & Wilkins Co., 1927–31.
Sauerbruch, Ferdinand. *Master Surgeon: Ferdinand Sauerbruch.* Translated by Fernand G. Renier and Anne Cliff. New York: Thomas Y. Crowell Co., 1954.
Saunders, J. B. de C. M., and O'Malley, Charles D. *The Illustrations from the Works of Andreas Vesalius of Brussels.* With annotations and translations. New York: World Publishing Co., 1950.
Scarborough, J. "Celsus on Human Vivisection at Ptolemaic Alexandria." *Clio Med.* 2 (1976): 25–38.
———. "Drug Lore of Asclepiades of Bythnia." *Pharm. Hist.* 17 (1975): 43–57.
———. *Facets of Hellenic Life.* Boston: Houghton Mifflin Co., 1976.
———. "Galen and the Gladiators." *Episteme* 5 (1971): 98–111.
———. "Nicander's Toxicology, I: Snakes." *Pharm. Hist.* 19, no. 51 (1977).
———. *Roman Medicine.* Ithaca: Cornell University Press, 1969.
———. "Some Notes on the Etruscan Heritage of Early Roman Medicine." *Episteme* 3 (1969): 160–66.
Schachner, August. *Ephraim McDowell, "Father of Ovariotomy" and Founder of Abdominal Surgery.* London and Philadelphia: J. B. Lippincott Co., 1921.
Schouten, J. *Rod and Serpent of Asklepios, Symbol of Medicine.* Amsterdam and London: Elsevier Publishing Co., 1967.
Schultz, A. "Notes on Diseases and Healed Fractures of Wild Apes and Their Bearing on the Antiquity of Pathological Conditions in Man." *Bull. Hist. Med.* 7 (1939): 571–82.
Selwyn, S. "Dr. Moffet and the Sixteenth Century Origins of Medical Microbiology." *Proc. Roy. Soc. Med.* 69 (1976): 558.

Shambaugh, G. E., Jr. *Surgery of the Ear*. Philadelphia: W. B. Saunders Co., 1959.

Shattuck, L. *The Report of the Sanitary Commission of Massachusetts*. 1850. Reprint. Cambridge, Mass.: Harvard University Press, 1948.

Shryock, Richard Harrison. *The Development of Modern Medicine: An Interpretation of the Social and Scientific Factors Involved*. New York: Alfred A. Knopf, 1947.

———. "The Medical Reputation of Benjamin Rush: Contrasts over Two Centuries." *Bull. Hist. Med.* 45 (1971): 507.

Siegel, Rudolph E. *Galen on Psychology, Psychopathology, and Functions and Diseases of the Nervous System*. Basel: S. Karger, 1973.

———. *Galen's System of Physiology and Medicine: His Doctrines and Observations on Blood Flow, Respiration, Humors, and Internal Diseases*. Basel and New York: S. Karger, 1968.

Sigerist, Henry E. *American Medicine*. Translated by Hildegard Nagel. New York: W. W. Norton & Co., 1934.

———. *Civilization and Disease*. Chicago: University of Chicago Press, 1962.

———. "An Elizabethan Poet's Contribution to Public Health: Sir John Harington and the Water Closet." *Bull. Inst. Hist. Med.* 13 (1943): 229.

———. *The Great Doctors: A Biographical History of Medicine*. Translated by Eder and Cedar Paul. Garden City, N.Y.: Doubleday & Co., Anchor Books, 1958.

———. "The Historical Aspects of Art and Medicine." *Bull. Inst. Hist. Med.* 4 (1936): 271–97.

———. *On the Sociology of Medicine*. Edited by M. I. Roemer. New York: MD Publications, 1960.

Simpson, E. B. *Sir James Y. Simpson*. Edinburgh and London: Oliphant Anderson & Ferrier, 1896.

Sims, James Marion. *The Story of My Life*. Edited by H. Marion-Sims. New York: D. Appleton & Co., 1886.

Sinclair, Sir William J. *Semmelweis: His Life and Doctrine*. Manchester: Manchester University Press, 1909.

Singer, Charles. *The Discovery of the Circulation of the Blood*. London: G. Bell & Sons, 1922.

———. *The Evolution of Anatomy and Physiology: From the Greeks to Harvey*. New York: Dover Publications, 1957.

———. *From Magic to Science: Essays on the Scientific Twilight*. New York: Boni & Liveright, 1928.

———. *Greek Biology and Medicine*. Oxford: Clarendon Press, 1922.

———. *A Short History of Medicine*. Oxford: Clarendon Press, 1928.

———, and Sigerist, H. E., eds. *Essays on the History of Medicine, Presented to Karl Sudhoff on the Occasion of His Seventieth Birthday, November 26, 1923*. London: Oxford University Press, 1924.

Slaughter, Frank G. *Immortal Magyar*. New York: Henry Schuman, 1950.

Smart, N. *The Religious Experience of Mankind*. New York: Charles Scribner's Sons, 1969.

Smith, Elizabeth C. "Heirs to Trotula: Early Women Physicians in the United States." *N. Y. State J. Med.*, June 1977, pp. 1142–65.

Smith, Wesley D. "Galen on Coans versus Cnidians." *Bull. Hist. Med.* 47 (1973): 569–85.

Smithcors, J. F. *Evolution of the Veterinary Art*. Kaiser City, Mo.: Veterinary Medicine Publishing Co., 1957.

Snapper, I. *Chinese Lessons to Western Medicine*. New York: Grune & Stratton, 1965.

Snow, J. *On Cholera*. 1856. Reprint. New York: Commonwealth Fund, 1936.

Soranus. *Gynecology*. Translated, with introduction by O. Temkin. Baltimore: Johns Hopkins University Press, 1956.

Speert, H. *Iconographia gyniatrica: A Pictorial History of Gynecology and Obstetrics*. Philadelphia: F. A. Davis, 1973.

Stark, Richard B. "The History of Plastic Surgery in Wartime." *Clinics in Plastic Surgery* 2 (1975): 509–15.

Starolinski, J. *Histoire de la Médecine*. Editions Rencontres, and Erik Nitsche, 1963.

Steuer, R. O. *Aetiological Principle of Pyaemia in Ancient Egyptian Medicine*. Baltimore: Johns Hopkins University Press, 1948.

Stevenson, L. A., and Multhauf, R. P., eds. *Medicine, Science, and Culture: Historical Essays in Honor of Oswei Temkin*. Baltimore: Johns Hopkins University Press, 1968.

Stevenson, L. G. "Suspended Animation and the History of Anesthesia." *Bull. Hist. Med.* 49 (1975): 482–511.

Still, George Frederic. "The History of Paediatrics: The Progress of the Study of Diseases of Children up to the End of the Eighteenth Century." London: Oxford University Press, 1931.

Stoddart, Anna M. *The Life of Paracelsus, Theophrastus von Hohenheim, 1493–1541*. London: John Murray, 1911.

Stone, E. *Medicine among the American Indians*. New York: Paul B. Hoeber, 1932.

Subba Rao, D. V., ed. *Western Epitomes of Indian Medicine*. With the collaboration of P. R. K. Murthy. Osmania: Osmania Medical College, 1966.

Sudhoff, Karl. "Guihelmus Fabricius Hildanus." *München Med. Wchnschr.* 57 (1910): 1410.

"Surgeons of the Sea." *MD Medical News Magazine* 2 (1958): 125–29.

Sushruta Samhita. 3 vols. Translated by K. K. L. Bhishagratna. Calcutta: J. N. Bose, 1907–16.

Sydenham, T. *Selected Works of Thomas Sydenham*. Translated by J. D. Comrie. London: John Bale, Sons & Danielsson, 1922.

Taton, René, ed. *Ancient and Medieval Science from the Beginnings to 1450*. New York: Basic Books, 1963.

———, ed. *The Beginnings of Modern Science from 1450 to 1800*. New York: Basic Books, 1964.

Temkin, L. *Four Treatises of Theophrastus von Hohenheim, Called Paracelsus*. Baltimore: Johns Hopkins University Press, 1941.

Temkin, Oswei. *The Falling Sickness: A History of Epilepsy from the Greeks to the Beginnings of Modern Neurology*. 2d rev. ed. Baltimore: Johns Hopkins University Press, 1971.

———. *Galenism: Rise and Decline of a Medical Philosophy*. Ithaca: Cornell University Press, 1973.

———. "History and Prophecy: Meditations in a Medical Library." *Bull. Hist. Med.* 49 (1975): 305–17.

Theophrastus. *Theophrastus' Enquiry into Plants*. 2 vols. Translated by Sir Arthur Hart. New York: G. P. Putnam's Sons, 1916.

Thomas, K. B. "John Snow." In *Dictionary of Scientific Biography*. 1975.

Thompson, C. J. S. *The History and Evolution of Surgical Instruments*. New York: Henry Schuman, 1942.

Thorndike, Lynn. *A History of Magic and Experimental Science*. New York: Macmillan Co., 1923.

Thorwald, Jurgen. *The Century of a Surgeon*. New York: Pantheon Books, 1956.

———. *Science and Secrets of Early Medicine*. Translated by Richard and Clara Winston. New York: Harcourt, Brace & World, 1963.

Toledo-Pereyra, L. H. "Galen's Contributions to Surgery." *J. Hist. Med. Allied Sci.* 28 (1973): 357–75.

Toole, H. "Asclepius in History and Legend." Pt. 1 in "Asclepius." *Surgery* 53 (1963): 387–419.

———. "Critical Analysis of the Records Attributed to Asclepius." Pt. 2 in "Asclepius." *Surgery* 53 (1963): 387–419.

Triaire, P. *Dominique Larrey et les campagnes de la Révolution et de l'Empire, 1768–1842*. Tours: Mame, 1902.

Tuttle, E. F. "The Trotula and Old Dame Trot: A Note on the Lady of Salerno." *Bull. Hist. Med.* 50 (1976): 61–72.

Underwood, E. Ashworth, ed. *Science, Medicine, and History: Essays on the Evolution of Scientific Thought and Medical Practice Written in Honour of Charles Singer*. London: Oxford University Press, 1953.

Vallery-Radot, René. *The Life of Pasteur*. New York: McClure, Phillips, 1906.

Veith, Ilza, trans. *Huang Ti nei ching su wên—The Yellow Emperor's Classic of Internal Medicine*. Baltimore: Williams & Wilkins, 1949.

Viets, H. R. *Brief History of Medicine in Massachusetts*. 1930. Reprint. New York: AMS Press, 1976.

Virchow, Rudolf. "The Influence of Morgagni on Anatomical Thought." *Lancet* 1 (1894): 843.

———. *Johannes Müller: Eine Gedächtnissrede*. Berlin: A. Hirschwald, 1858.

Vogel, Virgil J. *American Indian Medicine*. Norman: University of Oklahoma Press, 1970.

Wakefield, E. G., and Dellinger, S. C. "Possible Reasons for Trephining the Skull in the Past." *Ciba Symposia* 1, no. 6 (1939).

Walsh, Joseph. "Galen's Studies at the Alexandrian School." *Ann. Med. Hist.*, 1st ser. 9 (1927): 132–43.

———. "Refutation of the Charges of Cowardice Made against Galen." *Ann. Med. Hist.*, n.s. 3 (1931): 195–208.

Walton, Alice. *The Cult of Asclepios*. Cornell Studies in Classical Philology. Boston: Ginn & Co., 1894.

Wangensteen, O. H. "Has Medical History Importance for Surgeons?" *Surg. Gynecol. Obstet.* 140 (1975): 434–42.

———. "Surgeons and Wound Management: Historical Aspects." *Conn. Med.* 39 (1975): 568–74.

———, and Wangensteen, S. D. "The Surgical Amphitheatre: History of Its Origins, Functions, and Fate." *Surgery* 77 (1975): 403–18.

———, Wangensteen, S. D.; and Klinger, C. "Wound Management of Ambroise Paré and Dominique Larrey, Great French Military Surgeons of the Sixteenth and Nineteenth Centuries." *Bull. Hist. Med.* 46 (1972): 207–34.

Waterhouse, Benjamin. "American Pioneer." Editorial. *Ann. Med. Hist.* 9 (1927): 195.

Webb, Gerald B. *René Théophile Hyacinthe Laennec: A Memoir*. New York: Paul B. Hoeber, 1928.

Webster, Jerome P., and Gnudi, M. T. *The Life and Times of Gaspare Tagliacozzi*. New York: Herbert Reichner, 1950.

Weeks, J. H. *Among the Primitive Bakongo*. London: Seeley, Service & Co., 1914.

Weinberger, Bernhard Wolf. *An Introduction to the History of Dentistry*. St. Louis: C. V. Mosby Co., 1948.

Weiner, Dora B. "The French Revolution, Napoleon, and the Nursing Profession." *Bull. Hist. Med.* 46 (1972): 274–305.

Wells, C. "Ancient Obstetric Hazards and Female Mortality." *Bull. N.Y. Acad. Med.* 51 (1975): 1235–49.

Werner, D. *History of the Red Cross*. London: Cassell & Co., 1941.

Wershub, Leonard Paul. Book review of *Urology: From Antiquity to the Twentieth Century*. *Bull. Hist. Med.* 46 (1972): 312–13.

Wessler, C. *The American Indian*. 2d ed. New York and London, 1922.

Whipple, Allen O. "Role of the Nestorians as the Connecting Link between Greek and Arabic Medicine." *Ann. Med. Hist.*, n.s. 8 (1936): 313.

Wiese, E. Robert. "Guillaume Dupuytren." *Med. Life* 38 (1931): 477.

Williams, C. "The Tractors." *J. Hist. Med.* 30 (1975): 61.

Williams, H. U. "The Origin and Antiquity of Syphilis: The Evidence from Diseased Bones." *Arch. Path.* 13 (1932): 779–814, 931–83.

———. "The Origin of Syphilis: Evidence from Diseased Bones: A Supplementary Report." *Arch. Derm. Syph.* 33 (1936): 782 ff.

Wilson, R. McNair. *The Beloved Physician, Sir James Mackenzie*. London: John Murray, 1926.

Withington, Edward Theodore. *Medical History from the Earliest Times*. London: Scientific Press, 1894.

Wong, K. C., and Wu, L. T. *History of Chinese Medicine*. 2 vols. Shanghai: Gordon Press Publications, 1976.

Wreszinski, Walter. *Der grosse medizinische Papyrus des Berliner Museums*. Leipzig: J. C. Hinrichs, 1909.

———. *Der Londoner medizinische Papyrus und der Papyrus Hearst*. Leipzig: J. C. Hinrichs, 1912.

Wright, L. *Clean and Decent: The Fascinating History of the Bathroom and the Water Closet*. New York: Viking Press, 1960.

Wunderlich, C. A. *On Temperature in Diseases*. Translated by W. B. Woodman. London: Sydenham Society, 1871.

Wylie, W. Gill. *Hospitals: Their History, Organization, and Construction*. New York: D. Appleton & Co., 1877.

Wynder, E. L. "A Corner of History: John Graunt, 1620–1674, the Father of Demography." *Prev. Med.* 4 (1975): 85–88.

Young, J. H. *Medical Messiahs: A Social History of Medical Quackery in the Twentieth Century*. Princeton: Princeton University Press, 1967.

Zielonka, J. S. "A Man-Midwife." *J. Hist. Med.* 30 (1975): 259.

Zigrosser, C. *Medicine and the Artist*. New York: Dover Publications, 1970.

Zilboorg, Gregory, and Henry, George W. *A History of Medical Psychology*. New York: W. W. Norton & Co., 1941.

Zimmerman, Leo M. "Cosmas and Damian, Patron Saints of Surgery." *Am. J. Surg.* 33 (1936): 160–68.

———. "The Evolution of Blood Transfusion." *Am. J. Surg.* 55 (1942): 613–20.

INDEX

PHOTOGRAPHIC CREDITS

The authors and publisher wish to thank the libraries, museums, and private collectors for permitting the reproduction of works of art in their collections and for supplying the necessary photographs. Photographs from other sources are gratefully acknowledged below.

Air India/Karange: 189;
Alinari (including Anderson and Brogi), Florence: 247, 248, 259, 269, 273, 277, 278, 285, 289, 323, 324, 325, 326, 327, 341, 342, 352, 356, 361, 362, 400, 406, 431, 604, 605, 710, 766;
The American Journal of Roentgenology and Radium Therapy, April 1923: 979;
Paul Almasy (WHO) 31, 997;
Jessie Tarbox Beals: 1017;
Bibliothèque Nationale, Paris: 109, 110, 112, 198, 208, 217, 251, 261, 279, 307, 334, 420, 427, 435, 439, 441, 444, 448, 459, 465, 466, 467, 468, 469, 475, 476, 477, 480, 481, 482, 483, 484, 485, 501, 502, 503, 504, 505, 506, 507, 508, 510, 514, 515, 519, 520, 521, 524, 525, 546, 555, 576, 590, 622, 663, 668, 669, 689, 691, 723, 732, 917;
Bildarchiv Preussischer Kulturbesitz, Berlin: 194, 402;
Erwin Böhm, Mainz: 4, 91, 92, 161;
Bulloz, Paris: 736, 737;
Caisse Nationale des Monuments Historiques, Paris: 105, 150, 175, 227, 233, 351;
Canali, Rome: 412, 564, 573;
Chiolini, Pavia: 545;
Chuzeville, Malakoff: 118, 156;
Ciba-Geigy, Ltd., Basel: 163, 164;
Clayton: 235;
Clements, New York: 901;
Connaughton, New York: 874, 905;
Cooper-Bridgeman, London: 121, 725, 873;
Courtauld Institute, London: 417, 422, 638;
Wim Cox, Cologne: 426;

Lance Dane, Madras: 171;
J. L. Daniel and Robert Bagnell, Batelle Memorial Institute, Pacific Northwest Laboratories, Richland, Wash: 11;
Delval, Corbeil: 743, 744;
Department of the Environment, England: 415;
Deutsches Archaeologisches Institut, Athens: 249, 263, 264, 266, 268, 270, 293, 295, 312, 357, 382;
Deutsches Medizinischen Wochenschrift, no. 47, Art Supplement 25: 854;
Forsyth: 38;
Fotofast, Bologna: 388, 512;
Foto Fiorucci Giuliana, Pisa: 623–625;
Foto Fürbock, Graz: 28;
Foto Marburg, Marburg/Lahn: 539;
Foto Meyer, Vienna: 329;
Fototeca Unione, Rome: 316–318, 350, 353, 354, 358, 363, 569;
Freeman, London: 176;
Giraudon, Paris: 167, 168, 173, 262, 283, 292, 299, 331, 332, 370, 371, 509, 544, 547, 558, 574, 620;
Greek Government: 245;
Gunner, Wellesley: 847;
Guy's Hospital Reports, Thomas Guy, Publisher: 816;
Haase, Frankfurt: 688;
Hassia, Athens: 230;
Held, Ecublens: 29, 360;
Hewicker, Kaltenkirchen: 255;
Hirmer Verlag, Munich: 102, 154, 231, 232, 238, 239, 241, 253, 254, 260, 274, 275, 279, 280, 286, 290, 291, 296, 300, 310, 330, 338, 346, 347;
Joint Expedition to Ur: 165;
Dimitri Kessel, Paris: 281;
Lajoux, Editions d'Art Lucien Mazenod, Paris: 20, 21;
Lennart Larsen: 26;
Rev. T. Lewis, in Among the Primitive Bakongo by John H. Weeks, Seely, Service & Co.: 44;
Lichtbildwerkstatte, Alpenland, Vienna: 542;
Löbl, Bad Tölz: 419;
Mas, Barcelona: 14, 429, 699;
Leonard von Matt, Buochs: 344, 352, 355, 425, 918;

Mella, Milan: 314, 559;
Mexican Tourist Department: 55;
Mosechlin, Basel: 72;
Moodie, The Antiquity of Disease, University of Chicago Press: 7, 8;
Morrow, South Dakota: 809;
Musée d'Histoire de la Médecine, Paris: 662, 784, 787, 946;
O.E. Nelson, New York: 135, 159, 328;
Lennart Nilsson, Stockholm: 965
Orlandini, Modena: 470;
Pasquino (WHO): 51;
Josephine Powell, Athens: 229, 234, 236, 242–244;
Carlos Sanchez, Mexico: 39, 40, 45;
Scala/EPA, New York: 337, 611;
Roy Schwartz: 932;
Schweizerisches Landes Museum, Zurich: 19;
Service Photographique des Musées Nationaux, Paris: 17, 93, 96, 99, 101, 104, 107, 118, 125, 127, 156, 188, 237, 239, 240, 256, 294, 319, 393–395, 571, 612, 751, 917;
G.E. Smith, "Ancient Splints," British Medical Journal (1908): 152;
W. Starks, Kingston: 437;
Stierlin, Geneva: 124;
Szaszfai, New Haven: 721;
R.F. Turnbull: 879;
United Press International, New York: 952, 953, 959, 990;
University of Kansas Medical School Library, Lawrence: 80, 218, 267;
Manuel Usandizaga, Historia de la obstetricia y ginecología en España: 12, 13;
J. Vertut, Issy-les-Moulineaux: 123;
Roger Viollet, Paris: 95;
Larry Wainwright, New York: 157;
Webb, London: 572;
World Health Organization, Geneva: 31, 33, 51, 142, 147, 148, 189, 349, 373, 410, 411, 428, 458, 554, 577, 582, 583, 629, 636, 644, 660, 671, 698, 700, 702, 714, 735, 756, 786, 794, 824, 894, 904, 906, 914, 916, 962, 963, 989, 997, 1005, 1018;